ADMET FOR MEDICINAL CHEMISTS

ADMET FOR MEDICINAL CHEMISTS

A Practical Guide

Edited by

KATYA TSAIOUN

STEVEN A. KATES

WILEY

A JOHN WILEY & SONS, INC., PUBLICATION

Published by John Wiley & Sons, Inc., Hoboken, New Jersey
Published simultaneously in Canada

Library of Congress Cataloging-in-Publication Data:

ADMET for medicinal chemists : a practical guide / edited by Katya Tsaioun, Steven A. Kates.
p. ; cm.
Other title: Absorption, distribution, metabolism, excretion, toxicity for medical chemists
Includes bibliographical references and index.
ISBN 978-0-470-48407-4 (cloth)
1. Drug Development. I. Tsaioun, Katya. II. Kates, Steven A., 1961- III.
Title: Absorption, distribution, metabolism, excretion, toxicity for medical chemists.
[DNLM: 1. Drug Design. 2. Drug Toxicity. 3. Pharmaceutical Preparations–chemistry.
4. Pharmacokinetics. QV 744 A238 2011]
RM301.27.A36 2011
615′.19–dc22

2010021925

Printed in Singapore

eBook: 978-0-470-91509-7
oBook: 978-0-470-91511-0
ePub: 978-0-470-92281-1

10 9 8 7 6 5 4 3 2 1

CONTENTS

PREFACE

Medicinal chemistry and drug development have undergone a rapid evolution since the 1990s due to a much expanded biological and chemical toolbox allowing novel target identification and rapid synthesis of a large number of diverse chemical libraries. Despite this progress, substantial increases in R&D expenditures, and an ever-increasing number of molecules screened and synthesized every year, the pharmaceutical industry has found itself in a productivity paradox. While these improvements should have significantly increased the number of new molecular entities (NMEs) identified each year, the actual numbers in this period remained at a low and constant level with high attrition rates at both the early and the late stages of clinical development.

We believe a number of factors have contributed to this paradox.

One factor is the current system of academic training whose objectives of instructing scientists are not always aligned with the objectives of the pharmaceutical industry. The discovery of novel therapeutics is an inherently complex and interdisciplinary process, requiring close integration of scientists from several disciplines in an environment in which lessons are shared and taught across an organization. Current models of academic training emphasize specialization and insufficiently address the need to understand related subjects.

Not surprisingly, drug-discovery organizations frequently experience difficulties integrating the efforts of chemists, biologists, and preclinical and clinical development specialists. This leaves each discipline producing scientifically valid work that may often have little relevance for developing a commercial product. This book is a product of a collaborative work of a medicinal chemist and an ADMET scientist; however, the bulk of the content of this book was written by experts in specialized subsegments of these fields. The structure of this book mirrors the most successful organizational model for drug discovery: collaboration and communication among team members comprising a variety of specialties.

While medicinal chemists collaborate among themselves, successful programs depend upon these drug developers to interact with specialists from other disciplines to commercialize therapeutic agents. This is the key insight *ADMET for Medicinal Chemists* provides; the techniques are just a "*how-to*."

The acronym "ADMET" refers to "absorption, distribution, metabolism, excretion, and toxicity." These parameters, in addition to efficacy, are critical in determining whether an NME will become a clinical candidate and subsequently a commercially viable product. Depending on context, the acronym can refer either to the properties of a compound, the process of determining those properties, or the discipline that focuses on that process.

"Early ADMET" is a discipline that emerged in the late 1990s. The field has created a unique interdisciplinary interface between medicinal chemists, biologists, formulators, toxicologists, and preclinical development scientists. Consequently, for medicinal chemists, early ADMET is the ideal entry point for expanding the understanding to related disciplines.

The advent of early ADME profiling of drug candidates in a high-throughput fashion in conjunction with proof-of-principle biological efficacy optimization has reduced drug failures in clinical trials due to ADME/DMPK reasons from 40 to $<7\%$ during the 1980s–1990s to late 2000s. Even though drug-discovery productivity failed to improve during this period, the implementation of early ADMET was indisputably a major success. The goal of an ADMET program is to guide candidate selection through the early identification of molecules with suboptimal properties so that their corresponding technical issues could be addressed before large development costs have been incurred. The goal of this book is to guide medicinal chemists in how to implement early ADMET testing in their workflow in order to improve both the speed and efficiency of their efforts.

Many medicinal chemists are unfamiliar with the pharmacological pathway of a drug administered orally. Their chemical innovation can be improved by a better understanding of the digestive system which is provided in Chapter 1. Topics such as enterohepatic circulation, permeability, P-glycoproteins, microsomal stability, first-pass, and glomerular filtration are described.

Structure-based *in silico* ADMET screening models and software approaches are often used to guide medicinal chemistry efforts to design molecules with desired properties. Lipinski, Veber, and Oprea have developed rules that describe the relationship between a compound and its corresponding ADMET properties. These rules have been built into software. Chapter 2 outlines the key computer methods, such as rule-based methods, QSAR, and machine learning approaches. The chapter also discusses and compares the commercially available programs and demonstrates methods for implementation to prepare compound collections.

The physicochemical properties of a new chemical entity (NCE) can impact absorption and pharmacokinetics. Chapter 3 summarizes the strategies for applying *in silico* filters for optimization, and the impact of the solid state of the molecule on physicochemical properties of NCEs in medicinal chemistry.

Chapter 4 provides an overview of liver metabolic stability, plasma stability, solution stability, plasma protein binding, intestinal, blood–brain barrier, tissue distribution, permeability models, excretion (biliary and renal), CYP450 inhibition, and efflux and uptake transporters. These parameters are important because physiological phenomena and the properties of drug candidates in biological systems are based upon the disposition and metabolism of a NCE. The chapter also discusses the various preclinical tools that may be used to predict human performance, and strategies for prioritizing and conducting these assays in a lead optimization program.

Pharmacokinetics (PK) describes what the body does to the drug and is dependent on the dose administered, site of administration, and the physiological state of the organism. PK expresses the rates of disposition (movement) of a drug when administered to a living organism such as (A)bsorption, (D)istribution, (M)etabolism, and (E)xcretion (ADME). Chapter 5 provides a brief overview of basic pharmacokinetic principles such as T_{max}, C_{max}, V_{d} (volume of distribution), AUC (area under the curve), $t_{1/2}$ (half-life), bioavailability, extraction ratio, and metabolic clearance. The inevitable formulas that explicate the concepts are conceptually and pictorially described and explained.

Toxicity assays are the most critical tests of an NCE performed prior to its administration into humans. These tests are designed to ensure the safety of the first human subjects. The FDA requires many different assays for achieving this essential objective. These assays examine how a compound affects different aspects of human pharmacology. Chapter 6 discusses the fundamentals and mechanisms of cardiac safety including hERG, other ion channels, and nonion channel related cardiac toxicity. Chapter 7 outlines genetic toxicity, including AMES, micronucleus, and GreenScreen. Chapter 8 describes hepatic toxicity, including necrosis, steatosis, cholestasis, reactive metabolites, and covalent binding.

The FDA requires for an NCE *in vivo* toxicological assessment of typically two species: one rodent and one nonrodent. Chapter 9 considers the route of administration for the intended therapeutic (bolus versus infusion and potential inadvertent routes), and the compound requirements for toxicological studies as related to different species. Chapter 9 also covers formulation issues, such as overage, spillage, stability, reactivity/compatibility with glassware, infusion equipment, method validation, and sample analysis. IND-enabling studies and species selection for different therapeutic indications are also reviewed.

Preclinical candidate nomination and development are discussed in Chapter 10, which provides an overview of the late stages of the discovery process, including the process of selecting preclinical candidates, and designing appropriate preclinical studies to support an IND.

Novel approaches to drug design constantly evolve. Chapter 11 addresses fragment-based drug design, such as minimal pharmacophoric elements and fragment hopping, which are recent innovative tools developed for designing drug candidates.

We wish to thank the contributors to this book. They have succeeded in describing the importance for a medicinal chemist to understand ADMET. We are appreciative of their support and substantial effort in providing their expertise and thoughtfulness to this project.

We hope that this book provides readers with an appreciation for the complexity of designing and developing new therapeutic agents for human clinical trials and their subsequent approval into the marketplace. We are privileged to be able to work in a field with such boundless opportunities for reducing human suffering and it is our obligation to create the best of these opportunities.

Color representations of selected figures in this book can be found at ftp://ftp.wiley.com/public/sci_tech_med/admet

KATYA TSAIOUN
STEVEN A. KATES

Watertown, Massachusetts
Maynard, Massachusetts
October 2010

CONTRIBUTORS

Nils Bergenhem, Vice President & CSO, CPEX Pharmaceuticals, Inc., 2 Holland Way, Exeter, NH, USA

Anne-Claude Camproux, UMRS 973 Inserm-Paris Diderot, Paris, France

Po-Chang Chiang, Pfizer Inc., Chesterfield Parkway West, Chesterfield, Missouri

John P. Devine, Jr., Basi Mount Vernon, Indiana

Martin E. Dowty, Pfizer Inc., Chesterfield Parkway West, Chesterfield, Missouri

David Elder, GalaxoSmithKline Research and Development, Externalisation Group, PCD, Ware, United Kingdom

Keith Hoffmaster, Novartis Institutes for Biomedical Research, Cambridge, Massachusetts

Haitao Ji, Department of Chemistry, University of Utah, Salt Lake City, Utah, USA

Corinne Kay, Med-Simple, Hillside Farm, Keir, Dunblane, Scotland

Ralf Kettenhofen, AXIOGENESIS AG, Nattermannallee, Cologne, Germany

Leonid (Leo) Kirkovsky, Pfizer Inc., Chesterfield Parkway West, Chesterfield, Missouri

David Lagorce, UMRS 973 Inserm-Paris Diderot, Paris, France

Yurong Lai, Pfizer Inc., Chesterfield Parkway West, Chesterfield, Missouri

Dean M. Messing, Pfizer Inc., Chesterfield Parkway West, Chesterfield, Missouri

Maria A. Miteva, UMRS 973 Inserm-Paris Diderot, Paris, France

Christelle Reynes, UMRS 973 Inserm-Paris Diderot, Paris, France

Silke Schwengberg, AXIOGENESIS AG, Nattermannallee, Cologne, Germany

Jon Selbo, SSCI, A Division of Aptuit, West Lafayette, Indiana

Olivier Sperandio, UMRS 973 Inserm-Paris Diderot, Paris, France

Bruno O. Villoutreix, UMRS 973 Inserm-Paris Diderot, Paris, France

Richard M. Walmsley, Faculty of Life Sciences, University of Manchester, Manchester, United Kingdom

Jinghai James Xu, Merck Research Labs, West Point, Pennsylvania

Anup Zutshi, Pfizer Inc., Chesterfield Parkway West, Chesterfield, Missouri

1

INTRODUCTION

CORINNE KAY

1.1 INTRODUCTION

Absorption, distribution, metabolism, and excretion (ADME) properties have been and still are a significant reason for attrition in drug discovery. Paradoxically, medicinal chemists have to solve complex ADME issues with a solid organic chemistry background and scant anatomy or physiology training. In reality, drug metabolism is not any different from daily food digestion and understanding of human nutrition demystifies many drug metabolism reactions. Grasping the logical sequence of each step in the digestion process as well as the nature of the chemical reactions that occur in each organ contributes to the understanding of food digestion and drug metabolism.

The human digestive system processes on average 30 tons of food in a lifetime. Food digestion provides nutrients for the body's function and repair. Useful nutrients are stored in a form that is compatible with existing biological systems (e.g., fat, glycogen). It produces and recycles complex molecules such as bile acids and catabolizes fats. More importantly, the liver is set up to recognize and destroy toxic entities and does so with relentless efficiency.

In order to carry out such a vast array of chemical reactions in a highly compact space, the human body effectively runs the process in set stages corresponding to the various organs of the digestive system. Each organ possesses its own controlled pH. An associated battery of enzymes as well as coenzymes are activated at this pH but denatured at another pH at the next stage. Ingested food will spend from minutes (mouth) to hours (gut) in a single organ where it is effectively mechanically stirred at 37°C in an enzyme bath at a set pH. After all possible chemical transformations

ADMET for Medicinal Chemists: A Practical Guide, Edited by Katya Tsaioun and Steven A. Kates

have occurred in that organ, it then moves to the next organ in the digestive tract. Fascinatingly, the associated pH change causes the incoming enzymes to denature, thus exposing the partially processed food to a new set of reaction conditions and enabling new chemical transformations to take place. Little wonder that after meandering for 12–48 h through the 8–9 m length of the digestive track that most complex chemicals have been transformed (or metabolized) to their constituent building blocks. Since the purpose of eating is not to dispose of food waste but to bring nutrients to our body, these chemical building blocks (amino acids, sugars, etc.) are carried to and then stored in appropriate cells in the human body.

Not surprisingly, a drug entering the digestive system will be exposed to the same environment as food and will be subjected to the same battery of chemical reactions. For a patient ingesting a tablet, the constituent chemicals will be exposed to the same mechanical stirring at 37°C, the same pH as well as enzymes. The chemical transformations that occur during food digestion are free to act on the constituents of the drug. Since most drugs are presented to the body as solid or semisolid dosage forms, the drug particles must first be released from that form and dissolved. Furthermore, drug absorption, whether from the gastrointestinal (GI) tract or other sites, requires the passage of the drug in a molecular form across the barrier membrane. The drug will be required to possess the desirable biopharmaceutical properties enabling it to pass from a region of high concentration to a region of low concentration across the membrane into the blood, or general circulation.

Insight to this process is a key to understanding many drug metabolism concepts. This introduction chapter is not intended to be a physiology textbook. It demonstrates the link between nutrition and drug metabolism and thus provides a framework upon which medicinal chemists can apply their extensive organic chemistry knowledge to solve the ever occurring ADME issues. It has been said that "anyone can contribute solutions provided the problem is explained in a language they understand." Aspiring and even experienced medicinal chemists are encouraged to take basic nutrition and physiology courses to deepen their understanding of developed drugs exposure to these environments.

1.2 VOYAGE THROUGH THE DIGESTIVE SYSTEM

It takes 12–48 h for ingested food to complete its voyage through the digestive system. The food first arrives in the mouth (pH = 7) where it is chewed and exposed to its first set of enzymes, called salivary enzymes. Subsequently, the food travels down the esophagus to the stomach (pH = 1–2), which undergoes receptive relaxation as it fills to a capacity of 2 L or more (Figure 1.1). The next stage in the digestive system is the small intestine where chemical digestion continues and most nutrients are absorbed. The small intestine is made up of three parts: the duodenum where the contents of the stomach are neutralized to pH = 6 by pancreatic secretions ($NaHCO_3$), then the 2 m long jejunum (pH = 7–8), and finally the ileum (3 m long). Those substances which are not digestible or not absorbed join the large intestine, where leftovers are formed into semisolid masses ready for disposal. When digested nutrients are absorbed

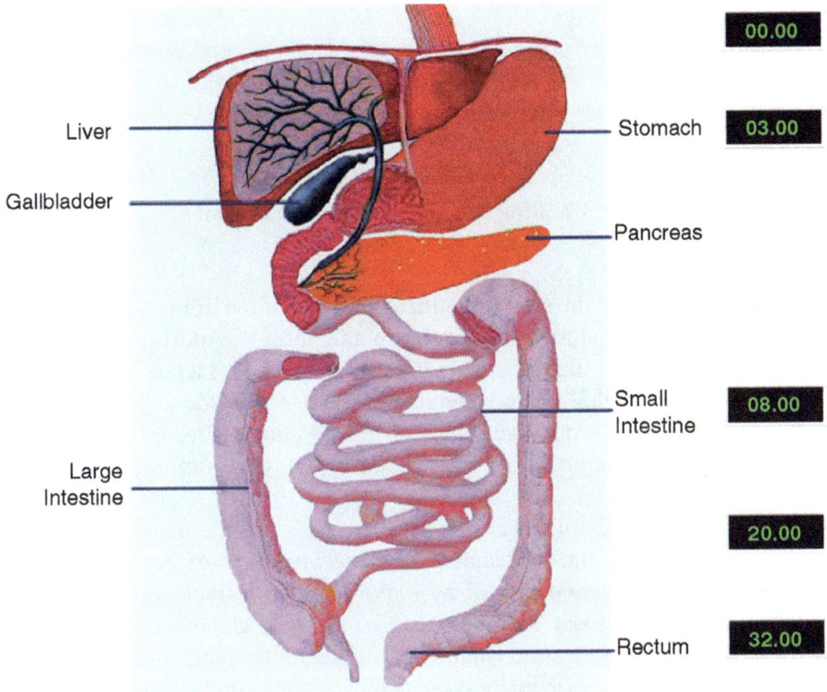

Figure 1.1 The digestive system. The numbers to the right of the diagram represent the elapsed time.

(i.e., exit the gut into the blood stream), they are ducted to the liver via the hepatic-portal vein (HPV) (pH = 7.4). Following metabolism in the liver, molecules can either be ducted back into the digestive system via the bile (enterohepatic cycling) or finally enter the general blood circulation. Finally, approximately 25% of total systemic blood flow is diverted through the kidneys, which act as an on-line filtration unit, and water-soluble waste is concentrated in the urine.

The various events occurring during drug metabolism are more easily understood by visualizing the sequence "mouth—esophagus—stomach—duodenum—gut—liver—kidneys" as well as understanding the chemical reactions taking place in each organ.

1.2.1 The Mouth

The mouth is the reception center of the digestive system and the place where food is initially processed before being passed onto the stomach via the esophagus. In the mouth, mechanical as well as chemical digestion occurs. On average 1 L of saliva is secreted at various points into the mouth through salivary glands. Saliva contains salivary enzymes, which include amylases, which break down complex carbohydrates into simple sugars such as maltose and glucose, and peroxidases. Some

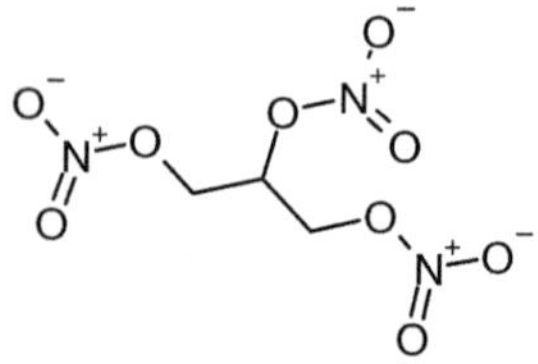

Figure 1.2 Structure of GTN (glycerin trinitrate).

lipases are also present in the saliva, resulting in some of the lipid (i.e., fat or dietary triglycerides) digestion starting to occur in the mouth. Additionally, aspartate aminotransferase (AST), alanineamino transferase (ALT), lactate dehydrogenase (LDH), and acidic and alkaline phosphatase have been reported to be released from the normal and especially damaged cells of periodontal tissues into saliva. Saliva also contains immunoglobin A (IgA), an antibody playing a minor role in human immunity.

Some nutrients are capable of crossing the mucosa and the membranes that line the cavity of the mouth and are captured by the profusion of capillaries to enter the bloodstream. This avenue is used by hypoglycemic patients to quickly deliver glucose to raise their glucose blood levels by placing a glucose tablet under their tongue. The same principle is used when small molecular weight, water-soluble drugs such as glycerin trinitrate, or nitroglycerin (GTN) (Figure 1.2) are given *via* the sublingual route to patients suffering from angina. This ensures the rapid entry of the drug into the bloodstream as well as bypasses the remainder of the digestive system including the liver where it would otherwise be extensively metabolized.

The same route of administration has been exploited by Generex Biotechnology Corporation [1] to develop Oral-lyn™. This formulation delivers insulin as a fine spray in the buccal (i.e., mouth) cavity. The peptide drug is rapidly absorbed through the mucosal lining of the mouth and enters the bloodstream, where it is reported to produce glucodynamic profiles comparable to that produced by injection of regular human insulin. This drug was first approved for use in Ecuador in 2005 [2] and recently received approval in a number of other countries. The buccal administration of insulin also assures that the drug does not enter the lungs and, therefore, is free of pulmonary side-effect associated with inhaled insulin products.

Similarly, the anticoagulant drug heparin, a polysaccharide not suitable for oral administration, is given to patients *via* the subcutaneous route. Its similarity to starch makes it an obvious target to amylases (Figure 1.3).

1.2.2 The Stomach

The food bolus is swallowed and enters the stomach where both chemical digestion as well as absorption (from the stomach into the bloodstream) occurs. The wall of the stomach is lined with millions of gastric glands, which together secrete 400–800 mL of gastric juice at each meal. Several types of cells are found in the gastric glands

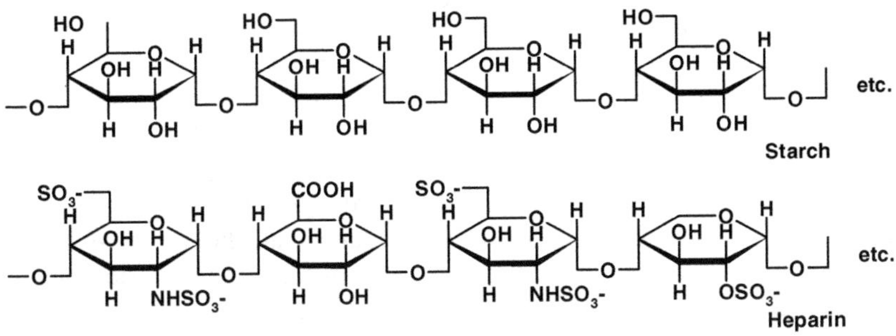

Figure 1.3 The similarities between the structures of starch and heparin.

including parietal cells, chief cells, mucus-secreting cells, and hormone-secreting (endocrine) cells.

1.2.2.1 Chemical Digestion Claude Bernard (1813–1878), known as the founder of experimental physiology, demonstrated that contrary to popular belief, little digestion occurs in the stomach. This organ only processes up to half the carbohydrates in a meal, one-tenth of the protein, and hardly any fat while the bulk of the digestion takes place in the intestines. The stomach effectively acts as a food mixer and acid-and-enzyme bath and the breadth of chemical reactions that ensue are of importance to the medicinal chemist. Every few minutes its strong, muscular walls undergo a spasm of squeezing to churn the food into semiliquid state called chyme. Parietal cells secrete hydrochloric acid (HCl) and intrinsic factor. Intrinsic factor is a protein that binds ingested vitamin B12 and enables it to be absorbed by the intestine. A deficiency of intrinsic factor, as a result of an autoimmune attack against parietal cells, causes pernicious anemia. Chief cells synthesize and secrete pepsinogen, the precursor to the proteolytic enzyme pepsin. Pepsin cleaves peptide bonds, favoring those on the C-terminal side of tyrosine, phenylalanine, and tryptophan residues. Its action breaks long polypeptide chains into shorter lengths. Secretion by the gastric glands is stimulated by the hormone gastrin, which is released by endocrine cells in the stomach in response to the arrival of food. Gastrin stimulates the production of hydrochloric acid (HCl), reducing the pH to 1–2, which inactivates amylases, swallowed with the saliva, and denatures ingested proteins, making them more vulnerable to attack by pepsins. Although most of the lipases are secreted from the pancreas into the duodenum, some lipases are present in the stomach and perform an ester bond hydrolysis on a limited range of lipids to produce fatty acids and glycerol.

This panoply of chemical reactions highlights the breadth and variety of the chemical transformations that can occur in the stomach and provide a warning to medicinal chemists attempting to design compounds of peptidic nature or containing multiple amide bonds and unhindered alkyl esters.

1.2.2.2 Absorption Only a limited range of substances are actually absorbed through the stomach lining into the blood. The stomach can absorb glucose and other simple sugars, amino acids, and some fat-soluble substances. A number of alcohols, including ethanol, are readily absorbed from the stomach. Water moves freely from the gastric contents across the gastric mucosa into the blood. In tracer experiments [3] using deuterium oxide, about 60% of the isotopic water placed in the stomach was absorbed into the blood in 30 min. The net absorption of water from the stomach is small because water readily moves from the blood across the gastric mucosa to the lumen of the stomach. The absorption of both water and alcohol can be slowed down if the stomach contains food, especially fat, presumably since gastric emptying is delayed and most water is absorbed from the jejunum.

From a medicinal chemistry point of view, the persistent issue associated with the stomach is that of solubility. Only compounds in solution are available for permeation across the gastric membrane and solubility of drug molecules at pH = 2 is often an issue. The following examples illustrate the significance of this problem.

Salicylic acid (pK_a 3.5 and 13.4) is weakly acidic and only 30% is ionized at pH = 2. Its insolubility precludes its absorption in the stomach (Figure 1.4). It is soluble in the intestine (pH = 6.4), but since it is present in its ionized form, it is unable to be effectively absorbed through the gut wall. Given that salicylic acid is also a stomach irritant, it is prepared as an ester prodrug to reduce the amount of acid actually in contact with the gut lining. When it reaches the blood where it is 50–90% plasma bound (depending on the concentration), it is processed by esterases and is converted back to its active form (salicylic acid).

Acid-reducing agents including omeprazole are widely used [4] by patients with HIV to treat acid reflux disease, heartburn, and stomach ulcers. In a recent study [5], 18 HIV-negative volunteers were given ritonavir-boosted saquinavir along with omeprazole for 15 days. Results showed that the addition of omeprazole caused an 82% increase in the levels of saquinavir (invirase) in the blood. It was argued that omeprazole is unlikely to increase saquinavir levels by its weak inhibition of the major liver enzyme CYP3A4 that breaks down saquinavir. However, the most plausible explanation was that saquinavir is dissolving more readily in a less-acidic environment.

The pH of the gastric contents controls the absorption of certain ionizable materials such as aspirin, which is readily absorbed in its unionized form when the stomach is acidic, but more slowly when gastric contents are neutral.

A number of solubility tests are available to assist in identifying this issue prior to drug administration to humans, and these are discussed in subsequent chapters. In addition to the usual solubility tests, many groups [6] have reported the use of the fasted and fed-state simulated gastric fluid (SGF) test [7] due to its more relevance to a physiological environment.

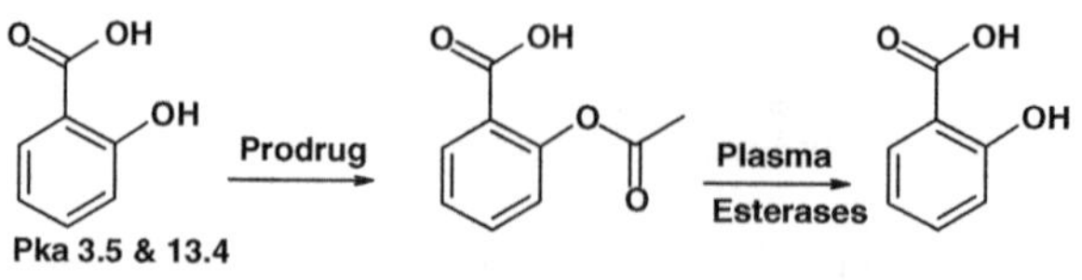

Figure 1.4 Aspirin—solubility and ionization.

1.2.3 The Small Intestine: Duodenum

Following stomach peristalsis and digestion, the pyloric sphincter relaxes and allows the food (and ingested drugs) to enter the first part of the small intestine, the duodenum. The duodenum [8] is a 20 cm long smooth muscle lined tube (Figure 1.5). Two ducts enter the duodenum: one of them drains the gallbladder and hence the liver, and the other drains the exocrine portion of the pancreas. Both organs produce secretions that enable further chemical digestion and have an impact on drug design. The pancreas consists of clusters of endocrine cells (the islets of Langerhans) and exocrine cells whose secretions drain into the duodenum.

1.2.3.1 Pancreatic Juices Since the pHs of the stomach and the intestine are very acidic and nearly neutral, respectively, the pancreas produces 1.5 L/day of alkaline juices (e.g., bicarbonate) to neutralize the partially acidic digested chyme. The neutralization is carried out at a slow, controlled rate and has the additional effect of denaturing incoming stomach enzymes and rendering them inactive. The secretion of pancreatic fluid is controlled by two hormones—secretin and cholecystokinin (CCK). Secretin mainly affects the release of sodium bicarbonate and CCK stimulates the release of the digestive enzymes.

Pancreatic fluid also contains a number of digestive enzymes. Most carbohydrate digestion occurs in the duodenum and is performed by pancreatic amylase, which hydrolyzes starch into a mixture of maltose and glucose. Pancreatic lipase hydrolyzes ingested fats into a mixture of fatty acids and monoglycerides. Its action is enhanced by the detergent effect of bile. In April 1999, the FDA approved orlistat as a treatment for obesity. Orlistat inactivates pancreatic lipase. About one-third of ingested fats fail to be broken down into absorbable fatty acids and monoglycerides and simply passes out in the feces.

The four "zymogens" (proteins that are precursors to active proteases) secreted from the pancreas are trypsin, chymotrypsin, elastase, and carboxypeptidase. These are immediately converted into the active proteolytic enzymes. Trypsin cleaves peptide bonds on the C-terminal side of arginine and lysine. Chymotrypsin cuts amide bonds on the C-terminal side of tyrosine, phenylalanine, and tryptophan

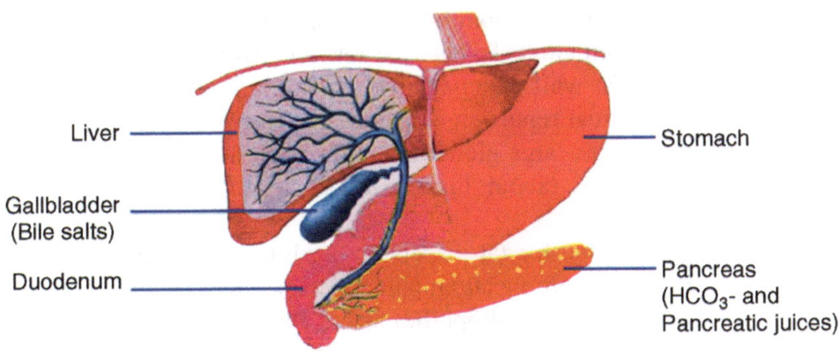

Figure 1.5 The duodenum receives input from the pancreas and the liver.

residues (the same bonds as pepsin, whose action ceases when $NaHCO_3$ raises the pH of the intestinal contents). Elastase cuts peptide bonds next to small, uncharged side-chains such as those of alanine and serine. Trypsin, chymotrypsin, and elastase are members of the family of serine proteases. Chymotrypsin precipitates hydrophilic kappa casein in milk by breaking the bond between phenylalanine (105) and methionine (106) to produce two insoluble fragments resulting in the milk curdling, thus slowing down its digestion. Finally, carboxypeptidase removes, one by one, the amino acids at the C-terminal of peptides. Carboxypeptidase A cleaves carboxyl terminal amino acids that have aromatic or aliphatic side-chains, and carboxypeptidase B cleaves carboxyl terminal amino acids that have basic side-chains. It is the presence of this wide array of enzyme proteases, which precludes the oral administration of protein or peptide drugs such as corticotrophin, vasopressin, and insulin. These would be rapidly degraded in the digestive tract and are not generally given orally. Some microencapsulation and nanoparticle formulation studies have been carried out in an attempt to circumvent these issues and are showing promise.

Diarrhea, a side-effect commonly associated with highly active antiretroviral therapy (HAART), has been ascribed to the inhibition of pancreatic lipases by protease inhibitors such as agenerase, norvir, and fortovase. An *in vitro* study [9] showed that the protease inhibitor agenerase formulated as a solution or a capsule exhibited complete inhibition of pancreatic lipase at physiological concentration. Norvir and fortovase produced 72% and 75% inhibition, respectively, at physiological concentration, as calculated from the plots to determine IC_{50} values.

Erythromycin stearate USP (ethryl) is the stearic acid salt of erythromycin. It is a crystalline powder that is practically insoluble in water. Similar to erythromycin base, the stearate is acid labile. It is thus film-coated [10] to protect it from acid degradation in the stomach and in the alkaline pH of the duodenum, where the free base is liberated from the stearate and absorbed.

1.2.3.2 Hepatic Bile The human liver produces 400–800 mL of hepatic bile each day. The bile (pH = 7.8–8.6) is then concentrated fivefold and stored in the gallbladder between meals. When food, especially containing fat, enters the duodenum, the release of the hormone CCK stimulates the gallbladder to contract and discharge its bile into the duodenum. The main constituents of bile are bile salts, bilirubin, bile pigments (end products of hemoglobin breakdown), and electrolytes. Bile salts are amphiphilic steroids, which emulsify ingested fat. The hydrophobic portion of the steroid dissolves in the fat while the negatively charged side-chain interacts with water molecules. The mutual repulsion of these negatively charged droplets keeps them from coalescing. Thus, large globules of fat (liquid at body temperature) are emulsified into tiny droplets (about 1 μm in diameter) that can be more readily digested and absorbed.

The molecules responsible for fat dispersion are bile salts such as glycocholic acid (Figure 1.6). Bile acids are facial amphipathic since they contain both hydrophobic (lipid soluble) and polar (hydrophilic) faces. The cholesterol-derived portion of a bile acid has one face that is hydrophobic (methyl groups) and one that is hydrophilic (hydroxyl groups); the amino acid conjugate is polar and hydrophilic.

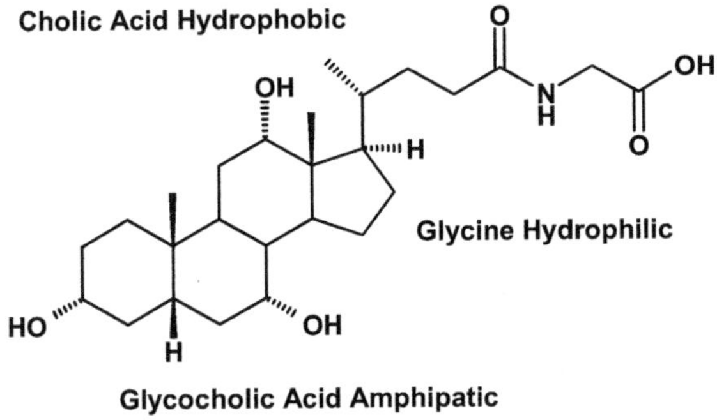

Figure 1.6 Glycocholic acid (conjugate of cholic acid and glycine) is facial amphipathic.

Their amphipathic nature enables bile acids to aggregate to form water-soluble micelles, with the hydrophobic and hydrophilic sides toward the center and outside, respectively. In the center of these micelles are dietary triglycerides, which are separated from a larger globule of lipid. Pancreatic lipase is then able to reach the molecules of triglyceride through gaps between the bile salts, providing a largely increased surface area for the digestion of fat.

Glycocholic acid is biosynthesized in the liver starting from cholesterol. Interestingly, the series of synthetic reaction steps are a mimic of the Phases 1 and 2 processes that take place in the metabolism of drug molecules and will be described in Section 1.3. Bile salts promote dissolution of lipophilic drugs and lipophilic drug formulations, enteric coatings, and waxy drug matrices. Bile salts may also promote membrane permeability of lipophilic molecules through micelle formation and solubilization. The brownish color of the bile pigments imparts the characteristic brown color of the feces.

1.2.4 The Small and Large Intestine: Jejunum, Ileum, Colon

Food and ingested drugs exit the duodenum and enter the second part of the small intestine, namely the jejunum. This has the dual role of digestion as well as absorption before food/drugs reach the ileum concerned mainly with absorption.

The actual process of digestion and absorption occurs in the villi, which line the inner surface of the small intestine (Figure 1.7). The crypts at the base of the villi contain stem cells that continuously divide by mitosis producing more stem cells and cells that migrate up the surface of the villus that differentiate into three types:

- Columnar epithelial cells responsible for digestion and absorption (these are the majority of the cells)
- Goblet cells which secrete mucus
- Endocrine cells which secrete a variety of hormones

Finally, Paneth cells secrete antimicrobial peptides that sterilize the contents of the intestine. All these cells replace older cells that continuously die by apoptosis.

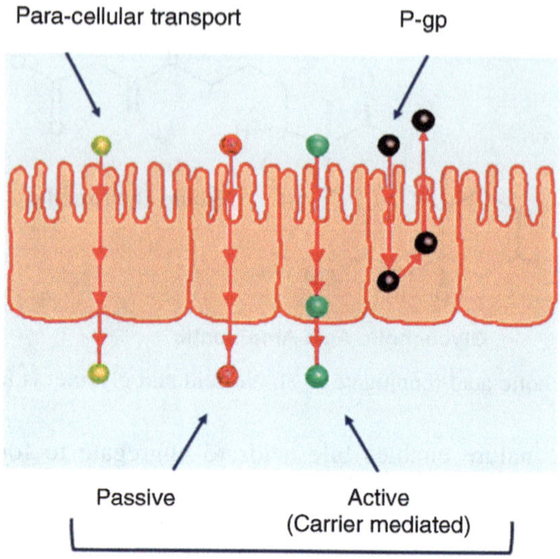

Figure 1.7 Routes for intestinal absorption.

The villi increase the surface area of the small intestine by a larger fold than if it were simply a tube with smooth walls. In addition, the apical (exposed) surface of the epithelial cells of each villus is covered with microvilli (also known as a "brush border"). Due to the microvilli, the total surface area of the intestine is almost 200 m^2 [16] (about the size of a tennis court) and approximately 100-fold the surface area of the exterior of the body.

Finally, undigested items such as cellulose along with other food wastes are passed into the large intestine (colon) and then the bowel for disposal as feces. The aim of food ingestion is not to produce waste but to provide the body with the nutrients and energy it requires to remain alive and function effectively. The digestive system is therefore equipped with a sophisticated system to ensure both digestion and absorption.

To ensure digestion, nutrients are maintained at 37°C at pH = 6.4–8.0 throughout the small intestine, and exposed to a comprehensive array of new enzymes such as maltase, lactase, intestinal lipases, and nucleases. Optimal exposure is further ensured by the peristaltic action of the gut, which slowly passes food along its 5 m length of convoluted tube while at the same time contracting in short segments to ensure thorough mixing.

Absorption ensures that molecules are transported through the gut wall into the blood circulation. This highly efficient process occurs *via* the paracellular or the transcellular route (Figure 1.7).

1.2.4.1 Paracellular Route The simplest exit from the gut is *via* the paracellular route namely through the interstitial space between cells (Figure 1.7). This exit route represents a relatively small area (only 0.01%) compared to the total cell surface area.

The tight junctions are studded with desmosomes (aka macula adherentes or macula adherens), cell structures specialized in cell-to-cell adhesion, limiting the transport of water, small polar molecules, and electrolytes. The restricted diameter of the aqueous pores (typically 3–6 Å in humans) indicates that hydrophilicity and molecular size are important factors in the ability of polar drug molecules to utilize this pathway. Paracellular absorption varies in different regions of the gastrointestinal tract due to varying pore size and frequency. Species differences in absorption have been attributed to variation in pore size, leading to varying efficiency of the paracellular pathway. It has been speculated that absorption of polar drugs are higher in the dog, compared to rat and human due to increased pore size in the dog [11]. Examples of drugs showing this species difference [12] include the α-adrenoceptor antagonists, atenolol, and xamoterol. Atenolol ($\log D_{7.4} = -1.9$, molecular weight 266) shows complete absorption (90%) in dog but only about 50% absorption in rat and human [18–20]. In contrast, absorption of the larger molecule xamoterol ($\log D_{7.4} = -1.0$, molecular weight 339) is lower overall, but remains higher in dog (about 36%) compared to rat (19%) or human (9%). Rat appears to be a better predictor than dog for paracellular transport regarding animal species modeling absorption in human.

1.2.4.2 Transcellular Route There are two main modes of transport available to molecules that use the transcellular route.

Active Transport The transcellular route is served by an array of ATP-powered active transporters for common nutrients such as glucose. Such molecules are absorbed by carrier-mediated cotransport with Na^+ ions. In this instance, the concentration difference of sodium ions (high in the intestinal lumen and low in the mucosa cells) drives the import of nutrients against a concentration gradient. Examples of drugs that utilize these transporters include methotrexate and L-DOPA [13]. However, the majority of drug molecules is not recognized by these transporters and has to be passively transported across the membrane causing the panoply of permeability issues that plague the medicinal chemist.

Passive Transport The more common transcellular route requires a molecule to passively cross the cell membrane, then cytoplasm before emerging at the other side of the enterocyte mucosa. To facilitate this unlikely process, the inside lining of the gut is covered with an extensive array of villi and microvilli. The surface area in the lumen is increased as the cellular surface of each villus is gathered into the "brush border." The brush borders of the intestinal lining have enzymes anchored into their apical plasma membrane as integral membrane proteins and these are located near the transporters that will then allow absorption.

The transport of a drug through a membrane depends largely on its relative solubility in water and lipids. If the drug is too water soluble, it will not enter the membrane, but if it is too lipid soluble it will enter but not leave the membrane. Good absorption requires that a drug's hydrophilic–lipophilic nature is in balance. The selection of a suitable carrier can be used to adjust this balance and consequently improve absorption of the drug.

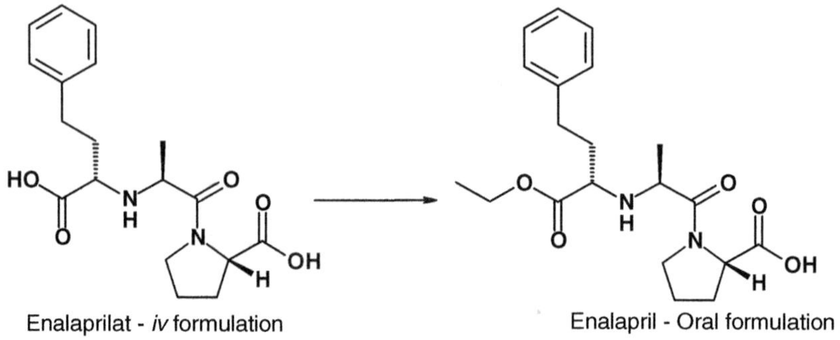

Figure 1.8 Enalaprilat for intravenous administration and enalapril for oral administration.

Enalaprilat possesses unfavorable ionization characteristics and is administered intravenously due to its poor oral bioavailability (Figure 1.8). However, esterification of the hydrophilic groups to give enalapril enhanced its transcellular diffusion and bioavailability.

Similarly, pivampicilin [14] and bacampicillin are both prodrugs of ampicillin and result from the esterification of the polar carboxylic group with a lipophilic, enzymatically labile ester. Both prodrugs are more lipid-soluble and absorbed more efficiently across the gut wall than the parent compound ampicillin. The serum levels attained following oral administration of bacampicillin are similar to those obtained after intramuscular injection of an equimolar amount of free ampicillin.

1.2.4.3 P-gp The surface area of the human gut is estimated to be 200 m^2 [15]. Unfortunately, such a large surface area is also available for the absorption of molecules that would potentially be harmful to the organism. Consequently, membrane efflux transporters such as P-glycoprotein (P-gp) act as a safety mechanism aimed at preventing toxins and xenobiotics from entering the general circulation by effectively pumping them back into the gut lumen. P-gp, a 170 kDa transmembrane glycoprotein, is a member of the adenosine triphosphate (ATP)-binding cassette (ABC) superfamily. It was discovered in 1976 [16] and was originally identified as a key reason for multidrug resistance in the treatment of certain cancers [17]. It is expressed in intestinal epithelia, hepatocytes, kidney proximal tubules, blood–brain barrier (BBB) endothelia, and placental trophoblast. Vinblastin, verapamil, quinidine, and omeprazole are known P-gp ligands [18], a property which has consequences for their oral absorption. Glibenclamide, a type-2 diabetes drug known to act at the sulfonyl urea receptor (SUR), is both a substrate and an inhibitor [19] of P-gp.

Many authors [20–22] have suggested that gut-wall CYP3A4 and P-glycoprotein act in concert to control the absorption of their substrates. This is based on the large overlap of substrates between the two and the proximity of their expression within the gut wall. It is proposed that P-glycoprotein effectively recycles its substrates allowing CYP3A4 several opportunities to metabolize compounds in the gut. A small amount of CYP3A4 in the gut wall (relative to the liver content) can exert a profound extraction of the compound. A study was conducted [23] with the gastrointestinal absorption of the HIV protease inhibitor saquinavir mesylate (Invirase®), whose oral bioavailability is low, variable, and significantly increased by coadministration with ritonavir. Both saquinavir and ritonavir were found to be P-gp substrates. Active efflux was temperature dependent, saturable, and inhibited by verapamil and cyclosporin A. Saquinavir and ritonavir decreased each other's secretory permeability and elevated their net transport by the absorptive pathway. Together with sensitivity to gut-wall metabolism by cytochrome CYP3A, it was proposed that this may partially account for the low and variable oral bioavailability of saquinavir in clinical studies and for its increased bioavailability after coadministration with ritonavir.

It has been shown that P-glycoprotein mRNA levels increase longitudinally along the intestine, with the lowest levels in the stomach and highest in the colon [24]. This observation has implications for controlled release technology.

1.2.5 Hepatic-Portal Vein

Following absorption in the small intestine, amino acids from protein digestion and the sugars from carbohydrates plus vitamins and important minerals such as calcium, iron, and iodine, as well as hydrophilic drugs, are absorbed directly into the blood capillaries in the villi. In contrast, glycerol, fatty acids, and dissolved vitamins enter the lacteals, are carried into the lymphatic system, and then released into the bloodstream at the lymphatic duct. Either way the nutrients (or drugs) exiting the GI tract are captured by the multitude of capillaries and blood vessels that line the outer surface of the digestive system (Figure 1.9). There is an abundance of blood vessels to ensure that all molecules absorbed through the intestinal wall are safely transported into the blood circulation. It has been estimated that a human being possesses 150,000 km of blood-carrying tubes with 98% containing microscopic capillaries for molecules exiting the gut to readily enter the bloodstream *via* a

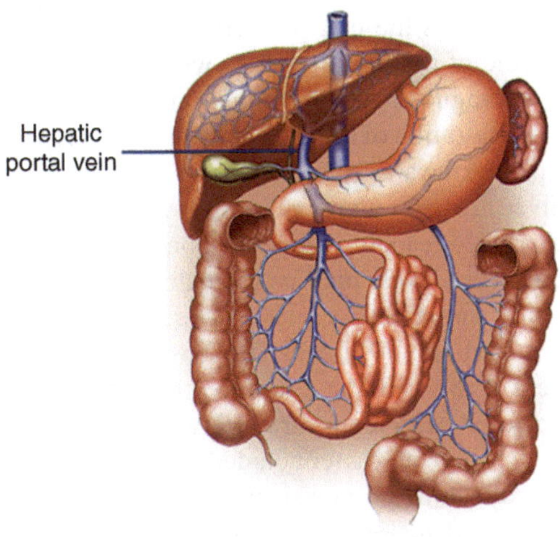

Figure 1.9 The hepatic-portal vein carrying nutrients from the gut to the liver.

neighboring capillary. After a meal, blood flow increases by 30–130% of basal flow and the hyperemia is confined to the segment if the intestine is exposed to the chyme. During periods of enhanced absorption or electrolyte secretion, blood is preferentially distributed to the mucosa. Nutrients and drugs do not exit into the general circulation once removed from the gut. The capillary beds of most tissues drain into veins that lead directly back to the heart. For the intestines, however, the draining veins lead to a second set of capillary beds in the liver, which serves as a gatekeeper between the intestines and the general circulation. This additional step ensures that useful substances are stored efficiently and that potentially harmful substances are metabolized for excretion.

The liver screens blood from the hepatic-portal system to ensure that its composition, when it leaves, will be close to normal for the body. This homeostatic mechanism functions in both directions. If the concentration of glucose in blood drops between meals, the liver converts its glycogen stores (glycogenolysis) or certain amino acids (gluconeogenesis) into glucose for release into the blood stream [25] (Figure 1.9). Glucose is removed and converted into glycogen. Other monosaccharides are removed and converted into glucose. Excess amino acids are removed and deaminated. The amino group is converted into urea. The residue can then enter the pathways of cellular respiration and be oxidized for energy.

Many nonnutritive molecules, such as ingested drugs, are removed by the liver and, often, metabolized to be detoxified and excreted through the kidneys. Since the liver is the main store of numerous nutrients and the organ responsible for a significant proportion of drug metabolism, it is not surprising that the multitude of capillaries and blood vessels that drain the digestive system converge into the HPV leading to the liver. The blood in the portal vein is relatively poor in oxygen, but rich in nutrients that have been absorbed from the GI tract. Upon entry into the liver, nutrients can be extracted by the liver cells for further metabolism. A significant proportion of a drug arriving into the liver will partition or be transported into the hepatocyte, where it may be metabolized by hepatic enzymes to inactive chemicals during the initial trip to the liver. This process is known as the first-pass effect.

Understanding the role of the portal vein as well as its position in the digestive system provides a key to diagnosing the plausible causes of "low oral bioavailability" of a compound. The concentration of a drug in the portal vein represents the amount of drug that has already passed the absorption and intestinal metabolism barriers but has not yet reached the liver [26]. A compound with low oral bioavailability and a low HPV level has issues prior to reaching the liver. Conversely, low oral bioavailability and good hepatic portal vein levels may be indicative of high liver metabolism.

This is illustrated in a comprehensive study carried out at Merck [27] on the design of $5HT_{1D}$ agonists. Compound 1 (Figure 1.10) showed low oral bioavailability and low hepatic portal vein levels (HPV < 5 ng/mL). Rigidification of the amino side chain gave much increased HPV exposure (HPV $= 558$ ng/mL at 0.5 h) and thus improved oral bioavailability. It was concluded that reducing the conformational mobility may have resulted in the compound being less susceptible to gut-wall metabolism. In addition, rigid analogues are simply more able to pass through the gut wall without conducting many entropically unfavorable conformational changes.

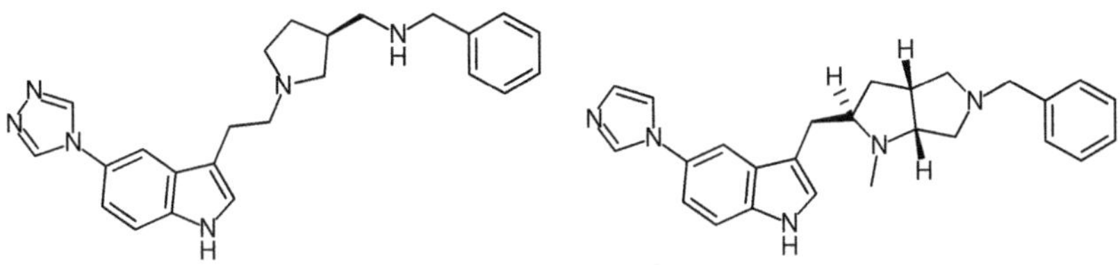

Compound 1 Compound 2

Figure 1.10 Compound 1: (HPV < 5 ng/mL). Rigidification of the amino side chain resulted in increased HPV exposure in Compound 2: (HPV = 558 ng/mL at 0.5 h).

1.3 THE LIVER METABOLISM

Nutrients and drug molecules arrive in the liver *via* the hepatic portal vein. The liver is a major organ, where nutrient storage, synthesis, and breakdown occur. It stores a multitude of substances, including glucose (in the form of glycogen), vitamin A (1–2 years' supply), vitamin D (1–4 months' supply), vitamin B12, iron, and copper. The liver is responsible for immunological effects. The reticuloendothelial system of the liver contains many immunologically active cells, acting as a "sieve" for antigens carried to it *via* the portal system. The liver produces albumin, the major osmolar component of blood serum. The liver synthesizes angiotensinogen, a hormone that is responsible for raising the blood pressure when activated by renin, a kidney enzyme that is released when the juxtaglomerular apparatus senses low blood pressure.

The liver performs several roles in carbohydrate metabolism including gluconeogenesis (the synthesis of glucose from certain amino acids, lactate or glycerol), glycogenolysis (the breakdown of glycogen into glucose), and glycogenesis (the formation of glycogen from glucose). The latter also occurs in the muscle. The liver is responsible for the mainstay of protein metabolism, synthesis, as well as degradation, and plays a major role in amino acid synthesis. The liver also performs several roles in lipid metabolism: cholesterol synthesis, lipogenesis, and the production of triglycerides (fats). This organ produces coagulation factors I (fibrinogen), II (prothrombin), V, VII, IX, X, and XI, as well as protein C, protein S, and antithrombin. The liver function changes from embryo to adult stage. In the first trimester fetus, the liver is the main site of red blood cell production, but by the 32nd week of gestation, the bone marrow has almost completely taken over that task. The liver produces and excretes bile (a greenish liquid) required for emulsifying fats. Some of the bile drains directly into the duodenum, and some is stored in the gallbladder. The liver also produces insulin-like growth factor 1 (IGF-1), a polypeptide protein hormone that plays an important role in childhood growth and continues to have anabolic effects in adults. The liver is a major site of thrombopoietin production. Thrombopoietin is a glycoprotein hormone that regulates the production of platelets by the bone marrow.

The breakdown of insulin and other hormones occurs in the liver. The liver breaks down hemoglobin, creating metabolites that are added to bile as pigment (bilirubin and biliverdin) and converts ammonia to urea.

Finally, the liver ensures that no toxic entities whether nutrients or drugs are released into the circulation. The process of breakdown of toxic substances and drugs is called drug metabolism and sometimes results in the formation of metabolites that are more toxic than its precursor. This is why understanding of liver metabolism is crucial at the earliest stages of drug discovery.

The metabolism process is best illustrated in the biosynthesis of bile acids from cholesterol, which takes place in the hepatocytes [28]. Cholesterol is ingested as part of the diet and converted into the bile acids chenodeoxycholic acid and cholic acid in a series of Phase 1 oxidation steps (Figure 1.11). The resulting carboxylic acid functionality is then conjugated to glycine or taurine in a Phase 2 conjugation step. The resulting water-soluble product is then actively secreted into tiny bile cannaliculi between liver cells that lead into bile duct that connects to duodenum and stored in the gallbladder.

Phase 1 oxidation steps are commonly catalyzed by cytochrome P450 enzymes (CYPs) [29] and introduce polar water-solubilizing groups such as –OH, –COOH, and $-SO_3H$ or unmask water-solubilizing groups already present in the molecule. These often provide a point of anchor for further conjugation (Phase 2) with suitable water-soluble fragments. The result is usually an increase in the polarity and a change in the biological activity or toxicity profile of the substance [30].

Phase 2 reactions (conjugate formation) couple substrates (bilirubin, metabolites of xenobiotics, drugs, and steroid hormones) to highly polar, water-solubilizing

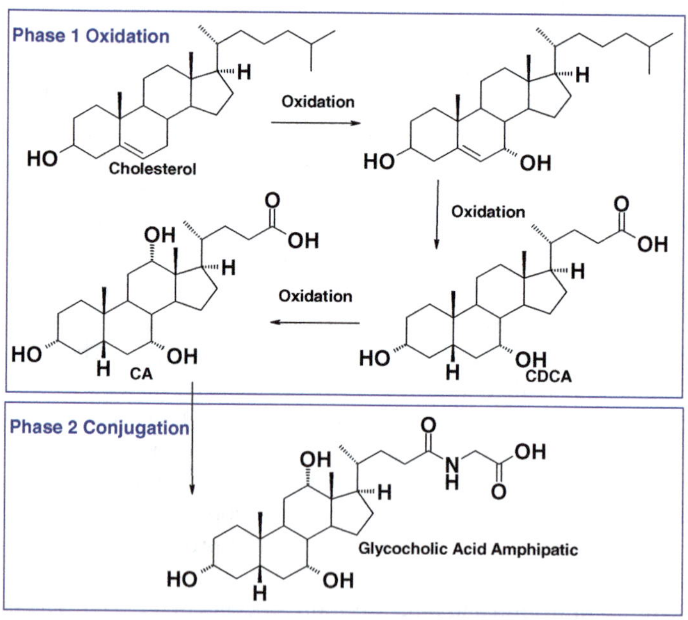

Figure 1.11 The biosynthesis of glycocholic acid in hepatocytes resulting from Phase 1 (oxidation) and Phase 2 (conjugation) processes.

amines (glycine, taurine), or alcohols (glucoronates) taken from the store of the liver. The enzymes involved are transferases.

1.3.1 CYP450 (CYPs)

"CYP" is a host of enzymes that use iron to oxidize xenobiotics, endogenous substances, and nutrients, often as part of the body's strategy to dispose of potentially harmful substances by making them more water soluble. More than half of known drugs are primarily cleared by CYPs. CYP catalyzes a variety of reactions including epoxidation, N-dealkylation, O-dealkylation, S-oxidation, and hydroxylation. A typical cytochrome P450 catalyzed reaction is

$$\text{NADPH} + \text{H}^+ + \text{O}_2 + \text{RH} \Rightarrow \text{NADP}^+ + \text{H}_2\text{O} + \text{R–OH}$$

The main organ in humans involved in drug and toxin removal is the small intestine even though most of the CYPs are found in the liver. CYP is usually found in the "microsomal" part of the cytoplasm (endoplasmic reticulum). Metabolic clearance of drugs is not the only function of CYP. Recently, it has been found that CYP is intimately involved in vascular autoregulation, particularly in the brain. CYP is vital to the formation of cholesterol, steroids, and arachidonic acid metabolites. There are over a thousand different CYPs, although the number in man is only about 50 (49 genes and 15 pseudogenes have been sequenced). It is likely that most of the human CYPs have already been discovered.

What's in a name?

Cytochrome P450 chemistry is fascinating. All chemists appreciate that the bond between the two atoms in an oxygen molecule is rather strong. This implies that a substantial amount of energy is required to break the bond. The energy is supplied by the addition of electrons to the iron atom of heme. These electrons come from the last protein in an "electron transfer chain." There are two such chains in cells that end up at P450. The first is in the endoplasmic reticulum (ER), and the protein involved is called NADPH cytochrome P450 reductase. Electrons pass from NADPH to FAD to FMN and finally to heme. The second chain is located within mitochondria. A complex chain of proteins transfers the electrons to heme. NADPH passes electrons to ferredoxin reductase, thence to ferredoxin (which itself has an iron–sulfur cluster), and finally to CYP.

1.3.1.1 CYP Isoforms

How do we classify CYP since there are numerous isoforms of cytochrome P450? An isoform is a CYP enzyme variant that derives from one particular gene. They are classified according to the similarities of their amino acid sequences. Such classification allows division of CYP isoforms into families. CYP families contain genes that have at least 40% sequence homology. There are at least 74 CYP families, but only about 17 of these have been described in man. Families are numbered such as *CYP2* and *CYP21*. Families are further subdivided into subfamilies in which members must have at least 55% identity. About 30 subfamilies are well characterized in man. Subfamilies are identified by a letter such as *CYP3A* and *CYP2D*. Finally, there are individual CYP genes. There are approximately 50 genes important in man. Individual genes are identified by a number such as *CYP2D6*.

Among the diverse human genes, several have been identified as particularly important in oxidative metabolism including

- *CYP3A4* (by far the most important, metabolizing ~40% of xenobiotics)
- *CYP2D6*
- *CYP*2C9
- *CYP*2C19

Other notable CYPs are *CYP2E1*, *CYP2A6*, and *CYP1A2*. On exposure to appropriate substrates, enzyme induction occurs with all of these CYPs, apart from CYP2D6.

What is polymorphism and why is it significant? The activity of CYP oxidases differs in different people and different populations. Genetic variation in a population is termed "polymorphism" when both gene variants exist with a frequency of at least 1%. Such differences in activity may have profound clinical consequences, especially when multiple drugs are given to a patient. There are profound racial differences in the distribution of various alleles. Data on a drug that behaves in one way in one population group cannot necessarily be extrapolated to another group. The explanations for the various polymorphisms are thought to be complex, but perhaps the most interesting is the high expression of *CYP2D6* in many persons of Ethiopian and Saudi Arabian origin. *2D6* is not inducible, so these people have developed a different strategy to cope with the presumably high load of toxic alkaloids in their diet—multiple copies of the gene. These CYPs break down a variety of drugs such as many antidepressants and neuroleptics, thus making them ineffective. Conversely, prodrugs such as codeine will be extensively activated and will be largely converted into morphine.

In contrast, many individuals lack functional *2D6*. These subjects will be predisposed to drug toxicity caused by antidepressants or neuroleptics, but will find codeine and tramadol to be inefficacious due to lack of activation. Other drugs that have caused problems in those lacking *2D6* include dexfenfluramine, propafenone, mexiletine, and perhexiline. Perhexiline was withdrawn from the market due to the neuropathy it caused in those *2D6*-inactive patients.

Another potentially disastrous polymorphism is the deficient activity of *CYP2C9*. Patients possessing this enzyme variant are ineffective in clearing (*S*)-warfarin to an extent that a 0.5 mg dose in a day results in full anticoagulation. Additionally, the same CYP is important in removal of phenytoin and tolbutamide, both potentially very toxic drugs in excess. Alternatively, the prodrug losartan will be poorly activated and inefficacious with *2C9* deficiency. Azole antifungals, sulphinpyrazone, and even amiodarone may cause a similar effect by inhibiting the enzyme.

Occasionally benefits are derived from an unusual CYP phenotype. Cure rates for peptic ulcer treated with omeprazole are substantially greater in individuals with defective *CYP2C19* due to sustained, high plasma levels of the drug.

CYP induction is another important concept. Most of the CYPs can be induced with CYP3A4 the most important and CYP2D6 the most notable exception. CYP3A4 is the most prevalent CYP in the body and metabolizes many substrates. The most important inducers of 3A4 are antimicrobials such as rifampicin, and anticonvulsants such as carbamazepine and phenytoin. Potent steroids such as dexamethasone may also induce 3A4. The long list of agents metabolized by the enzyme includes opioids, benzodiazepines, and local anesthetics, as well as erythromycin, cyclosporine, haloperidol, calcium-channel blockers, cisapride, and pimozide. Oral contraceptives are also metabolized, and their efficacy may be impaired when an inducer such as rifampicin is administered.

The inhibitors of 3A4 are even more important than the inducers of 3A4 and include azole antifungals, HIV protease inhibitors, calcium-channel blockers, some macrolides such as troleandromycin and erythromycin, and the commonly used "SSRI" antidepressants. Lethal clinical consequences can result from combining 3A4 inhibitors with drugs that are metabolized by this cytochrome. Non-sedating antihistamines have resulted in fatal arrhythmias, as has occurred with cisapride administration in combination with an inhibitor. Erythromycin in combination with theophylline may cause toxicity due to the latter.

There is an interesting association between some CYPs and the important transmembrane pump protein, P-glycoprotein (the product of the *MDR1* gene). Generally, if P-glycoprotein is present, then CYP3A4 is also found. This presumably is due to a concerted strategy by the body to eliminate xenobiotics. The P-glycoprotein pumps out as much xenobiotics as possible and CYP3A removes the remainder! This association contributes to even more interesting drug interactions such as calcium-channel blockers and drugs as diverse as azole antifungals, immunosuppressants, and macrolides interacting with the membrane pump and the CYP.

CYP metabolism is so critical that predominant degradation of a drug by one of the polymorphic CYPs is often enough to terminate further research on that compound during discovery.

Although most of the CYP metabolism occurs in the liver, with a minor contribution from the intestine, some isoforms are found throughout the body such as CYP51. Other isoforms are limited to one specific tissue such as CYP11B2, found mainly if not exclusively in the glomerulosa zone of the adrenal gland. Differential expression of some CYPs in different organs may also have clinical consequences, especially where the unfortunate side-effect of "degradation" of a drug produces a more toxic product. The degradation of paracetamol by CYP2E1 results in a highly active intermediate product, which in sufficient quantities can result in fulminant liver failure. Antioxidants protect against this catastrophe. In contrast, chronic ethanol consumption induces CYP2E1 and may increase the likelihood of toxicity.

Drug molecules that are not recognized by liver enzymes and considered toxic are subjected to a similar reaction sequence as illustrated in the liver metabolism of aspirin [31] (Figure 1.12). Phase 1 oxidation introduces a number of solubilizing hydroxyl groups. In the Phase 2 steps, the hydroxyl moiety is glucoronidated, while the carboxylic acid functionality is conjugated with the amine group in glycine. This produces a range of water-soluble products suitable for elimination.

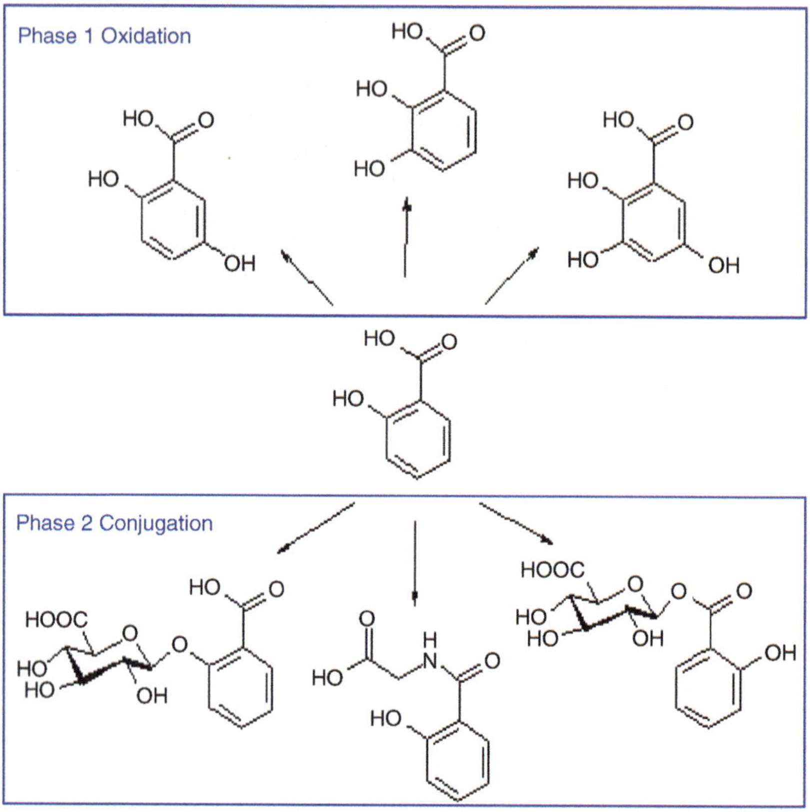

Figure 1.12 The metabolism of aspirin in hepatocytes with Phase 1 (oxidation) and Phase 2 (conjugation) resulting in water-soluble products.

The metabolism of aromatic carboxylic acids involves the conjugation of the acid with glycine (a Phase 2 conjugation reaction) *via* an acetyl coenzyme-A intermediate. The resulting hippuric acid (Figure 1.13) conjugate is very water soluble and readily excreted through the kidneys. Thus a reduced concentration of hippuric acid in the urine indicates the possibility of liver damage and this formed the basis of a test for checking [32] the detoxification function of the liver.

Many factors may affect liver metabolism. Dietary factors such as lack of vitamins or a low protein diet can cause decreased oxidative drug metabolism. Drugs and some foods (e.g., grapefruit juice) that are known inhibitors, inducers, or substrates for

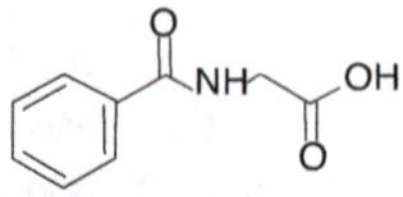

Figure 1.13 Hippuric acid produced in the liver from a Phase 2 conjugation reaction with glycine.

CYPs can potentially interact with the metabolism of coadministered drugs affecting its AUC and rate of clearance.

Variable expression of CYP has substantial clinical consequences, not only in different people and different race groups, but also in individuals as they progress from infancy to old age. Age affects the expression of metabolizing enzymes leading to potentially fatal situations. The antibacterial drug chloramphenicol, which is no longer used for premature babies, relies on the presence of Phase 2 glucoronyl transferase to eliminate the oxamyl chloride intermediate produced from Phase 1 as its soluble glucoronide conjugate [33]. Since infants lack this Phase 2 enzyme, the highly reactive oxamyl chloride is free to produce an *N*-nitroso-derivative, which causes fatal aplastic anemia in neonates. CYP1A2 is not expressed in neonates and so they are particularly susceptible to toxicity from substance such as caffeine.

Some disease states cause patients to develop impaired liver function, liver cirrhosis, or hepatoma, which can present altered hepatic blood flow and decreased number of functional hepatocytes (CYPs). This has serious consequences for the administration of drugs that display or rely on high liver clearance.

Understanding CYP metabolism has been used productively in AIDS therapy. As discussed previously, saquinavir (Invirase®) is a potent HIV protease inhibitor with oral bioavailability limited by extensive first-pass metabolism mediated primarily by CYP3A4 [34]. While saquinavir is a weak CYP3A4 inhibitor [35], its exposure is enhanced [36] when combined with a low (subtherapeutic) dose of ritonavir [37], a potent inhibitor of CYP3A4.

In summary, once a drug has completed a route from the mouth through the stomach, duodenum, jejunum, ileum, hepatic portal vein and the liver, first pass metabolism is complete. During this process, a portion of the drug is lost before it reaches the systemic circulation.

Not all the drug substances that have been processed in the liver reach the blood circulation. Some drugs such as steroid hormones, digoxin, and some cancer chemotherapeutic agents are secreted from the liver back into the bile and reenter the digestive system *via* the bile duct. The secretion is effected [38] by members of ABC superfamily of transporters, which include seven families of proteins such as the multidrug resistance (MDR) family. In many cases, these drugs undergo enterohepatic circulation, in which they are reabsorbed in the small intestine and reenter the liver *via* the hepatic portal vein.

1.4 THE KIDNEYS

The final filters in the voyage of a drug are the kidneys and 25% of cardiac output is directed to these organs. The kidneys act as an "on-line filtration unit" and provide the primary route of excretion for many drugs such as vancomycin, atenolol, and ampicillin. These drugs can accumulate to toxic levels in patients with compromised renal function and in elderly patients. Blood has a cellular (45% organic) and plasma (55% aqueous) component. Cellular blood component consists of red blood cells (erythrocytes), monocytes, white blood cells, etc. The plasma is composed of water, small solutes, and proteins such as albumin and $\alpha 1$ acid glycoprotein that adsorb acidic and basic molecules, respectively. An initial liquid–liquid separation takes the aqueous part of the blood in the nephron where it is filtered, cleansed, and its composition readjusted. It is then gradually reunited with the organic phase and the resulting reconstituted "cleansed" blood emerges in the afferent vein while the waste products are excreted in the urine. From the 1100–2000 L of blood that flows through the human kidneys each day, the nephron processes about 180 L of filtrate, but excretes only about 1.5 L of urine. The rest of the filtrate, including about 99% of the water, is reabsorbed into the blood.

The renal medulla is studded with an excess of one million nephrons, which are the basic functional filtering units. Blood arrives into the Bowman capsule via a cluster of porous capillaries called the glomerulus (Figure 1.14). The high hydrostatic pressure inside the capillaries causes the aqueous part to separate from the blood and enter the proximal tubule through the pores. This process is known as *glomerular filtration.* Most drug particles pass easily through the spaces of the capillary walls into the urine in the proximal tubule. Large particles, such as cells, proteins, or drug molecules bound to protein remain in the capillaries and exit the renal corpuscle *via* afferent arterioles.

Efferent arterioles wrap themselves around the structure of the nephron and will collect cleansed water and ions as they are produced by the remainder of the nephron apparatus. Next, the proximal tubule actively reabsorbs up to two-thirds of the valuable substances such as glucose, vitamins chloride ions *via* ATP-powered pumps, which use Na^+ as the cotransporter (Figure 1.14). Water follows by osmosis and together they enter blood vessels near the tubule and are thus returned to the body. The filtrate that emerges from the proximal tubule, which is high in wastes and low in nutrients, now enters a U-shaped region of the nephron named the

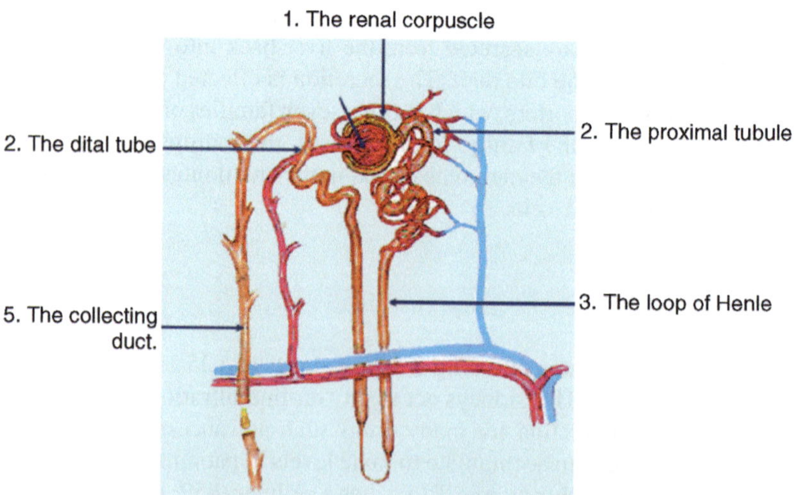

Figure 1.14 A nephron made up of five regions. 1. The renal corpuscle. 2. The proximal tubule. 3. The loop of Henle. 4. The distal tube. 5. The collecting duct.

loop of Henle. The wall of the descending limb is impermeable to solutes but permeable to water, which is removed by osmosis into the tissue fluid surrounding this section of the loop. The thick region of the ascending limb of the loop of Henle is highly permeable to Na^+ and Cl^- but impermeable to water and contains chloride pumps, which remove sodium and chloride ions from the fluid in the lumen by active transport. The fluid in the two limbs of the loop of Henle flows in opposite directions, and the active removal of ions from the ascending limb and their constant inflow in the descending limb create an osmotic gradient along the length of the loop of Henle, which is known as a counter current multiplier system. The peritubular capillaries that surround the loop of Henle passively absorb the water and the ions that have been removed. The filtrate enters the distal tubule where electrolytes and water are reabsorbed under hormonal control (aldosterone and arginine vasopressin (AVP), also known as vasopressin, argipressin or antidiuretic hormone (ADH)). Urea, uric acid, creatinine, and other substances are finally collected as waste and released in the urine.

Urinary excretion occurs through glomerular filtration, active tubular secretion, and passive tubular reabsorption. The glomeruli filter unbound xenobiotics in a manner that is not saturable and at a rate that depends on renal blood flow [39]. Most drugs are filtered from blood in the glomerular unless they are tightly plasma protein bound or have been incorporated into red blood cells. From a medicinal chemistry point of view, the overall renal excretion is controlled by what happens in the tubules, namely, active tubular secretion and passive tubular reabsorption.

1.4.1 Active Tubular Secretion

Active transport systems in the renal tubule move some drugs from the blood to urine. The secretory mechanisms are not generally specific to drugs. Drug secretion takes advantage of molecular similarities between the drug and naturally occurring substances such as organic anions (transported by OAT family proteins) and cations (transported by OCT family proteins). Penicillin (Figure 1.15) is an example of a drug that is eliminated largely by active transport in the proximal tubule [40]. The extent of plasma protein binding appears to have a relatively small effect on drug secretion into the proximal tubule, because the highly efficient transporters that mediate active tubular secretion rapidly remove free (unbound) drug from the peritubular capillaries, thereby altering the equilibrium between free and protein-bound drug at these sites.

Since tubular secretion is an active process, it may be subject to saturation and drug interactions. The clearance of penicillin G [41] in normal individuals occurs predominantly *via* the kidney. It is extremely rapid and is the result of glomerular filtration and active tubular transport, with the latter route predominating [42]. Urinary recovery is reported to be 58–85% of the administered dose. Coadministration of probenecid, a drug normally administered to treat gout, competes with the same acid transporter and blocks the renal tubular secretion of penicillin resulting in slower rate of excretion of penicillin G and increased serum concentrations. It has been shown that probenecid also alters the distribution of penicillins to various

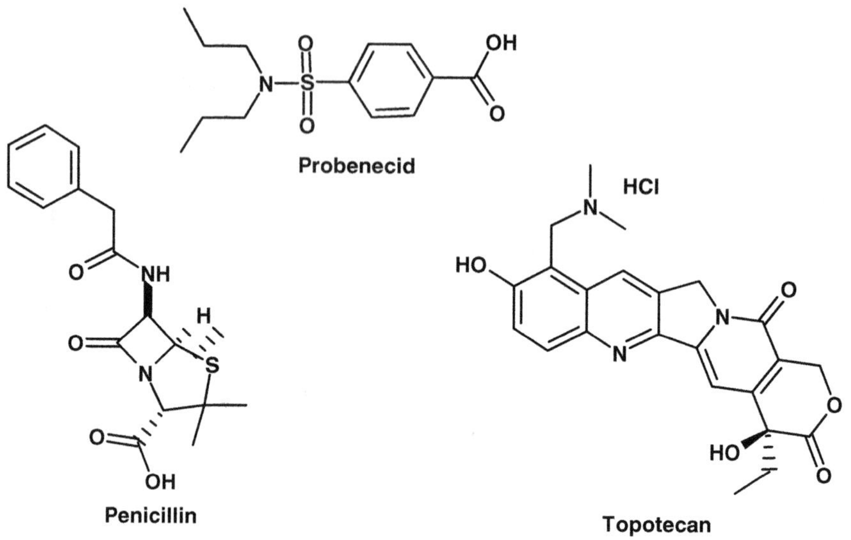

Figure 1.15 Structures of penicillin, probenecid, and topotecan. Three acidic molecules competing for the acid transporter.

tissues causing more drug to distribute out of plasma, causing even less to be eliminated.

The topoisomerase 1 inhibitor topotecan (Hycamtin®) is an antineoplastic chemotherapy drug. It is primarily eliminated by the kidneys, with 60–70% of the dose recovered as topotecan total in the urine. Coadministration [43] of topotecan lactone or hydroxy acid in combination with probenecid resulted in decreased topotecan lactone, total, and hydroxy acid systemic clearance, and total renal clearance. By inhibiting renal tubular secretion, probenecid decreased renal and systemic clearance, which led to an increase in topotecan systemic exposure.

1.4.2 Passive Tubular Reabsorption

Passive tubular reabsorption accounts for the reabsorption of noncharged, lipid-soluble xenobiotics. A concentration gradient exists with more drug particle in the urinary tubule than in the bloodstream because much of the water in the filtrate has been reabsorbed. The concentration gradient is in the direction of reabsorption. Drugs in the renal tubules have a tendency to transfer back into the blood by passive reabsorption. Like other passive diffusion processes, passive reabsorption is controlled by the drug's lipid solubility, degree of ionization, and pH of both the blocked and tubular filtrate. If the compound is nonionized, it will have a greater tendency to be reabsorbed. If the compound is charged, it will tend to be excreted. These changes can be quite significant as urine pH can vary from 4.5 to 8.0 depending on the diet (meat can cause a more acidic urine) or drugs (which can increase or decrease urine pH). The pH of the renal tubules can be therapeutically manipulated to increase the excretion of drugs. In the case of an overdose from the weak acid phenobarbital [44], increasing the pH of the urine will cause an increase in the rate of excretion of the drug. This process is called forced alkaline diuresis. In addition, changing the rate of urine flow through the tubules can also modify the rate of drug reabsorption, since an increased rate of urine output tends to dilute the drug concentration in the tubule and to decrease the amount of time during which facilitated diffusion can occur. Aspirin is a weak acid that is excreted by the kidney. Aspirin overdose is treated [45] by administering sodium bicarbonate to alkalinize the urine (and trap aspirin in the tubule) and by increasing the urine flow rate (and thus dilute the tubular concentration of the drug). Both of these clinical maneuvers result in faster elimination of the drug. Conversely, the excretion of weak bases can sometimes be increased by acidification of the urine using ammonium chloride.

1.5 CONCLUSIONS

Understanding the process of digestion allows for the appreciation of the various routes of administration. Although drugs administered by intravenous by-pass the digestive system, they are still exposed to the liver or kidneys and metabolized. While the suppository route of administration relies on permeability through the large intestine, this part of the gut is not normally involved in absorption and can lead to low plasma levels. Oral administration of salbutamol alleviates symptoms associated with asthma, whereas intravenous administration delivers a muscle relaxant systemically and is used to avert premature labor. Finally, administration of local anesthetic to the bone can lead to temporary tachycardia, as adrenaline (vasoconstrictant used to reduce bleeding) can leak into a neighboring blood vessel.

Drugs undergo the same metabolic processes as food. The most important issue that medicinal chemists encounter is that of solubility, followed by the intricacies of permeability, which are complicated by the intervention of P-gp efflux. Finally, the perennial issues of metabolism in the liver and other organs (mainly by the CYPs) often plague drug development. Diagnosing drug metabolism issues will assist medicinal chemists in solving recurrent problems encountered in the course of drug development.

REFERENCES

1. Generex Gets Approval for Oral-Lyn Phase ii Trial, (2005). *Diabetes in Control, On Line Newsletter, 260*, 17 May.
2. Oral-lyn Insulin: First Non-Injectable Insulin Gets Released this Month, (2005). *Diabetes in Control, On Line Newsletter, 287*, 22 November.
3. Washington, N., Washington, C., and Wilson, C. *Physiological Pharmaceutics: Barriers to Drug Absorption*, CRC Press, Boca Raton, FL, 2000, p. 85.
4. Singh, K., Dickinson, L., Chaikan, A., Back, D., Fletcher, C., Pozniak, A., Moyle, G., Nelson, M., Gazzard, B., Herath, D., and Boffito, M. Pharmacokinetics and safety of

saquinavir/ritonavir and omeprazole in HIV-infected subjects. *Clin. Pharmacol. Ther.* 2008, *83(6)*, 867–872.

5. Winston, A., Back, D., Fletcher, C., Robinson, L., Unsworth, J., Tolowinska, I., Schutz, M., Pozniak, A. L., Gazzard, B., and Boffito, M. Effect of omeprazole on the pharmacokinetics of saquinavir-500 mg formulation with ritonavir in healthy male and female volunteers. *AIDS* 2006, *20*, 1401–1406.
6. Collins, J. L., Blanchard, S. G., Boswell, E., Charifson, P. S., Cobb, J. E., Henke, B. R., Hull-Ryde, E. A., Kazmierski, W. M., Lake, D. H., Leesnitzer, L. M., Lehmann, J., Lenhard, J. M., Orband-Miller, L. A., Gray-Nunez, Y., Parks, D. J., Plunkett, K. D., and Tong, W.-Q. *N*-(2-Benzoylphenyl)-l-tyrosine PPARγ agonists. 2. Structure–activity relationship and optimization of the phenyl alkyl ether moiety. *J. Med. Chem.* 1998, *41*, 5037–5054.
7. Brooks, D. A. PPAR alpha and PPAR gamma Co-agonists for Treatment of Type 2 Diabetes and Cardiovascular Risk Factors. *221st ACS Symposium – San Diego, California, 2001.*
8. Netter, F. H. *Atlas of Human Anatomy*, Saunders, Philadelphia, PA, 2006, p. 320.
9. Wignot, T. M., Stewart, R. P., Schray, K. J., Das, S., and Sipos, T. 3, 4 *In vitro* studies of the effects of HAART drugs and excipients on activity of digestive enzymes. *Pharm. Res.* 2004, *21(3)*, 420–427.
10. Wilson, C. O., Block, J. H., Gisvold, O., Marlowe, J., and Wilson, B. *Gisvold's Textbook of Organic Medicinal and Pharmaceutical Chemistry*, Lippincott Williams and Wilkins, Baltimore, MD, 2004, p. 331.
11. Marten, T. R., Bourne, G. R., Miles, G. S., Shuker, B., Rankine, H. D., and Dutka, V. N. The metabolism of ICI 118,587, a partial agonist of alpha1-adrenoceptors, in mice, rats, rabbits, dogs and humans. *Drug Metab. Dispos.* 1984, *12*, 652–660.
12. Bastain, W., Boyce, M. J., Stafford, L. E., Morton, P. B., Clarke, D. A., and Marlow, H. F. Pharmacokinetics of xamoterol after intravenous and oral administration to volunteers. *Eur. J. Clin. Pharmacol.* 1988, *34*, 469–473.
13. Fraga, S., Sampaio-Maia, B., Serrao, M. P., and Soares-Da-Silva, P. Regulation of apical transporter of L-DOPA in human intestinal Caco-2 cells. *Acta Physiol. Scand.* 2002, *175(2)*, 103–111.
14. Shek, E., Higushi, T., and Bodor, N. Improved delivery through biological membranes. 2. Distribution, excretion and metabolism of *N*-methyl-1,6-dihydropyridine-2-carbaldoxime hydrochloride, a prodrug of *N*-methylpyridinium-2-carbaldoxime chloride. *J. Med. Chem.* 1976, *19*, 108–112.
15. Van Asperen, J., Van Tellingen, O., and Beijnen, J. H. The pharmacological role of P-glycoprotein in the intestinal epithelium. *Pharm. Res.* 1998, *37*, 429–435.
16. Juliano, R. L. and Ling, V. A surface glycoprotein modulating drug permeability in Chinese hamster ovary cell mutants. *Biochim. Biophys. Acta* 1976, *455*, 152–162.
17. Gottesman, M. M., Pastan, I., and Ambudkar, S. V. P-glycoprotein and multidrug resistance. *Curr. Opin. Genet. Dev.* 1996, *6*, 610–617.
18. Pajeva, I. K. and Wiese, M. Pharmacophore model of drugs involved in P-glycoprotein multidrug resistance: explanation of structural variety (hypothesis). *J. Med. Chem.* 2002, *45*, 5671–5686.
19. Golstein, P. E., Boom, A., van Geffel, J., Jacobs, P., Masereel, B., and Beauwens, R. P-glycoprotein inhibition by glibenclamide and related compounds. *Pflügers Arch. – Eur. J. Physiol.* 1999, *437*, 652–660.

20. Hebert, M. F. Contributions of hepatic and intestinal metabolism and P-glycoprotein to cyclosporine and tacrolimus oral drug delivery. *Adv. Drug Deliv. Rev.* 1997, *27*, 201–214.
21. Hall, S. D., Thummel, K. E., Watkins, P. B., Lown, K. S., Benet, L. Z., Paine, M. F., Mayo, R. R., Turgeon, D. K., Bailey, D. G., Fontana, R. J., and Wrighton, S. A. Molecular and physical mechanisms of first pass extraction. *Drug Metab. Dispos.* 1999, *27*, 161–166.
22. Lown, K. S., Mayo, R. R., Leichtman, A. B., Hsiao, H., Turgeon, D. K., Schmiedlin-Ren, P., Brown, M. B., Guo, W., Rossi, S. J., Benet, L. Z., and Watkins, P. B. Role of intestinal P-glycoprotein (mdr1) in interpatient variation in the oral bioavailability of cyclosporine. *Clin. Pharmacol. Ther.* 1997, *62*, 248–260.
23. Alsenz, J., Steffen, H., and Alex, R. Active apical secretory efflux of the HIV protease inhibitors saquinavir and ritonavir in Caco-2 cell. *Pharm. Res.* 1998, *15(3)*, 423–428.
24. Wacher, V. J., Silverman, J. A., Zhang, Y., and Benet, L. Z. Role of P-glycoprotein and cytochrome P450 3A in limiting oral absorption of peptides and peptidomimetics. *J. Pharm. Sci.* 1998, *87*, 1322–1330.
25. Washington, N., Washington, C., and Wilson, C. *Physiological Pharmaceutics: Barriers to Drug Absorption*, CRC Press, Boca Raton, FL, 2000, p. 113.
26. Sills, A. K., Williams, J. I., Tyler, B. M., Epstein, D. S., Sipos, E. P., and Davis, J. D. Intraoperative cytodiagnosis for detecting a minute invasion of the portal vein. *Curr. Opin. Oncol.* 1999, *11(6)*, 219.
27. Russel, M. G. N., Beer, M. S., Stanton, J. A., Sohal, B., Mortishire-Smith, R. J., and Castro, J. L. 2,7-Diazabicyclo [3.3.0] octanes as novel h5-HT1D receptor agonists. *Bioorg. Med. Chem. Lett.* 1999, *9(17)*, 2491–2496.
28. Koolman, J. and Rohm K.-H. *Color Atlas of Biochemistry*, Thieme, New York, Please insert if available (search online) 1996, pp. 290–293.
29. Vaz, R. J. and Klabunde, T. *Antitargets. Prediction and Prevention of Drug Side Effects*, Wiley-VCH Verlag GmbH, Wienhiem, 2008, p. 267.
30. Foye, W. O., Lemke, T. L., and Williams D.A. *Principles of Medicinal Chemistry*, Williams and Wilkins, Baltimore, MD, 1995, pp. 83–140.
31. Thomas, G. *Medicinal Chemistry – An Introduction*, Wiley, New York, 2000, pp. 336–360.
32. Borsook, H. and Dubnoff, J. W. The biological synthesis of hippuric acid *in vitro*. *J. Biol. Chem.* 1940, *132(1)*, 307–324.
33. Sills, M. R. and Boenning, D. Chloramphenicol. *Pediatr. Rev.* 1999, *20*, 357–358.
34. Ogden, R. C. and Flexner, C. W. *Protease Inhibitors in AIDS Therapy*, Informa Health Care, 2001, pp. 27–48.
35. Malaty, L. I. and Kuper, J. J. Drug interactions of HIV protease inhibitors. *Drug Saf.* 1999, *20*, 147–169.
36. Eagling, V. A., Back, D. J., and Barry, M. G. Differential inhibition of cytochrome p450 isoforms by the protease inhibitors, ritonavir, saquinavir and indinavir. *Br. J. Clin. Pharmacol.* 1997, *44*, 190–194.
37. Merry, C., Barry, M. G., and Mulcahy, F. Saquinavir pharmacokinetics alone and in combination with ritonavir in HIV-infected patients. *AIDS* 1997, *11*, 29–33.
38. Golan, D. E., Tashjian, A. H., Armstrong, E. J., and Armstrong, A. W. *Principles of Pharmacology: The Pathophysiologic Basis of Drug Therapy*, Lippincott Williams and Wilkins, Baltimore, MD, 2007, p. 42.

39. Goldfrank, L. R., Flomenbaum, N. E., Howland, M. A., and Hoffman, R. S., *Goldfrank's Toxicologic Emergencies*, McGraw-Hill Professional, New York, 2006, p. 174.
40. Golan, D. E., Tashjian, A. H., Armstrong, E. J., and Armstrong, A. W. *Principles of Pharmacology: The Pathophysiologic Basis of Drug Therapy*, Lippincott Williams and Wilkins, Baltimore, MD, 2007, p. 40.
41. Rang, H. P. *Pharmacology*, Churchill Livingstone, Edinburgh, 2003, p. 112.
42. VanWert, A. L., Bailey, R. M., and Sweet, D. H. Organic anion transporter 3 (Oat3/Slc22a8) knockout mice exhibit altered clearance and distribution of penicillin G. *Am. J. Physiol. – Renal Physiol.* 2007, *293*, 1332–1341.
43. Zamboni, W. C., Houghton, P. J., Johnson, R. K., Hulstein, J. L., Crom, W. R., Cheshire, P. J., Hanna, S. K., Richmond, L. B., Luo, X., and Stewart, C. F. Probenecid alters topotecan systemic and renal disposition by inhibiting renal tubular secretion. *J. Pharmacol. Exp. Ther.* 1998, *284(1)*, 89–94.
44. O'Leary, J. P., Tabuenca, A., and Capote, L. R. *The Physiologic Basis of Surgery*, Lippincott Williams and Wilkins, Baltimore, MD, 2007, p. 268.
45. Aschenbrenner, D. S. and Venable. S. J. *Drug Therapy in Nursing*, Lippincott Williams and Wilkins, Baltimore, MD, 2008, pp. 46–47.

2

IN SILICO ADME/Tox PREDICTIONS

David Lagorce, Christelle Reynes, Anne-Claude Camproux,
Maria A. Miteva, Olivier Sperandio, and Bruno O. Villoutreix

2.1 INTRODUCTION

Partial decline in the productivity of pharmaceutical R&D departments threaten the sustainability of the current business model. During many years, the drug discovery process involved chemical synthesis and *in vivo* testing with optimization of the compounds' pharmacokinetic, metabolic, and toxic properties postponed to later stages. In recent years, there has been increasing awareness about the importance of predicting and optimizing the absorption, distribution, metabolism, excretion, and toxicity (ADME/Tox) properties of chemical compounds along the discovery process rather than at the final stages. Several *in vitro* and *in silico* approaches have been devised to predict some key ADME/Tox properties. In this chapter, we focus on methods pertaining to the field of *in silico* ADME/Tox prediction.

In Section 2.2, we introduce the field of drug discovery and comment on key computer methods available to carry out ADME/Tox predictions. These encompass rule-based methods, QSAR (quantitative structure–activity relationship), and machine learning approaches among others. In Section 2.3, examples to profile a compound library using *in silico* approaches, key commercial and public compound collections, freely available and commercial computer packages, examples of implementation of *in silico* methods in the private sector, and the main statistical methods used in the field of *in silico* ADME/Tox profiling are discussed.

ADMET for Medicinal Chemists: A Practical Guide, Edited by Katya Tsaioun and Steven A. Kates

2.2 KEY COMPUTER METHODS FOR ADME/Tox PREDICTIONS

2.2.1 Drug Discovery

Today's innovative drug discovery projects are very costly and time-consuming, with very few novel therapeutics making it to the market place [1]. In modern drug discovery campaign, the process usually starts from an unmet clinical need (disease), followed by target identification and validation, high-throughput screening (HTS) and/or *in silico–in vitro* screening to identify hit compounds, hit-to-lead and lead optimizations, clinical trials up to the approved drug (Figures 2.1 and 2.2) [2–4].

The overall process takes an average of 12–15 years, costs about $1 billion, and has a low success rate [5–8]. For example, from an analysis program at Pfizer, over a 10 year period, nearly 100 small molecule discovery campaigns had to be initiated to result in the identification of a single new chemical entity (NCE, Figure 2.3) [9].

Similar observations were made in all pharmaceutical companies [10]. A study in the 1990s showed that several reasons may explain why drugs were failing in development (Table 2.1). At that time, NCEs were essentially dropped because of poor pharmacokinetic properties, lack of efficacy, and toxicity [11, 12]. In fact, approximately 75% of the total cost of drug development was attributed to the

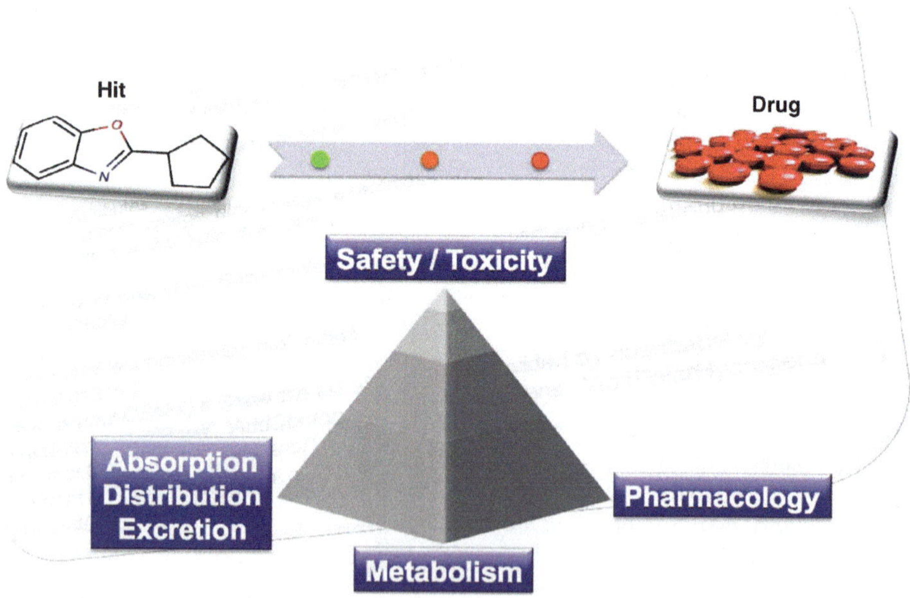

Figure 2.1 ADME/Tox concepts in the context of drug discovery and development. This figure illustrates the key pharmacokinetic concepts (ADME) that are commonly used in the public and private sectors during the course of a drug development project. It is also of utmost importance to consider toxicity and pharmacodynamic events along with the process and, when possible, at a very early stage of development.

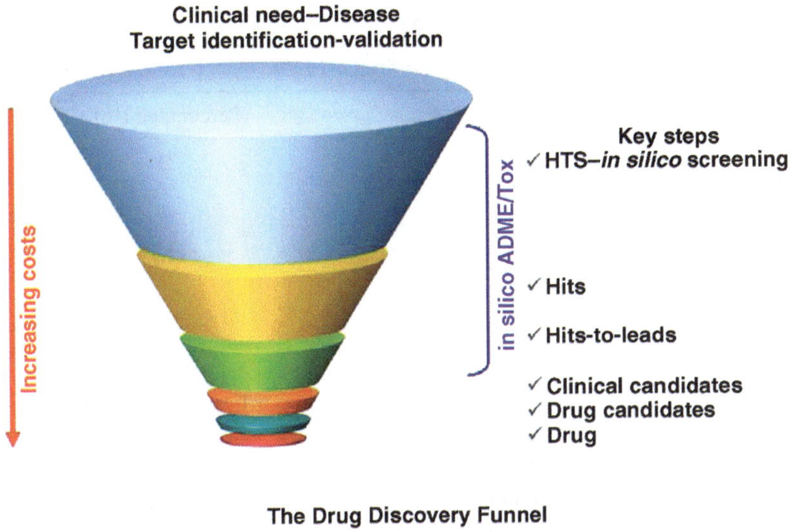

Figure 2.2 The drug discovery funnel. Stages of drug discovery underlining that the process becomes more and more expensive and that in the early phases, *in silico* ADME/Tox approaches can be used.

development failures. The assignment of failure to a distinct category might itself be misleading, as factors such as efficacy, toxicity, solubility, and pharmacokinetics are all inter-related. For instance, toxicity might be cited as the ultimate reason for the termination of a compound in development, but the pertinent factors might actually be prolonged and unnecessary systemic exposure (i.e., poor pharmacokinetics) or the

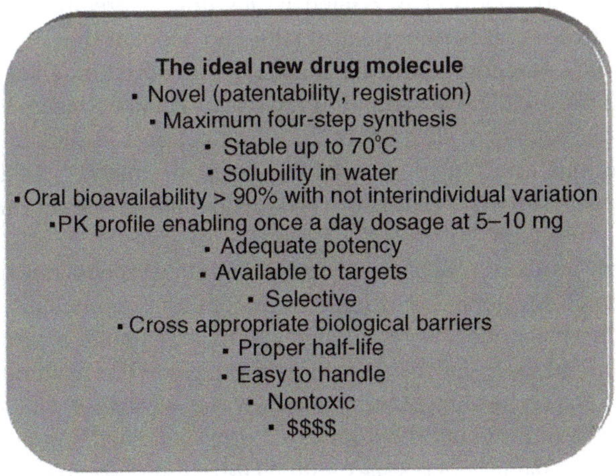

Figure 2.3 NCE development requires simultaneous optimization of several parameters and should bring return on investment. Some of these data can be predicted *in silico*.

TABLE 2.1 Drug Discovery Failures in the 1990s

Drug Discovery in the 1990s	
Reasons for Failures	Percentage (%)
Toxicity	25
Lack of efficacy	30
Market reasons	5
Pharmacokinetics	40

need to administer high doses because of low potency (i.e., poor efficacy) [13, 14]. Independently of numbers (i.e., values can change according to authors, depending on the molecules assessed, some authors include all NCEs while others exclude anti-infective compounds) and as a result of these observations, major initiatives were undertaken by the pharmaceutical industry in order to address absorption, distribution, metabolism, excretion, toxicity issues early during the drug discovery process [14–16].

Today, a promising molecule may still be dismissed at each and every step, starting from the hit/lead phase, along the preclinical investigations, during clinical trials, and even years after its successful market launch. The reasons for failures are still manifold: wrong target, poor pharmacokinetics, animal toxicity, lack of clinical efficacy, contraindication with other drugs, commercial reasons, formulation issues and most severe, adverse reactions in humans [17]. Recent analysis suggests that over 90% of failures are now due to toxicity, with hepatotoxicity and cardiovascular implications alone causing two out of three market withdrawals [18]. Termination of drug development in clinical phases is mainly caused by inadequate efficacy that supersedes the pharmacokinetic reasons of the 1990s. This may be due to the increased attention to ADME/Tox related issues during preclinical development. Yet as mentioned above, it is important to take into account that the assignment of failure to a distinct category could be misleading. These so-called adverse drug reactions are gaining broad public attention and rise to a major concern in recent years. Estimate suggests that every year, about 2 million patients in the United States are affected by a serious drug reaction, resulting in approximately 100,000 fatalities, making such events the fourth leading cause of death, not far behind cancer and heart diseases [19]. Similar numbers have also been estimated for other western countries.

Drug discovery professionals have reacted to these low success rates and economic pressure toward the development of higher quality compounds, thus, the quest for ADME/Tox prediction models were initiated and included both, *in vitro* and *in silico* methods [2, 10, 17, 20–54]. One turning point example was due to compounds such as fluconazole (a triazole antifungal drug used in the treatment and prevention of superficial and systemic fungal infections, oral drug launched around 1991), which achieved an excellent balance of potency with ADME/Tox properties. This compound was optimized for both potency and ADME/Tox early during the discovery process, illustrating the advantages of *in vitro* technologies to reduce time and cost while

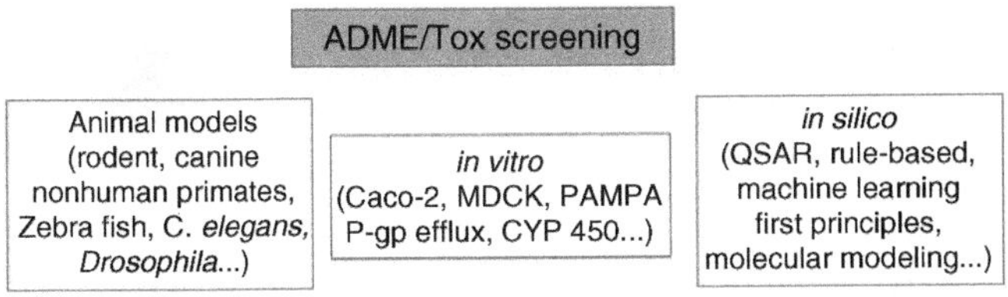

Figure 2.4 Some current ADME/Tox screening technologies (P-gp, P-glycoprotein; MDCK, Madin–Darby canine kidney; PAMPA, parallel artificial membrane permeability assay; CYP 450, cytochrome P450 enzymes; Caco-2 cells, immortalized line of heterogeneous human epithelial colorectal adenocarcinoma cells) [56]. *In silico* models attempt to predict solubility, intestinal absorption, plasma protein binding, blood–brain-barrier permeability, metabolism by individual CYP 450 enzymes, affinity to transporters, renal clearance, among others. Numerous experimental methods for screening human ADME/Tox properties can be found in a review by Li including intestinal absorption, drug metabolism, drug–drug interactions, and toxicity [36, 57].

developing a "better molecule" [55]. Standard methods to address such problems *in vitro* involve the application of preclinical *in vitro* safety profiling where compounds are tested using *in vitro* biochemical and cellular assays. Various animal models are also used. Some of the key events that one would like to estimate are presented in Figures 2.4–2.6, some of these properties can be predicted using *in silico* methods.

In this context and with regard to computer predictions, the well-known rule-of-5 can be seen as a milestone of *in silico* models, comprising sets of rules, for orally administered drugs. This pragmatic approach to gain an understanding of the balance of physical properties that leads to a suitable pharmacokinetic profile for oral administration was investigated by Lipinski and coworkers [59], at Pfizer, in part due to observations about the increasing MW and lipophilicity of compounds added to the HTS screening collections. These authors profiled a range of properties leading to

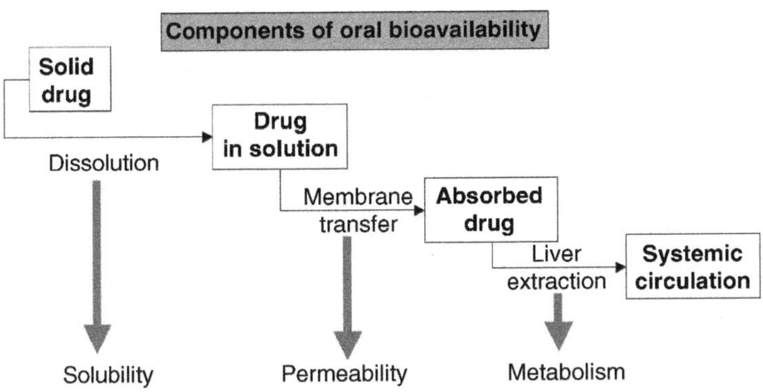

Figure 2.5 Examples of properties that one wishes to predict (adapted from Abou-Gharbia [1]).

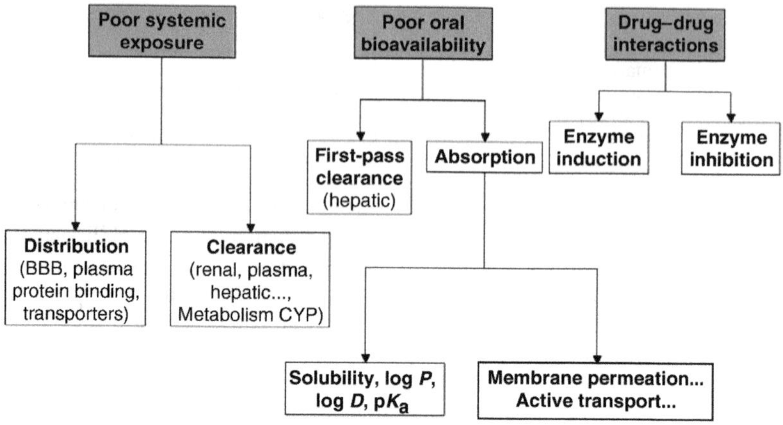

Figure 2.6 Overview of key ADME/Tox processes. Various events that would need to be estimated *in vitro–in vivo* or predicted (see Beresford et al. [58] and Eddershaw et al. [13]).

the "rule-of-5." This work was based on the results of calculated physical properties on a set of 2245 compounds chosen from the World Drug Index because it was presumed that they would have suitable solubility and permeability for oral administration. This Pfizer's team found after cleaning the collection that approximately 90% of the compounds had molecular weight less than 500, calculated log *P* less than 5, sum of hydrogen bond donors (as a sum of NH and OH) less than 5, and sum of hydrogen-bond acceptors (as a sum of N and O) less than 10 (*note*: four rules, not five, see below). Thus, they proposed that poor absorption and permeation are more likely when one or more of these limits are exceeded. The approach has been revisited numerous times and the overall output of these new investigations supports Lipinski's findings, although anti-infectious drugs, some anticancer drugs, and natural compounds tend to escape these rules [9, 60]. Further investigations led to the lead-like concept (rule-of-3: MW < 300, log $P < 3$) [61, 62].

Although this type of analysis and concepts about compound library profiling are still under debates, several studies suggest that a paradigm shift in drug discovery has occurred. The key challenge is now to include in most design and drug discovery campaigns (high-throughput and *in silico* screening) and whenever appropriate depending on the target/disease types, potency, selectivity and ADME/Tox properties and thus to simultaneously optimize binding affinity/selectivity, pharmacokinetic properties while avoiding toxicity (Figure 2.7). Comparing property profiles of development and marketed oral drugs certainly can assist the process. Increasing the numbers of available and validated test sets for *in silico* computations should also help in this endeavor. Pharmacokinetic and the pharmacodynamic profiles are complex functions of properties; however, one might expect that at some points, after years of chemogenomics and systems chemical biology research, the drug discovery community will fully understand relationships between physical properties of compounds and *in vitro–in vivo* behaviors [9, 60, 63–71].

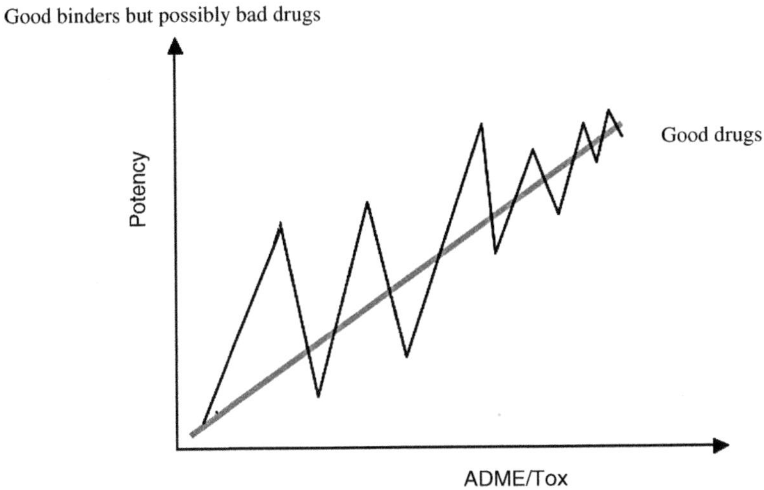

Figure 2.7 Paradigm shift in drug discovery. For many years, the attention was focused on potency with emphasis on ADME/Tox variables at the end of the process (jagged line). In this approach, potency is optimized first with a realization that ADME/Tox properties are declining. The process is repeated many times before hopefully finding an optimum in multiple property spaces [64]. Currently, it is suggested to optimize both in parallel, potency, and ADME/Tox properties (straight gray line).

2.2.2 Applying or Not ADME/Tox Predictions, Divided Opinions

Academic research groups and pharmaceutical industries are both interested in reducing the risk of failure during drug development [58]. ADME/Tox modeling can certainly play a role in this process but it is also reasonable to question how reliable these *in silico* predictions are. Considering the complexity of the human body and the fact that some chemical reactions are not fully understood yet, some scientists suggest that deriving rules based upon simple descriptors (molecular weight, number of hydrogen bond acceptors and donors, etc.) or complex ones cannot allow for a good appreciation of the therapeutic potential of a chemical compound. When complex statistical methods are used to develop *in silico* predictive filters, it can be argued that the training sets are

- not sufficiently diverse,
- too large with too many outliers,
- too small, not sufficiently validated, or
- that the model is not interpretable by medicinal chemists,

and therefore of little use for finding solutions through the next rounds of chemical syntheses [24, 25, 72–76]. Clearly, as with all reductionist approaches, simplifications introduced in *in silico* modeling (even in *in vitro*) of ADME/Tox properties are clearly imperfect. Proponents of *in silico* methods claim when properly used that it is possible to do much better even with simple rules than a seasoned medicinal chemist. Opponents point out that there are many exceptions to the rules and that the fate of xenobiotics in the human body cannot be predicted accurately. It is understandable that some scientists believe that when screening a compound collection with *in silico* high-throughput ADME/Tox prediction models, there is always a chance that the next blockbuster drug be disregarded from the list. Yet, the cost for optimization of molecules containing "nasty groups" must certainly be considered even though the burden eventually may fall on patients (high dosage, intravenous route, etc.). Also, the strategy will depend on the stage and nature of the project

- if one is looking for a hit or is trying to optimize molecules,
- if the goal is to probe a molecular function,
- if the project aims at inhibiting protein–protein or other types of macromolecular interactions.

As such, one may decide to screen all compounds, assuming that medicinal chemists and formulation scientists can solve the problem later. Conversely, one might argue that hit molecules should be simple, clean, and as much as possible free of reactive functional groups (Figure 2.8).

The debate about experimental and *in silico* artifacts in ADME/Tox profiling, who and which approaches are right and who is wrong, is not closed [2, 25, 34, 46, 77]. As pointed out by Beresford et al., there will be mistakes with the example of the Pfizer Ltd antihypertensive amlodipine drug that has made billions of dollars and is highly bioavailable; however, it is predicted to be poorly bioavailable though QSAR modeling [25]. Yet, it is important to note that the risk of incorrectly classifying a compound as good or bad based on an *in silico* predictive model may not be greater than the risk inherent from using *in vitro* or *in vivo* tests, since these ones also have limitations. A possible solution to this conundrum could be to remove compounds from a screening collection that are too far away from a softly defined drug-like space (e.g., high MW usually not appropriate for oral administration) and to flag molecules with problematic groups without removing them (e.g., compound with a nitro group, see below). Certainly, avoiding some chemicals or functional groups in preclinical discovery does not guarantee success, but most likely including them increases the

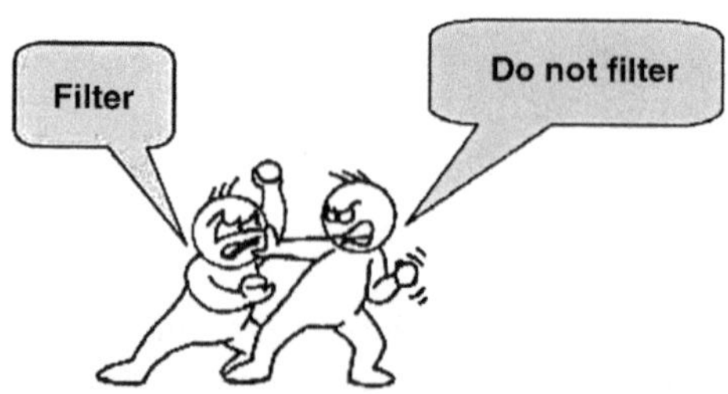

Figure 2.8 Polemics about applying predictive ADME/Tox models to filter compound collections or prior to synthesis.

chances of problems later in clinical development and beyond. Several studies continue to show that the compounds lacking the rule-of-5 compliance have low chances of survival [9]. Although not all medicinal chemists will consider the exact same substructures as problematic [78], some chemical functions have to be avoided while most people agree that a good lead molecule has low MW and log *P* and chemical features that are amenable to optimization. In general, clear risks are associated with selecting compounds for the development that possess poorer physicochemical properties.

DEFINITIONS

The term ADME originally referred to as *in vivo* processes that govern pharmacokinetics (PK). It has been expended to include *in vitro* physicochemical and biochemical properties that affect *in vivo* PK. In general, suitable ADME properties are essential to both success of *in vitro* assays and of *in vivo* studies.

Pharmacokinetic is a branch of pharmacology dedicated to the determination of the fate of substances administered externally to a living organism. Pharmacokinetic is often studied in conjunction with pharmacodynamics. Pharmacodynamics explores what a drug does to the body, whereas pharmacokinetics explores what the biological system does to the drug [79]. Pharmacokinetics includes the study of the mechanisms of absorption and distribution of an administered drug, the rate at which a drug action begins and the duration of the effect, the chemical changes of the substance in the body (e.g., by enzymes), and the effects and routes of excretion (of the metabolites) of the drug.

Among the ADME/Tox issues, absorption, distribution, and excretion are relevant to the journey of the compound from the application point to the site of action. The other issues, metabolism and toxicity can be considered of a somewhat different nature in terms of mechanisms and can be treated separately although all these issues are inter-related. The structure and physical properties of a compound determine its PK behavior in the body. ADME/Tox plays a major role in the design of new molecular entities (NMEs, warning, NMEs can be small molecules, as discussed in this chapter, but the term also applies to therapeutic proteins and even viral delivery agents). The ADME/Tox methods presented here cannot be used for peptides or therapeutic proteins, while numerous challenges are associated with these molecules e.g., peptides can bind to many proteins, are usually unstable with short *in vivo* half-life and usually require large or frequent dosages, in general they can not be given orally [80].

The term off-target is commonly used in the ADME/Tox field. Off-target activity is often referred to as activity of a particular compound toward a target that was not anticipated during the design and that can be beneficial or detrimental (e.g., sildenafil or Viagra, was initially developed by Pfizer to treat angina, but its side effect on male volunteers led to a change in the therapeutic area of the drug). However, this term also means antitarget activity, and binding to antitargets is considered to be detrimental for the progression of a compound toward a drug. Antitargets involve, for instance, hERG, CYPs, some GPCRs, P-gp, and PRX, among others.

PHARMACOKINETICS

Pharmacokinetics is the study of the time course of a drug within the body and it incorporates the ADME processes. The study of absorption, distribution, metabolism, and excretion of a molecule results in the generation of a number of pharmacokinetic parameters that characterize that compound. The PK parameters are based on the measurement of drug concentrations in blood or plasma. Several important PK terms are investigated such as volume of distribution, clearance, and half-life.

Effective intestinal permeability, P_{eff}, measures how fast a compound crosses apical membrane of the intestine and enters the cytosol. The fraction or percentage of the dose absorbed (*A* or *FA*, fraction absorbed) is a measure of extent of oral absorption (includes all processes from the dissolution to its transport across the apical membrane of the epithelial barrier of the intestine). Bioavailability (*F*) is the fraction or percentage of the dose available in the systemic circulation and is equal to *FA* only if metabolism terms are zero. Drugs that are targeted to the central nervous system (CNS) also need to cross the blood–brain barrier (BBB). The volume of distribution (V_d) is a theoretical concept that relates the administered dose with the initial concentration (C_0) present in the circulatory system.

$$V_d = \text{Dose}/C_0$$

Clearance (*Cl*) of the drug from the body mainly takes place via the liver (by hepatic clearance or metabolism, and by biliary excretion) and the kidney (by renal excretion). When plotting the plasma concentration against time, the area under the curve (AUC) relates to dose, bioavailability, and clearance.

$$\text{AUC} = F \times \text{Dose}/Cl$$

The combined parameter half-life ($t_{1/2}$), the time taken for the drug concentration in the plasma to reduce by 50%, is a function of the clearance and volume of distribution, and reflects how often a drug needs to be administered.

$$\text{Human } t_{1/2} = 0.693\ V_d/Cl$$

METABOLISM

Most drugs cannot be eliminated from the body without previous biotransformation to metabolites. The key sites in the body for metabolism are the gut wall and the liver. Metabolic alteration of xenobiotics is traditionally subdivided into two main phases: Phase I (oxidation, often via cytochrome P450 enzymes, reduction, and hydrolysis) results in the introduction of new functional groups, while in Phase II (conjugation reactions), highly hydrophilic moiety such as sulfate or glucuronide is attached to make the compounds more water-soluble and to prepare for excretion through urine and bile. The most important enzymes involved in metabolism in humans are the cytochrome P450s: CYP3A4, CYP2D6, CYP2C9, and CYP2C19. Metabolism is species-dependent and therefore animal studies may not be fully predictive for humans. Today, it is generally accepted that prior to Phase I, Phase 0 takes place (uptake), mediated by transport proteins belonging to the SLC (solute carrier) transporter superfamily. Phase II is followed by Phase III (export); this efflux is mediated mostly by the members of the ABC (ATP-binding cassette, e.g., P-gp) transporter superfamily.

2.2.3 *In Silico* ADME/Tox Methods and Modeling Approaches

ADME/Tox properties are very difficult to predict, that is, human intestinal absorption or metabolic stability arises from multiple physiological mechanisms difficult to model. To manage this biological complexity, simplifications have to be introduced and numerous methods have been developed during these past years in an attempt to predict some of these properties.

In silico modeling of ADME/Tox properties can be performed using many different approaches. These range from the so-called *rules of thumb* (e.g., rule-of-5, polar surface area) to quantitative prediction approaches: QSAR and quantitative structure–property relationship (QSPR) up to classification models, and similarity searches, molecular modeling (structure-based approaches such as ligand–protein docking, pharmacophore modeling, substructure, quantum mechanics) and physiologically based pharmacokinetic (PBPK) modeling [74, 75, 81–83] (Figures 2.9–2.11). While PBPK models have received a lot of attention because they may provide valuable information on how various factors influence PK, they are not be discussed because these methods usually need experimental data and cannot be developed solely from the molecular structures of the compounds (see for instance Ref. 84). The assumption with many of these approaches is that there is always a function that correlates biological properties with chemical structure.

Molecular modeling approaches can be used when the underlying ADME/Tox mechanisms are relatively well understood (e.g., docking into a CYP experimental structure or docking compounds into an hERG, human ether-a-go-go channel, 3D structure built by comparative modeling methods). QSAR modeling includes several steps (e.g., see Figure 2.9): data collection (a training set), descriptor generation and selection (e.g., descriptors to characterize compounds such as molecular properties, fingerprints, etc.), a statistical model (multiple linear regression, neural networks, etc.) to relate the target property (e.g., solubility) to the descriptors, generation of the model and finally, validation of the model on a test set. To illustrate this point, one can take a theoretical example of QSAR modeling. In this situation, several descriptors

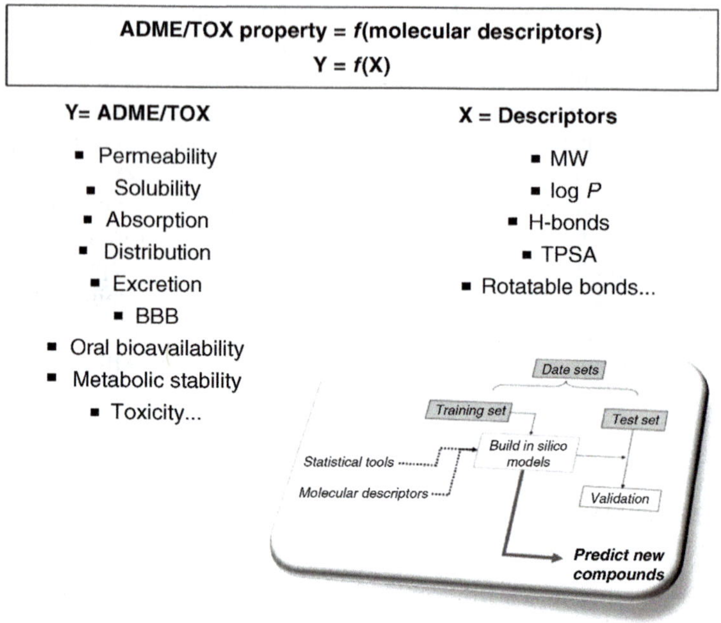

Figure 2.9 *In silico* ADME/Tox modeling. Top: Key concepts to model ADME/Tox properties. In this case, information regarding molecular structures and biological responses are known and relationships between the two are derived. Bottom: Diagram of the main elements used to build *in silico* models.

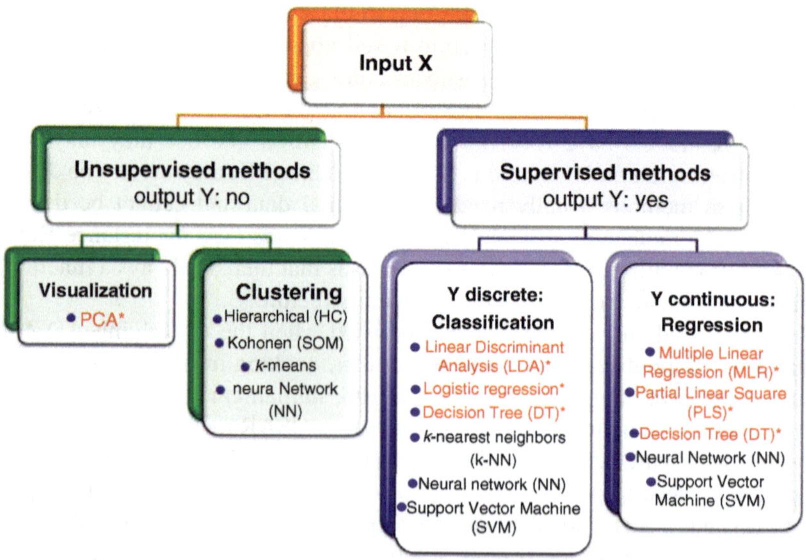

Figure 2.10 Typology of the learning methods (asterisk denotes methods interpretable in terms of the impact of input descriptors over the model or output values).

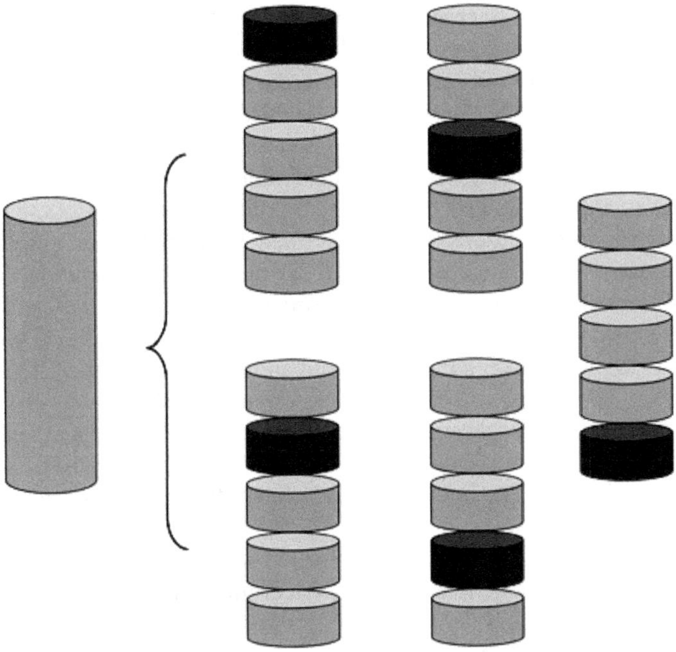

Figure 2.11 Overview of a fivefold cross-validation scheme. Partition of a sample of data into subsets, iteratively, one part becomes a test set (black) the others are learning sets (gray). Analysis is performed on the training/learning sets and test sets.

describing the molecular structure (denoted *X*, input variable) are related to the observed activity (denoted *Y*, output variable) [75]. The parameters of the model relating *Y* to *X* are fitted from a set of molecules for which experimental data are available. This is commonly referred to as the training set. In general, models can only reliably predict for molecules similar to those in the training set. This is sometimes referred to as either the chemical space of the model or domain of applicability. A statistical regression tool is used to derive linear models between *X* and *Y*. Multiple linear regression model (MLR) and PLS approaches are commonly used but nonlinear classification techniques tend to be used more and more at present. For instance, multiple biological mechanisms usually contribute to a single ADME/Tox property but the relations are seldom linear, and in this situation, it might be more appropriate to use nonlinear methods (see below).

Classification modeling operates similar to QSAR modeling. Thus reliable data that translate in the field of ADME/Tox to a set of molecules for which ADME/Tox properties have been determined experimentally are needed. There are over 6000 molecular descriptors that can be used for *in silico* modeling [85–87]. Some descriptors contain information about the conformation of a compound and can be defined by the dimensionality of the structural representation. Descriptors fall into a number of classes such as physicochemical, geometrical, topological, electropological, quantum chemical, and molecular fingerprints. One challenge is to use descriptors that are capable of mechanistic interpretation and that can be translated to the bench [46].

Molecular descriptors are grouped according to their dimensionality as 0D, 1D, 2D, 3D, and 4D [85]. Zero-dimensional-descriptors are independent from molecular connectivity and conformations and refer to atom and bond type counts. 1D-descriptors contain information about fragment counts, and their calculation is independent of information on molecule structure. 2D-descriptors, called graph invariants or topologic descriptors, are derived from molecular graphs, and are conformationally independent. In contrast, 3D-descriptors depend on the geometrical coordinates of the atoms of molecules (quantum chemistry, molecular surface, volumes, etc.). 4D-descriptors are energetic descriptors obtained by computing the energy of interaction between the compound and molecular probes. The definition of descriptors, according to Roberto Todeschini and Viviana Consonni, is the following: "The molecular descriptor is the final result of a logic and mathematical procedure which transforms chemical information encoded within a symbolic representation of a molecule into a useful number or the result of some standardized experiment."

Once all the descriptors are computed for the studied dataset, they are used in a model aiming at obtaining information concerning ADME/Tox properties. The general workflow for the modeling and process conception is presented below and schematically represented in Figure 2.9.

To perform an efficient analysis, preliminary processing of the data, such as selecting molecular descriptors (X) most related to the output variable Y in a large dataset, has a large effect on the quality of the final solution. Analyses such as principal component analysis can assist the process to reduce the dimensionality of the data, to check the diversity of molecules in the training dataset, or to eliminate outliers. Then, the challenge is the selection of the learning technique(s) that is most suitable for modeling the property under investigation. The "learning problem" can be roughly categorized as either supervised or unsupervised (Figure 2.10 and Section 2.3 of this chapter).

In unsupervised learning, there is no output measure Y and the goal is to describe the association and patterns among a set of input descriptors X. The features are only observed and the task is to describe how the data are organized and clustered. These methods are particularly useful for features extraction, data clustering, and visualization. They include hierarchical clustering, k-means, unsupervised neural networks, Kohonen self-organizing mapss (SOMs) methods, and principal component analysis (PCA).

In supervised learning, the goal is to predict the value of one or more output measure(s) Y based on a number of input measures X. The methods are called "supervised" because of the presence of the output variable(s) that guide the learning process. The outputs vary in nature; they can be discrete (categorical or qualitative) or continuous (quantitative). This distinction in output types has led to a naming convention for the prediction tasks: classification and regression when one predicts qualitative and continuous outputs, respectively.

Statistical regression is primarily a tool for deriving models between inputs X and output Y, and has been applied in many ADME models, including the calculation of whole molecules physicochemical properties. Regression methods correspond to supervised methods. The most commonly used are multiple linear regression model, partial least square (PLS), recursive partitioning or decision tree (DT), artificial neural networks (ANN), and support vector machines (SVM). Classification methods, employed to assign the property of a molecule to one of two or more classes, mainly include linear discriminant analysis (LDA), k-nearest-neighbors, decision trees, artificial neural networks, and support vector machine. Classification and regression tasks have some commonality and methods, such as ANN, DT, SVM, can be applied to both.

UNSUPERVISED

Hierarchical Clustering [88] and *k*-Means [89]

Cluster analysis, also called data segmentation, groups a collection of objects into "clusters," such that those within each cluster are more closely related to one another than objects assigned to other clusters. The measure of similarity is central to the cluster analysis and has to be appropriately chosen. For hierarchical classification, objects then clusters are successively grouped between themselves to form a hierarchical classification. For k-means, the number of clusters k is first chosen and objects are clustered around k centroids.

PCA

The goal of principal component analysis [90] is to project data into a subspace made of linear combinations of the original descriptors so that this subspace is the best-simplified image, in a small dimension, of the original data in terms of variation (see Section 2.3).

UNSUPERVISED AND SUPERVISED

Neural networks are based on neurons (computational elements) connected to a framework. The two most important subtypes are Kohonen self-organizing maps and artificial neural networks. SOM are examples of unsupervised NNs, particularly useful for features extraction, data classification, clustering, and visualization. Artificial neural networks is a pattern recognition approach [91], fitting nonlinear function relating a discrete or continuous output Y and a set of inputs for a training set of molecules. Once memorized, this network can then be used to make predictions for molecules for which Y is unknown (see Section 2.3).

SUPERVISED

Classification

Linear Discriminant Analysis is conceptually close to PCA, but linear combinations of descriptors are performed to optimize the prediction of the discrete outcome variable. It calculates discriminant functions or hyperplanes that partition the space of chemical descriptors to give the best separation between classes [92].

k-nearest-neighbors (*k*NN) identifies the *k* molecules in the training set that lies closest to the molecules for which the prediction is being made [93]. Measure of structural similarity between molecules is assessed using Tanimoto index or Euclidean distance in the space of descriptors. The unknown molecule is then assigned by a voting procedure among the *k*-nearest-neighbors.

Regression

Multiple linear regression model is one of the oldest methods to find a linear relationship between the observed activities and a set of descriptors [94]. A problem with this approach is that it is generally considered as requiring more molecules in the training set than descriptors (roughly five times more). Moreover, correlated descriptors or descriptors with skewed distribution (i.e., low variance) will result in poor regression models. MLR is close to partial least square but concerns the prediction of only one quantitative output using the best linear combination of descriptors and without any use of graphical representations and thus poorer interpretation.

Partial least square has become a standard in ADME/Tox as it overcomes most of the previously mentioned problems [95]. A large number of descriptors can be used, even larger than the number of molecules in the training set, and the descriptors that influence the most the model can be conveniently identified. More complex nonlinear relationship can be treated by nonlinear PLS [96] (see Section 2.3).

Classification or Regression

Decision tree creates a branching structure in which the branch taken at each intersection is determined by a rule related to the descriptors splitting the local molecule set into two more homogeneous subsets. Each "leaf" of a tree is assigned to a class or a value [97] (see Section 2.3).

Support vector machine is one of the most popular kernel methods, initially introduced by Vapnik in 1995 [98]. Owing to its outstanding performance in nonlinear structures, the application has spread rapidly over the past decade (see Section 2.3).

With this large range of available methods, it is not always easy to decide which strategies to use [47]. The reliability of the methods will obviously depend on several factors such as noise, size of the data, and output types. Performance of the models can be quantified in terms of accuracy (such as good classification rate, sensitivity, specificity for classification, and sum-of-squares errors for regression) but also in terms of interpretability. Concerning accuracy of predictions, there is a need to find a balance between oversimplified and complicated models. An oversimplified model could ignore complicated features and noise, thus its predictive performance could be poor. On the other hand, if one uses a complicated model that interpolates the data exactly, the prediction error on the training data can become close to zero. However, such complicated models tend to have poor generalization performance, that is, the models make poor prediction on new test data points not similar to any of the existing training data points. Such poor generalization performance is called overfitting. This overfitting phenomenon can be avoided by using a cross-validation technique [99]. When training data are used for constructing the model and also for assessing its performance, they tend to overfit the model. Hence, it is necessary to assess an external validation data set that should be large and diverse enough, and which overlaps as less as possible with the training set while remaining in the domain of application. Cross-validation is an effective technique to avoid overlaps with the learning set. First, the training data are partitioned into k parts, in which one part is used for the test set and the remaining $k - 1$ parts are used for modeling. The process is iterated k times. This process is called k-fold cross-validation (Figure 2.9).

When k is equal to the number of molecules, it is called leave-one-out (LOO) cross-validation. In general, the most unbiased estimates can be obtained by LOO, but it often produces high variance and is computationally intensive [100]. A recommended approach to estimate true accuracy of a model, when sufficient data are available, is to add an independent test set of molecules to which the model is never fitted. If the model is not overfitted, the correlation between predicted and experimental values for the test should be comparable to that of the training set. Concerning interpretability, some models tend to be "black boxes" (i.e., the chemical structure is taken as input and a prediction is returned with little or no possibility of understanding the connection between the two). This lack of interpretability is a problem for chemists and drug designers as it is difficult to propose potential solutions. For example, some nonlinear models are more appropriate for early stages of lead identification, as they are often "black-box" techniques that derived little information about their prediction. Linear correlation has to be preferred during lead optimization when more comprehensible and interpretable models are desired. Therefore, a good prediction must represent a balance between accuracy and interpretability. The integration of different methods or consensus modeling can be a valid solution to optimize the prediction and its interpretability, allowing to overcome the limitations of a single method [101]. In fact, a combination of two or more models for the same property, based on different principles, may provide higher confidence in the results obtained for which they agree.

In practice, ADME/Tox filtering usually initially uses simple counting methods (e.g., rule-of-5) combined with some structural alert checks (e.g., identification of reactive groups). Subsequently, more CPU demanding and/or complex statistical methods can be applied.

2.2.4 Physicochemistry, Pharmacokinetics, Drug-Like and Lead-Like Concepts

Drug molecules generally act on specific targets, and upon binding to the receptors, hopefully exert a desirable alteration of the target/cellular activities. Before interacting with the receptor, drug molecules must travel from the entry point through the body to reach the site of action at the desired concentration and with sufficient duration. After executing their activities, drug molecules should be eliminated from the organism. For most drugs, the preferred route of administration is by oral ingestion. Compounds have to be soluble and possess an appropriate level of lipophilicity. The latter is critical to achieve cell permeability, a prerequisite for oral bioavailability. Such observations have prompted drug discovery researchers as early as in the 1960s to search for properties (e.g., MW, log *P* [partition coefficient determined by the logarithm of the concentration ratio of a nonionized solute in two different solvents (generally water and octanol)], among others) that drug molecules should display as compared to nondrugs. At about the same time, the quest for the design of molecular descriptors that could correlate with the so-called drug-like profile was initiated [40, 46, 52, 102–105]. If one examines the journey of a drug in the human body, the entire process can be broadly described by several subevents such as absorption, distribution, metabolism, and excretion. This area of research aiming at understanding the fate a molecule in the body is often referred to in the literature as DMPK drug metabolism and pharmacokinetics [52]. The key questions that this research is trying to address involve, for example, the following:

- Is it possible to define some specific features that match with these subprocesses?
- Is it possible to find specific characteristics in known drugs that are missing or different in nondrugs?
- How to mathematically model these reactions, which level of complexity, and which stage of the drug discovery process one should act upon?
- How reliable such predictions could be?

As mentioned above, one of the first attempts to address some of these questions is the "rule-of-5" devised by Lipinski and coworkers at Pfizer [59]. The rule-of-5 is specifically related to the permeability and solubility of the compounds and thus to the absorption of therapeutic agents but has also other implications. Lipinski et al. analyzed the physicochemical properties of over 2200 compounds from the World Drug Index because it was presumed that they would have suitable solubility and permeability (the compounds were supposed to have entered Phase 2 clinical trials). They found that in a high proportion of compounds, a series of four rules was generally true. These rules state that an orally active drug has in general no more than one violation of the following criteria:

- hydrogen-bond donors ≤ 5
- hydrogen-bond acceptors ≤ 10

- molecular mass ≤ 500 Da
- log *P* (the method used was C log *P*, see for instance www.daylight.com) ≤ 5.

If the molecule has more than one violation, it may be poorly absorbed. First, one notes that all numbers are multiples of five, which is the origin of the rule's name. In that work, any oxygen and nitrogen atoms are defined as hydrogen-bond acceptors and N–H and O–H groups are considered to be hydrogen-bond donors. Interestingly, all the rule-of-5 descriptors can be derived from the structure of the compound while the log *P* is in fact a QSAR-fitted descriptor method. The authors underlined that the majority of drugs that violate the rule-of-5 are antibiotics, antifungal agents, vitamins, natural products among others, yet these compounds are often orally available, suggesting that they act as substrates for transporters [20, 106]. The rule-of-5 concept has been extended along the following line, it describes molecular properties important for a drug's pharmacokinetics in the human body, not only absorption but also distribution, metabolism, and excretion. However, the rule-of-5 does not predict if a compound is pharmacologically active. The rule-of-5 can thus be considered as necessary conditions but not sufficient for a molecule to become a drug, it tends to avoid false negatives at the expense of false positives. Obviously, simplicity may also lead to the lack of discrimination.

Sakaeda et al. have analyzed the rule-of-5 and reported similar exclusion criteria (MW ≥ 500 and log $P \geq 5$) that differentiated poorly absorbed drugs from good drug candidates after investigation of over 200 marketed oral drugs [107]. Similar investigations were carried out by several other groups [9, 60, 108] and usually supported the view of Lipinski and collaborators. The rule-of-5 was also further validated by Ghose and coworkers [109]. These authors examined the computed physical properties of over 6000 molecules taken from the Comprehensive Medicinal Chemistry Database. Ranges were established for log *P* values (computed with *A* log *P*), molecular refractivity, MW, and number of atoms (e.g., most of the compounds have MW values ranging from 200 to 400 and log *P* values running from 0 to 4). A large percentage of high MW compounds were either antibacterials or antineoplastics. Many compounds with high log *P* values were from classes considered to be CNS active (anti-Parkinsonian, antipsychotic, and antidepressant), consistent with the fact that CNS compounds tend to be more lipophilic than other biologically active small molecules [110, 111]. Veber and colleagues [112] investigated the concept further. This group assembled a database of over 1000 drug candidates with extensive animal data such as rat oral bioavailability, and, from many computed molecular properties such as rotatable bond, H-bond acceptors and donor, log *P*, and molecular weight. The authors found that reducing the number of rotatable bonds had the largest impact on determining oral bioavailability in rats. They proposed that compounds with 10 or fewer rotatable bonds and a polar surface area below 140 $Å^2$ will have a higher chance of displaying good bioavailability. Vieth et al. have studied a large collection of marketed drugs in order to uncover optimal physicochemical parameters associated with compounds that are presumed to have good pharmacokinetic properties (e.g., those assumed to have poorer properties would be infused molecules or topical drugs) [113]. They found that on average, intravenous drugs have significantly higher MW, greater number of H-bond acceptors/donors, rotatable bonds and rings than orally available molecules.

The rule-of-5 concept was recently reinvestigated, but this time, with the goal of designing drugs that will be administered via the inhaled/intranasal routes. After analysis of 81 marketed respiratory drugs, Ritchie et al. found that these molecules have significantly higher hydrogen bonding and polar area, significantly higher MW (yet, the significance disappears if glucocorticoids are excluded), a trend toward lower lipophilicity but no difference in rotatable bonds and total ring count [114]. Overall, the rule-of-5 descriptors are intuitively appealing. For instance, log *P* is an important physicochemical parameter for oral absorption, since it relates to solubility and influences the ability of a compound to permeate through cell membranes including those of the intestinal epithelial cells. Too hydrophilic compounds (negative log *P*) are not able to pass through membranes, as they hardly enter the hydrophobic interior (mimicked by the octanol phase in the octanol/water system) of the lipophilic bilayer. Too lipophilic compounds (high log *P*) tend to be insoluble and also poorly permeate through membranes, as they get stuck in the lipophilic bilayer. Molecular weight is an important parameter indicating the size of the molecule. Too large molecules have obviously difficulties to passively diffuse through membranes. A recent analysis of antibacterial compounds was reported and indicates that these molecules occupy a unique property space different as compared to drugs of other therapeutic areas. The rule-of-5 do not apply to these molecules [115].

Several opposing arguments have been given against these rule-based counting methods. For example, one argument against the rule-of-5 was that the property profile of existing successful drugs only highlights a historical artifact. Analysis of reported drugs provide information about properties of more "simple drugs of the past" aimed at acting on more tractable targets that are not representative of the greater complexity of modern drugs, required to interact with more challenging biological targets. Also, an ambiguity that fueled further the debate against the rule-of-5 was that the Lipinski's dataset contained compounds that did make it to the market along with compounds that failed in Phase 2 or 3. Further, do preclinical and Phase 1 or 2 studies truly eliminate compounds with poorer ADME characteristics? Also, the work assumed that passive diffusion was the dominant process for passage across membranes, while in many cases, specific transporters play a role. Although these simple rules can be criticized, they still tend to be supported today as the descriptors used to profile the compounds capture some of the essential futures of the ADME/Tox issues [60, 66]. However, the relationship between log *P* and ADME/Tox properties may be the result of false perceptions, lack of knowledge, or oversimplifications [77]. Therefore, these rules are guidelines to help selecting molecules with desirable physical properties. They are not intended to form a dogma and have to be tailored according to the project, target and therapeutic area, and enhanced with new approaches and concepts as our awareness over ADME/Tox matters increases. Yet, with our present knowledge about formulation, it does seem, independent of the underlying molecular mechanisms, that the fate of compounds with excessive molecular weight (>500) or log *P* (>5) tends to be heavily disfavored in the latter stages of clinical development [9].

TABLE 2.2 Default Values for the REOS Filtering Tool

Property	Minimum	Maximum
MW	200	500
log *P*	−5	5
Hydrogen-bond donors	0	5
Hydrogen-bond acceptors	0	10
Formal charge	−2	2
Number of rotatable bonds	0	8
Number of heavy atoms	15	50

Using simple counting methods to predict drug-likeness is often used in the literature (e.g., see a recent review by Ritchie and Macdonald about counting aromatic rings [116]). The structural and physicochemical properties of a compound may determine its pharmacokinetic and metabolic behavior in the body (Table 2.2). For example, the REOS system is a hybrid computer method that combines a set of functional group filters (see Sections 2.2.11 and 2.3) with some simple counting schemes similar to those used in the rule-of-5 [108]. Several parameters result from modifications of the rule-of-5, while others, such as formal charges, come from observations that benzamidine moiety (e.g., positively charged) tends to prevent absorption, thus formal charges are often investigated. Number of heavy atoms can also be important and the value range usually comes from the analysis of drugs present on the market.

Several computer packages perform similar investigations (see Section 2.3) including FAF-Drugs2 [117], Screening-Assistant [118, 119], or Filter (OpenEye Scientific Software).

It is important to note that different authors are using the term "drug-like" slightly differently [35]. Drug-likeness literally means similarity to known drugs. Considering the diversity of mechanisms of action and properties of the known drugs and the different administration routes, it is not surprising that the drug-like term is difficult to define precisely and that there are multiple approaches to its assessment. Walters and Murcko define "drug-like" compounds as "molecules that contain functional groups and/or have physical properties consistent with the majority of known drugs" [24]. Lipinski defines drug-like "as those compounds that have sufficiently acceptable ADME properties and sufficiently acceptable toxicity properties to survive through the completion of human Phase 1 clinical trials." In addition to favorable physical properties that should translate into good absorption, distribution, metabolism, excretion, and toxicity profiles of drug-like molecules, the synthetic accessibility of the compound and its analogs is also considered an important aspect of drug-like molecules. Further, the filtering techniques described above provide a convenient and efficient means for identifying compounds that an experienced medicinal chemist would tend to avoid. However, these methods do not necessarily identify molecules that could be considered as interesting hits/leads. Thus, for numerous projects, in addition to eliminating molecules containing undesirable fragments, it is also

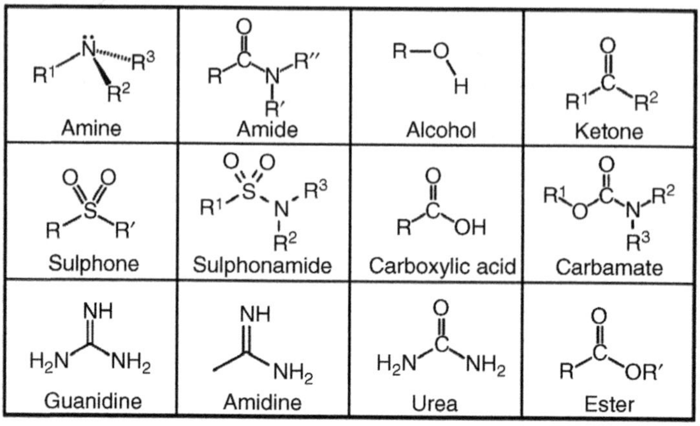

Figure 2.12 Chemical groups commonly found in drugs.

important to ensure that molecules in a screening collection contain functionality known to impart biological activity. One example of this concept reported by Muegge and coworkers [120] involves the idea of privileged structures. In this work, each molecule was assigned a score on the basis of the presence of structural fragments typically found in drugs; the fragments used in this study are shown in Figure 2.12. A molecule is given one point for each nonoverlapping fragment. Molecules with a score between two and seven are classified as drugs, otherwise they are classified as nondrugs.

Lead-likeness versus drug-likeness is another key concept. Drug-likeness is a property that is most often used to characterize compound libraries that are screened to find novel hit/lead chemicals. Yet drugs are typically the endpoints of a medicinal chemistry optimization program. Teague et al. pointed out that hits/leads may be classified into three categories: (i) low-affinity compounds with low MW and log *P*, (ii) high affinity and high MW including peptides and natural products that need improved pharmacokinetic profiles, and (iii) low affinity with MW between 300 and 500 and log *P* between 3 and 5 [61]. Most of the HTS hits belong to category (iii). Optimization of these hits/leads is difficult because most often, hydrophobic groups are added during the optimization to increase potency of the compounds. Thus, in general, lead compounds become larger and more lipophilic during the optimization process. Teague et al. estimate that the MW increases by up to 200 Da while the log *P* increases by 0.5–4 U during the optimization. Taking these observations into account, it may be more desirable to bias libraries toward "lead-like" compounds rather than toward fully optimized drug-like compounds [121–125]. These authors suggested to bias screening libraries to have MW < 350 Da and computed log *P* between 1 and 3. Congreve et al. [62] suggested the following values to profile a compound collection toward "hit discovery," MW < 300, HBD ≤ 3; HBA ≤ 3, calculated log $P = 3$ with some authors suggesting a polar surface area around 60 $Å^2$ and a few rotatable bonds.

There are differing philosophies as to the introduction of filtering methods (drug-like, lead-like, ... etc.) in the drug-discovery process. One idea suggests that as compounds undergo significant changes during the lead-optimization process, it might be premature to use predictive ADME/Tox in compound selection at the screening stage. However, analyses of the progress of a number of drug-discovery programs have indicated that drug candidates are typically larger and more lipophilic than the initial lead. On the basis of these observations, it may be beneficial to select screening compounds that are predicted to be soluble and orally bioavailable.

As discussed above, properties implicit to the drug-likeness of molecules such as oral bioavailability or membrane permeability have often been connected to simple molecular descriptors such as log *P*, MW, or the counts of hydrogen-bond acceptors and donors. Other simple counting criterion for drug-likeness is an atom filter. Typically, compounds with atoms other than C, N, O, S, H, P, Cl, Br, F, I, Na, K, Mg, Ca, Li are removed from a compound selection (some authors tend also to avoid Br). This criterion discriminates, for example, against antineoplastics, antiacids, or vitamins that contain Pt, As, Al, Si, Fe, or Co. Some authors combine several of the rules mentioned above; these are then generally referred to as the extended rule-of-5. These counting methods are generally used to filter or clean a collection and tend to give a yes/no answer or binning as poor/medium/good. More complex models build through mathematical modeling or docking/scoring and can be used at later stages of the drug discovery process [108]. In most cases, the above-mentioned rules were developed by translating the collected knowledge of scientists involved in drug discovery into a computer program. An alternative approach is to use two sets of compounds—one labeled as drugs and the other as nondrugs—and allow the method to learn to distinguish the two classes (see above the different classification methods and Section 2.3). This method is less dependent on experts' point of view, but the outputs also have to be analyzed with care to ensure that the models are meaningful (see below).

2.2.5 Lipophilicity

Assessing the pharmacokinetic structure–activity relationships throughout these past 30 years identified several essential physicochemical properties to control in drug development, including the numbers of hydrogen bond-donors and acceptors, polar surface area, the number of rotatable bonds, molecular weight, and lipophilicity. These parameters are often interrelated although arguably lipophilicity is the most wide reaching [64].

The IUPAC (International Union of Pure and Applied Chemistry) definition of lipophilicity is "Lipophilicity represents the affinity of a molecule or part of it for a lipophilic environment. It is commonly measured by its distribution behavior in a biphasic system, either liquid-liquid (e.g., partition coefficient in octanol/water)." A small amount of lipophilicity is required in almost all drugs to facilitate their passage from aqueous environments (e.g., gastric fluid, blood, extra-cellular fluid) into tissue compartments and cells. Lipophilicity is implicated in numerous biological events (e.g., decreased metabolic stability in liver microsomes when log *P* is increasing).

Lipophilicity for organic compound is often expressed as a partition or distribution coefficient (P, log P, or log D) between octanol (usually octan-1-ol) and aqueous phases. The partition coefficient P is a ratio of concentrations of unionized compound between these two solutions. To measure the partition coefficient of ionizable solutes, the pH of the aqueous phase is adjusted such that the predominant form of the compound is unionized. The logarithm of the ratio of the concentrations of the unionized solute in the solvents is called log P and is commonly used in drug discovery.

The distribution coefficient D is defined as the overall ratio of a compound (ionized and nonionized) between the two phases. This value log D is pH-dependent, and hence one must specify the pH at which the log D is measured. For unionizable compounds, log P = log D at any pH.

Lipophilicity significantly impacts ADME/Tox properties and is widely used in drug discovery for quantitative SAR and quantitative structure–property relationship studies. Highly lipophilic compounds (log $P > 5$) tend to have high potency due to nonspecific binding, but they are also more vulnerable to metabolism, leading to high hepatic clearance, they have low solubility, erratic oral absorption and high plasma protein binding, and they are more likely to bioaccumulate [56]. A compound with moderate lipophilicity (log P between 0 and 3) has a good balance between solubility and permeability and is optimal for oral absorption, cell-membrane permeation in cell-based assays, is generally good for BBB penetration, and has usually low metabolic liability. Hydrophilic compounds (log $P < 0$) have good solubility, but poor permeability for gastrointestinal (GI) or BBB penetration, and are more susceptible to renal clearance. Lipophilicity can be enhanced by increasing the molecular size and decreasing the hydrogen-bonding capacity.

It is necessary to account for the ionic state of the compound when describing the lipophilicity of a potential drug. Ionization results in decreased lipophilicity with respect to the neutral state. The changing pH environment in the body indicates that the compounds will often be found as a mixture of ionic species. While biochemical mechanisms maintain the pH of blood at 7.4, the pH along the GI tract varies from the stomach (fasted pH 1–2, fed pH 3–7) to the colon (pH 5–8). Oral drug absorption occurs in the small intestine at pH around 5.5. As such, it has been suggested to use log D in place of log P when filtering compounds via the rule-of-5 and other drug-likeness tools [126].

In a recent review, Mannhold et al. benchmarked most of the existing *in silico* methods to compute log P [127]. Numerous methods can be used, including substructure-based methods in which molecules are cut into fragments (fragmental methods) or down to the single-atom level (atom-based methods), and a final summing of the substructure contributions gives the final log P (i.e., problems arise when fragments are missing or when atomic contributions cannot be parameterized properly). Property-based approaches can also be used. These methods utilize descriptions of the entire molecule and comprise (i) empirical approaches and methods that use 3D structure representation and (ii) methods based on topological descriptors, using diverse types of statistical approaches. Some of these tools to predict log P (and log D and log S (see below) [128]) are listed in Table 2.3.

TABLE 2.3 Examples of *In Silico* Tools to Predict log *P* (and log *D*) and Other ADME Values: Solubility (Sol), HIA, Caco-2 (C2), Oral Bioavailability (OB)

Programs	log *P*	log *D*	Sol	HIA	C2	OB	URL
AB/log *P*	Y[a]						http://www.ap-algorithms.com
ABSOLV, LSER	Y						http://www.ap-algorithms.com
ACD/log *P*	Y	Y	Y				http://www.acdlabs.com
ADME Boxes	Y	Y	Y	Y	Y	Y	http://www.ap-algorithms.com
ADMEWORKS	Y		Y	Y			http://www.fqs.pl/life_science/admeworks_predictor
ALOGP	Y	Y					http://www.talete.mi.it
Discovery Studio	Y		Y	Y			http://www.accelrys.com
ALOGPS	Y		Y				http://www.vcclab.org
Chemaxon	Y	Y					http://www.chemaxon.com
CLOGP	Y						http://www.biobyte.com, http://www.daylight.com
COSMOFrag	Y						http://www.cosmologic.de
CSLogP	Y						http://www.chemsilico.com
HINT	Y						http://www.edusoft-lc.com
KowWIN	Y						http://www.syrres.com
KnowItAll	Y	Y	Y	Y		Y	http://www.knowitall.com
MiLogP	Y						http://www.molinspiration.com
MLOGP	Y						http://www.talete.mi.it
MLOGP(SR)	Y						http://www.simulations-plus.com
MolLogP	Y						http://www.molsoft.com
NCR + NHET	Y						http://www.vcclab.org
OsirisP	Y						http://www.actelion.com
PreADME	Y		Y	Y	Y		http://camd.ssu.ac.kr/adme
QikProp	Y	Y	Y		Y		http://www.schrodinger.com
Quantum Pharmaceuticals	Y	Y	Y			Y	http://q-pharm.com
SRlogP, ADMET predictor	Y	Y	Y	Y			http://www.simulations-plus.com
SLIPPER-2002	Y						http://camd.ipac.ac.ru
SPARC	Y	Y					http://ibmlc2.chem.uga.edu
TLOGP	Y						http://www.upstream.ch
VEGA	Y						http://www.ddl.unimi.it
VLOGP	Y						http://www.accelrys.com
Volsurf/Volsurf+	Y		Y		Y		http://www.moldiscovery.com
XLOGP2	Y						ftp://ftp2.ipc.pku.edu.cn
XLOGP3	Y						http://sioc-ccbg.ac.cn

[a] Y means the tool performs this prediction.

2.2.6 pK_a

pK_a is the ionization constant of a compound [129]. More than 60% of marketed drugs are ionizable. pK_a affects solubility, permeability, log *D*, and oral absorption by modulating the distribution of neutral and charged species. Acidic compounds tend to be more soluble and less permeable at high pHs and basic compounds tend to be more soluble and less permeable at low pH. pK_a impacts biological activity and metabolism through electrostatic interaction. For example, CYP2D6 typically metabolizes nitrogen-containing bases where the basic nitrogen is 5–7 Å from the site of metabolism.

Prediction can be done through applying a mechanistic perturbation method to estimate the pK_a value based on a number of models that account for electronic effects, solvation effects, hydrogen-bonding effects, and the influence of temperature (e.g., SPARC). One of the most common techniques used in pK_a prediction is quantitative structure activity/property relationships deriving their fit equations from partial least squares or multiple linear regression. Other methods include neural networks, quantum mechanical continuum, solvation models, and anticonnectivity models (see a recent review by Meloun and Bordovska [130]). Unfortunately, these authors note that to date no reliable method for predicting pK_a values over a wide range of molecular structures has been made available, although some recent tools could be more efficient but independent benchmarking is missing.

There are several available packages for the prediction of pK_a values (Table 2.4).

Two of the software programs are freely usable online (SPARC and VCCLAB). A decision tree model based on a novel set of SMARTS strings has also been recently reported [132]. Protonation states can also be assigned using simple rules in the OpenBabel open source package (http://openbabel.org/) and with SPORES [133]. A recent Web application for studying the protonation states of protein–ligand complexes (and also the free energy of binding) has been reported (http://hinttools.isbdd.vcu.edu/CT). This method should assist in investigating molecules and preparing files for ADME/Tox predictions and virtual screening computations [134].

2.2.6.1 Absorption, Solubility, Permeability, Bioavailability The oral *absorption* of a drug depends on the free concentration in the gastric fluid and the subsequent

TABLE 2.4 Software Available for pK_a Value Prediction

Software	Website
ACD/Labs	www.acdlabs.com
ADME Boxes	www.ap-algorithms.com
MOE	www.chemcomp.com
ADMET Predictor	www.simulationsplus.com
ChemAxon	www.chemaxon.com
CS pK_a	www.chemsilico.com
PALLAS	www.compudrug.com
Pipeline Pilot	www.scitegic.com
Epik	www.schrodinger.com [131]
QikProp	www.schrodinger.com
SPARC	ibmlc2.chem.uga.edu/sparc
MoKa	www.moldiscovery.com
VCCLAB	www.vcclab.org

membrane permeation to reach the blood. Overall, it is commonly accepted that solubility, permeability, and bioavailability are all related and interdependent [50]. The definitions for intestinal absorption, permeability, fraction absorbed, and bioavailability are used interchangeably [135]. Several *in silico* models and computer tools are available to predict oral absorption. These models can be relatively simple and involve only a few descriptors, such as log P, log D, or polar surface area. Alternatively, they can make use of complex mathematical modeling and even docking/scoring into some specific receptors, while pharmacophore modeling, ligand-based approaches, and simulation of diffusion across a biological membrane at atomic resolution (Table 2.3) can also be applied. Many reactions/events have to be considered, such as active transport (transporters), efflux pumps (e.g., P-gp), cell permeability predictions (Caco-2, PAMPA), as well as physicochemical properties such as pK_a, size, polar surface area, rotatable bonds, and H-bond donors and acceptors. Predictions are extremely difficult even at this stage. Computer packages typically assume that the compounds are passively absorbed, while methods considering active transport or efflux are still under development.

The rule-of-5 is considered to relate to intestinal absorption and can thus be used for this purpose. For instance, using QSPR approaches and 17 diverse drug compounds, the following equation was proposed (see reviews such as [20, 136, 137]):

$$\log \text{Permeability} = [0.008(\text{MW})] - [0.043(\text{PSA})] - 5.165$$

Absorption–simulation programs, such as GastroPlus (www.simulations-plus.com), are valuable tools in lead optimization as they require only a limited number of *in vitro* input data [20, 26, 138]. The OraSpotter program (www.zyxbio.com) uses only information about the molecular structures, which are transformed into SMILES strings. The descriptors are then evaluated from the SMILES data.

Solubility *Solubility* affects both *in vitro* assay results and *in vivo* oral bioavailability. Compounds with poor aqueous solubility may precipitate during *in vitro* assays and result in lower concentration than was anticipated. Insoluble compounds tend to give erratic assay results. Poor aqueous solubility is also one of the major causes for low systemic exposure and, consequently, lack of *in vivo* activity. Therefore, screening of solubility early in drug discovery is of great importance [56, 139]. Different methods can be used to model solubility such as fragment-based models that sum substructure contributions and models based on log P, on solvation properties, and hybrid models (e.g., neural network models using log P in combination with topological and quantum chemical descriptors [140]) (Table 2.3) [141, 142]. Empirically, it appears that most drugs have a log S ranging from -1 to -5, reflecting a compromise between the polarity needed for reasonable aqueous solubility and the hydrophobicity needed for acceptable diffusion across the membrane [142]. Possible ways to improve solubility involve adding ionizable groups, hydrogen bonding/polar groups, and reduce log P and MW. A Web application [143] to predict pH-dependent aqueous solubility of drug-like molecules (pHSol) is available at http://www.cbs.dtu.dk/services/pHSol/.

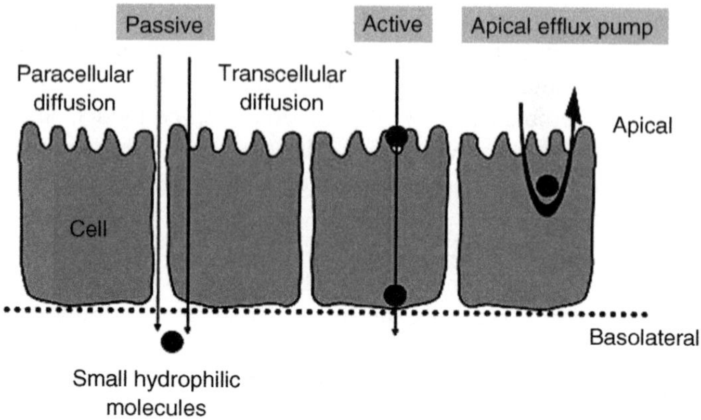

Figure 2.13 Simplified view of some permeability mechanisms.

Permeability *Permeability* is an important factor for passage through cell membranes in cell-based assays, absorption through the GI tract, and penetration through the blood–brain barrier and through other physiological barriers (Figure 2.13). There are several transport mechanisms involved for small molecules: transcellular passive diffusion, paracellular passive transport, and active/carrier-mediated and efflux [144]. The two most important pathways for drug absorption are transcellular passive diffusion and efflux transport by P-gp or multidrug-resistant proteins. Transcellular diffusion is driven by the concentration gradient, while efflux transport is energy-driven. The paracellular route is only available in the small intestine, while transcellular absorption can take place throughout the length of the GI tract. The GI tract also contains drug metabolism enzymes (e.g., CYP3A4, sulfotransferases) and efflux pumps (in particular P-gp) that decrease the absorption of compounds. Investigation of these mechanisms is complex, *in vitro* assays, such as Caco-2 cells (include transporters) and PAMPA (parallel artificial membrane permeability assay analyzes passive transports) have been developed for this purpose and can be somewhat simulated *in silico*. P-gp-efflux is an important mechanism that nature uses to prevent entrance of toxic substances. P-gp is abundant in cells with protective barriers. It plays a key role in drug resistance in chemotherapy, BBB penetration, and oral absorption. It also plays an important role in metabolism, where P-gp and CYP3A4 work in concert to eliminate certain drugs. This is named "efflux-metabolism alliance" in which both act on a wide variety of xenobiotics and overlap for substrate specificity and tissue location. There is a strong relationship between solubility and lipophilicity—when log P increases, solubility tends to decrease [145]. In general, when one has to choose between improving solubility or permeability, preference should be given to permeability, because solubility can often be improved through formulation [23, 146, 147]. Permeability can be improved by modification of structure or by prodrug approaches.

Prediction of effective permeability can be performed through the use of different methods (Table 2.3). The rule-of-5 and different types of polar surface area models can be used (e.g., well-absorbed compounds have a log P between -1 and 5.9 and a polar surface area between 0 and 132 $Å^2$) [144]. One study reported that

$$\text{Permeability} = -2.546 - 0.011(\text{PSA}) - 0.278(\text{HBD}) \ [136]$$

Models using both linear and nonlinear relationships have also been used to model intestinal permeability [144]. Possible ways to improve permeability involve the removal of ionizable groups, adding hydrophobic groups, reduce size, hydrogen bonding, and polarity (high PSA suggests many hydrogen bonds to water and may hinder facile passage into membranes).

Bioavailability The oral *bioavailability* of a molecule is a complex PK parameter that comprises absorption (solubility, permeability) and clearance. For all these factors, ionization of the molecules tends to play an important role, but this state is difficult to predict *in silico* [50]. Many methods have been developed and reviewed to predict solubility [137, 141, 142, 148], permeability [144, 149], and/or absorption [43, 84, 150–153] (Table 2.3). In 2002, Veber et al. reported the findings from a study of rat availability data, acquired by GlaxoSmithKline, for 1100 drug candidates [112]. They found that molecules possessing fewer than 10 rotatable bonds and having a polar surface area less than 140 $Å^2$ (or H-bond count less than 12) generally showed oral bioavailability in rats exceeding 20%. In 2004, Lu and coworkers examined the relationship of rotatable bond count and polar surface area (PSA) with the oral bioavailability in rats for 434 compounds and found that the correlations were dependent on the calculation methods [154]. Martin proposed a score to predict bioavailability based on several molecular properties, including polar surface area, rule-of-5, and molecular charged state [155]. Generally, the work of Veber, Lu, and Martin support the same conclusion that bioavailability may be well predicted by simple molecular properties. However, Hou et al. found that the prediction of intestinal absorption was possible with "rule-based" and counting methods and cautioned the prediction of human bioavailability with these approaches [156]. They also suggested that statistical methods could provide better results. Often, prediction models of oral bioavailability are based on QSAR/QSPR analysis [47]. A possible method to evaluate bioavailability according to Van der Waterbeemd [20, 21] is

$$\text{Oral bioavailability} = f\,(\log D,\ \text{molecular size, H-bond capacity})$$

Distribution Distribution of drugs throughout the body is important since it determines whether the molecule will elicit a pharmacological response. Distribution parameters that can be investigated *in silico* include blood–brain barrier permeability, plasma protein binding (PPB), volume of distribution, and transporters. BBB is an essential property for drugs that target the CNS such as anxiolytics and antidepressants. The protein human serum albumin is present in many tissues and is responsible for unspecific drug binding (PPB). Yet, other proteins (low-density lipoprotein, high-density lipoprotein, α1-acid glycoprotein, myosin, actin, etc.) are known to also bind drugs in a nonspecific manner. Nonspecific protein binding should be carefully considered in drug design because only the free drug concentration determines the pharmaceutical activity. Transport proteins are found in most organs involved in the uptake and elimination of endogenous compounds and xenobiotics including drugs. An attempt to predict binding to these proteins is very important. The volume of distribution is a nonphysiological term that is a measure of drug distribution and together with clearance determines the half-life of a drug and thus affects its dosing regimen.

BBB Permeability Several recent reviews have been reported about BBB and *in silico* modeling [28, 157–168]. CNS acting drugs have to overcome physical barriers before reaching their drug target in the form of the blood–brain barrier. The BBB is formed by the microvasculature of the brain that exhibits selective permeability for substances [169]. The brain capillary endothelium forms tight junctions that surround the cell margin circumferentially. This results in the BBB being essentially impermeable to hydrophilic compounds. The BBB has developed carrier systems or transporters for the uptake of larger, hydrophilic, or charged compounds. These transporters play a role in transporting amino acids, monocarboxylic acids, peptides, and organic cations across the BBB. BBB transporters include the organic cation transporters (OCT), organic anion transporters (OAT), and nucleoside transport system (Table 2.5). There are transporters located at the BBB interface also involved in the removal (efflux) of drugs from the CNS such as P-glycoprotein. P-gp is a part of the multidrug resistance (MDR) gene and has a key role as a result of tight junctions between the cells.

TABLE 2.5 Blood–Brain Barrier Transporters

BBB Transporters [165]	
Energy	GLUT1 MCT1 CRT
Amino acids	LAT1, CAT1, EAAT, TAUT System beta ASCT2 System T
Neurotransmitters	GAT/BGT SERT NET
Organic cation and anion	OCTN2 CHT1 OAT3 Oatp
ABC	ABCB1 ABCC1 ABCG2

In silico methods have been developed to establish predictive models for the uptake of drugs into the CNS. Observations of simple descriptors underline that molecules with MW < 300 have a favorable brain/blood ratio as compared to drug with MW > 700 (analysis of 3059 diverse molecules with CNS penetration data) [145]. Ionization state is also critical with basic molecules typically more CNS penetrant than neutral molecules, followed by zwiterrions. Acidic molecules are the least CNS penetrant compounds [145].

Multiple linear regression or partial least squares methods have been used to determine brain permeation models (log BBB) [20]. From these studies, several "rules of thumb" have arisen for passive BBB permeability (in the absence of active transport), similar to Lipinski's rule-of-5 for intestinal absorption. These include, if the sum of the nitrogen and oxygen (N + O) atoms in a molecule is less than five (some studies report six) and if $C \log P - (N + O) > 0$, then compounds are likely to penetrate the BBB [170]. Additionally, the polar surface area should be less than 90 Å^2 (some studies suggest PSA < 70 Å^2), the MW < 450, and the $\log D$ between 1 and 3.

The degree of hydrogen-bonding capacity of the molecule also plays a significant role in facilitating BBB permeability. Generally, increasing the hydrogen-bonding capacity of a molecule leads to decreased BBB permeability, as observed from highly polar/strong hydrogen-bonding molecules that do not cross the BBB readily [164]. Using these rules and tuning software packages that compute rule-of-5 values, it is possible to filter compound collections to determine which compounds are excluded from the CNS due to low predicted BBB permeability. Most computational models predicting BBB are based on experimental log BB values, the logarithmic ratio between the concentrations of a substance in the brain to that in the blood (log ([brain]/[blood])). Experimental log BB data are relatively time-consuming to obtain and surrogate measures are often performed. Molecules that show and do not show activity at a CNS target are CNS+ and CNS−, respectively. The measure of permeability (log PS) by vascular perfusion methods are relatively rapid to determine and can also be used. In general, *in silico* log BB models have been derived assuming passive diffusion and equilibrium conditions. In contrast to $\log P$, log BB covers a much narrower range, in general between −2 and 1. Compounds with log BB > 0.3 cross the BBB readily, while values <−1 indicate minor penetration [17]. PLS, *k*-nearest-neighbor, decision trees, neural networks, and SVM have been used for qualitative classification of compounds, CNS+ for those that are readily available to the CNS, and CNS−, for the molecules that are unlikely to penetrate the brain [17]. Comparison of relevant descriptors in QSAR equations for log BB to those in CNS+/− classification algorithms is complicated. It has been suggested that CNS+ agents should contain less than three H-bond donors and no carboxylic acids unless they mimic neurotransmitters. Overall, compared to non-CNS drugs, CNS+ molecules tend to be more lipophilic, more rigid, have fewer HBD, fewer formal charges, and lower PSA (<80 Å^2) (Figure 2.14).

Little structural knowledge is available for many BBB transporters, limiting the design of compounds that will interact with these transporters as well as understanding mechanisms for increasing BBB permeability of neuroactive compounds. Thus the use of docking/scoring, comparative modeling, and related approaches is difficult.

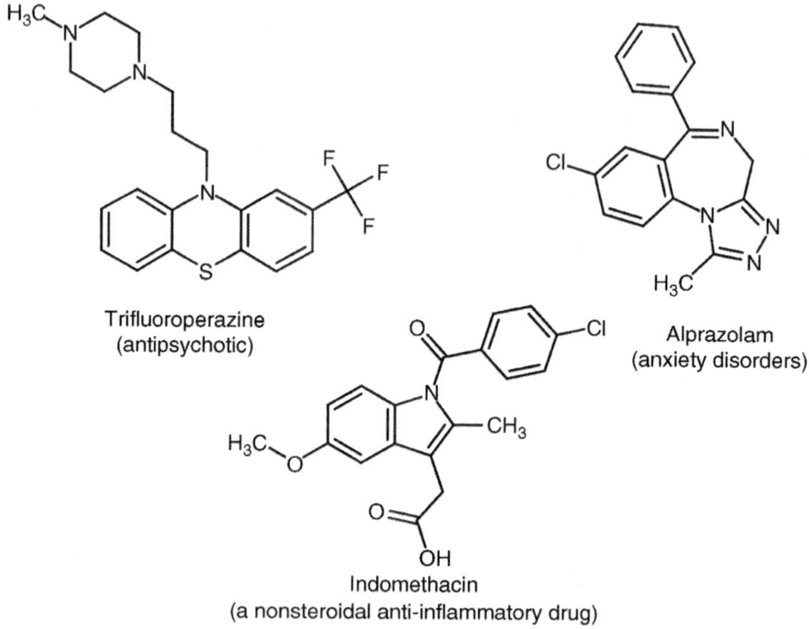

Figure 2.14 Trifluoroperazine is a good brain permeator (log BB = 1.44) with calculated properties slightly within the guidelines for CNS compounds (MW = 407.5, PSA = 16, log D = 4.04, N + O count = 3). Alprazolam partitions equally between the brain and the blood, with a log BB = 0.04 (MW = 308, PSA = 49.5, log D = 2.5, N + O count = 4) possibly because the balance between hydrogen bonding and lipophilicity is not ideal. Indomethacin is a poor brain permeator, with a log BB = − 1.26 (MW = 357, PSA = 78, log D = 0.3, N + O count = 5). The lack of penetration seems to be due to the carboxylic moiety, while the hydrogen-bonding/lipophilicity balance is also against brain penetration [164, 171].

Ligand-based methods can be used but are indirect since the transporter is inferred from a series of ligands with experimentally derived affinity for a certain target. These methods included QSAR, and techniques such as pharmacophore modeling [172–174] using programs such as Catalyst (Accelrys, San Diego, CA) and DISCOtech (Tripos). Also the popular 3D-QSAR technique of the SYBYL program (Tripos, St. Louis, MO), comparative molecular field analysis (CoMFA) [175] is used. Homology modeling has been applied to predict the structure of transporters such as the P-glycoprotein structure, which was modeled by using the MsbA lipid transporter experimental structure. The resulting 3D model of the protein has been criticized because it is certainly not very accurate and therefore should have low predictive value [176]. A dopamine transporter (DAT), serotonin (SERT), and noradrenalin (NET) models were defined using the crystal structure of Aquifex aeolicus LeuT(Aa) [177]. Cocaine was docked into one binding pocket of DAT (corresponding to the leucine-binding site in LeuT(Aa)), which involved several transmembrane helices (TMHs). Clomipramine was docked into another binding pocket of DAT, corresponding to the clomipramine-binding site in the crystal structure of a

TABLE 2.6 Packages for the Prediction of BBB

Software Package	Website
ADME Boxes (P-gp)	www.ap-algorithms.com
ACD/ADME suite	www.acdlabs.com
ADMET Predictor	www.simulationsplus.com
QikProp	www.schrodinger.com
KnowItAll	www.biorad.com
Volsurf	www.moldiscovery.com
ChemSilico	www.chemsilico.com

LeuT(Aa)–clomipramine complex. The structures of the proposed cocaine- and tricyclic antidepressant-binding sites were of particular interest for the design of novel DAT interacting ligands.

Some packages for the prediction of BBB are listed in Table 2.6.

2.2.7 Transport Proteins

The exchange between body compartments often uses active transporters. Several types have been identified and are not discussed in this chapter. About 40 proteins that belong to the ABC and SLC superfamilies that influence absorption, distribution, and excretion of drugs and xenobiotics are known. These transporters can modify PK and PD parameters but also effect toxicity. In the ABC family (multidrug resistance, ATP-binding cassette), P-gp is considered of significant importance. The multi-specific solute carrier transporters are the other main superfamily of proteins that play a key role in the human body. Transporters are integral membrane proteins with primarily 12 transmembrane domains (some have some extra or less helices). The classification also accounts for the type of energy source and the direction of the transport. The energy source can be the hydrolysis of ATP or use of a voltage and/or ion gradient to transport both ions and solutes. The coordination between transporters and metabolic enzymes is important [43]. One of the best-studied transporters is P-gp, encoded by human *MDR1* gene, a member of the ABC superfamily of transport proteins. The overexpression of P-gp is associated with a multidrug resistance phenotype in various forms of cancer that cause a suboptimal efficacy of many molecules. P-gp plays a significant role in the absorption, distribution, metabolism, and excretion processes of a wide range of drugs [178]. For instance, P-gp has been shown to limit oral absorption of paclitaxel and docetaxel, modulate hepatic, renal or intestinal elimination, and restrict CNS entry of certain drugs (e.g., cyclosporin A, digoxin, indinavir, ritonavir, saquinavir). Molecules can be substrates, inhibitors, or inducers of P-gp. A better understanding of the relationships between the structure of P-gp binders (substrate or inhibitor) has been obtained using QSAR, pharmacophore, and protein modeling, yet, data are still missing to fully capture the functioning of this protein. Models are not sufficiently sophisticated to fully rationalize earlier observations for well-known P-gp substrates in terms of MW, lipophilicity, hydrogen bonding, presence of a basic nitrogen, but are useful to assist some of the drug design steps [179, 180]. One study made use of the MolSurf program to generate descriptors to build a PLS model to predict P-gp-associated ATPase activity [181]. This model identified the main contributing descriptors for predicting ATPase activity as the size of the molecular surface, polarizability, and hydrogen-bonding potential. In general, as MW increases, the P-gp efflux ratio increases (MW > 400). As molecules become larger, the permeability, on average, decreases, limiting oral and/or brain exposure, and P-gp efflux becomes an additional complication-reducing exposure [145]. Ionization state plays only a minor role in determining the efflux when compared to MW. Increasing the number of hydrogen bond acceptors appears to confer increasing likelihood of P-gp efflux. Log *P* values have a weak nonlinear effect. Example of programs able to predict P-gp binders are implemented in ADME Boxes (www.ap-algorithms.com) and ACD/ADME suite (www.acdlabs.com). A machine learning method, SVM, was explored for the prediction of P-gp substrates. About 120 substrates and 80 nonsubstrates were collected from the literature and 22 final descriptors were used to develop the model [182]. Although the prediction accuracies were reasonably good, the structural features responsible for discriminating the two groups of molecules could not be identified. An unsupervised machine learning approach based on the Kohonen self-organizing maps was explored to classify drugs as P-gp substrates or inhibitors [183]. As for the SVM model, the P-gp SOM model was unable to provide hints on structural modifications that should be pursued to modify P-gp binding. The X-ray structure of multidrug efflux pump P-gp was recently reported (mouse P-gp solved at 3.8 Å resolution, PDB entry 3G60) by Aller et al. [184]. The relatively low resolution and as a nucleotide-free state suggest that the structure may represent a crystallization artifact or a nonfunctional conformation that has only very transient existence, impeding its use for ADME/Tox prediction [185] (Figure 2.15). Other transporters potentially involved in limiting the oral uptake of drugs include the MDR-associated proteins MRP1 and MRP2, and the recently discovered breast-cancer-resistance protein (BCRP). It will be important to expand our knowledge about these transporters in order to understand their effects on pharmacokinetics, pharmacodynamics, and toxicity. Currently, knowledge about these transport systems is relatively poor compared to P-gp.

2.2.8 Plasma Protein Binding

The binding of drugs to plasma proteins and to human serum albumin (HSA) in particular has ADME/Tox implications affecting clearance, volume of distribution, and efficacy. Drugs can bind to a variety of particles in the blood, including red blood cells, leukocytes, and platelets, as well as proteins HSA (particularly acidic drugs), α1-acid glycoprotein (AAG) (basic drugs), lipoproteins (neutral and basic drugs), erythrocytes, and α,β,γ-globulins. From a recent analysis of 2939 diverse drugs with *in vitro* plasma protein binding data, it has been shown that as MW increases, plasma protein binding on average increases (molecules with MW between 500 and 700 are 98.2% bound) [145]. In terms of ionization state, binding to plasma proteins follow the trend acids > neutrals > zwiterrions > bases. Lipophilicity is a key contributor to the extent of binding.

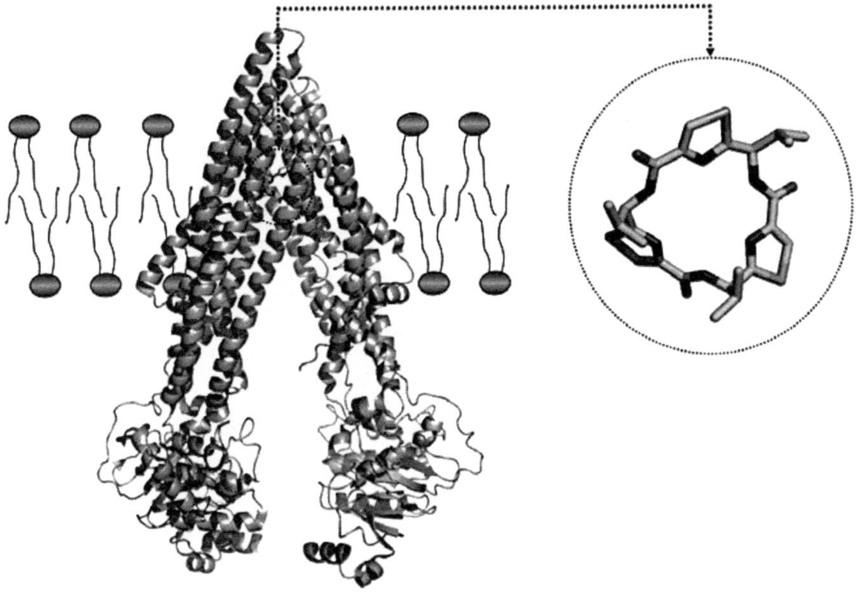

Figure 2.15 Ribbon drawing of mouse P-gp embedded in a membrane bilayer (PDB file 3G60). The inhibitor QZ59-SSS bound in the transmembrane region is shown as a stick model (in circle).

HSA binding has been intensively investigated [41, 186, 187]. HSA is a single-chain protein that contains several binding sites for drugs, including site I and site II (indole-benzodiazepine site) (Figures 2.16 and 2.17). Site I compounds seem to be dicarboxylic acids and/or bulky heterocyclic molecules with a negative charge localized in the middle of the structure. The site appears to be large and can accommodate large ligands such as bilirubin. Site II seems to be smaller, and ligands are often aromatic carboxylic acids with a negatively charged acidic group at one end of the molecular removed from a hydrophobic center.

Blood levels for plasma proteins are increased or decreased under different conditions. The level of AAG is increased in neoplasms, while HSA is markedly depressed in progressive malignancies [187].

The experimental structure of AAG has been solved recently at 1.8 resolution (PDB file 3BX6) [188]. This protein belongs to the lipocalin family in which the beta-barrel, built up from eight antiparallel β-strands encloses a central cavity (Figure 2.18). The AAG cavity is divided into three distinct pockets—the central, deep hydrophobic site and the two adjacent smaller and negatively charged sites. The cavity allows for the binding of both apolar and basic ligands. AAG binds to more than 300 pharmaceutical agents. The majority are basic compounds such as beta-blockers, but neutral and acidic molecules such as steroid hormones or the anticoagulant coumarin molecules may also bind. Genetic variability of AAG adds even more variability to its ligand-binding properties [187].

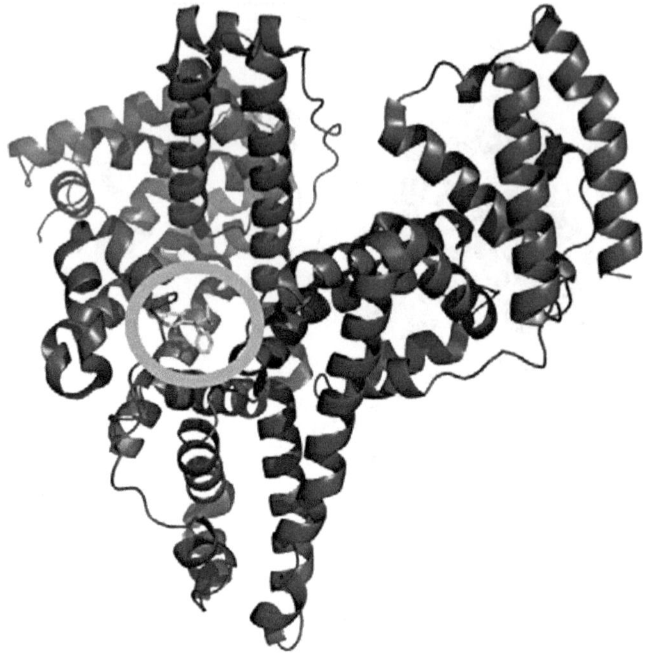

Figure 2.16 Warfarin bound to the site I of HSA (PDB file 1H9Z).

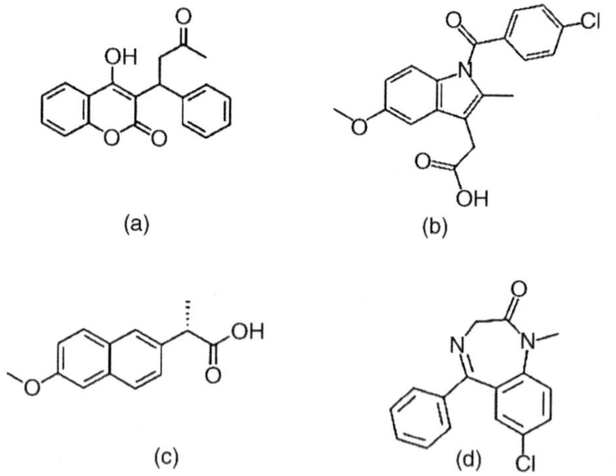

Figure 2.17 Examples of molecules binding to HSA. Site I (a) warfarin (anticoagulant); (b) indometacin (nonsteroidal anti-inflammatory drug, NSAID). Site II (c) naproxen (NSAID); (d) diazepam (valium).

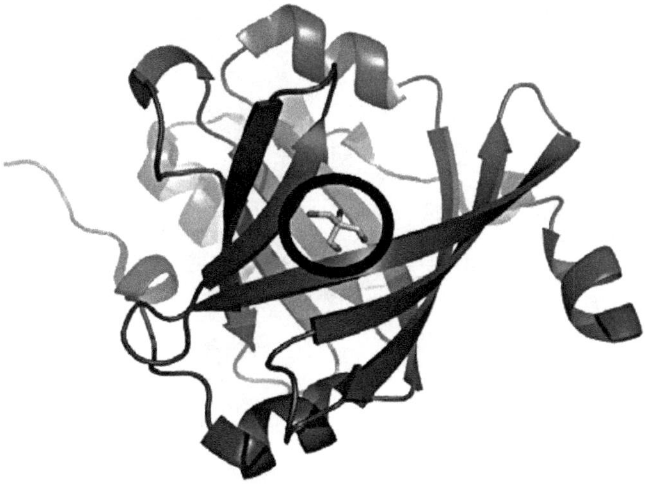

Figure 2.18 Cartoon diagram of AAG in complex with 2-amino-2-hydroxymethyl-propane-1,3-diol (tris) highlighting the relatively large binding cavity.

TABLE 2.7 Packages for the Prediction of Plasma Protein Binding

Software Package	Website
ChemSilico	www.chemsilico.com
ACD/Labs	www.acdlabs.com
ADMET Predictor	www.simulationsplus.com
ADME Boxes	www.ap-algorithms.com
QikProp	www.schrodinger.com
KnowItAll	www.biorad.com
DSMedChem	www.accelrys.com
q-Albumin	QuantumLead, www.q-lead.com

Several studies were reported that attempt to predict HSA binding using known HSA binders and QSAR [189, 190]. Several software packages known to predict binding to plasma proteins are listed in Table 2.7.

2.2.9 Metabolism

Drug metabolism is traditionally divided into Phase I and Phase II processes. This classical division while useful is neither absolute nor definitive. Phase I enzymes include cytochrome P450 monooxygenase (CYPs), azo and nitro group reductase, monoamine oxidase, while Phase II enzymes involve *N*- and *O*-methyl transferases, D-glucuronic acid transferase, glutathione transferase, and sulfate transferase. CYP enzymes have been extensively investigated because they play a pivotal role in drug

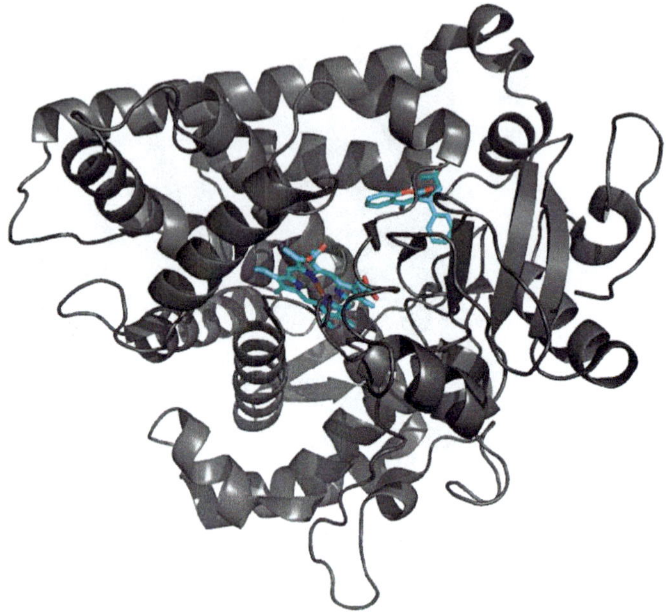

Figure 2.19 CYP2C9 cocrystallized with warfarin (PDB file 1OG5). The substrate-binding pocket is essentially hydrophobic and the compound is at about 10 Å from the heme group. See insert for color representation of this figure.

metabolism. CYP is a heme-containing superfamily of enzymes consisting of isoenzymes and catalyze several oxidation reactions (Figure 2.19). The most important forms in man are CYP2D6, CYP2C9, CYP3A4, CYP1A1, CYP2C19, and CYP2E1. More than 90% of all marketed drugs are subjected to metabolic reactions by at least one of the CYP enzymes. The abundance of CYPs in many organs/tissues is established in the gut and intestinal tissues. Genetic diversity issues have been reported for this family usually causing decreased or missing enzymatic activity. Gene duplication can occur and lead to increased activity [191]. Thus, it is becoming imperative to recognize individuals who could have such genetic diversities. Certain substances can induce increased expression of CYPs via binding to nuclear receptors. For example, known inducers of CYP3A4 bind to RXR receptor tamoxifen. Conversely, xenobiotics may block specific CYPs and cause drug–drug interactions. Numerous X-ray structures of CYPs have been reported and will assist to rationalize compound binding to these proteins [17, 192].

Simple CYP alerts have been developed over the years and may assist the hit-finding stage but not during optimization. CYP3A4 usually binds lipophilic molecules and has a large flexible binding site. CYP2D6 has bases with aromatic groups 5–7 Å removed from the basic center similar to tricyclic antidepressants. CYP2C9 tend to interact with amphipathic molecules and favor acidic compounds like some nonsteroidal anti-inflammatory agents. Numerous computer studies have been performed on diverse CYP enzymes using small datasets of compounds [17, 145, 193].

TABLE 2.8 Packages for the Prediction of CYP Metabolism

Software Package	Website
MetabolExpert	www.compudrug.com
META multicase	www.multicase.com
MetaSite	www.moldiscovery.com
KnowItAll	www.biorad.com
Meteor	www.lhasalimited.org
MDL database Metabolite	www.mdl.com
SimCYP	www.simcyp.com

Several *in silico* packages and databases to predict CYP metabolism are listed in Table 2.8.

2.2.10 Elimination

Elimination of drugs usually occurs *via* the liver and the kidney but the lungs, skin, and so on, also play a role. Typically, lipophilic compounds tend to be eliminated by the liver, whereas hydrophilic molecules undergo renal clearance. There has been very little *in silico* modeling or prediction of excretion. Passive excretion can theoretically be predicted using some of the approaches described above for tissue distribution since similar physicochemical and physiological properties (blood flow, protein binding, lipophilicity, pK_a) with different limits (glomerular filtration and molecular weight) may be used. *In silico* packages to predict drug clearance with only molecular structure input data are still under development.

2.2.11 Toxicity

In the pharmaceutical industry, there is a concern that close to 20% (and possibly more) of drug attrition during preclinical and clinical development is due to toxicity issues. Because of the relatively small number of patients enrolled in clinical trials, it is statistically difficult to detect rare adverse reactions. Thus, all toxicity issues are not noticed during clinical trials, thereby causing major problem in today's drug discovery endeavors [32, 53].

Toxicity *effects* can be divided in at least four categories according to the pathological effect induced:

- cell death (apoptosis and necrosis) and tissue injury, which is probably the most common response;
- cancer;
- altered phenotype/function relating to cell alterations;
- immunological hypersensitivity, causing downregulation of the immune system or producing autoimmunity to native proteins [194].

Numerous types of toxicities occur including hepatic, hematological, cardiovascular, carcinogenicity, teratogenicity, reproductive toxicity, cytotoxicity, and phospholipidosis.

Another possible classification is to break down toxicity into the following:

- pharmacophore-induced toxicity (CYP inhibition and drug–drug interaction or hERG binding);
- structure-related toxicity (structural features and physicochemical properties of the compound or metabolite allowing interactions at sites distinct from the intended target);
- metabolism-induced toxicity (drug altered to a reactive metabolite such as electrophiles can react with nucleophilic functions in proteins, Cys, Lys, Ser, His, and nucleic acids causing organ toxicity including carcinogenicity (epoxides, quinine imines, thiophenes, thioureas, chloroquinolines) [20, 21].

Toxicity is a subtle issue since most chemicals become toxic at high doses. To minimize patient risk during the drug discovery process, a compound may be admitted as drug only if its efficacy and nontoxicity are demonstrated by pharmacological and clinical trials. During preclinical development, toxicologists calculate the "Therapeutic index" (the ratio of toxic dose to the therapeutic dose), the "safety window" (the range between the effective concentration and the toxic concentration), and the "maximum tolerated dose" (MTD) or "no observable adverse effect level" (NOAEL) (the maximum concentration of a drug at which no toxics effects are observed) [54].

TOXICITY DEFINITIONS [54]

Acute toxicity is the toxic effects from a substance resulting from a single exposure or several exposures during less than 24 h from a single dose, occurring within 14 days after administration.

Carcinogenicity is toxicity due to agents that promote cancer and/or increase its propagation.

Clastogenicity refer to a form of mutagenicity due to chromosome breakage.

Chronic toxicity is the toxic effects from repeated exposures to a substance over a long-term dosing (months or years).

Cytotoxicity is toxicity against the cells promoting cell death, which could drive to the whole organ toxicity (e.g., hepatoxicity).

Drug–drug interaction is the fact that a pharmaceutical or dietary agent affects the metabolism, clearance, or safety of another molecule.

Genotoxicity is toxicity capable to induce DNA damage and thus inducing mutations and cancer.

Idiosyncratic toxicity is an adverse reaction that occurs rarely (less than 1 in 1000) and unpredictably among the population, caused by reactive metabolites. Patient enzyme irregularities or polymorphisms may be implicated.

Immunotoxicity is toxicity due to an immune reaction initiated by the drug administered or its metabolites, which react as an antigen.

Metabolite-mediated toxicity is toxicity due to the formation of reactive metabolites or electrophilic metabolites that could bind covalently to proteins and DNA, driving to genotoxicity, target organ toxicity, and idiosyncratic toxicity.

Mutagenicity is DNA damage that is considered to initiate carcinogenicity.

Organ toxicity is an organ-specific form of toxicity that alters an organ (e.g., liver, kidney, heart) in its integrity and then its function.

Phospholipidosis is an adverse drug reaction in response to cationic amphiphilic drugs that drive to a lipid storage disorder due to the accumulation of polar phospholipids in cells.

Primary pharmacology or target-based toxicity is toxicity directly from modulation of the drug target.

Reproductive toxicity is adverse effects on sexual function and fertility, including developmental toxicity in the offspring.

Safety pharmacology studies the effects of a compound on normal physiological functions. Well-known studies are the assessment of hERG potassium channel binding and/or hERG blockade. Blocking this channel may be predictive for QT interval prolongation and ultimately to potential life-threatening drug-induced ventricular tachyarrhythmia.

Teratogenicity is embryo toxicity conducting to abnormalities of physiological development and birth defects.

Toxicogenomics is a combination of toxicology and genomics. It represents the study of structure and function of the genome, in addition to interindividual variations across the genome depending on responses to xenobiotic exposures.

2.2.11.1 Toxicity Mechanisms In general, toxicity mechanisms are classified into five categories [194]:

- on-target
- hypersensitivity and immunological reactions
- off-target
- biological activation
- idiosyncratic toxicity

Statins are a well-known example of on-target toxicity (Figure 2.20). These molecules are employed to regulate synthesis of cholesterol. Extensive data support the use of 3-hydroxy-3-methylglutaryl coenzyme A reductase inhibitors (statins) for both primary and secondary prevention of myocardial infarction, revascularization procedures, stroke, and peripheral vascular disease. Yet, toxicity may occur because statins inhibit the target HMG-CoA reductase in muscles leading to myopathy and kidney damage.

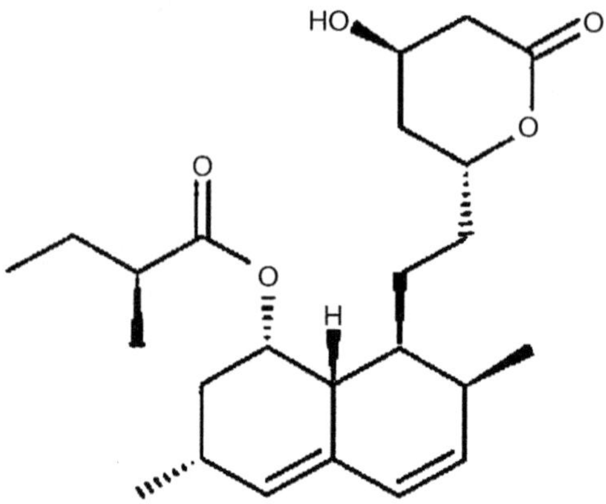

Figure 2.20 Lovastatin, the first statin to be marketed.

Hypersensitivity, immunological reactions, and allergic reactions may be immediate (IgE antibodies), cytotoxic and immune complex reactions (IgG or IgM), or delayed (T-lymphocytes). It has also been reported that covalent binding of reactive metabolites to tissue proteins can play a role in this toxicity. Penicillins and other beta-lactam antibiotics are examples of these autoimmune responses.

Off-target activities can be beneficial or detrimental and involve interactions with a target that was not expected. Antitargets are targets that are detrimental to the progression of a compound. Off-target toxicity such as binding to CYP or hERG is related to pharmacophore-induced toxicity. Drug–drug interaction can occur when patients receive several medications, at the same time potentially leading to a competition for the same metabolizing enzyme such as CYP3A4. Consumption of grapefruit or grapefruit juice inhibits the metabolism of statins, which increases the risk of dose-related adverse effects including myopathy/rhabdomyolysis. Furanocoumarins in grapefruit inhibit the cytochrome P450 enzyme CYP3A4, which is involved in the metabolism of most statins.

Cardiac arrhythmias characterized by a prolongation of the QT-interval [195] are measured by electrocardiogram on the surface of the heart tissue. hERG channel blockade can cause this adverse event. This reaction seems to be a consequence of a drug binding within a water cavity inside the transmembrane region of the channel presumably preventing required conformational changes [17] (Figure 2.21). Terfenadine, an antihistamine formerly used for the treatment of allergic conditions, is a known example. It was marketed under various brand names and removed from the market in the 1998 due to the risk of cardiac arrhythmia (Figure 2.22). When considering safety margins for hERG and cardiac issues, free plasma concentrations and plasma protein binding are important (e.g., fluoroquinolone antibiotics and antipsychotics) [195].

Biological activation includes structure-related toxicity (toxic structural features and physicochemical properties) and metabolism-induced toxicity (CYP induction [rifampicin, carbamazepine, nevirapine, probenicid] or inhibition [erythromycin,

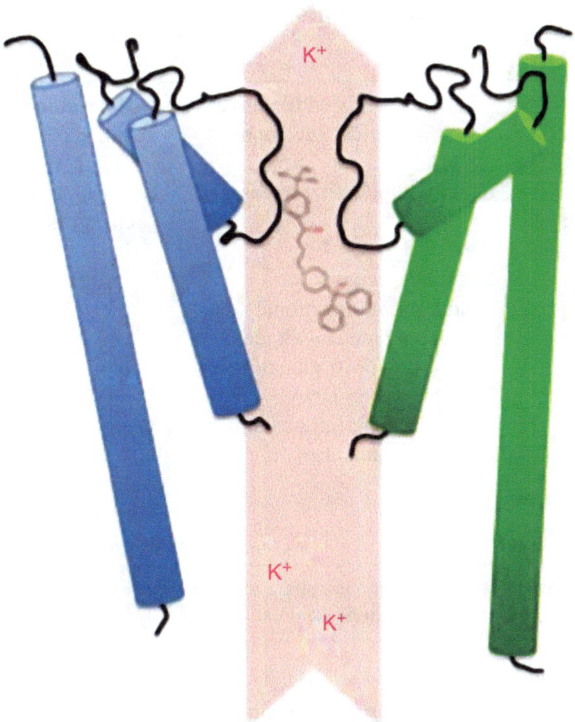

Figure 2.21 Putative interactions between a small compound and the hERG potassium channel.

tamoxifen, ritonavir]), pregnane X receptor, and drug altered to a reactive metabolites. The latter can react with nucleophilic functions in proteins and nucleic acids causing organ toxicity, including carcinogenicity (e.g., epoxides, quinine imines, thiophenes, thioureas, chloroquinolines). Over the years, several authors [33, 38, 39, 196, 197]

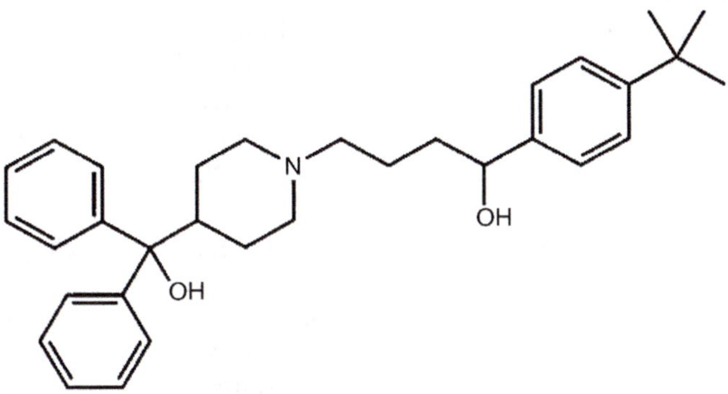

Figure 2.22 Drug withdrawn due to QT prolongation concerns. Terfenadine (antihistamine) binds to hERG and removed from the market in 1998.

TABLE 2.9 Known Unacceptable Toxicophore Moieties[a]

Classification	Reactivity	Chemical Function
Electrophilic reactive molecules	React covalently with proteins and biological nucleophiles	α-Haloketones, boronic acids, aldehydes, and 1,2-dicarbonyls
Tight-binding or metal-chelating molecules	React with metalloproteases	Hydroxamate, oxime, and thiol chelators
Redox/thiol	Michael acceptors, undesirable functional group which can alkylate thiol groups of glutathione, proteins, and DNA	Quinones
DNA intercalating agents	Strong binding (intercalation) causing mutations	Acridine
Others		Aldehydes, soft electrophiles as aliphatic ketones and cyclohexanones

[a] See Section 2.3 for examples of reactive groups, please see some other examples of chemical structures in drugs that can become toxic metabolites in Nassar et al. [198].

have focused on identifying chemical compounds or moieties (structural alerts), which have been associated with toxicity issues such as covalent binding, and intercalation to DNA. Some of these known unacceptable moieties (toxicophores) are categorized in Table 2.9.

In general, some drugs containing such groups can be considered safe if the dose does not exceed 10 mg day^{-1}, but this observation has to be investigated on a case-by-case basis.

Idiosyncratic toxicities are due in most situations to reactive metabolites. Subsequent the complex, protein–metabolite conjugate triggers an immune response. This is difficult to reproduce and predict and seldom occurs [199]. Bromfenac, an NSAID that was withdrawn from the market in 1998 due to reports of idiosyncratic hepatoxicity, is one example (Figure 2.23). This molecule contains several toxicophores including an aniline ring that has the potential to form a reactive nitroso group. The molecule appears to bind to endogenous protein, which is then recognized as a nonself protein and initiates an immune response [200].

2.2.11.2 In Silico Models for Toxicity Overall, the existing packages to forecast toxicity are categorized into two groups [20, 31, 201] (see Section 2.3). The first is data-driven or structure-based that relies on the generation of descriptors from the chemical structure and statistical analysis of the relationships between these descriptors and the toxicological effect. Gepp and Hutter have been using a decision trees to predict putative hERG blockers [202]. Other classification models have also been used to predict the cardiotoxicity of drug molecules [203] and one approach

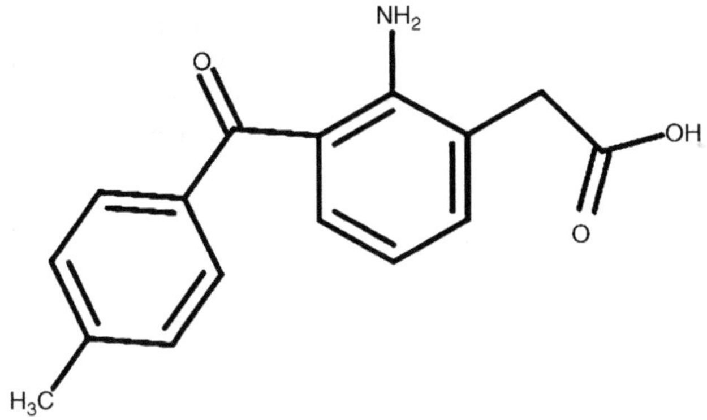

Figure 2.23 Bromfenac (NSAID) and idiosyncratic toxicity.

TABLE 2.10 Packages for the Prediction of Toxicity *In Silico*

Software Package	Website
MCASE	www.multicase.com
Discovery Studio TOPKAT	www.accelrys.com
DEREK	www.lhasalimited.org
Lazar	http://lazar.in-silico.de
Leadscope Solutions	www.leadscope.com
PreADMET	http://preadmet.bmdrc.org
Q-Lead	www.q-lead.com
Hazard-Expert	www.compudrug.com

[202] is available online at http://www.cbs.dtu.dk/services/hERG/. The second package is based on expert system approaches, which synthesize and formalize the knowledge present in the scientific literature and of human experts.

Although complex, it is possible to attempt to predict toxicity [204] using the *in silico* packages listed in Table 2.10. Development of new mathematical models and better understanding of toxicity are greatly assisted by the storage of information in databases. At present, several key publicly available toxicity databases can be consulted to gain insights about toxicity mechanisms and to assist decision making [205].

2.3 PREPARATION OF COMPOUND COLLECTIONS AND COMPUTER PROGRAMS, CHALLENGING ADME/Tox PREDICTIONS AND STATISTICAL METHODS

2.3.1 Preparation of Compound Collections and Computer Programs

The nature/composition of a compound collection has a significant impact in determining both the quantity and quality of identified hits/leads and ultimately of the overall success of a screening project [206]. The different types of screening collections and different ways to prepare them depending on the projects, targets, and goals can be used for HTS campaigns or virtual screening. Available electronic compound collections (over 40 million compounds in total in 2009) are categorized as follows (some collections fit into several categories):

- combinatorial chemistry libraries
- collections for cherry picking
- focused-libraries (either bioactive collections containing compounds with well-characterized biological function or target-specific collections)
- fragment or building block libraries
- diversity sets
- collections containing only marketed experimental drugs
- collections containing natural products.

In general, the first step toward the preparation of a screening library suitable for hit discovery projects is to assemble several public/commercial/proprietary collections. At least two different scenarios occur, either the library is used without additional intervention or it can go through series of gradual *in silico* filtering steps. For the latter, there are no perfect filters and filters can be tailored according to the project and/or stage of the project (according to target location in the human body, target types, project stage [hit discovery or compound optimization, etc.]). Some scientists believe that the screening library should be as large as possible to explore more chemical space even if it becomes less "drug-like," expecting that medicinal chemists will be able to fix the problems later. Conversely, others might argue that the first hit compounds must be as "clean" as possible to provide suitable development candidates easier to handle by chemists avoiding difficult formulation strategies [24]. There are still major debates about how to design a compound collection. Both the private sector and academic groups increasingly agree that collections should be "filtered" in order to remove undesirable molecules/groups [9, 33, 39, 56]. It is well documented that to avoid costly failures in screening projects, ADME/Tox properties should be considered at an early stage [58, 63]. As a result, currently, most libraries are at least crudely rule-of-5 compliant.

In the following paragraphs, we suggest possible avenues to design a generic compound collection and also give examples of strategies implemented in pharmaceutical companies. We provide URL links to several compound collections, databases [207], and computer packages that should facilitate the work. There are several types of computer methods helping to filter a collection including methods that are rule-based (Lipinski's rule-of-5) or knowledge-based. The process is better described as "cleaning" a collection since the human body is immensely complex and the available tools cannot yet handle this intricacy. The latter usually uses machine-learning approaches (e.g., neural networks, support vector machines) that can yield models with higher predictive accuracy as compared to rule-based strategies. This improvement is often costly since the chemical compound is retained (or rejected) in (from) the collection with little or no possibility of understanding why [25, 208]. This lack of interpretability hinders chemists' efforts to identify the causes and solutions of the problem. Thus, while statistical methods are of great value, they have to be used with care. A good compound collection filtering or profiling model or descriptor must represent a balance between accuracy and interpretability. For simplicity, we will focus on rule-based methods, while many reviews referring to machine-learning approaches are provided throughout the chapter.

2.3.2 Preparing a Compound Collection: Materials and Methods

One concept regarding ADME/Tox *in silico* filters is that the physicochemical properties of a compound are expected to determine its pharmacokinetic and metabolic behavior in the body. In general, molecules with inadequate initial properties (ADME/Tox profile) usually increase the development costs and tend to put significant burden to patients even if they do not fail in clinical trials. Further, a compound collection may be prepared for a chemical biology project or for drug discovery, and in these cases, one may need molecules with a more "lead-like" or "drug-like" profile [45, 61, 209]. Experimental ADME/Tox measurements are still very difficult since there are many different levels of complexity such as crossing physiological barriers, group reactivity, and metabolism. Different experimental assays have been developed over the years to attempt to assess/predict ADME/Tox properties, but *in silico* ADME/Tox computations can also be carried out. These calculations provide valuable information that can then be further investigated experimentally [25]. Well-known methods for evaluating the drug-like or lead-like properties of a compound were implemented in several library design programs and are routinely used in the pharmaceutical industry. Such rules are the so-called rule-of-5 [210], a set of four property values that were derived from classifying the key physicochemical properties of drug compounds. These properties are defined by the values of the log P (ratio of concentrations, at equilibrium, of a compound in the two phases of mixture of two immiscible solvents, commonly octanol and water), the molecular weight, the number of hydrogen bond donors (expressed as the sum of OHs and NHs), and the number of hydrogen bond acceptors (expressed as the sum of N and O). Furthermore, screening processes are often clouded if selected molecules contain reactive functional groups [211] that interfere and aggregate in biochemical assays [212, 213] or are frequent hitters (defined as compounds that are biologically active across a range of targets and often causing serious problems in drug discovery projects) [214]. Over the years, many additional rules have thus been proposed [112, 215] and can be smartly combined with "rule-of-5." The polar surface area, roughly defined as the surface sum over all polar atoms (O and N) and the number of flexible bonds, can be proposed as extended rules (Section 2.2). Likewise, the selection of compounds based on substructure features or similarity measures could be managed by encoding molecules in a bit-string technology or "fingerprints" [104]. Their structural similarity can be evaluated using Tanimoto coefficient. Other physicochemical properties, BBB, HSA binding, or toxicity predictions can be carried out (Section 2.2).

In order to design a compound collection, one needs to search and select appropriate databases and computer programs. Several outstanding commercial packages have been developed and can be used to perform this filtering. Free computer tools are also available, either as standalone software or online. Compound collections distributed by chemical vendors are typically in 2D. If 3D structures are required to compute descriptors, commercial or open source packages are available. Below are some major tools in the field and a practical approach to design a compound collection.

2.3.2.1 Databases Chemical compounds are stored in databases in different electronic formats. For chemists, the easiest representation of a molecule is a 2D diagram. Since 2D representation is not fully adapted to computational operations, several formats have been developed over the years. A commonly used format is the atom–bond connection table [31] that mimics the chemical structure as a graph containing a set of vertices (atoms) linked by edges (bonds). Examples include SDF (structure-data-file) and MOL (created by MDL and now owned by Symyx) file formats [216] (Figure 2.24). Other types of formats are often referred to as line format since one molecule can be described by one line of strings. Examples include SMILES (simplified molecular input line entry specification) [217], SMARTS (Smiles ARbitrary Target Specification) [218] (Daylight Chemical Information Systems), and the InChI (IUPAC International Chemical Identifier, provided by the IUPAC) formats [219].

SMILES ASCII strings define a typographical standard representation of molecular structure of compound using common letters and numbers. Depending on the canonicalization algorithm used to obtain the string sequence for one molecule, Canonical SMILES can be cited when this string sequence describe and ensure the uniqueness of the compound. Finally, Isomeric SMILES term is employed when structure, connectivity, and chirality properties are specified in the sequence. SMARTS are also one-line notation but specify substructural features and atom typing in molecule. IUPAC InChI describes the standard for formula representation of a molecule but is more difficult to read.

2.3.2.2 Free and Open-Access Online Chemistry Databases Tables 2.11 and 2.12 list free compound libraries. DrugBank, PubCHem, and ZINC are briefly discussed with more detailed information found at www.vls3d.com.

DrugBank DrugBank (http://www.drugbank.ca) [232] is hosted at the University of Alberta, Canada, and supported by Genome Alberta & Genome Canada, a private, nonprofit Corporation. In 2009, the database contained nearly 4800 drug entries including around 1350 FDA approved drugs, and more than 3200 experimental drugs.

PubChem Currently, PubChem (http://pubchem.ncbi.nlm.nih.gov) [247] is the largest freely available public molecular information database. PubChem consists of three databases (PubChem Compound, PubChem Substance, and PubChem BioAssay) and contains more than 18 million unique chemical structures and more than

a. **b.**

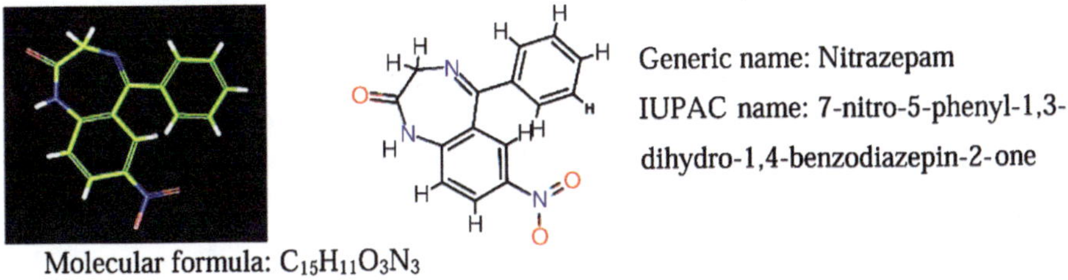

c.

```
1595


 32 34  0      0  0  0  0  0  0999 V2000
    2.8367    3.1429    0.0000 O   0  0  0  0  0  0  0  0  0  0  0  0
    2.2628   -3.1429    0.0000 O   0  5  0  0  0  0  0  0  0  0  0  0
    3.9895   -3.0068    0.0000 O   0  0  0  0  0  0  0  0  0  0  0  0
    2.6471    1.4601    0.0000 N   0  0  0  0  0  0  0  0  0  0  0  0
./.
1 15  2  0  0  0  0
  2  6  1  0  0  0  0
  3  6  2  0  0  0  0
  4  8  1  0  0  0  0
  4 15  1  0  0  0  0
./.
M  CHG  2   2  -1   6   1
M  END
> <DRUGBANK_ID>
DB01595

> <DRUGBANK_GENERIC_NAME>
Nitrazepam

$$$$
```

header block; count lines; atom block; bond block; properties block; data items; delimiter — connection table; non-structural datas — compund

d.

InChI: 1/C15H11N3O3/c19-14-9-16-15(10-4-2-1-3-5-10)12-8-11(18(20)21)6-7-13(12)17-14/h1-8H,9H2,(H,17,19)/f/h17H

Isomeric SMILES : [O-][N+](=O)C1=CC2=C(NC(=O)CN=C2C2=CC=CC=C2)C=C1

Canonical SMILES : [O-][N+](=O)C1=CC2=C(NC(=O)CN=C2C2=CC=CC=C2)C=C1

Figure 2.24 Nitrazepam represented in different formats: (a) 2D stick representation, (b) chemical structure diagram, denomination, and molecular formula, (c) SDF file format, (d) different line formats. See insert for color representation of this figure.

38 million substances. It provides biological property information for each compound and is hosted by the National Center for Biotechnological Information (NCBI). The PubChem Compound database is a repository of individual compounds. The PubChem substance database contains descriptions of chemical samples. This database is linked to the PubMed citation engines and with PubChem BioAssay information. PubChem BioAssay is a collection of bioassay data from several HTS campaigns.

TABLE 2.11 Free Chemistry Databases

Database	URL	Reference
ACToR	http://actor.epa.gov/actor/faces/ACToRHome.jsp	[220]
AKos	http://www.akosgmbh.de/AKosSamples/index.html	[221]
Allergen Atlas	http://tiger.dbs.nus.edu.sg/ATLAS/	[222]
Animal Toxin Database	http://protchem.hunnu.edu.cn/toxin/index.jsp	[223]
Brenda	http://www.brenda-enzymes.info/	[224]
Biometa	http://biometa.cmbi.ru.nl/	[225]
ChEBI	http://www.ebi.ac.uk/chebi/	[226]
ChemBank	http://chembank.broad.harvard.edu/	[227]
ChemSpider	http://www.chemspider.com	[228]
Clan Tox	http://www.clantox.cs.huji.ac.il/	[229]
Ditop	http://bioinf.xmu.edu.cn/databases/ADR/index.html	[230]
DSSTox	http://www.epa.gov/ncct/dsstox/index.html	[231]
DrugBank	http://www.drugbank.ca/	[232]
DUD	http://dud.docking.org/	[233]
eMolecules	http://www.emolecules.com/	[234]
EMBL Databases	http://www.ebi.ac.uk/FTP/	[235]
HaptenDB	http://www.imtech.res.in/raghava/haptendb/	[236]
Human Metabolome Database	http://www.hmdb.ca/	[237]
KEGG Drug	http://www.genome.jp/kegg/drug/	[238]
KEGG Ligand	http://www.genome.jp/kegg/ligand.html	[238]
Ligand Expo	http://ligand-expo.rcsb.org/	[239]
LigandInfo	http://www.ligand.info/	[240]
MDPI	http://www.mdpi.org/molmall/	[241]
Metabolic Site Predictor	http://www-ucc.ch.cam.ac.uk/msp/htdocs/	[242]
MMsINC	http://mms.dsfarm.unipd.it/MMsINC.html	[243]
MDSI	http://www.msdiscovery.com/downloads.html	[244]
US NCI Database	http://cactus.nci.nih.gov/ncidb2/download.html	[245]
US National Toxicology Program	http://ntp.niehs.nih.gov/	[246]
PubChem	http://pubchem.ncbi.nlm.nih.gov/	[247]
Querychem	http://llama.med.harvard.edu/~jklekota/QueryChem.html	[248]
Relibase	http://www.ccdc.cam.ac.uk/free_services/free_downloads/	[249]
Screening Browser	http://cimlcsext.cim.sld.cu:8080/screeningbrowser	[250]
SuperNatural Database	http://bioinformatics.charite.de/supernatural	[251]
SuperDrug	http://bioinf.charite.de/superdrug/	[252]
SuperHapten	http://bioinformatics.charite.de/superhapten/	[253]
SuperLigands	http://bioinformatics.charite.de/superligands/	[254]
SuperToxic	http://bioinformatics.charite.de/supertoxic	[255]
TimTec	http://www.timtec.net/	[256]

TABLE 2.11 (*Continued*)

Database	URL	Reference
TOXNET	http://toxnet.nlm.nih.gov	[257]
Toxicity Datasets	http://cheminformatics.org/datasets/index.shtml#tox	[258]
UCI ChemDB	http://cdb.ics.uci.edu/	[259]
VITIC	http://www.lhasalimited.org/index.php?cat=2&sub_cat=72	[260]
ZINC	http://zinc.docking.org/	[261]

PubChem continues to grow in stature, content, and capability and will take a prominent role in the field of chemical biology and drug discovery.

ZINC ZINC (http://zinc.docking.org/) [261] is a free database of commercially available compounds ready for virtual screening computations. The library contains over 8 million molecules in 3D, most often annotated with molecular properties. ZINC allows a user to create a subset based on physicochemical properties and is

TABLE 2.12 Commercial Databases and Compound Libraries

Database	URL
4SC	http://www.4sc.de
ACB blocks	http://www.acbblocks.com
Akos	http://www.akosgmbh.com
Ambinter	http://www.ambinter.com/
AnalytiCon discovery	http://www.ac-discovery.com
Arkive	http://ark.chem.ufl.edu/pages/arkive.htm
Array BioPharma	http://www.arraybiopharma.com
Asinex	http://www.asinex.com
Aurora	http://www.aurora-feinchemie.com
BioFocus	http://www.biofocus.com/
CEREP	http://www.cerep.fr/Cerep/Users/index.asp
ChemBridge	http://www.chembridge.com/
Chemical Diversity	http://www.chemdiv.com/
Chemical Block	http://www.chemical-block.com
Combi-Blocks	http://www.combi-blocks.com/
Comprehensive Medicinal Chemistry	http://www.symyx.com/products/databases/bioactivity/cmc/index.jsp
ChemStar	http://www.chemstar.ru
ComGenex	http://www.rdchemicals.com/targeted-compound-libraries/comgenex.html
EMC	http://www.microcollections.de/
Enamine	http://www.enamine.relc.com
IFLab	http://www.iflab.kiev.ua
InterBioScreen	http://www.ibscreen.com
iResearch Library	http://www.chemnavigator.com/cnc/products/IRL.asp

(*Continued*)

TABLE 2.12 Commercial Databases and Compound Libraries (*Continued*)

Database	URL
Key organics Ltd	http://www.keyorganics.ltd.uk
Leadscope	http://www.leadscope.com/
Maybridge	http://www.maybridge.com
MDDR	http://www.symyx.com/products/databases/bioactivity/mddr/index.jsp
MDPI	http://www.mdpi.org/molmall/
MDL ACD	http://www.symyx.com/
MSDiscovery	http://www.msdiscovery.com
Nanosyn	http://www.nanosyn.com
Pharmacopeia	http://www.pharmacopeia.com/
Pharmeks	http://www.pharmeks.com
Polyphor	http://www.polyphor.com/
Prestwick	http://www.prestwickchemical.com
StARLITe	http://www.admensa.com/StARLITe/Index.htm
Sigma-Aldrich	http://www.sigma-aldrich.com
Specs	http://www.specs.net
SPRESI	http://infochem.de/en/products/databases/spresi.shtml
TimTec	http://www.timtec.net
TOSLab	http://www.toslab.com
Tranzyme	http://www.tranzyme.com/
Tripos	http://leadquest.tripos.com
VitasMLab	http://www.vitasmlab.com/
WOMBAT	http://www.sunsetmolecular.com/index.php
Worldmolecules	http://www.worldmolecules.com/

target-dependent. ZINC is provided by the Shoichet Lab, in the Department of Pharmaceutical Chemistry at the University of California, San Francisco (UCSF).

2.3.2.3 Free Tools to Filter Compound Libraries

Standalone Versions

(a) *FAF-Drugs2*
http://www.mti.univ-paris-diderot.fr/fr/downloads.html
FAF-Drugs2 [262] is a free adaptable tool for the ADME/Tox filtering of electronic compound collections. FAF-Drugs2 is a command-line utility program (e.g., written in Python) based on the open source chemistry toolkit OpenBabel. FAF-Drugs2 performs various physicochemical calculations, identifies key functional groups such as some toxic and unstable molecules/functional groups, and can provide, via Gnuplot, several distribution diagrams of major physicochemical properties of the screened libraries. Within FAF-Drugs2, numerous physicochemical and substructure searching filtering rules can be easily tuned, depending on the projects and aims.

(b) *CLEVER*
http://datam.i2r.a-star.edu.sg/clever/
CLEVER [263] (Chemical Library Editing, Visualizing and Enumerating Resource) is a free platform- independent, standalone Java application. It supports chemical library creation and manipulation, combinatorial chemical library enumeration using user-specified chemical components, and chemical format conversion and visualization. CLEVER analyses and filters compound libraries with respect to drug-likeness, lead-likeness, and fragment-likeness based on computed physicochemical properties.

(c) *Screening-Assistant*
http://www.univ-orleans.fr/icoa/screeningassistant/
Screening-assistant [118] is designed to manage chemical databases and select a set of compounds for screening tests. Drug-like properties are computed and molecules that are predicted to be nondrug-like are highlighted.

(d) *ToxTree*
http://ecb.jrc.ec.europa.eu/qsar/qsar-tools/index.php?c=TOXTREE
ToxTree [264] is a free application developed by Ideaconsult Ltd. The program can categorize and predict various kinds of toxic effects by applying decision tree approaches, such as the Cramer [265] classification scheme for skin and eye irritation, and the Benigni–Bossa rule based models [29] for mutagenicity and carcinogenicity.

(e) *sMol Explorer*
http://www.biotec.or.th/ISL/SMOL/
sMOL Explorer [266] is a web-based open source integrated suite that provides necessary tools for chemists to design and mine a compound library either by drawing molecules or uploading (query) data files. The user's database created by the software can be analyzed, structural similarity search can be performed, and results can be compared to existing external public databases, such as PubChem and DrugBank. Users can mine the database with programming language R (designed for statistical computing) and Weka software (Java written toolkit of machine learning algorithms designed for data mining). The packages are included inside sMol Explorer with the aim of finding frequent substructures, cluster compounds using molecular fingerprints, and defining a classification model compatible with a desired biological activity.

(f) *XLOGP3*
http://www.sioc-ccbg.ac.cn/software/xlogp3/
This toolkit provides functionalities to screen a compound library including log P computation [267]. XLOGP3 can remove compounds that do not satisfy "drug-likeness" properties such as Lipinski's RO5, number of rotatable bonds, and number of rings.

Online Tools>

(a) *VCCLAB Servers*
http://vcclab.org/lab/alogps/

VCCLAB [86] provides several on-line tools, which are able to compute log P, log S, pK_a, and more than 1600 molecular descriptors from the DRAGON software. These tools can be useful for computational chemistry, ADME/Tox predictions via the calculation of molecular properties, and the analysis of relationships between chemical structure and properties.

(b) *ChemMine*
http://bioweb.ucr.edu/ChemMineV2/
ChemMine [268] is a compound mining database that facilitates drug and agrochemical discovery and chemical genomics screens.

(c) *ChemXSeer*
http://chemxseer.ist.psu.edu/
ChemXSeer [269] is an integrated digital library and database allowing for intelligent search of documents in the field of chemistry and data obtained from chemical kinetics.

(d) *Chemaxon*
http://www.chemaxon.com/
Through the company website, Chemaxon provides several online toolkits pertaining to the field of chemoinformatics and allowing compound profiling.

(e) *eMolecules*
http://www.emolecules.com/
eMolecules is a free online database and perhaps the most comprehensive openly accessible search engine for chemical structures. eMolecules offer over 7 million unique chemical structures supplied by over 150 suppliers.

(f) *Lazar Toxicity Predictions*
http://lazar.in-silico.de/
The Lazar [270] system allows to predict some aspects of toxicity. It is possible to draw a query compound and perform a similarity search across compounds with experimentally determined toxicity data.

(g) *Molinspiration*
http://www.molinspiration.com/
Molinspiration is an online molecular processing and property calculation toolkit that allows users to analyze chemical compounds.

(h) *MolSoft*
http://www.molsoft.com/mprop/
MolSoft is an online drug-likeness and molecular property prediction toolkit.

(i) *OSIRIS*
http://www.organic-chemistry.org/prog/peo/index.html
OSIRIS [271] allows users to draw a molecule and compute instantly various drug-relevant properties, high risks for undesired effects such as mutagenicity, or a poor intestinal absorption.

(j) *PK/DB*
http://miro.ifsc.usp.br/pkdb/

PK/DB [272] is a free database for pharmacokinetic properties designed to create online databases for pharmacokinetic studies and *in silico* ADME/Tox prediction.

(k) *RoadRunner*
http://nmmlsc.health.unm.edu/rrnmmlsc/
Roadrunner is a free online access of properties and bioactivities to over 220,000 unique compounds, which allows user compound searches by similarity or to obtain experimental assays related to the compound of interest.

(l) *RPBS*
http://bioserv.rpbs.jussieu.fr
RPBS [273] (Ressource Parisienne en Bioinformatique Structurale) is a web server that provides several tools for database preparation, test sets for virtual ligand screening and basic ADME/Tox filtering via FAFDrugs1 online version, salts removal, file format conversion, or compound collections in 3D. Online ligand-based methods are available and searches against libraries of toxic molecules and drug-like compounds using wwLigCSRre can be performed [274].

(m) *SuperDrug*
http://bioinformatics.charite.de/superdrug/
SuperDrug [252] allows user to access 2396 compounds with 108,198 conformers and manage 2D similarity searching.

(n) *XLOGP3*
http://www.sioc-ccbg.ac.cn/software/xlogp3/
XLOGP3 [267] software can also be accessible online and can predict basic drug-likeness chemical rules.

(o) *ISIDA*
http://infochim.u-strasbg.fr/recherche/isida/index.php
ISIDA *In Silico* Design and Data Analysis is a project devoted to the development of new methods and original software tools for structure–property modeling and computer-aided design of new compounds, from ligand screening to ADME/Tox predictions [275].

Commercial Packages Table 2.13 presents a list of commercial software packages to predict ADMET properties.

2.3.3 Cleaning and Designing the Compound Collection

It is beneficial to process and filter a compound library in order to retain as much as possible "lead-like" or "drug-like" compounds and reject undesirable molecules. Several commercial packages have been developed to perform collection filtering (e.g., ChemAxon [287], OpenEye [279], or the Chemical Computing Group [286]). These filter-based approaches should not be used as "black-boxes." In general, users have to "clean-up" the collection by first removing salts/counterions and duplicates from the library. The compound library must be in a computer-acceptable standard

TABLE 2.13 Commercial Software Packages to Predict ADMET Properties

Software	Description	Predictions	References
DEREK	Knowledge-based systems	C^c,M^m,G^g,S^s, T^{tt},H^h,N^n	[276]
METEOR		Mt^{mt}	
www.lhasalimited.org			
META/MCASE/CASETOX	Knowledge-based systems	Mt/C/A^a/C/M	[277]
www.multicase.com			
ADMENSA Interactive	Proprietary ToolBox	A	[278]
www.admensa.com			
OpenEye Filter	Proprietary ToolBox	A	[279]
www.eyesopen.com			
Schrödinger QikProp	Proprietary ToolBox	A	[280]
https://www.schrodinger.com			
Discovery Studio 2.0	Proprietary ToolBox		[281]
www.accelrys.com			
ADMET Descriptors	Knowledge-based system	A/H	
TOPKAT	QSAR-based system	C/M/S/A	
VolSurf+	Molecular descriptors	D^d/A	[282]
MokA	Statistical model for pK_a predictions		[283]
http://www.moldiscovery.com/index.php			
OncoLogic	Knowledge-based system	C	[284]
Quantum Pharmaceutical Suite	Knowledge-based system	A/D	[285]
http://q-pharm.com			
MOE	Proprietary Toolbox	A/D	[286]
http://www.chemcomp.com	Molecular Descriptors		
OncoLogic	Knowledge-based system	C	[284]

[a]ADME/Tox optimization, [d]DMPK, [c]Carcinogenicity, [m]Mutagenicity, [g]Genotoxicity, [s]Skin Sensitisation, [tt]Teratogenicity, [h]Hepatotoxicity, [n]Neurotoxicity, [mf]Metabolism fate.

format (e.g., user must check for wrong entries, bad connection tables, incorrect chiral centers, etc.). Cleaning and filtering the database can also be performed at a later stage, for example, after a first *in silico* screening step. Overall, users must note that compound physicochemical properties have to be considered before preparing a collection and take into account

- the biological nature/type of the target,
- the anatomic region and the disease/pathology to treat, and
- the administration route.

One can apply both simple rules such as the Lipinski's "rule-of-5" [210], as well as additional filters that assess the presence of functional groups known to be toxic or that are reactive or unstable. Many such rules have been proposed [211, 212, 214] in the past few years. Problematic structure or groups can be specified by using SMARTS [218] pattern matching. Such an approach has been exploited at Bayer [120] by tagging molecules that contain specific fragments. Possible values for some descriptors to generate a drug-like collection could be as follows:

- no more than one violation of RO5 ($200 \leq MW \geq 500$, $\log P \leq 5$, $HBD \leq 5$, $HBA \leq 10$).
- tPSA no more than 160
- no more than 10 rotatable bonds
- no more than 50 rigid bonds
- no more than four ring system
- no more than 35 heavy atoms
- no more 20 atoms in a system ring
- no more than 35 carbon atoms
- no more than 20 heteroatoms
- formal charge within 0–3
- sum of formal charges within −2 to 2
- eliminate compounds having undesirable atom types and unacceptable functional groups (Figure 2.25).

2.3.4 Searching for Similarity

Medicinal chemists usually assume that similar compounds are likely to have similar properties. Subsequently, it is interesting to compare compounds present in a collection and marketed, active, experimental molecules as well as to withdrawn drugs or even natural products. For this purpose, numerous approaches could be employed [104] depending on the choice of molecular descriptors, weighting procedure(s), and similarity coefficient (e.g., Tanimoto) [104]. In addition, several recognition methods of specific frameworks designed for similarity (dissimilarity) measures are also available [17, 111, 120, 288–290].

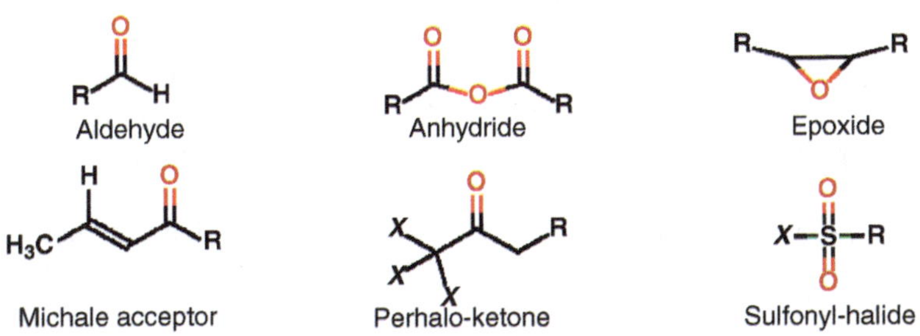

Figure 2.25 Examples of functional groups known to be reactive or toxic [215].

2.3.5 Generating 3D Structures

In silico screening methods based on ligand 3D structures (ligand-based screening computations or structure-based screening methods) have become essential tools to facilitate the drug discovery process. The structure of each ligand has to be generated since compounds are usually distributed in 2D file format. Some descriptors involved in several ADME/Tox prediction models also require the 3D structures of the molecules. The user has the choice between free toolkits or commercial packages. For the latter, Molecular Networks CORINA, Tripos CONCORD®, or OpenEye OMEGA are cited. Several free standalone or online tools are also available. Balloon [291] (http://users.abo.fi/mivainio/balloon/), smi2sdf (http://www.chembiogrid.org/cheminfo/smi23d/#ack), The Dundee PRODRG2 Server [292] (http://davapc1.bioch.dundee.ac.uk/prodrg/), FROG [293] (http://bioserv.rpbs.jussieu.fr/cgi-bin/Frog), and DG-AMMOS (http://www.vls3d.com/DGAMMOS/DG-AMMOS.tar.gz) are cited.

2.4 ADME/Tox PREDICTIONS WITHIN PHARMACEUTICS COMPANIES

Below is the list of different types of *in silico* filtering tools pharmaceutical companies have used to process their compound collections.

2.4.1 Actelion Pharmaceuticals Ltd.

Actelion uses chemoinformatics strategies as opposed to conventional approaches (use of expensive commercial packages) since they implemented their own internal system. Actelion developed the OSIRIS procedure [271] and implemented a toxicity alert system.

2.4.2 Bayer

At Bayer HealthCare Pharma, chemoinformatics tools and *in silico* ADME/Tox predictions are usually used in the early hit discovery phase and during the hit-to-lead optimization steps [123, 294]. These techniques are employed just after the screening hits have been validated and prior to *in vitro* and *in vivo* characterization. Bayer has developed an in-house system to flag compounds, named TLs for "traffic lights" and where different values are summed to derive an *in silico* oral PhysChem score ranging from 0 to 10. The lower the values, the more the compounds are suitable for oral administration. The traffic lights involve TL Microsomal Clearance Alert, TL CYP Inh Alert, TL hERG Inh Alert, TL Undesirable Groups, the PhysChem score derived from the values of TL Solubility score ($\geq$50, 10–50, $\leq$10), TL C log P ($\leq$3, 3–5, $\geq$5), TL MWcorr ($\leq$400, 400–500, $\geq$500), TL PSA ($\leq$120, 120–140, $\geq$140), TL RotBonds ($\leq$7, 8–10, $\geq$11), and the TL Caco-2 score built from a decision tree that involves H-bond acidity and basicity, PSA, MW, and charges. Bayer has recently developed CypScore [295], an *in silico* tool able to predict the likely sites of cytochrome P450-mediated metabolism of drug-like organic molecules.

2.4.3 Bristol-Myers Squibb

Data collected during the HTS process are stored and analyzed. The company applies empirical methods to help validate the filter tool. According to Pearce et al. [296], Bristol-Myers Squibb applies Lipinski-type property filters as part of an HTS triage carried out at a later stage rather than at the beginning of the screening process. During the filtering step, a compound is flagged if it has two or more violations over these following values, MW > 639, the number of hydrogen bond donors >5, the number of hydrogen bond acceptors > 9, the number of rotatable bonds >14, and the C log *P* is between 3.0 and 5.5. Earlier in the HTS process, an in-house SMARTS-based chemical functional groups filtering process intended for compound removal is applied. The Promiscuity Ratio Index (PRI), an observed/expected functional group filter hit rate, and the Promiscuity Strength Index (PSI), the strength of that hit rate across multiple assays, are measured. These were combined with a statistical analysis of in-house assay data to provide confidence intervals that link the filters to a promiscuity category (high, medium, and low).

2.4.4 Hoffmann-La Roche Ltd.

At Roche, computer-assisted methods are directly integrated in the medicinal chemistry department and their use is defined by the screening strategy [31, 297]. A proprietary filtering procedure based on lead generation divided into four phases—hit evaluation, hit validation, lead generation, and lead expansion—is used [298]. ADME/Tox is performed early during hit evaluation and validation involving the selection of compounds with suitable physicochemical properties according to the common "desirable" substructures and/or undesired structural features employing commercial tools. The company also developed proprietary *in silico* tools—CAFCA and RADDAR [298, 299]. The former was for the calculation of molecule's amphiphilic properties and the latter for the design of virtual libraries. Using the commercial software Leadscope, a computer-based method [214] for rapid and automatic identification of potential "frequent hitters" (compounds with nonspecific activity, promiscuous) or that are disturbing the assays was developed.

2.4.5 Neurogen Corporation

At Neurogen, an internal analysis [122] on oral drugs launched from 1984 to 2002 suggested that physicochemical ranges could be scaled according to Lipinski RO5 and demonstrated that some physicochemical properties were increasing during the optimization phase. To improve the success, an in-house virtual library, named PriVLib (Privileged Virtual Library), was developed. PriVLib has several desirable properties including low molecular weight, low lipophilicity, relatively high solubility, and high likelihood of synthetic success and immediate availability of synthesis. To share and to standardize internal information in the aim to help in the design of drugs, a proprietary chemoinformatic language, NDL (Neurogen Data Language), which is coupled to a web-based data display system, was developed.

2.4.6 Novartis

Novartis applies computer-aided methods to support the lead discovery process [300]. The *in silico* group is integrated into the global lead-finding department and is used to work in parallel with the HTS process with the aim of improving the quality of the output. In some cases, *in silico* processes can successfully replace HTS experiments. Novartis procedures focus on designing screening libraries with greater ring diversity, low molecular weight (<700), low hydrophobicity ($\log P < 7.5$), and good permeability (PSA < 200 Å). The Lipinski RO5 seems to be further applied during lead optimization. Natural products are not excluded since such compounds can act as excellent molecular probes or inspire chemical synthesis.

2.4.7 Schering AG

At Schering AG, a dedicated hit-to-lead team exists and uses chemoinformatics to assist the lead generation step [301]. Besides improving the lead process by evaluating and implementing software tools for property predictions, the team provides the following guidelines to design drug-like libraries: suitable molecular properties such as MW between 200 and 500, log *P*/log *D* between −1 and 5, H-bond donors between 0 and 5, H-bond acceptors <10, favorable pharmacodynamics and kinetics (*in vivo*, *in vitro*, and *in silico*) properties like permeability in Caco2 cells $>100\,\mathrm{cm\,s^{-1}} \times 10^{-7}$, rat plasma clearance $<50\,\mathrm{mL\,min^{-1}\,kg^{-1}}$, rat oral bioavailability >25%, toxicity assessed by the commercial DEREK package, good chemical optimization potential, and patentability.

2.4.8 Vertex Pharmaceuticals

Chemoinformatics approaches are used at Vertex and the company has published several methods. Drugs are distinguished from nondrugs by using machine learning methods [111] such as decision trees that help the hit-to-lead decision process. The REOS (rapid elimination of swill) program to filter out molecules that might be problematic was developed [24, 108, 110]. REOS combines a set of SMARTS-based chemical functional group filters and a set of RO5-like physicochemical property filter. The default values for the property filter are MW 200–500, log *P* (from −5 to 5), HBD 0 to 5, HBA 0 to 10, formal charge between − 2 and 2, rotatable bonds 0–8, and 15–20 heavy atoms.

2.5 CHALLENGING ADME/Tox PREDICTIONS

Several drugs have been withdrawn from the market in past few years such as Astemizole or Glafenine for hERG blocking, or Mibefradil responsible of hepatoxicity via the CYP450 enzymatic system [18, 302]. Below is an illustration for the utility of ADME/tox prediction for the investigations of a compound and some assistance to decision-making.

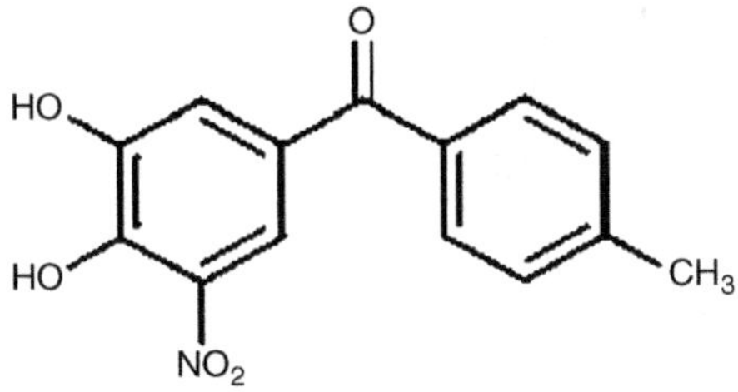

Figure 2.26 Tolcapone. Molecular weight = 273.24; X Log $P3$ = 3.3; tPSA = 97.51; H-bond donors = 2; H-bond acceptors = 5; rotatable bond = 3; rigid bond = 14.

2.5.1 Tolcapone

Tolcapone (tasmar, Figure 2.26) is an inhibitor of catechol-*O*-methyltransferase (COMT) and can be used as anti-Parkinsonian agent. This molecule has the ability to cross the blood–brain barrier and exerts its COMT inhibitory effects in the CNS as well as in the periphery. During the clinical trials, the molecule showed acute hepatotoxicity with three fatalities. Due to significant hepatotoxicity, the drug's therapeutic utility is limited to a drug of last resort. Tolcapone possesses one nitro group, which has been reported to be hepatotoxic and hepatocarcinogen [303]. Nitroaromatics can be reduced to form reactive, nitroanion radical, nitroso intermediate, and *N*-hydroxy derivatives [304]. These reactive metabolites are usually not desired in drug discovery projects and molecules containing nitroaromatic groups are in general removed from a compound collection [198].

2.5.2 Factor V Inhibitors

Inhibitors of blood coagulation can be serine protease inhibitors, molecules blocking the catalytic site of coagulation enzymes such as factor Xa or thrombin. A prospective study was undertaken by Segers et al. [305] in order to find potential inhibitors of the coagulation factor Va–membrane interaction. The prothrombinase complex, the macromolecular system that generates thrombin, is essential to the process. This mechanism requires transient interactions with the cell membrane. To discover small molecules that could impede factor Va–membrane interaction, a structure-based virtual ligand screening study was performed. More than 300,000 molecules were docked into factor Va C2 domain and seven hits were identified. The molecules were shown to bind directly to the right factor Va domain using surface plasmon resonance (SPR). *In vitro* experiments indicated that those compounds do not inhibit FVa procoagulant activity in a plasma-based assay system. Further experiments confirmed by SPR analysis showed that as albumin concentration increased, the inhibitory activity of the compound gradually decreased. Retrospectively, by using the commercial software q-Mol, marketed by Quantum Pharmaceuticals and capable to predict human serum albumin binding for the most potent compound was confirmed (Figure 2.27).

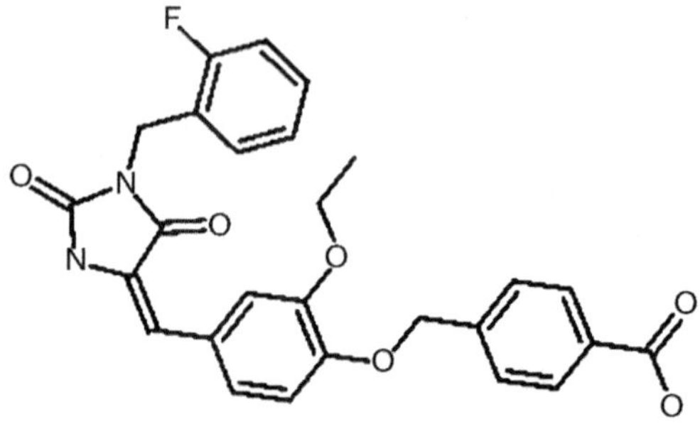

Figure 2.27 Coagulation factor V–membrane interaction inhibitor. MW = 490.48; *X* Log *P*3 = 4.19; tPSA = 105.17; H-bond donors = 2; H-bond acceptors = 6; rotatable bond = 9; rigid bond = 27.

2.5.3 CRF-1 Receptor Antagonists

In 2003, at Neurogen Corporation, Hodgetts et al. described the development, synthesis, and structure–activity study for discovering a novel series of 2-arylpyrimidin-4-ones as CRF-1 receptor antagonists [306] (Figure 2.28). The group showed that chemical optimization of the compounds could lead to potent CRF-1 antagonists and commented about the interest of using early ADME/Tox predictions. ADME/Tox properties such as log *P* and polar surface area were calculated to design CNS agents with appropriate physical properties. Compounds were optimized with physical chemistry values within the range that lead to a reasonable membrane permeability and brain penetration.

2.6 STATISTICAL METHODS

2.6.1 Principal Component Analysis

2.6.1.1 Aim The goal of PCA [90] is to project the data into a subspace made of linear combinations of the original descriptors so that this subspace is the best-

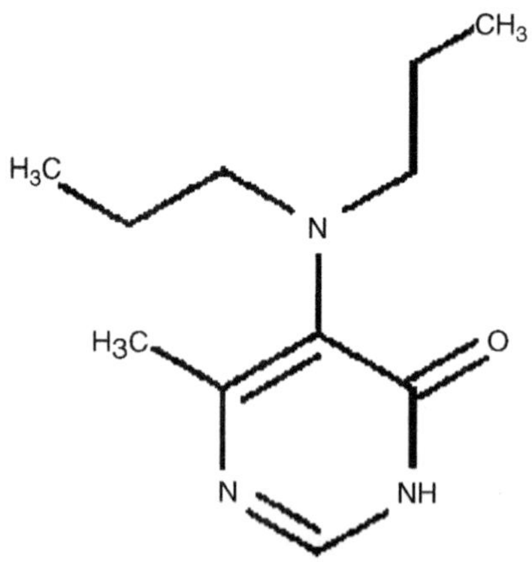

Figure 2.28 CRF-1 receptor antagonist. MW = 376.54; *X* Log *P*3 = 4.32; tPSA = 48.05; H-bond donors = 1; H-bond acceptors = 2; rotatable bond = 8; rigid bond = 13.

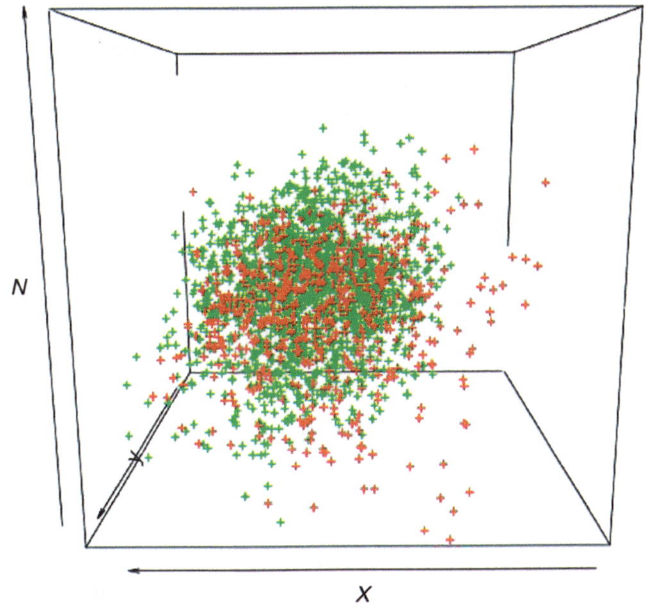

Figure 2.29 Illustration of chemical space coverage between learning compounds (in green) and test compounds (in red). See insert for color representation of this figure.

simplified image, in a small dimension, of the original data in terms of variation (i.e., a projection that best represents the data). Data may then be explored in a small space spanning the most informative view (according to data variance) of the original features. Visually, according to the final chosen dimensions, successive 2D or 3D graphics can be obtained. In this space, the new axes (called components) are orthogonal to each other. This space can be used to globally study for possible outliers, clusters of individuals, and coverage between descriptor spaces of several groups of observations (Figure 2.29). One goal would be to use fewer principal components for subsequent data analysis than in the original high-dimensional space.

In a second step and if required (in clustering studies, for example), the axes of the new space (called components) can be interpreted in terms of the original data according to the correlations between these axes and the original descriptors.

Examples of ADME/Tox Applications PCA can be used in several ways in ADME/Tox studies; PCA can be used to study redundancy between descriptors because there is a connection between PCA components and original descriptors [307]. As components are orthogonal, if two components are correlated to different descriptors, those descriptors are unlikely to provide the same information. If two descriptors are highly correlated to the same component, their correlation has to be studied. Orthogonality of components as well as dimension decrease allows PCA to become a good preliminary step to classification or regression methods requiring uncorrelated features as input variables (logistic regression for example). In the study of Benigni and Bossa, PCA [308] was applied to obtain 160 principal components (explaining

94% of the total variance), which were used in stepwise linear discriminant analysis aiming at predicting chemical carcinogenicity of different compounds. As PCA can provide a low-dimensional image of quite complex data, the first components can be used to study the global space of studied data, which can be linked to the applicability domain. Kortagere et al. [309] predicted BBB using support vector machine models. As several datasets were available (learning and test sets), applying PCA on one sample and projecting the second one in the same space allowed to study the coverage between the chemical space of the training set and the space spanned by the test compounds. As the first two components accounted for 79% of variability, a 2D representation provided a good qualitative way to graphically compare those spaces. If the test observations were outside the chemical space of the learning material, any prediction is quite unreliable.

Usage Warning The most important point to consider before any use of PCA results is the amount of variability provided by the successive components. This is particularly important when reducing the space dimension. Using all the components provided by PCA ensures that all the information is not loss. Usually 80–90% of the components are considered as a good representativeness of the global information. In the case of complex data with numerous descriptors and depending on the objective, a smaller amount of global variability can be considered.

In order to obtain meaningful principal components, if descriptors have different variances, scaling the data is required. However, careful study of descriptors is necessary, for example to remove noise variables before giving them the same importance as important variables.

Finally, PCA remains a representation in the space of descriptors. The new components are only linear combinations of the original variables, no new information is provided.

2.6.1.2 Technical Description

Input Data This method is based on the description of n individuals by p descriptors collected in a matrix having n rows and p columns.

Output New coordinates for each individual in the new subspace are provided. The coordinates are collected into a matrix having k columns (where k is the dimension of the new subspace) and called scores. PCA also produces the coefficients, called loadings or components, applied to the original descriptors to obtain the successive new descriptors spanning the new subspace.

Description Principal components are linear combinations of the original descriptors obtained so that the first principal component is the linear combination best explaining the data total variance. The second principal component is orthogonal and describes the remaining variance. It aims at maximizing the amount of variance explained by the second linear combination.

These components are obtained by diagonalization of the matrix giving the variances of the original descriptors (in diagonal) and the covariances between them. The diagonalization of this matrix provides both eigenvectors and eigenvalues. These eigenvalues represent the empirical variances of the successive components. Once sorted in decreasing order, the highest eigenvalue represents the variance associated with the first component. The corresponding successive eigenvectors are the loadings or coefficients applied to the original variables in the successive linear combinations.

The final number of components, k, is chosen so that a reasonable amount of variation is explained on the k axes (80–90%). The decomposition of the total variance is a breaking point in the histogram of eigenvalues and can be an indication of where to stop. If graphical representation is the main objective, two or three components can be considered if enough variation is accounted.

2.6.1.3 Possible Extensions PCA can be applied in a nonlinear way to provide more complex combinations between original variables. This is performed by transforming the original descriptors (more or less explicitly) to nonlinear transformations (e.g., product of descriptors) and by applying PCA on the new obtained variables. Kernel-PCA [310] uses a kernel to implicitly project original descriptors in a higher dimension space (just as in support vector machine) before applying classical PCA.

2.6.2 Partial Least Square

2.6.2.1 Aim Partial least square regression [311] is a technique allowing the prediction of one or more response variables generally accounting for numerous descriptors. It is adapted when the dataset contains more descriptors than observations and multicollinearity between descriptors. It is one of the rare methods that allow for the prediction of more than one variable at the same time. PLS generalizes and combines features from both PCA and multiple regression. Linear combinations of descriptors are used to build new factors (identical to PCA) called latent variables. The objective is not to maximize variance but to obtain the best predictive power. PLS finds the linear combinations of predictors having the maximum covariance with the response variables. The obtained decomposition of the descriptors is used to predict the response values. Similar to PCA, the number of components can be chosen to explain enough variation of descriptors and responses while avoiding overfitting. This choice can be performed through cross-validation or use of a test dataset.

Both a prediction of the response values and graphical interpretation tools are provided. It is possible to study correlations between the original variables (descriptors and responses) and the latent ones. Figure 2.30 represents this type of correlation for descriptors ($X1, \ldots, X5$) and responses ($Y1$, $Y2$). The first latent variable (PLS1) is mainly predictive of $Y1$ values, which are highly related to $X2$ and $X3$ (more specifically $Y1$ tends to increase with $X2$ and when $X3$ decreases). The second latent variable (PLS2) mostly accounts for $Y2$ prediction, which is essentially due to $X1$ and $X5$. $Y2$ tends to increase when $X1$ and $X5$ decrease. Descriptor $X2$ provides information on $Y2$. This theoretical example shows the interpretation possibilities offered by PLS. Observations can be plotted in the new space to discover clusters and outliers.

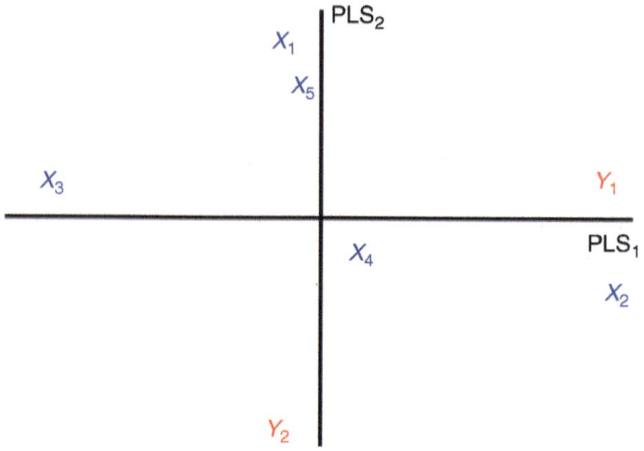

Figure 2.30 Example of simultaneous representation of correlation between the latent variables and original variables (descriptors are X_1–X_5 and responses are Y_1 and Y_2).

Examples of ADME/Tox Applications PLS is mostly used to predict the values of one continuous response variable. The interpretation of latent variables helps to understand which predictors are most involved in the prediction accuracy. In Chohan et al. [312], PLS is used among other regression methods to predict Cytochrome P450 1A2 inhibition (pIC_{50}) from in-house computed descriptors accounting for topological, geometrical, and electronic features of molecules. Feature selection (according to variance, redundancy, and predictivity) was performed before PLS application. The final model is based on two components (chosen by minimizing the cross-validation error rate). Interpretation of correlations between the latent variables and original variables (pIC_{50} and the descriptors) suggested that lipophilicity and aromaticity were the most important features to describe CYP1A2 inhibition. A more precise link can be derived showing that decreasing these two features should decrease inhibition.

In Luco [313], PLS is used to predict brain–blood distribution through computation and investigation of 25 structural descriptors. The variable importance for the projection (VIP) has been used to select the most relevant descriptors while strong outliers were removed. Three components (accounting for 85% of the variance in log BB) were retained (threefold cross-validation). A validation set was used with a careful verification of the applicability domain. The BBB and aqueous solubility in Obrezanova [314] was also modeled through PLS.

PLS is used in ADME/Tox context to perform discrimination. In Kriegl et al. [315], a classification model was trained on 2D, 3D, and quantum-mechanical descriptors to predict two (low versus high) or three (low, medium, high) classes of human cytochrome P450 3A4 inhibitors. PLS was shown to be less efficient than real discrimination methods.

Usage Warning The amount of variability provided by the successive latent variables has to be taken into consideration. The user should choose fewer components to obtain a model that could be generalized to new data for predictions. Using a few latent variables provides graphical representations of the chosen ones. Interpretation of coefficients is not possible as descriptors are generally not independent.

PLS is often used to perform classification. It is simply obtained by providing the group labels as response variable. As PLS is a regression method designed to predict continuous variables, the qualitative side of group labels will not be taken into account. This can lead to negative values. Thresholds have to be defined to obtain the predicted groups. Group labels have to be coded into a dummy matrix containing as many columns as groups and filled with zeros and ones.

Although PLS can handle more variables than observations, more predictive models are obtained when irrelevant descriptors have been removed. Before applying PLS, careful preprocessing of data is needed.

2.6.2.2 *Technical Description*

Input Data This method is based on the description of n individuals by p descriptors collected in a matrix having n rows and p columns, called X, and of the values of q response values measured on the same n individuals and collected in Y.

Output The prediction of Y is provided. New coordinates for each individual in the new subspace are given and are collected into a matrix having k columns (where k is the dimension of the new subspace) and called latent variables. PLS produces the coefficients applied to X and Y to build these latent variables.

Description PLS is a stepwise algorithm where at each step, one latent variable is provided. At the first step, one linear combination is defined for X and another for Y so that the covariance between them is maximum. This result is obtained via an iterative algorithm. The obtained new feature is called the first latent variable. It is possible to compute the proportion of variance of X and Y explained by the first latent variable. Information by the first latent variable is subtracted from both X and Y (or equivalently only from X) and new linear combinations are obtained in the same way, operating on the deflated matrices. The same process is repeated until the covariance is null.

PLS provides both graphical representation of the data and prediction of the response values. Graphical representations allow for both observations and predictors to be viewed on the same graph. The relative position of observations with regard to the different predictors is readily explained. Correlations between response and latent variables can be represented.

The choice of the number of latent variables to be used can be obtained through cross-validation or use of a test dataset. The objective is to obtain a precise prediction while avoiding overfitting (difficulties in generalizing to new observations). The optimal number of latent variables is the one resulting in the best prediction error.

Possible Extensions Most extensions of PLS use nonlinear regressions to introduce more complex combinations of predictors (see ASPLS [316] using spline functions to perform regression). Multiblock PLS where blocks of variables (or observations) are applied to the same operations during the latent variables construction is also possible.

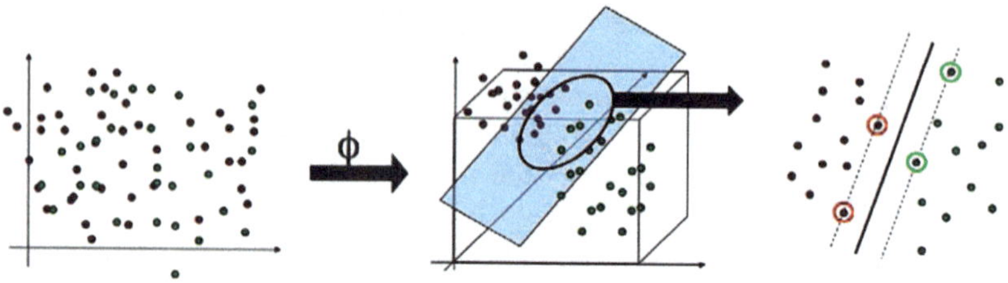

Figure 2.31 Illustration of SVM principle. Starting from the left, observations are illustrated in their original space, and then are projected into the new space and finally separated by the maximum-margin hyperplane (circled points are called support vectors). See insert for color representation of this figure.

2.6.3 Support Vector Machine

2.6.3.1 Aim The support vector machine classifier [98] was originally designed to perform discrimination between two groups (Figure 2.31). It has been extended to classify more than two groups and to perform regression (i.e., modeling one continuous variable). SVM is supported by two main ideas. A transformation performed by means of a function called kernel. The kernel projects the observations into a new space (generally of higher dimension than the original one) where the two groups are likely to be (or almost be) linearly separable. Second, building the best linear rule (a hyperplane) separating the two groups in the new space. In SVM, according to the Vapnik–Chervonenkis theory, this hyperplane is chosen so that the distance between it and the nearest observations on either side is maximized. It is called the maximum-margin hyperplane. Observations located on the margins are called support vectors.

2.6.3.2 Examples of ADME/Tox Applications Vapnik introduced SVM in 1995 with emergence to ADME/Tox work in the early 2000s. SVM can be used when several predictors (usually quantitative but there are some kernels to deal with qualitative ones) are used to predict one other variable. The predictive variable can be qualitative or quantitative.

For qualitative data, the objective is to predict membership of groups. A recent application of SVM is described by Hou et al. [317]. The goal was to predict HIA by defining two levels of absorption according to a fractional absorption threshold value. The prediction issue was converted into a binary classification problem that particularly fits SVM use. One SVM model was built with each of the 10 chosen descriptors as input. This allowed to investigate individual performances of the descriptors and to rank them according to their predictive power (evaluated by a validation process recursively splitting the sample into learning and test ones). The usefulness of descriptor combinations was addressed. Systematic search was performed to find the best combination. In this work, SVM parameters (kernels, error penalty, etc.) were very carefully chosen by a validation process. A very good prediction rate was achieved for both classes (100% for the poor-absorption class and 97.8% for the good-absorption class).

For quantitative data, any continuous (or discrete with really numerous values) variable can be chosen to be predicted. In Kortagere et al. [309], an SVM model was applied with shape signatures descriptors to predict BBB.

Usage Warning The main issue with SVM is to choose the different parameters. The kernel obviously is the first one. Despite some known recommendations, it is not an easy task and depends on the goals. When using new data, several kernels should be tried or an original one can be designed. The problem is exactly the same for kernel parameters even if some advices have been posted. A cross-validation choice has to be performed most of the time. The same work has to be done for the error penalty parameter that controls balance between overfitting (very precise modeling of the learning sample) and generalization error (ability to generalize the model to new observations). By setting an adequate value, it is always possible to make a perfect classification of the learning dataset. This is likely due to overtraining and no satisfactory results will be obtained on a test set. Any parameter choice has to be done through cross-validation. Eventually, obtaining a precise and robust model requires several choices that involve advanced analyses. As the transformed space is never explicitly known, it is not possible to have any interpretation of the original descriptors results. As numerous descriptors are often available, knowledge of the descriptors that account for the explanation of the predicted variable would be of interest. In the case of a "black box" method such as SVM, prior work on feature selection is required for any interpretation. To conclude, SVM is a powerful but not straightforward method allowing to model quite complex relationships.

2.6.3.3 Technical Description

Input Data SVM requires two objects, the description of n individuals by p descriptors and the vector of length n containing the data to be predicted (either group numbers or any continuous variable).

Output The modeling of the vector to be predicted contains either the predicted groups or the predicted values of the target variable.

Description This description will focus on the original SVM issue, the discrimination of two groups.

The first step is the kernel transformation. The goal is to project data into a higher dimension space where linearly dividing the data into two groups is easier. The kernel function allows combining original features leading to a new space describing the data in a higher dimension. According to the chosen transformation, the dimension can even be infinite. In the new space, computations may become difficult or even impossible. The so-called kernel trick indicates that if the kernel fulfils some properties, distances in the new space can be handled without computing the coordinates of its observations. Many different kernels can be used and the most common ones include the linear kernel (especially used in the case of large sparse data, such as found in text categorization), the Gaussian radial basis kernel (general-purpose kernel to be used in the case of no particular prior knowledge), the polynomial kernel (mostly used in image analysis) and the hyperbolic tangent kernel [318] (that often plays the role of proxy in neural networks).

Once the kernel has been chosen, the best hyperplane to separate the two groups has to be determined. In SVM, the maximum-margin hyperplane is chosen. This hyperplane is the best one with regard to the Vapnik–Chervonenkis theory. This is limiting overfitting (i.e., making a very precise definition of the learning sample but losing any ability to generalize to new data), which is a risk when involved with very high dimensional spaces.

A tolerance to misclassifications on either side of the hyperplane has to be introduced since it is rare to have perfectly linearly separable observations. This is performed through the introduction of an error penalty, which is chosen by the user and allows a trade-off between a large margin and a small number of errors. This is called the soft margin. The final optimization issue is a classical one solved by usual optimization algorithms.

Possible Extensions SVM can be extended to classify more than two groups. Generalizing a method designed to classify two groups consists in reducing the multiclass problem into several two-class problems. There are two approaches: the one-versus-one where each group is compared to each other and the one-versus-all comparing each group to the other ones. The former one is the most frequently used. In this approach, each comparison outputs a vote for one class and the majority class is assigned. SVM can also be used to perform regression. SVM principle has been used in several other contexts to perform nonlinear transformations before applying other methods (kernel-PCA, kernel-PLS, etc.).

2.6.4 Decision Trees

2.6.4.1 Aim A decision tree is a simple supervised model, which explains and predicts one response variable (discrete or continuous) taking into account numerous descriptors/features. DTs are based on tree diagrams where leaves or nodes represent classifications and branches represent conjunctions of features that lead to those classifications. DTs correspond to a binary recursive partitioning process since parent nodes are split into two child nodes and recursive because it can be repeated by treating each child node as a parent. The first step of DT is splitting each parent node in two children nodes using some split index, and then deciding when a tree is complete. A splitting rule showing maximal index value is regarded as the best rule among possible splitting rules. Each terminal node of the tree is assigned to a class outcome or predicted value. Pruning can be used to avoid overfitting. Pruning cuts deepest subtrees of the built decision tree according to their potential generalization performance.

Classification tree analysis is possible when the predicted outcome is the class to which the data belong (discrete outcome, e.g., active versus inactive compounds). Regression tree analysis is when the predicted outcome can be considered as a real number (continuous outcome as solubility, permeability values of drugs). Classification and regression tree (CART) analysis, first introduced by Breiman et al. [319], is used to refer to both the above procedures. Figure 2.32 represents an example of

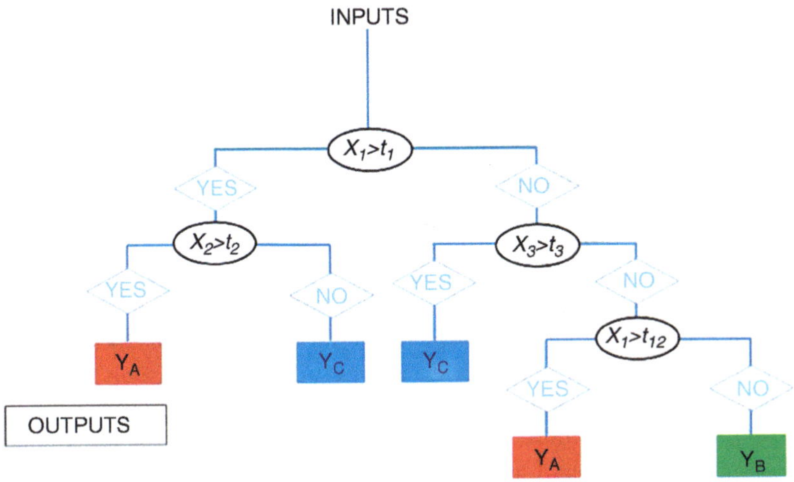

Figure 2.32 DT example. Diagram tree predict molecules of three types $Y = (Y_A, Y_B, Y_C)$ using three descriptors (X_1, X_2, X_3). First discriminant descriptor is X_1, related to threshold t_1; for branch $X_1 > t_1$: discriminant descriptor is X_2, related to threshold t_2, allowing to predict $Y_A(X_2 > t_2)$ else $Y_C(X_2 \leq t_2)$; for other branch ($X_1 \leq t_1$): descriptor X_3, related to t_3, predict $Y_c(X_3 > t_3)$; and else ($X_3 \leq t_3$), descriptor X_1 predict $Y_A(X_1 > t_{12})$, either $Y_B(X_1 \leq t_{12})$.

a diagram tree to predict molecules of three types $Y = (Y_A, Y_B, Y_C)$ using three descriptors (X_1, X_2, X_3). DT creates a branching structure in which the branch at each intersection is determined by a rule relating to one of the three descriptors for the molecules and final leaves are assigned to the dominant type among the observations falling in each leaf. DT is a simple method, easy to understand and interpret.

2.6.4.2 Examples of ADME/Tox Application DT approach has been applied in combinatorial library design, prediction of "drug-likeness" as a general property, prediction of specific biological activities, and on some specific compound profiling.

With discrete outcome, decision trees are used for the identification of substructures that discriminate activity from nonactivity within a given collection of compounds [320–323]. DT approach allows to estimate the conditional probability of activity given the combination of substructures present (or absent) in a given collection of compounds while accounting for the abundance of substructures within the library [323]. Once identified, each of these discriminating substructures are tested statistically for enriched activity and compared to the privileged substructures reported in the literature. DTs are also used for the classification of chemical compounds into drug and nondrugs [111, 324]. In Schneider et al., DT interpretation suggested the main criteria for separating drugs from nondrugs. These were a molecule weight higher than 230 Da, a molar refractivity higher than 40, and the presence of ring(s) as well as one or more functional groups. This approach resulted in at least 39% of the nondrugs filtered out, while retaining more than 83% of the actual drugs.

With continuous outcome, decision trees are also used to predict ADME/Tox properties such as absorption properties [317, 325], solubility or permeability of drugs [326], distribution properties [327], P-glycoprotein [328] or BBB penetration [329], and metabolic stability [330]. For toxicity properties, DTs are used to predict hERG inhibition [202] and toxicity involving cytochrome P450 such as six CYP isoforms [331], 2D6 and 1A2 isoforms [193, 312], or the 3A4 isoform [332].

2.6.4.3 Usage Warning The main issue with DT is to choose the "best" appropriate index to split parent node into two child nodes and to decide when a tree is complete. If the target is a classification outcome, different measures of node impurity for splitting nodes and pruning the tree can be used as misclassification errors. Gini index and cross-entropy or deviance are the most common measures of error [88]. For regression, the squared-error node impurity measure can be used.

The preferred strategy for pruning is to grow a large tree T0, stopping the splitting process only when some minimum node size is reached. The large tree is pruned using cost-complexity pruning. By using five- or ten-fold cross-validation, the subtree (obtained by pruning T0 that is collapsing any number of the internal nodes) is established, which minimizes the cost complexity.

One major problem with trees is their high variance. Often a small change in the data can result in a very different series of splits, complicating the interpretation. This instability is due to the hierarchical nature of the process: the effect of an error in the top split is propagated down to all the splits below.

DTs are valuable even with complex data or with a few observations (pruning). It is an appropriate choice from even a very large set of input descriptors due to the recursive partitioning strategy. It results in a descriptive means for calculating conditional probabilities and does not need any preselection of informative variables. To conclude, decision trees are conceptually simple yet powerful and, easy to understand. Classification scheme can be easily interpretable with the most significant descriptors usually appearing at early decision nodes.

2.6.4.4 Technical Description

Input Data Data come in records of the form $(x, y) = (x_1, x_2, x_3, \ldots, x_p, y)$: the description of n individuals by p descriptors $(x_1, x_2, x_3, \ldots, x_p)$ and the vector y of length n containing the data to be predicted (either discrete or any continuous variable).

Output The dependent variable, y, is the target variable to understand, classify, or predict. To follow the decision tree (with binary decisions obtained on most significant descriptors) allows assigning one y value to each leaf, indicating either the predicted group or the predicted value of the target variable. DT can describe or predict continuous output or discrete one (for two or more groups).

Description The goal is to create a model that predicts the value of a target variable based on several input variables. Each interior node is split according to a dichotomous decision based on one of the input variables. There are two edges to children for each of the possible types of values of that input variable. Each leaf is assigned a value that is the predicted one for observations following the path leading to this leaf. A tree can be "learned" by splitting the source set into subsets based on an attribute value test.

A decision criterion based on maximal purity results in a mixture of classes in the children nodes that are lower than in the parent node. To construct the tree, the "best" division in term of purity criterion is chosen for the p descriptors x. The descriptor (associated to its best division), which results in the best decision in term of purity criterion among all descriptors, is chosen for the first branching. A splitting rule showing a maximal Gini index value is regarded as the best. This process is repeated on each derived subset or node in a recursive manner and is called recursive partitioning. The recursion is completed when the subset at a node has the same value as the target variable, or when splitting no longer adds value to the predictions. Each node of the tree is assigned to a class outcome or predicted value regression. To avoid excessive partitioning, there exist some techniques of pruning to optimize the tree. The pruning component of CART is analogous to the backward elimination approach in regression analysis. This idea provides a control for tree sizes, thus reducing the prediction error of the tree for new data not seen in the learning process. In the CART pruning process, Breiman et al. [333] use a linear combination of the expected loss of the decisions by the tree and the total number of the terminal nodes of the tree. A new observation follows the tree with a particular path and is affected to the corresponding final node.

Possible Extension The other popular methodology is C5.0, which uses a different scheme for deriving rule sets resulting in simpler trees [334]. A random forest combines many decision trees, in order to improve the classification rate. It is a relatively new technique introduced by Breiman in 2001 [335]. In random forest, training data are randomly selected for replacement from the original training data. The forest chooses the most popular class having most votes over all the trees in the forest.

2.6.5 Neural Networks

2.6.5.1 Aim Neural network (NN) attempts to mimic a network or circuit of biological neurons [336]. Each unit represents a neuron, and the connections represent synapses. The modern usage of the term often refers to artificial neural networks, which are composed of interconnecting artificial neurons or nodes (programming constructs that mimic the properties of biological neurons). NN result in powerful nonlinear statistical models. The central idea of NN is to extract linear combinations of the inputs as derived features, and then model the target as a nonlinear function of these features. An NN is a two-stage regression or classification model, typically represented by a network diagram (Figure 2.33). Derived features Z_m are created from linear combinations of the inputs, and then the target Y_q is modeled as a nonlinear function of Z_m, using an activation function. This function performs a linear

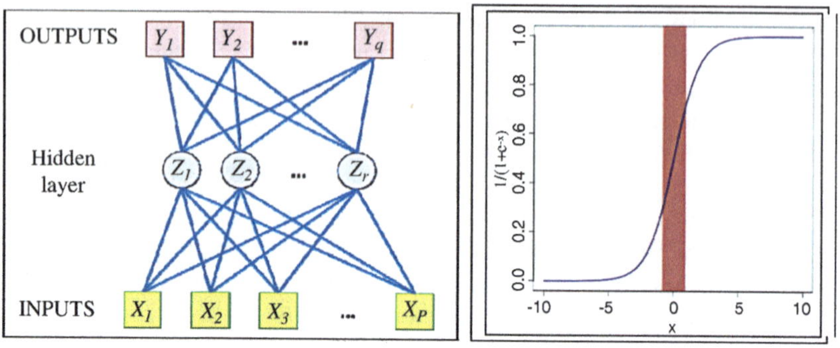

Figure 2.33 Left: Schematic representation of a single hidden layer, feed-forward neural network. Right: The sigmoid function, the red zone shows that for x values near from 0, the sigmoid function is approximately linear.

transformation for small coefficients but progressively implies nonlinear transformation when the coefficient values increase. The units in the middle of the networks, computing the derived features Z_m, are called hidden units because the values Z_m are not directly observed. In general there can be more than one hidden layer. The result is a powerful learning method with widespread applications in many fields. It is often difficult to decode the final model to identify the changes to molecular structure needed to obtain a desired property. NNs also have a tendency to "memorize" rather than learn and are particularly susceptible to overfitting, especially if the training data are noisy.

2.6.5.2 Examples of ADME/Tox Applications The application of NNs in the field of ADME/Tox predictions was initiated in the 1990s to predict physicochemical properties of molecules such as aqueous solubility [337] and lipophilicity [338]. In the early 2000s, more sophisticated NN techniques have gradually emerged and been applied to this area [339]. With discrete outcome, filter programs have been established that use large databases of drug and nondrugs [111, 340]. These programs used NN approaches together with topological descriptors to encode the molecular structures. In these papers, the NN classification method has been found to discriminate between drug-like chemical matter (represented by databases such as CMC, MDDR, WDI) and nondrug-like chemical matter (represented by dataset such as ACD). The result was 80–90% of the compounds were correctly classified as drugs or nondrugs.

With continuous outcome, NNs are used for prediction of lipophilicity and aqueous solubility of chemical compounds [341]. The ALOGPS 2.1 package, based on associative neural networks, combines k-nearest-neighbor and ANN methods on several datasets to carefully analyze the associative neural network parameters. The predictive ability of associative neural network for the training sets was estimated using the leave-one-out method.

For ADME/Tox properties, NN have been used to predict solubility, distribution [327], P-glycoprotein [183], for QSAR modeling of human serum protein binding [342], or absorption [343, 344]. For Toxicity properties, NN have been used to predict P450 1A2 inhibition [312], P450 2D6 [345], P450 3A4 inhibition [346, 347], and to predict whenever a compound might be cytotoxic [348].

2.6.5.3 Usage Warning Training neural networks is quite an art. As NNs are iterative processes, initialization of the coefficients is required. Usually, small coefficients are initially provided leading to a model that is not far from the linear one. It aims at providing a simple model that is not overfitting the training data. More complex transformations are derived during the training process if regularization is well controlled. In order to facilitate the coefficient initialization, a prior scaling of inputs (leading to zero mean and unit variance) is recommended (see PCA for more details about data scaling). In addition, the objective function often possesses many local minima. Different initializations can lead to different solutions. Several initial parameter sets to obtain a more reliable final solution should be attempted.

The number of hidden layers and of units generally has to be provided by the user. With too few hidden units, the model might not have enough flexibility to capture the nonlinearities in the data. Too many hidden layers are likely to produce overfitting models. However if regularization is well controlled, useless layers will simply reproduce the results obtained in the previous ones. Choosing a high number of hidden layers should not be a problem if the required work on regularization has been performed (see Section 2.6.5.4 for more details). Typically the number of hidden units is in the range of 5–100, with the number increasing with the number of inputs and number of training cases. Choice of the number of hidden layers is guided by background knowledge and experimentation.

Finally, neural networks are complex models but they are likely to be very efficient if well tuned. The model is generally overparameterized, and the optimization problem is nonconvex and unstable unless certain guidelines are followed. Similar to SVMs, NN models cannot be interpreted in terms of relationships between input and output variables.

These tools are especially effective in problems with a high signal-to-noise ratio and settings where prediction without interpretation is the goal. They are not effective to describe a process and the roles of individual inputs. Each input enters the model in many places in a nonlinear fashion.

2.6.5.4 Technical Description

Input Data This method is based on the description of n individuals by p descriptors collected in a matrix having n rows and p columns, called X, and of the values of q response variables measured on the same n individuals and collected in Y.

Output The predicted values of Y are provided. The final coefficients applied to each input variable and internal node are generally given.

Description NNs are a wide category of methods aiming at performing nonlinear regression and classification. In general, they tend to imitate biological neurons behavior. Simple units receive information and produce other information in order to achieve a given goal.

Figure 2.33 outlines the main features of a very simple NN. Input variables are combined in one layer of hidden units via linear combinations. Inside these hidden nodes, an activation function is applied to the result of the linear combination producing one value. This activation function is typically a sigmoid one (or sometimes radical basis function). As shown in Figure 2.33 (right), the sigmoid function is approximately linear at approximately zero. If the norm of the vectors containing the coefficients applied in the linear combination is not far from zero (i.e., if all the coefficients are small), the corresponding hidden unit can be considered as only performing linear transformation. To the contrary, higher coefficients imply a nonlinear transformation. The values provided by the hidden layers are linearly combined in each output variable and the obtained value is transformed by the output function. This function is usually the identity function for regression (the value remains unchanged) and the softmax function for classification (allowing one to obtain a probability for each class). There may be several hidden layers performing successive transformations.

In order to train a neural network an objective function is required. For regression, the sum of squared differences between the true and predicted values is used. The same method can be applied in classification as well as other functions such as cross-entropy (which measures the quantity of disagreement between true and predicted values). In order to minimize these objective functions, back propagation (also called gradient descent) is used. It consists in adapting the coefficients applied to each hidden unit (to obtain the output values) according to their contribution to the global error. It is possible to propagate these contributions to the linear combinations implying the input variables and to perform similar coefficient corrections. This process is repeated until convergence (there are no more changes in the coefficients) or a user-defined maximum number of iterations is reached. In this correction step, a penalty is applied to control regularization (the ability to generalize to new observations). This consists in penalizing high coefficients, which lead to highly nonlinear functions and thus to potential overfitting. This tuning parameter is often chosen through cross-validation.

Possible Extensions Many extensions have been proposed. They generally rely on changes concerning topology of connections between units (cycles can be allowed), using combination functions (weighted linear combinations, for example), activation and output functions, and learning algorithm.

2.7 CONCLUSIONS

In summary, although many currently developed molecules tend to challenge known rules, the alliance of medicinal chemistry and drug-metabolism pharmacokinetics-ADME/Tox has made a substantial impact on quality of drug candidates [125]. As new regions of the chemical space are explored, there will be a need to continue to explore the boundaries of the drug-like chemical space in order to be able to rationally design and balance the physicochemical properties of a drug candidate. Here, *in silico* tools greatly assist the decision-making process [198, 349, 350]. A major challenge is to forge a comparable partnership with preclinical pharmacology such that concentration–effect relationships equal the pharmacokinetic structure–activity relationships in lead optimization. Many other obstacles await such as designing better drugs for children and the elderly using ADME/Tox issues [351–353] and better assessment of interindividual variability [354, 355]. Pharmacogenomics, genotyping, toxicogenomics, proteomics, metabonimics and metabolomics, chemogenomics, structural biology, chemical systems biology, mapping adverse drug reactions in chemical space, integration and annotation of the data, merging chemical and biological space, generation of drug–target networks, new algorithms, will all play a key role in understanding drug responses in different patients relative to their genetic constitution and in improving the predictive character of *in silico* methods [151, 356–362]. New experimental approaches and computer technologies will contribute to this process [67, 191, 363]. Better understanding of serious adverse drug reactions (SADRs) already allows for the development of the web-hosted tool such as SePreSA [364] http://sepresa.bio-x.cn/. SADRs are caused by unexpected drug–human protein interactions, and some polymorphisms within binding pockets make these populations more susceptible to drug attack (e.g., Vioxx, 2004 or Avandia, 2007). While automating every modeling task, it will be important to not transform the *in silico* processes into black boxes. Ultimately, new predictive methods will be developed in the coming years integrating new experimental data and theoretical concepts. Mutations or single nucleotide polymorphisms in drug-metabolizing enzymes and for other ADME/Tox involved proteins, age, pathology-dependent variations will be considered. From a patient and clinician perspective, it is imperative that new predictive methods are pursued to administer inherently less toxic drugs coupled to the identification of genetically susceptible patient groups. All these will take time and require important financial investment. Further, this should be accomplished while limiting as much as possible animal experimentations. We do hope that this chapter provides the readers with a global picture of different concepts currently used or emerging in the field of *in silico* ADME/Tox predictions. Definitively, this area will remain a challenge for at least the next 20–50 years.

REFERENCES

1. Abou-Gharbia, M. Discovery of innovative small molecule therapeutics. *J. Med. Chem.* 2009, *52*, 2–9.
2. Vistoli, G., Pedretti, A., and Testa, B. Assessing drug-likeness—what are we missing? *Drug Discov. Today* 2008, *13*, 285–294.
3. Phatak, S. S., Clifford, C. C., and Cavasotto, C. N. High-throughput and *in silico* screenings in drug discovery. *Expert. Opin. Drug Discov.* 2009, *9*, 947–959.
4. Kolb, P., Ferreira, R. S., Irwin, J. J., and Shoichet, B. K. Docking and chemoinformatic screens for new ligands and targets. *Curr. Opin. Biotechnol.* 2009, *20(4)*, 429–436.
5. Dickson, M. and Gagnon, J. P. Key factors in the rising cost of new drug discovery and development. *Nat. Rev. Drug Discov.* 2004, *3*, 417–429.
6. Schmid, E. F. and Smith, D. A. Pharmaceutical R&D in the spotlight: why is there still unmet medical need? *Drug. Discov. Today* 2007, *12*, 998–1006.

7. Smith, D. A. and Schmid, E. F. Drug withdrawals and the lessons within. *Curr. Opin. Drug Discov. Devel.* 2006, *9*, 38–46.
8. Schmid, E. F. and Smith, D. A. Keynote review: Is declining innovation in the pharmaceutical industry a myth? *Drug Discov. Today* 2005, *10*, 1031–1039.
9. Blake, J. F. Identification and evaluation of molecular properties related to preclinical optimization and clinical fate. *J. Med. Chem.* 2005, *1*, 649–655.
10. Grass, G. M. and Sinko, P. J. Physiologically-based pharmacokinetic simulation modelling. *Adv. Drug. Deliv. Rev.* 2002, *54*, 433–451.
11. Prentis, R. A., Lis, Y., and Walker, S. R. Pharmaceutical innovation by the seven UK-owned pharmaceutical companies (1964-1985). *Br. J. Clin. Pharmacol.* 1988, *25*, 387–396.
12. Kennedy, T. Managing the drug discovery/development interface. *Drug. Discov. Today* 1997, *2*, 436–444.
13. Eddershaw, P. J., Beresford, A. P., and Bayliss, M. K. ADME/PK as part of a rational approach to drug discovery. *Drug. Discov. Today* 2000, *5*, 409–414.
14. Kerns, E. H. and Di, L. Pharmaceutical profiling in drug discovery. *Drug Discov. Today* 2003, *8*, 316–323.
15. Hann, M. M. and Oprea, T. I. Pursuing the leadlikeness concept in pharmaceutical research. *Curr. Opin. Chem. Biol.* 2004, *8*, 255–263.
16. Kola, I. and Landis, J. Can the pharmaceutical industry reduce attrition rates? *Nat. Rev. Drug Discov.* 2004, *3*, 711–715.
17. Hutter, M. C. *In silico* prediction of drug properties. *Curr. Med. Chem.* 2009, *16*, 189–202.
18. Schuster, D., Laggner, C., and Langer, T. Why drugs fail—a study on side effects in new chemical entities. *Curr. Pharm. Des.* 2005, *11*, 3545–3559.
19. Scheiber, J., Chen, B., Milik, M., Sukuru, S. C., Bender, A., Mikhailov, D., Whitebread, S., Hamon, J., Azzaoui, K., Urban, L., Glick, M., Davies, J. W., and Jenkins, J. L. Gaining insight into off-target mediated effects of drug candidates with a comprehensive systems chemical biology analysis. *J. Chem. Inf. Model* 2009, *49(2)*, 308–317.
20. van de Waterbeemd, H. and Gifford, E. ADMET *in silico* modelling: towards prediction paradise? *Nat. Rev. Drug. Discov.* 2003, *2*, 192–204.
21. van de Waterbeemd, H. and Jones, B. C. Predicting oral absorption and bioavailability. *Prog. Med. Chem.* 2003, *41*, 1–59.
22. van De Waterbeemd, H., Smith, D. A., Beaumont, K., and Walker, D. K. Property-based design: optimization of drug absorption and pharmacokinetics. *J. Med. Chem.* 2001, *44*, 1313–1333.
23. Di, L. and Kerns, E. H. Biological assay challenges from compound solubility: strategies for bioassay optimization. *Drug Discov. Today* 2006, *11*, 446–451.
24. Walters, W. P. and Murcko, M. A. Prediction of 'drug-likeness'. *Adv. Drug Deliv. Rev.* 2002, *54*, 255–271.
25. Beresford, A. P., Segall, M., and Tarbit, M. H. *In silico* prediction of ADME properties: are we making progress? *Curr. Opin. Drug Discov. Devel.* 2004, *7*, 36–42.
26. Davis, A. M. and Riley, R. J. Predictive ADMET studies, the challenges and the opportunities. *Curr. Opin. Chem. Biol.* 2004, *8*, 378–386.
27. Keseru, G. M. and Makara, G. M. The influence of lead discovery strategies on the properties of drug candidates. *Nat. Rev. Drug Discov.* 2009, *8*, 203–212.

28. Vastag, M. and Keseru, G. M. Current *in vitro* and *in silico* models of blood–brain barrier penetration: a practical view. *Curr. Opin. Drug Discov. Devel.* 2009, *12*, 115–124.

29. Benigni, R. and Bossa, C. Structure alerts for carcinogenicity, and the *Salmonella* assay system: a novel insight through the chemical relational databases technology. *Mutat. Res.* 2008, *659*, 248–261.

30. Guha, R. and Schurer, S. C. Utilizing high throughput screening data for predictive toxicology models: protocols and application to MLSCN assays. *J. Comput. Aided Mol. Des.* 2008, *22*, 367–384.

31. Muster, W., Breidenbach, A., Fischer, H., Kirchner, S., Muller, L., and Pahler, A. Computational toxicology in drug development. *Drug Discov. Today* 2008, *13*, 303–310.

32. Erve, J. C. Chemical toxicology: reactive intermediates and their role in pharmacology and toxicology. *Expert Opin. Drug Metab. Toxicol.* 2006, *2*, 923–946.

33. Axerio-Cilies, P., Castaneda, I. P., Mirza, A., and Reynisson, J. Investigation of the incidence of "undesirable" molecular moieties for high-throughput screening compound libraries in marketed drug compounds. *Eur J. Med. Chem.* 2009, *44*, 1128–1134.

34. DeWitte, R. S. Avoiding physicochemical artefacts in early ADME-Tox experiments. *Drug Discov. Today* 2006, *11*, 855–859.

35. Muegge, I. Selection criteria for drug-like compounds. *Med. Res. Rev.* 2003, *23*, 302–321.

36. Li, A. P. Screening for human ADME/Tox drug properties in drug discovery. *Drug Discov. Today* 2001, *6*, 357–366.

37. Li, A. P. Human-based *in vitro* experimental systems for the evaluation of human drug safety. *Curr. Drug Saf.* 2007, *2*, 193–199.

38. Rishton, G. M. Failure and success in modern drug discovery: guiding principles in the establishment of high probability of success drug discovery organizations. *Med. Chem.* 2005, *1*, 519–527.

39. Rishton, G. M. Nonleadlikeness and leadlikeness in biochemical screening. *Drug Discov. Today* 2003, *8*, 86–96.

40. Ekins, S., Mestres, J., and Testa, B. *In silico* pharmacology for drug discovery: methods for virtual ligand screening and profiling. *Br. J. Pharmacol.* 2007, *152*, 9–20.

41. Colmenarejo, G. *In silico* prediction of drug-binding strengths to human serum albumin. *Med. Res. Rev.* 2003, *23*, 275–301.

42. Vedani, A., Dobler, M., and Lill, M. A. The challenge of predicting drug toxicity *in silico*. *Basic Clin. Pharmacol. Toxicol.* 2006, *99*, 195–208.

43. Szakacs, G., Varadi, A., Ozvegy-Laczka, C., and Sarkadi, B. The role of ABC transporters in drug absorption, distribution, metabolism, excretion and toxicity (ADME-Tox). *Drug Discov. Today* 2008, *13*, 379–393.

44. Richard, A. M. Future of toxicology–predictive toxicology: an expanded view of "chemical toxicity". *Chem. Res. Toxicol.* 2006, *19*, 1257–1262.

45. Oprea, T. I., Davis, A. M., Teague, S. J., and Leeson, P. D. Is there a difference between leads and drugs? A historical perspective. *J. Chem. Inf. Comput. Sci.* 2001, *41*, 1308–1315.

46. Dearden, J. C. *In silico* prediction of ADMET properties: how far have we come? *Expert Opin. Drug Metab. Toxicol.* 2007, *3*, 635–639.

47. Hou, T. and Wang, J. Structure–ADME relationship: still a long way to go? *Expert Opin. Drug Metab. Toxicol.* 2008, *4*, 759–770.

48. Xu, J. and Stevenson, J. Drug-like index: a new approach to measure drug-like compounds and their diversity. *J. Chem. Inf. Comput. Sci.* 2000, *40*, 1177–1187.
49. Jorgensen, W. L. The many roles of computation ion drug discovery. *Science* 2004, *303*, 1813–1818.
50. Fostel, J. Predictive ADME-Tox London, UK, 27–28 April 2005. *Expert Opin. Drug Metab. Toxicol.* 2005. *1*, 565–570.
51. Pavan, M. and Worth, A. P. Publicly-accessible QSAR software tools developed by the Joint Research Centre. *SAR QSAR Environ. Res.* 2008, *19*, 785–799.
52. Summerfield, S. and Jeffrey, P. Discovery DMPK: changing paradigms in the eighties, nineties and noughties. *Expert Opin. Drug Discov.* 2009, *4*, 207–218.
53. Merlot, C. *In silico* methods for early toxicity assessment. *Curr. Opin. Drug Discov. Devel.* 2008, *11*, 80–85.
54. Kramer, J. A., Sagartz, J. E. and Morris, D. L. The application of discovery toxicology and pathology towards the design of safer pharmaceutical lead candidates. *Nat. Rev. Drug Discov.* 2007, *6*, 636–649.
55. Tarbit, M. H. and Berman, J. High-throughput approaches for evaluating absorption, distribution, metabolism and excretion properties of lead compounds. *Curr. Opin. Chem. Biol.* 1998, *2*, 411–416.
56. Di, L. and Kerns, E. H. Profiling drug-like properties in discovery research. *Curr. Opin. Chem. Biol.* 2003, *7*, 402–408.
57. Hämäläinen, M. D. and Frostell-Karlsson, A. Predicting the intestinal absorption potential of hits and leads. *Drug Discov. Today* 2004, *1*, 397–405.
58. Selick, H. E., Beresford, A. P., and Tarbit, M. H. The emerging importance of predictive ADME simulation in drug discovery. *Drug Discov. Today* 2002, *7*, 109–116.
59. Lipinski, C. A., Lombardo, F., Dominy, B. W., and Feeney, P. J. Experimental and computational approaches to estimate solubility and permeability in drug discovery and development settings. *Adv. Drug Deliv. Rev.* 1997, *46*, 3–26.
60. Wenlock, M. C., Austin, R. P., Barton, P., Davis, A. M., and Leeson, P. D. A comparison of physiochemical property profiles of development and marketed oral drugs. *J. Med. Chem.* 2003, *46*, 1250–1256.
61. Teague, S. J., Davis, A. M., Leeson, P. D., and Oprea, T. The design of leadlike combinatorial libraries. *Angew Chem. Int. Ed. Engl.* 1999, *38*, 3743–3748.
62. Congreve, M., Carr, R., Murray, C., and Jhoti, H. A 'rule of three' for fragment-based lead discovery? *Drug Discov. Today* 2003, *8*, 876–877.
63. Kubinyi, H. Drug research: myths, hype and reality. *Nat. Rev. Drug Discov.* 2003, *2*, 665–668.
64. Oprea, T. I. and Matter, H. Integrating virtual screening in lead discovery. *Curr. Opin. Chem. Biol.* 2004, *8*, 349–358.
65. Rester, U. From virtuality to reality—Virtual screening in lead discovery and lead optimization: a medicinal chemistry perspective. *Curr. Opin. Drug Discov. Devel.* 2008, *11*, 559–568.
66. Blake, J. F. Chemoinformatics—predicting the physicochemical properties of 'drug-like' molecules. *Curr. Opin. Biotechnol.* 2000, *11*, 104–107.
67. Oprea, T. I., Tropsha, A., Faulon, J. L., and Rintoul, M. D. Systems chemical biology. *Nat. Chem. Biol.* 2007, *3*, 447–450.

68. Van Drie, J. H. Computer-aided drug design: the next 20 years. *J. Comput. Aided Mol. Des.* 2007, *21*, 591–601.

69. Bajorath, J., Peltason, L., Wawer, M., Guha, R., Lajiness, M. S., and Van Drie, J. H. Navigating structure–activity landscapes. *Drug Discov. Today* 2009, *14(13–14)*, 698–705.

70. Betz, U. A. How many genomics targets can a portfolio afford? *Drug Discov. Today* 2005, *10*, 1057–1063.

71. Betz, U. A., Farquhar, R., and Ziegelbauer, K. Genomics: success or failure to deliver drug targets? *Curr. Opin. Chem. Biol.* 2005, *9*, 387–391.

72. Sakiyama, Y. The use of machine learning and nonlinear statistical tools for ADME prediction. *Expert Opin. Drug Metab. Toxicol.* 2009, *5*, 149–169.

73. Tetko, I. V., Bruneau, P., Mewes, H. W., Rohrer, D. C., and Poda, G. I. Can we estimate the accuracy of ADME-Tox predictions? *Drug Discov. Today* 2006, *11*, 700–707.

74. Gedeck, P. and Lewis, R. A. Exploiting QSAR models in lead optimization. *Curr. Opin. Drug Discov. Devel.* 2008, *11*, 569–575.

75. Butina, D., Segall, M. D., and Frankcombe, K. Predicting ADME properties *in silico*: methods and models. *Drug Discov. Today* 2002, *7*, S83–S88.

76. Kirchmair, J., Distinto, S., Schuster, D., Spitzer, G., Langer, T., and Wolber, G. Enhancing drug discovery through *in silico* screening: strategies to increase true positives retrieval rates. *Curr. Med. Chem.* 2008, *15*, 2040–2053.

77. Jacob, A., Pratuangdejkul, J., Buffet, S., Launay, J. M., and Manivet, P. *In silico* platform for xenobiotics ADME-T pharmacological properties modeling and prediction. Part II: The body in a Hilbertian space. *Drug Discov. Today* 2009, *14*, 406–412.

78. Lajiness, M. S., Maggiora, G. M., and Shanmugasundaram, V. Assessment of the consistency of medicinal chemists in reviewing sets of compounds. *J. Med. Chem.* 2004, *47*, 4891–4896.

79. Testa, B., Vistoli, G., and Pedretti, A. Musings on ADME predictions and structure–-activity relations. *Chem. Biodivers.* 2005, *2*, 1411–1427.

80. Lin, J. H. Pharmacokinetics of biotech drugs: peptides, proteins and monoclonal antibodies. *Curr. Drug Metab.* 2009, *10(9)*, 661–691.

81. Yamashita, F. and Hashida, M. *In silico* approaches for predicting ADME properties of drugs. *Drug Metab. Pharmacokinet.* 2004, *19*, 327–338.

82. Gedeck, P., Rohde, B., and Bartels, C. QSAR—how good is it in practice? Comparison of descriptor sets on an unbiased cross section of corporate data sets. *J. Chem. Inf. Model* 2006, *46*, 1924–1936.

83. Villar, H. O., Hansen, M. R., and Kho, R. Substructural analysis in drug discovery. *Curr. Comput. Aided Drug Des.* 2007, *3*, 59–67.

84. Huang, W., Lee, S. L., and Yu, L. X. Mechanistic approaches to predicting oral drug absorption. *AAPS J.* 2009, *11(2)*, 225–237.

85. Helguera, A. M., Combes, R. D., Gonzalez, M. P., and Cordeiro, M. N. Applications of 2D descriptors in drug design: a DRAGON tale. *Curr. Top. Med. Chem.* 2008, *8*, 1628–1655.

86. Tetko, I. V., Gasteiger, J., Todeschini, R., Mauri, A., Livingstone, D., Ertl, P., Palyulin, V. A., Radchenko, E. V., Zefirov, N. S., Makarenko, A. S., Tanchuk, V. Y., and Prokopenko, V. V. Virtual computational chemistry laboratory—design and description. *J. Comput. Aided Mol. Des.* 2005, *19*, 453–463.

87. Zheng, S., Luo, X., Chen, G., Zhu, W., Shen, J., Chen, K., and Jiang, H. A new rapid and effective chemistry space filter in recognizing a druglike database. *J. Chem. Inf. Model* 2005, *45*, 856–862.
88. Hastie, T., Tibshirani, R., and Friedman, J. *The Elements of Statistical Learning: Data Mining, Inference, and Prediction*, 2nd Edition, Springer Series in Statistics. Springer, Berlin, 2009.
89. Hartigan, J. A. *Clustering Algorithms*, Wiley New York, 1975.
90. Jolliffe, I. T. *Principal Component Analysis*, ed. Statistics, S. S. i., 2002.
91. Hopfield, J. J. Neural networks and physical systems with emergent collective computational abilities. *Proc. Natl. Acad. Sci. USA* 1982, *79*, 2554–2558.
92. Anderson, T. W. *An Introduction to Multivariate Statistics*. Wiley Series in Probability and Statistics, Wiley, New York, 2003, p. 752.
93. Cover, T. M. and Hart, P. Nearest neighbor pattern classification. *Proc. IEEE—Trans. Inform. Theory* 1967, *IT-11*, 21–27.
94. Draper, N. R. and Smith, H. *Applied Regression Analysis*, Wiley New York, 1966, p. 407.
95. Wold, S. PLS in Chemistry. In *The Encyclopedia in Chemistry*, Wiley New York, 1999.
96. Wold, S. Nonlinear partial least squares modelling II. *Chem. Intell. Lab. Syst.* 1992, *14*, 71–84.
97. Quinlan, J. Induction of decision trees. *Mach. Learn.*, 1986, *1*, 81–106.
98. Vapnik, V. *The Nature of Statistical Learning Theory*, 2nd Edition, Wiley-Interscience, New York, 2000.
99. Stone, M. Cross-validatory choice and assessment of statistical predictions. *J. Roy. Statist. Soc.* 1974, *36*, 111–147.
100. Efron, B. Estimating the error rate of a prediction rule: improvement on cross-validation. *JASA* 1983, *78*, 316–331.
101. Balakin, K. V., Ivanenkov, Y. A., Savchuk, N. P., Ivashchenko, A. A., and Ekins, S. Comprehensive computational assessment of ADME properties using mapping techniques. *Curr. Drug Discov. Technol.* 2005, *2*, 99–113.
102. Barbosa, F. and Horvath, D. Molecular similarity and property similarity. *Curr. Top. Med. Chem.* 2004, *4*, 589–600.
103. Baskin, I. and Varnek, A. Building a chemical space based on fragment descriptors. *Comb. Chem. High Throughput Screen* 2008, *11*, 661–668.
104. Willett, P. Chemoinformatics—similarity and diversity in chemical libraries. *Curr. Opin. Biotechnol.* 2000, *11*, 85–88.
105. Jonsdottir, S. O., Jorgensen, F. S., and Brunak, S. Prediction methods and databases within chemoinformatics: emphasis on drugs and drug candidates. *Bioinformatics* 2005, *21*, 2145–2160.
106. Lombardo, F., Gifford, E., and Shalaeva, M. Y. *In silico* ADME prediction: data, models, facts and myths. *Mini. Rev. Med. Chem.* 2003, *3*, 861–875.
107. Sakaeda, T., Okamura, N., Nagata, S., Yagami, T., Horinouchi, M., Okumura, K., Yamashita, F., and Hashida, M. Molecular and pharmacokinetic properties of 222 commercially available oral drugs in humans. *Biol. Pharm. Bull.* 2001, *24*, 935–940.
108. Walters, W. P. and Namchuk, M. Designing screens: how to make your hits a hit. *Nat. Rev. Drug Discov.* 2003, *2*, 259–266.

109. Ghose, A. K., Viswanadhan, V. N., and Wendoloski, J. J. A knowledge-based approach in designing combinatorial or medicinal chemistry libraries for drug discovery. 1. A qualitative and quantitative characterization of known drug databases. *J. Comb. Chem.* 1999, *1*, 55–68.

110. Charifson, P. S. and Walters, W. P. Filtering databases and chemical libraries. *Mol. Divers.* 2002, *5*, 185–197.

111. Ajay, A., Walters, W. P., and Murcko, M. A. Can we learn to distinguish between "drug-like" and "nondrug-like" molecules? *J. Med. Chem.* 1998, *41*, 3314–3324.

112. Veber, D. F., Johnson, S. R., Cheng, H. Y., Smith, B. R., Ward, K. W., and Kopple, K. D. Molecular properties that influence the oral bioavailability of drug candidates. *J. Med. Chem.* 2002, *45*, 2615–2623.

113. Vieth, M., Siegel, M. G., Higgs, R. E., Watson, I. A., Robertson, D. H., Savin, K. A., Durst, G. L., and Hipskind, P. A. Characteristic physical properties and structural fragments of marketed oral drugs. *J. Med. Chem.* 2004, *47*, 224–232.

114. Ritchie, T. J., Luscombe, C. N., and Macdonald, S. J. Analysis of the calculated physicochemical properties of respiratory drugs: can we design for inhaled drugs yet? *J. Chem. Inf. Model* 2009, *49*, 1025–1032.

115. O'Shea, R. and Moser, H. E. Physicochemical properties of antibacterial compounds: implications for drug discovery. *J. Med. Chem.* 2008, *51*, 2871–2878.

116. Ritchie, T. J. and Macdonald, S. J. The impact of aromatic ring count on compound developability—are too many aromatic rings a liability in drug design? *Drug Discov. Today* 2009, *14(21–22)*, 1011–1020.

117. Lagorce, D., Sperandio, O., Galons, H., Miteva, M. A., and Villoutreix, B. O. FAF-Drugs2: free ADME/tox filtering tool to assist drug discovery and chemical biology projects. *BMC Bioinformatics* 2008, *9*, 396.

118. Monge, A., Arrault, A., Marot, C., and Morin-Allory, L. Managing, profiling and analyzing a library of 2.6 million compounds gathered from 32 chemical providers. *Mol. Divers.* 2006, *10*, 389–403.

119. Dubois, J., Bourg, S., Vrain, C., and Morin-Allory, L. Collections of compounds—how to deal with them? *Current Comput. Aided Drug Des.* 2008, *4*, 156–168.

120. Muegge, I., Heald, S. L., and Brittelli, D. Simple selection criteria for drug-like chemical matter. *J. Med. Chem.* 2001, *44*, 1841–1846.

121. Muegge, I. Synergies of virtual screening approaches. *Mini. Rev. Med. Chem.* 2008, *8*, 927–933.

122. Manly, C. J., Chandrasekhar, J., Ochterski, J. W., Hammer, J. D., and Warfield, B. B. Strategies and tactics for optimizing the hit-to-lead process and beyond—a computational chemistry perspective. *Drug Discov. Today* 2008, *13*, 99–109.

123. Wunberg, T., Hendrix, M., Hillisch, A., Lobell, M., Meier, H., Schmeck, C., Wild, H., and Hinzen, B. Improving the hit-to-lead process: data-driven assessment of drug-like and lead-like screening hits. *Drug Discov. Today* 2006, *11*, 175–180.

124. Leeson, P. D. and Springthorpe, B. The influence of drug-like concepts on decision-making in medicinal chemistry. *Nat. Rev. Drug Discov.* 2007, *6*, 881–890.

125. Gill, A. L., Verdonk, M., Boyle, R. G., and Taylor, R. A comparison of physicochemical property profiles of marketed oral drugs and orally bioavailable anti-cancer protein kinase inhibitors in clinical development. *Curr. Top. Med. Chem.* 2007, *7*, 1408–1422.

126. Bhal, S. K., Kassam, K., Peirson, I. G., and Pearl, G. M. The Rule of Five revisited: applying log *D* in place of log *P* in drug-likeness filters. *Mol. Pharm.* 2007, *4*, 556–560.

127. Mannhold, R., Poda, G. I., Ostermann, C., and Tetko, I. V. Calculation of molecular lipophilicity: State-of-the-art and comparison of log *P* methods on more than 96,000 compounds. *J. Pharm. Sci.* 2009, *98*, 861–893.

128. Kah, M. and Brown, C. D. Log *D*: lipophilicity for ionisable compounds. *Chemosphere* 2008, *72*, 1401–1408.

129. Mitra, R., Shyam, R., Mitra, I., Miteva, M. A., and Alexov, E. Calculating the protonation states of proteins and small molecules: implications to ligand–receptor interactions. *Curr. Comput. Aided Drug Des.* 2008, *4*, 169–179.

130. Meloun, M. and Bordovska, S. Benchmarking and validating algorithms that estimate pK_a values of drugs based on their molecular structures. *Anal. Bioanal. Chem.* 2007, *389*, 1267–1281.

131. Shelley, J. C., Cholleti, A., Frye, L. L., Greenwood, J. R., Timlin, M. R., and Uchimaya, M. Epik: a software program for pK_a prediction and protonation state generation for drug-like molecules. *J. Comput. Aided Mol. Des.* 2007, *21*, 681–691.

132. Lee, A. C., Yu, J. Y., and Crippen, G. M. pK_a prediction of monoprotic small molecules the SMARTS way. *J. Chem. Inf. Model* 2008, *48*, 2042–2053.

133. Ten Brink, T. and Exner, T. E. Influence of protonation, tautomeric, and stereoisomeric states on protein–ligand docking results. *J. Chem. Inf. Model* 2009, *49(6)*, 1535–1546.

134. Bayden, A. S., Fornabaio, M., Scarsdale, J. N., and Kellogg, G. E. Web application for studying the free energy of binding and protonation states of protein–ligand complexes based on HINT. _*J. Comput. Aided Mol. Des.* 2009, *23*, 621–632.

135. Burton, P. S., Goodwin, J. T., Vidmar, T. J., and Amore, B. M. Predicting drug absorption: how nature made it a difficult problem. *J. Pharmacol. Exp. Ther.* 2002, *303*, 889–895.

136. Clark, D. E. and Pickett, S. D. Computational methods for the prediction of 'drug-likeness'. *Drug Discov. Today* 2000, *5*, 49–58.

137. Johnson, S. R. and Zheng, W. Recent progress in the computational prediction of aqueous solubility and absorption. *AAPS J.* 2006, *8*, E27–E40.

138. Boobis, A., Gundert-Remy, U., Kremers, P., Macheras, P., and Pelkonen, O. *In silico* prediction of ADME and pharmacokinetics. Report of an expert meeting organised by COST B15. *Eur. J. Pharm. Sci.* 2002, *17*, 183–193.

139. Kerns, E. H., Di, L., Petusky, S., Kleintop, T., Huryn, D., McConnell, O., and Carter, G. Pharmaceutical profiling method for lipophilicity and integrity using liquid chromatography-mass spectrometry. *J. Chromatogr. B Analyt. Technol. Biomed. Life Sci.* 2003, *791*, 381–388.

140. Goller, A. H., Hennemann, M., Keldenich, J., and Clark, T. *In silico* prediction of buffer solubility based on quantum-mechanical and HQSAR- and topology-based descriptors. *J. Chem. Inf. Model* 2006, *46*, 648–658.

141. Faller, B. and Ertl, P. Computational approaches to determine drug solubility. *Adv. Drug Deliv. Rev.* 2007, *59*, 533–545.

142. Jorgensen, W. L. and Duffy, E. M. Prediction of drug solubility from structure. *Adv. Drug Deliv. Rev.* 2002, *54*, 355–366.

143. Hansen, N. T., Kouskoumvekaki, I., Jorgensen, F. S., Brunak, S., and Jonsdottir, S. O. Prediction of pH-dependent aqueous solubility of druglike molecules. *J. Chem. Inf. Model* 2006, *46*, 2601–2619.

144. Egan, W. J. and Lauri, G. Prediction of intestinal permeability. *Adv. Drug Deliv. Rev.* 2002, *54*, 273–289.

145. Gleeson, M. P. Generation of a set of simple, interpretable ADMET rules of thumb. *J. Med. Chem.* 2008, *51*, 817–834.

146. Di, L. and Kerns, E. H. Application of pharmaceutical profiling assays for optimization of drug-like properties. *Curr. Opin. Drug Discov. Devel.* 2005, *8*, 495–504.

147. Di, L. and Kerns, E. H. Solution stability—plasma, gastrointestinal, bioassay. *Curr. Drug Metab.* 2008, *9*, 860–868.

148. Eros, D., Keri, G., Kovesdi, I., Szantai-Kis, C., Meszaros, G., and Orfi, L. Comparison of predictive ability of water solubility QSPR models generated by MLR, PLS and ANN methods. *Mini. Rev. Med. Chem.* 2004, *4*, 167–177.

149. Hou, T., Wang, J., Zhang, W., Wang, W., and Xu, X. Recent advances in computational prediction of drug absorption and permeability in drug discovery. *Curr. Med. Chem.* 2006, *13*, 2653–2667.

150. Lennernas, H. Modeling gastrointestinal drug absorption requires more *in vivo* biopharmaceutical data: experience from *in vivo* dissolution and permeability studies in humans. *Curr. Drug Metab.* 2007, *8*, 645–657.

151. Ekins, S., Nikolsky, Y., and Nikolskaya, T. Techniques: application of systems biology to absorption, distribution, metabolism, excretion and toxicity. *Trends Pharmacol. Sci.* 2005, *26*, 202–209.

152. Hurst, S., Loi, C. M., Brodfuehrer, J., and El-Kattan, A. Impact of physiological, physicochemical and biopharmaceutical factors in absorption and metabolism mechanisms on the drug oral bioavailability of rats and humans. *Expert Opin. Drug Metab. Toxicol.* 2007, *3*, 469–489.

153. Dokoumetzidis, A., Valsami, G., and Macheras, P. Modelling and simulation in drug absorption processes. *Xenobiotica* 2007, *37*, 1052–1065.

154. Lu, J. J., Crimin, K., Goodwin, J. T., Crivori, P., Orrenius, C., Xing, L., Tandler, P. J., Vidmar, T. J., Amore, B. M., Wilson, A. G., Stouten, P. F., and Burton, P. S. Influence of molecular flexibility and polar surface area metrics on oral bioavailability in the rat. *J. Med. Chem.* 2004, *47*, 6104–6107.

155. Martin, Y. C. A bioavailability score. *J. Med. Chem.* 2005, *48*, 3164–3170.

156. Hou, T., Wang, J., Zhang, W., and Xu, X. ADME evaluation in drug discovery. 6. Can oral bioavailability in humans be effectively predicted by simple molecular property-based rules? *J. Chem. Inf. Model* 2007, *47*, 460–463.

157. Mensch, J., Oyarzabal, J., Mackie, C., and Augustijns, P. *In vivo, in vitro* and *in silico* methods for small molecule transfer across the BBB. *J. Pharm. Sci.* 2009, *98(12)*, 4429–4468.

158. Palmer, A. M. and Stephenson, F. A. CNS drug discovery: challenges and solutions. *Drug News Perspect.* 2005, *18*, 51–57.

159. Ecker, G. F. and Noe, C. R. *In silico* prediction models for blood–brain barrier permeation. *Curr. Med. Chem.* 2004, *11*, 1617–28.

160. Goodwin, J. T. and Clark, D. E. *In silico* predictions of blood–brain barrier penetration: considerations to "keep in mind." *J. Pharmacol. Exp. Ther.* 2005, *315*, 477–483.

161. Abbott, N. J., Dolman, D. E., and Patabendige, A. K. Assays to predict drug permeation across the blood–brain barrier, and distribution to brain. *Curr. Drug Metab.* 2008, *9*, 901–910.

162. Podlogar, B. L. and Muegge, I. "Holistic" *in silico* methods to estimate the systemic and CNS bioavailabilities of potential chemotherapeutic agents. *Curr. Top. Med. Chem.* 2001, *1*, 257–275.

163. Hitchcock, S. A. Blood–brain barrier permeability considerations for CNS-targeted compound library design. *Curr. Opin. Chem. Biol.* 2008, *12*, 318–323.

164. Clark, D. E. *In silico* prediction of blood–brain barrier permeation. *Drug Discov. Today* 2003, *8*, 927–933.

165. Allen, D. D. and Geldenhuys, W. J. Molecular modeling of blood–brain barrier nutrient transporters: *in silico* basis for evaluation of potential drug delivery to the central nervous system. *Life Sci.* 2006, *78*, 1029–1033.

166. Feng, M. R. Assessment of blood–brain barrier penetration: *in silico, in vitro* and *in vivo*. *Curr. Drug Metab.* 2002, *3*, 647–657.

167. Lobell, M., Molnar, L., and Keseru, G. M. Recent advances in the prediction of blood–brain partitioning from molecular structure. *J. Pharm. Sci.* 2003, *92*, 360–370.

168. Ekins, S. and Tropsha, A. A turning point for blood–brain barrier modeling. *Pharm. Res.* 2009, *26*, 1283–1284.

169. Eyal, S., Hsiao, P., and Unadkat, J. D. Drug interactions at the blood–brain barrier: fact or fantasy? *Pharmacol. Ther.* 2009, *123*, 80–104.

170. Norinder, U. and Bergstrom, C. A. Prediction of ADMET Properties. *ChemMedChem.* 2006, *1*, 920–937.

171. Rose, K., Hall, L. H., and Kier, L. B. Modeling blood–brain barrier partitioning using the electrotopological state. *J. Chem. Inf. Comput. Sci.* 2002, *42*, 651–666.

172. Chang, C., Ekins, S., Bahadduri, P., and Swaan, P. W. Pharmacophore-based discovery of ligands for drug transporters. *Adv. Drug Deliv. Rev.* 2006, *58*, 1431–1450.

173. Gozalbes, R., Barbosa, F., Nicolai, E., Horvath, D., and Froloff, N. Development and validation of a pharmacophore-based QSAR model for the prediction of CNS activity. *ChemMedChem* 2009, *4*, 204–209.

174. Chang, C., Bahadduri, P. M., Polli, J. E., Swaan, P. W., and Ekins, S. Rapid identification of P-glycoprotein substrates and inhibitors. *Drug Metab. Dispos.* 2006, *34*, 1976–1984.

175. Ekins, S., Ecker, G. F., Chiba, P., and Swaan, P. W. Future directions for drug transporter modelling. *Xenobiotica* 2007, *37*, 1152–1170.

176. Seigneuret, M. and Garnier-Suillerot, A. A structural model for the open conformation of the mdr1 P-glycoprotein based on the MsbA crystal structure. *J. Biol. Chem.* 2003, *278*, 30115–30124.

177. Ravna, A. W., Sylte, I., and Dahl, S. G. Structure and localisation of drug binding sites on neurotransmitter transporters. *J. Mol. Model.* 2009, *15(10)*, 1155–1164.

178. Fenner, K. S., Troutman, M. D., Kempshall, S., Cook, J. A., Ware, J. A., Smith, D. A., and Lee, C. A. Drug–drug interactions mediated through P-glycoprotein: clinical relevance and *in vitro–in vivo* correlation using digoxin as a probe drug. *Clin. Pharmacol. Ther.* 2009, *85*, 173–181.

179. Crivori, P., Reinach, B., Pezzetta, D., and Poggesi, I. Computational models for identifying potential P-glycoprotein substrates and inhibitors. *Mol. Pharm.* 2006, *3*, 33–44.

180. Cianchetta, G., Singleton, R. W., Zhang, M., Wildgoose, M., Giesing, D., Fravolini, A., Cruciani, G., and Vaz, R. J. A pharmacophore hypothesis for P-glycoprotein substrate recognition using GRIND-based 3D-QSAR. *J. Med. Chem.* 2005, *48*, 2927–2935.

181. Osterberg, T. and Norinder, U. Theoretical calculation and prediction of P-glycoprotein-interacting drugs using MolSurf parametrization and PLS statistics. *Eur J. Pharm. Sci.* 2000, *10*, 295–303.

182. Xue, Y., Yap, C. W., Sun, L. Z., Cao, Z. W., Wang, J. F., and Chen, Y. Z. Prediction of P-glycoprotein substrates by a support vector machine approach. *J. Chem. Inf. Comput. Sci.* 2004, *44*, 1497–1505.

183. Wang, Y. H., Li, Y., Yang, S. L., and Yang, L. Classification of substrates and inhibitors of P-glycoprotein using unsupervised machine learning approach. *J. Chem. Inf. Model* 2005, *45*, 750–757.

184. Aller, S. G., Yu, J., Ward, A., Weng, Y., Chittaboina, S., Zhuo, R., Harrell, P. M., Trinh, Y. T., Zhang, Q., Urbatsch, I. L., and Chang, G. Structure of P-glycoprotein reveals a molecular basis for poly-specific drug binding. *Science* 2009, *323*, 1718–1722.

185. Gottesman, M. M., Ambudkar, S. V., and Xia, D. Structure of a multidrug transporter. *Nat. Biotechnol.* 2009, *27*, 546–547.

186. Kragh-Hansen, U., Chuang, V. T., and Otagiri, M. Practical aspects of the ligand-binding and enzymatic properties of human serum albumin. *Biol. Pharm. Bull.* 2002, *25*, 695–704.

187. Zsila, F., Fitos, I., Bencze, G., Keri, G., and Orfi, L. Determination of human serumalpha (1)-acid glycoprotein and albumin binding of various marketed and preclinical kinase inhibitors. *Curr. Med. Chem.* 2009, *16*, 1964–1977.

188. Schonfeld, D. L., Ravelli, R. B., Mueller, U., and Skerra, A. The 1.8-A crystal structure of alpha1-acid glycoprotein (Orosomucoid) solved by UV RIP reveals the broad drug-binding activity of this human plasma lipocalin. *J. Mol. Biol.* 2008, *384*, 393–405.

189. Estrada, E., Uriarte, E., Molina, E., Simon-Manso, Y., and Milne, G. W. An integrated *in silico* analysis of drug-binding to human serum albumin. *J. Chem. Inf. Model* 2006, *46*, 2709–2724.

190. Gunturi, S. B., Narayanan, R., and Khandelwal, A. *In silico* ADME modelling 2: computational models to predict human serum albumin binding affinity using ant colony systems. *Bioorg. Med. Chem.* 2006, *14*, 4118–4129.

191. Grossman, I. ADME pharmacogenetics: current practices and future outlook. *Expert Opin. Drug Metab. Toxicol.* 2009, *5*, 449–462.

192. de Groot, M. J., Wakenhut, F., Whitlock, G., and Hyland, R. Understanding CYP2D6 interactions. *Drug Discov. Today* 2009, *14(19–20)*, 964–972.

193. Burton, J., Ijjaali, I., Barberan, O., Petitet, F., Vercauteren, D. P., and Michel, A. Recursive partitioning for the prediction of cytochromes P450 2D6 and 1A2 inhibition: importance of the quality of the dataset. *J. Med. Chem.* 2006, *49*, 6231–6240.

194. Liebler, D. C. and Guengerich, F. P. Elucidating mechanisms of drug-induced toxicity. *Nat. Rev. Drug Discov.* 2005, *4*, 410–420.

195. Raschi, E., Ceccarini, L., De Ponti, F., and Recanatini, M. hERG-related drug toxicity and models for predicting hERG liability and QT prolongation. *Expert Opin. Drug Metab. Toxicol.* 2009, *5(9)*, 1005–1021.

196. Mayer, J., Cheeseman, M. A., and Twaroski, M. L. Structure-activity relationship analysis tools: validation and applicability in predicting carcinogens. *Regul. Toxicol. Pharmacol.* 2008, *50*, 50–58.

197. Ashby, J. and Tennant, R. W. Prediction of rodent carcinogenicity for 44 chemicals: results. *Mutagenesis* 1994, *9*, 7–15.
198. Nassar, A. E., Kamel, A. M., and Clarimont, C. Improving the decision-making process in structural modification of drug candidates: reducing toxicity. *Drug Discov. Today* 2004, *9*, 1055–1064.
199. Shenton, J. M., Chen, J., and Uetrecht, J. P. Animal models of idiosyncratic drug reactions. *Chem. Biol. Interact.* 2004, *150*, 53–70.
200. Williams, D. P. and Park, B. K. Idiosyncratic toxicity: the role of toxicophores and bioactivation. *Drug Discov. Today* 2003, *8*, 1044–1050.
201. Greene, N. Computer systems for the prediction of toxicity: an update. *Adv. Drug Deliv. Rev.* 2002, *54*, 417–431.
202. Gepp, M. M. and Hutter, M. C. Determination of hERG channel blockers using a decision tree. *Bioorg. Med. Chem.* 2006, *14*, 5325–5332.
203. Aronov, A. M. Predictive *in silico* modeling for hERG channel blockers. *Drug Discov. Today* 2005, *10*, 149–155.
204. Benz, R. D. Toxicological and clinical computational analysis and the US FDA/CDER. *Expert Opin. Drug Metab. Toxicol.* 2007, *3*, 109–1024.
205. Yang, C., Benz, R. D., and Cheeseman, M. A. Landscape of current toxicity databases and database standards. *Curr. Opin. Drug Discov. Devel.* 2006, *9*, 124–133.
206. Shelat, A. A. and Guy, R. K. The interdependence between screening methods and screening libraries. *Curr. Opin. Chem. Biol.* 2007, *11*, 244–251.
207. Wren, J. D. and Bateman, A. Databases, data tombs and dust in the wind. *Bioinformatics* 2008, *24*, 2127–2128.
208. Zvinavashe, E., Murk, A. J., and Rietjens, I. M. Promises and pitfalls of quantitative structure–activity relationship approaches for predicting metabolism and toxicity. *Chem. Res. Toxicol.* 2008, *21(12)*, 2229–2236.
209. Lyne, P. D. Structure-based virtual screening: an overview. *Drug Discov. Today* 2002, *7*, 1047–1055.
210. Lipinski, C. A., Lombardo, F., Dominy, B. W., and Feeney, P. J. Experimental and computational approaches to estimate solubility and permeability in drug discovery and development settings. *Adv. Drug Deliv. Rev.* 2001, *46*, 3–26.
211. Rishton, G. M. Reactive compounds and *in vitro* fake positives in HTS. *Drug Discov. Today* 1997, *2*, 382–384.
212. Seidler, J., McGovern, S. L., Doman, T. N., and Shoichet, B. K. Identification and prediction of promiscuous aggregating inhibitors among known drugs. *J. Med. Chem.* 2003, *46*, 4477–4486.
213. McGovern, S. L., Helfand, B. T., Feng, B., and Shoichet, B. K. A specific mechanism of nonspecific inhibition. *J. Med. Chem.* 2003, *46*, 4265–4272.
214. Roche, O., Schneider, P., Zuegge, J., Guba, W., Kansy, M., Alanine, A., Bleicher, K., Danel, F., Gutknecht, E. M., Rogers-Evans, M., Neidhart, W., Stalder, H., Dillon, M., Sjogren, E., Fotouhi, N., Gillespie, P., Goodnow, R., Harris, W., Jones, P., Taniguchi, M., Tsujii, S., von der Saal, W., Zimmermann, G., and Schneider, G. Development of a virtual screening method for identification of "frequent hitters" in compound libraries. *J. Med. Chem.* 2002, *45*, 137–142.

215. Oprea, T. I. Property distribution of drug-related chemical databases. *J. Comput. Aided Mol. Des.* 2000, *14*, 251–264.

216. SD File format. Available at http://www.mdl.com/downloads/public/ctfile/ctfile.pdf, 2007, MDL—Symix.

217. Daylight Chemical Information Systems, Inc. *SMILES™—Simplified Molecular Input Line Entry System.* 2009.

218. Daylight Chemical Information Systems Inc, *SMARTS™—A Language for Describing Molecular Patterns.* 2007. Aliso Viejo, CA.

219. InChI™ *The IUPAC International Chemical Identifier.* 2009.

220. Judson, R., Richard, A., Dix, D., Houck, K., Elloumi, F., Martin, M., Cathey, T., Transue, T. R., Spencer, R., and Wolf, M. ACToR—Aggregated Computational Toxicology Resource. *Toxicol. Appl. Pharmacol.* 2008, *233*, 7–13.

221. AKos. Consulting & Solutions GmbH—Screening Compound Business. 2009.

222. Tong, J. C., Lim, S. J., Muh, H. C., Chew, F. T., and Tammi, M. T. Allergen Atlas: a comprehensive knowledge center and analysis resource for allergen information. *Bioinformatics* 2009, *25*, 979–980.

223. He, Q. Y., He, Q. Z., Deng, X. C., Yao, L., Meng, E., Liu, Z. H., and Liang, S. P. ATDB: a uni-database platform for animal toxins. *Nucleic Acids Res.* 2008, *36*, D293–D297.

224. Chang, A., Scheer, M., Grote, A., Schomburg, I., and Schomburg, D. BRENDA, AMENDA and FRENDA the enzyme information system: new content and tools in 2009. *Nucleic Acids Res.* 2009 *37*, D588–D592.

225. Ott, M. A. and Vriend, G. Correcting ligands, metabolites, and pathways. *BMC Bioinformatics* 2006, *7*, 517.

226. Degtyarenko, K., de Matos, P., Ennis, M., Hastings, J., Zbinden, M., McNaught, A., Alcantara, R., Darsow, M., Guedj, M., and Ashburner, M. ChEBI: a database and ontology for chemical entities of biological interest. *Nucleic Acids Res.* 2008, *36*, D344–D350.

227. Seiler, K. P., George, G. A., Happ, M. P., Bodycombe, N. E., Carrinski, H. A., Norton, S., Brudz, S., Sullivan, J. P., Muhlich, J., Serrano, M., Ferraiolo, P., Tolliday, N. J., Schreiber, S. L., and Clemons, P. A. ChemBank: a small-molecule screening and cheminformatics resource database. *Nucleic Acids Res.* 2008, *36*, D351–D359.

228. Williams, A. J. A perspective of publicly accessible/open-access chemistry databases. *Drug Discov. Today* 2008, *13*, 495–501.

229. Naamati, G., Askenazi, M., and Linial, M. ClanTox: a classifier of short animal toxins. *Nucleic Acids Res.* 2009, *37*, W363–W368.

230. Zhang, J. X., Huang, W. J., Zeng, J. H., Huang, W. H., Wang, Y., Zhao, R., Han, B. C., Liu, Q. F., Chen, Y. Z., and Ji, Z. L. DITOP: drug-induced toxicity related protein database. *Bioinformatics* 2007, *23*, 1710–1712.

231. Richard, A. M. and Williams, C. R. Distributed structure-searchable toxicity (DSSTox) public database network: a proposal. *Mutat. Res.* 2002, *499*, 27–52.

232. Wishart, D. S., Knox, C., Guo, A. C., Shrivastava, S., Hassanali, M., Stothard, P., Chang, Z., and Woolsey, J. DrugBank: a comprehensive resource for *in silico* drug discovery and exploration. *Nucleic Acids Res.* 2006, *34*, D668–D672.

233. Huang, N., Shoichet, B. K., and Irwin, J. J. Benchmarking sets for molecular docking. *J. Med. Chem.* 2006, *49*, 6789–801.

234. eMolecules. Del Mar, CA, USA. Available at http://www.emolecules.com, 2008.

235. Warr, W. A. ChEMBL. An interview with John Overington, team leader, chemogenomics at the European Bioinformatics Institute Outstation of the European Molecular Biology Laboratory (EMBL-EBI). *J. Comput. Aided Mol. Des.* 2009, *23*, 195–198.
236. Singh, M. K., Srivastava, S., Raghava, G. P., and Varshney, G. C. HaptenDB: a comprehensive database of haptens, carrier proteins and anti-hapten antibodies. *Bioinformatics* 2006, *22*, 253–255.
237. Wishart, D. S., et al. HMDB: the Human Metabolome Database. *Nucleic Acids Res.* 2007, *35*, D521–D526.
238. Kanehisa, M. The KEGG database. *Novartis Found. Symp.* 2002, *247*, 91–101; discussion 101–103, 119–128 244–252.
239. Feng, Z., Chen, L., Maddula, H., Akcan, O., Oughtred, R., Berman, H. M., and Westbrook, J. Ligand depot: a data warehouse for ligands bound to macromolecules. *Bioinformatics* 2004, *20*, 2153–2155.
240. von Grotthuss, M., Pas, J., and Rychlewski, L. Ligand-Info, searching for similar small compounds using index profiles. *Bioinformatics* 2003, *19*, 1041–1042.
241. MDPI. *MDPI molecules*. 2009.
242. Boyer, S., Arnby, C. H., Carlsson, L., Smith, J., Stein, V., and Glen, R. C. Reaction site mapping of xenobiotic biotransformations. *J. Chem. Inf. Model* 2007, *47*, 583–590.
243. Masciocchi, J., Frau, G., Fanton, M., Sturlese, M., Floris, M., Pireddu, L., Palla, P., Cedrati, F., Rodriguez-Tome, P., and Moro, S. MMsINC: a large-scale chemoinformatics database. *Nucleic Acids Res.* 2009, *37*, D284–D290.
244. MDSI. *MicroSource Discovery Systems, Inc. database*. 2009.
245. Sitzmann, M., Filippov, I. V., and Nicklaus, M. C. Internet resources integrating many small-molecule databases. *SAR QSAR Environ. Res.* 2008, *19*, 1–9.
246. NTP U. *National Toxicology Program (NTP) database.* 2009. Available at http://ntp.niehs.nih.gov/.
247. Wheeler, D. L., et al. Database resources of the National Center for Biotechnology Information. *Nucleic Acids Res.* 2006, *34*, D173–D180.
248. Klekota, J., Roth, F. P., and Schreiber, S. L. Query Chem: a Google-powered web search combining text and chemical structures. *Bioinformatics* 2006, *22*, 1670–1673.
249. Hendlich, M., Bergner, A., Gunther, J., and Klebe, G. Relibase: design and development of a database for comprehensive analysis of protein–ligand interactions. *J. Mol. Biol.* 2003, *326*, 607–620.
250. Diago, L. A., Morell, P., Aguilera, L., and Moreno, E. Setting up a large set of protein–ligand PDB complexes for the development and validation of knowledge-based docking algorithms. *BMC Bioinformatics* 2007, *8*, 310.
251. Dunkel, M., Fullbeck, M., Neumann, S., and Preissner, R. SuperNatural: a searchable database of available natural compounds. *Nucleic Acids Res.* 2006, *34*, D678–D683.
252. Goede, A., Dunkel, M., Mester, N., Frommel, C., and Preissner, R. SuperDrug: a conformational drug database. *Bioinformatics* 2005, *21*, 1751–1753.
253. Gunther, S., Hempel, D., Dunkel, M., Rother, K., and Preissner, R. SuperHapten: a comprehensive database for small immunogenic compounds. *Nucleic Acids Res.* 2007, *35*, D906–D910.
254. Michalsky, E., Dunkel, M., Goede, A., and Preissner, R. SuperLigands—a database of ligand structures derived from the Protein Data Bank. *BMC Bioinformatics* 2005, *6*, 122.

255. Schmidt, U., Struck, S., Gruening, B., Hossbach, J., Jaeger, I. S., Parol, R., Lindequist, U., Teuscher, E., and Preissner, R. SuperToxic: a comprehensive database of toxic compounds. *Nucleic Acids Res.* 2009, *37*, D295–D299.

256. TimTec. *TimTec LLC databases.* 2009.

257. Wexler, P. TOXNET: the National Library of Medicine's toxicology database. *Am. Fam. Physician* 1995, *52*, 1677–1678.

258. Toxicity, Datasets. Chemoinformatics.org website. Available at http://cheminformatics.org/datasets/index.shtml#tox, 2009.

259. ChemDB. *ChemDB: The UC Irvine ChemDB datasets.* 2009.

260. Briggs, K. A. Vitic—a data source for (quantitative) structure–activity relationship modelling. *Toxicol. Abstr.* 2007.

261. Irwin, J. J. and Shoichet, B. K. ZINC—a free database of commercially available compounds for virtual screening. *J. Chem. Inf. Model* 2005, *45*, 177–182.

262. Lagorce, D., Sperandio, O., Galons, H., Miteva, M., and Villoutreix, B. FAF-Drugs2: free ADME/tox filtering tool to assist drug discovery and chemical biology projects, 2008.

263. Song, C. M., Bernardo, P. H., Chai, C. L., and Tong, J. C. CLEVER: pipeline for designing *in silico* chemical libraries. *J. Mol. Graph. Model* 2009, *27*, 578–583.

264. ToxTree, *Toxtree—Ideaconsult Ltd.* 2009.

265. Cramer, G. M., Ford, R. A., and Hall, R. L., Estimation of toxic hazard—a decision tree approach. *Food Cosmet. Toxicol.* 1978, *16*, 255–276.

266. Ingsriswang, S., and Pacharawongsakda, E., sMOL Explorer: an open source, web-enabled database and exploration tool for Small MOLecules datasets. *Bioinformatics* 2007, *23*, 2498–2500.

267. Cheng, T., Zhao, Y., Li, X., Lin, F., Xu, Y., Zhang, X., Li, Y., Wang, R., and Lai, L., Computation of octanol–water partition coefficients by guiding an additive model with knowledge. *J. Chem. Inf. Model* 2007, *47*, 2140–2148.

268. Girke, T., Cheng, L. C., and Raikhel, N., ChemMine. A compound mining database for chemical genomics. *Plant Physiol.* 2005, *138*, 573–577.

269. Bolelli, L., Lu, X., Liu, Y., Jaiswal, A., Bai, K., Councill, I., Mitra, P., Wang, J. Z., Mueller, K., Kubicki, J., Garrison, B., Bandstra J., and Giles, C. L. ChemXSeer: A Chemistry Web Portal for Scientific Literature and Datasets In *Open Repositories Conference,* San Antonio, TX, 2007.

270. Helma, C. Lazy structure–activity relationships (lazar) for the prediction of rodent carcinogenicity and *Salmonella* mutagenicity. *Mol. Divers.* 2006, *10*, 147–158.

271. Sander, T., Freyss, J., von Korff, M., Reich, J. R., and Rufener, C. OSIRIS, an entirely in-house developed drug discovery informatics system. *J. Chem. Inf. Model* 2009, *49(2)*, 232–246.

272. Moda, T. L., Torres, L. G., Carrara, A. E., and Andricopulo, A. D. PK/DB: database for pharmacokinetic properties and predictive *in silico* ADME models. *Bioinformatics* 2008, *24*, 2270–2271.

273. Alland, C., Moreews, F., Boens, D., Carpentier, M., Chiusa, S., Lonquety, M., Renault, N., Wong, Y., Cantalloube, H., Chomilier, J., Hochez, J., Pothier, J., Villoutreix, B. O., Zagury, J. F., and Tuffery, P. RPBS: a web resource for structural bioinformatics. *Nucleic Acids Res.* 2005, *33*, W44–W49.

274. Sperandio, O., Petitjean, M., and Tuffery, P. wwLigCSRre: a 3D ligand-based server for hit identification and optimization. *Nucleic Acids Res.* 2009, *37*, W504–W509.

275. Varnek, A., Fourches, D., Horvath, D., Klimchuk, O., Gaudin, C., Vayer, P., Solov'ev, V., Hoonakker, F., Tetko, I. V., and Marcou, G. ISIDA—platform for virtual screening based on fragment and pharmacophoric descriptors. *Curr. Comput. Aided Drug Des.* 2008, *4*, 191–198.

276. Sanderson, D. M. and Earnshaw, C. G. Computer prediction of possible toxic action from chemical structure; the DEREK system. *Hum. Exp. Toxicol.* 1991, *10*, 261–273.

277. Klopman, G., Chakravarti, S. K., Zhu, H., Ivanov, J. M., and Saiakhov, R. D. ESP: a method to predict toxicity and pharmacological properties of chemicals using multiple MCASE databases. *J. Chem. Inf. Comput. Sci.* 2004, *44*, 704–715.

278. Inpharmatica. ADMENSA INTERACTIVE™. Available at http://www.admensa.com/admensa_old.htm, 2009.

279. FILTER. OpenEye Scientific Software. Available at http://www.eyesopen.com/products/applications/filter.html, 2009.

280. Schrödinger. *QikProp*, 2009.

281. Accelrys. Discovery Studio 2.0. Available at http://accelrys.com/products/discovery-studio/, 2009.

282. Discovery, M., VolSurf+. Available at http://www.moldiscovery.com, 2009.

283. Milletti, F., Storchi, L., Sforna, G., and Cruciani, G. New and original pK_a prediction method using grid molecular interaction fields. *J. Chem. Inf. Model* 2007, *47*, 2172–2181.

284. Woo, Y. T., Lai, D. Y., Argus, M. F., and Arcos, J. C. Development of structure–activity relationship rules for predicting carcinogenic potential of chemicals. *Toxicol. Lett.* 1995, *79*, 219–228.

285. q-pharm. Quantum Pharmaceuticals. Available at http://q-pharm.com/, 2009.

286. MOE. Chemical Computing Group. Available at http://www.chemcomp.com, 2009.

287. ChemAxon. Available at www.chemaxon.com, 2009.

288. Bemis, G. W. and Murcko, M. A. The properties of known drugs. 1. Molecular frameworks. *J. Med. Chem.* 1996, *39*, 2887–2893.

289. Bemis, G. W. and Murcko, M. A. Properties of known drugs. 2. Side chains. *J. Med. Chem.* 1999, *42*, 5095–5099.

290. Krier, M. and Hutter, M. C. Bioisosteric similarity of molecules based on structural alignment and observed chemical replacements in drugs. *J. Chem. Inf. Model* 2009, *49(5)*, 1280–1297.

291. Vainio, M. J. and Johnson, M. S. Generating conformer ensembles using a multiobjective genetic algorithm. *J. Chem. Inf. Model* 2007, *47*, 2462–2474.

292. Schuttelkopf, A. W. and van Aalten, D. M. PRODRG: a tool for high-throughput crystallography of protein–ligand complexes. *Acta Crystallogr. D Biol. Crystallogr.* 2004, *60*, 1355–1363.

293. Leite, T. B., Gomes, D., Miteva, M. A., Chomilier, J., Villoutreix, B. O., and Tuffery, P. Frog: a FRee Online druG 3D conformation generator. *Nucleic Acids Res.* 2007, *35*, W568–W572.

294. Lobell, M., Hendrix, M., Hinzen, B., Keldenich, J., Meier, H., Schmeck, C., Schohe-Loop, R., Wunberg, T., and Hillisch, A. *In silico* ADMET traffic lights as a tool for the prioritization of HTS hits. *ChemMedChem.* 2006, *1*, 1229–1236.

295. Hennemann, M., Friedl, A., Lobell, M., Keldenich, J., Hillisch, A., Clark, T., and Goller, A. H. CypScore: quantitative prediction of reactivity toward cytochromes P450 based on semiempirical molecular orbital theory. *ChemMedChem.* 2009, *4*, 657–669.

296. Pearce, B. C., Sofia, M. J., Good, A. C., Drexler, D. M., and Stock, D. A. An empirical process for the design of high-throughput screening deck filters. *J. Chem. Inf. Model* 2006, *46*, 1060–1068.

297. Stahl, M., Guba, W., and Kansy, M. Integrating molecular design resources within modern drug discovery research: the Roche experience. *Drug Discov. Today* 2006, *11*, 326–333.

298. Alanine, A., Nettekoven, M., Roberts, E., and Thomas, A. W. Lead generation–enhancing the success of drug discovery by investing in the hit to lead process. *Comb. Chem. High Throughput Screen* 2003, *6*, 51–66.

299. Fischer, H. CAFCA a novel tool for the calculation of amphiphilic properties of charged drug molecules. *Chimia* 2000, *54*, 640–645.

300. Davies, J. W., Glick, M., and Jenkins, J. L. Streamlining lead discovery by aligning *in silico* and high-throughput screening. *Curr. Opin. Chem. Biol.* 2006, *10*, 343–351.

301. Steinmeyer, A. The hit-to-lead process at Schering AG: strategic aspects. *ChemMed-Chem.* 2006, *1*, 31–36.

302. Giacomini, K. M., Krauss, R. M., Roden, D. M., Eichelbaum, M., Hayden, M. R., and Nakamura, Y. When good drugs go bad. *Nature* 2007, *446*, 975–977.

303. Gultekin, F. and Hicyilmaz, H. Renal deterioration caused by carcinogens as a consequence of free radical mediated tissue damage: a review of the protective action of melatonin. *Arch. Toxicol.* 2007, *81*, 675–681.

304. Metosh-Dickey, C. A., Mason, R. P., and Winston, G. W. Nitroarene reduction and generation of free radicals by cell-free extracts of wild-type, and nitroreductase-deficient and -enriched *Salmonella typhimurium* strains used in the umu gene induction assay. *Toxicol. Appl. Pharmacol.* 1999, *154*, 126–134.

305. Segers, K., Sperandio, O., Sack, M., Fischer, R., Miteva, M. A., Rosing, J., Nicolaes, G. A., and Villoutreix, B. O. Design of protein membrane interaction inhibitors by virtual ligand screening, proof of concept with the C2 domain of factor V. *Proc. Natl. Acad. Sci. USA* 2007, *104*, 12697–12702.

306. Hodgetts, K. J., Yoon, T., Huang, J., Gulianello, M., Kieltyka, A., Primus, R., Brodbeck, R., De Lombaert, S., and Doller, D. 2-Aryl-3, 6-dialkyl-5-dialkylaminopyrimidin-4-ones as novel crf-1 receptor antagonists. *Bioorg. Med. Chem. Lett.* 2003, *13*, 2497–2500.

307. Egan, W. J., Merz, K. M., Jr., and Baldwin, J. J. Prediction of drug absorption using multivariate statistics. *J. Med. Chem.* 2000, *43*, 3867–3877.

308. Benigni, R. and Bossa, C. Predictivity of QSAR. *J. Chem. Inf. Model* 2008, *48*, 971–980.

309. Kortagere, S., Chekmarev, D., Welsh, W. J., and Ekins, S. New predictive models for blood–brain barrier permeability of drug-like molecules. *Pharm. Res.* 2008, *25*, 1836–1845.

310. Schölkopf, B., Smola, A., and Muller, K. R. Nonlinear component analysis as a kernel eigenvalue problem. *Neural Comput.* 1998, *10*, 1299–1319.

311. Rosipal, R. and Kramer, N. Overview and recent advances in partial least squares, in subspace, latent structure and feature selection techniques. *Lect. Notes Comput. Sci.*, 2006, 34–51.

312. Chohan, K. K., Paine, S. W., Mistry, J., Barton, P., and Davis, A. M. A rapid computational filter for cytochrome P450 1A2 inhibition potential of compound libraries. *J. Med. Chem.* 2005, *48*, 5154–5161.

313. Luco, J. M. Prediction of the brain-blood distribution of a large set of drugs from structurally derived descriptors using partial least-squares (PLS) modeling. *J. Chem. Inf. Comput. Sci.* 1999, *39*, 396–404.

314. Obrezanova, O., Gola, J. M., Champness, E. J., and Segall, M. D. Automatic QSAR modeling of ADME properties: blood–brain barrier penetration and aqueous solubility. *J. Comput. Aided Mol. Des.* 2008, *22*, 431–440.

315. Kriegl, J. M., Eriksson, L., Arnhold, T., Beck, B., Johansson, E., and Fox, T. Multivariate modeling of cytochrome P450 3A4 inhibition. *Eur J. Pharm. Sci.* 2005, *24*, 451–463.

316. Durand, J.-F. and Sabatier, R. Additive splines for partial least squares regression. *J. Am. Stat. Assoc.* 1997, *92*, 1546–1554.

317. Hou, T., Wang, J., and Li, Y. ADME evaluation in drug discovery. 8. The prediction of human intestinal absorption by a support vector machine. *J. Chem. Inf. Model* 2007, *47*, 2408–2415.

318. Karatzoglou, A., Meyer, D., and Hornik, K. *Support Vector Machines in R*, Research Report Series, Wirstchaftuniversitat Wien, 2005.

319. Breiman, L., Friedman, J., Olshen, R., and Stone, C. *Classification and Regression Trees*, New edition (1-1-1984) ed, ed Hall/CRC, Boca Raton, FL, 1984, p. 368.

320. Young, S. S. and Hawkins, D. M. Analysis of a 2(9) full factorial chemical library. *J. Med. Chem.* 1995, *38*, 2784–2788.

321. Rusinko, A., 3rd, Farmen, M. W., Lambert, C. G., Brown, P. L., and Young, S. S. Analysis of a large structure/biological activity data set using recursive partitioning. *J. Chem. Inf. Comput. Sci.* 1999, *39*, 1017–1026.

322. van Rhee, A. M. Use of recursion forests in the sequential screening process: consensus selection by multiple recursion trees. *J. Chem. Inf. Comput. Sci.* 2003, *43*, 941–948.

323. Klekota, J. and Roth, F. P. Chemical substructures that enrich for biological activity. *Bioinformatics* 2008, *24*, 2518–2525.

324. Schneider, N., Jackels, C., Andres, C., and Hutter, M. C. Gradual *in silico* filtering for druglike substances. *J. Chem. Inf. Model* 2008, *48*, 613–628.

325. Deconinck, E., Zhang, M. H., Coomans, D., and Vander Heyden, Y. Classification tree models for the prediction of blood–brain barrier passage of drugs. *J. Chem. Inf. Model* 2006, *46*, 1410–1419.

326. Lamanna, C., Bellini, M., Padova, A., Westerberg, G., and Maccari, L. Straightforward recursive partitioning model for discarding insoluble compounds in the drug discovery process. *J. Med. Chem.* 2008, *51*, 2891–2897.

327. Gleeson, M. P., Waters, N. J., Paine, S. W., and Davis, A. M. *In silico* human and rat vs. quantitative structure–activity relationship models. *J. Med. Chem.* 2006, *49*, 1953–1963.

328. de Cerqueira Lima, P., Golbraikh, A., Oloff, S., Xiao, Y., and Tropsha, A. Combinatorial QSAR modeling of P-glycoprotein substrates. *J. Chem. Inf. Model* 2006, *46*, 1245–1254.

329. Mente, S. R. and Lombardo, F. A recursive-partitioning model for blood–brain barrier permeation. *J. Comput. Aided Mol. Des.* 2005, *19*, 465–481.

330. Sakiyama, Y., Yuki, H., Moriya, T., Hattori, K., Suzuki, M., Shimada, K., and Honma, T. Predicting human liver microsomal stability with machine learning techniques. *J. Mol. Graph Model* 2008, *26*, 907–915.

331. Yamashita, F., Hara, H., Ito, T., and Hashida, M. Novel hierarchical classification and visualization method for multiobjective optimization of drug properties: application to structure-activity relationship analysis of cytochrome P450 metabolism. *J. Chem. Inf. Model* 2008, *48*, 364–369.

332. Arimoto, R., Prasad, M. A., and Gifford, E. M. Development of CYP3A4 inhibition models: comparisons of machine-learning techniques and molecular descriptors. *J. Biomol. Screen* 2005, *10*, 197–205.

333. Breiman, L., Friedman, J., Olshen, R. A., and Stone, C. J. *Classification and Regression Trees*, Wadsworth and Brooks, Florence, KY, 1984.

334. Quinlan, J. R. C4.5: Programs for machine learning. *Mach. Learn.* 1993, *16*, 235–240.

335. Breiman, L. Random forests. *Mach Learn.* 2001, *45*, 5–32.

336. Rosenblatt, F. *Principles of Neurodynamics,* 1960. Spartan Books, Washington, DC, 1962.

337. Huuskonen, J., Salo, M., and Taskinen, J. Neural network modeling for estimation of the aqueous solubility of structurally related drugs. *J. Pharm. Sci.* 1997, *86*, 450–454.

338. Devillers, J., Domine, D., Guillon, C., and Karcher, W. Simulating lipophilicity of organic molecules with a back-propagation neural network. *J. Pharm. Sci.* 1998, *87*, 1086–1090.

339. Bruneau, P. Search for predictive generic model of aqueous solubility using Bayesian neural nets. *J. Chem. Inf. Comput. Sci.* 2001, *41*, 1605–1616.

340. Sadowski, J. and Kubinyi, H. A scoring scheme for discriminating between drugs and nondrugs. *J. Med. Chem.* 1998, *41*, 3325–3329.

341. Tetko, I. V. and Tanchuk, V. Y. Application of associative neural networks for prediction of lipophilicity in ALOGPS 2.1 program. *J. Chem. Inf. Comput. Sci.* 2002, *42*, 1136–1145.

342. Votano, J. R., Parham, M., Hall, L. M., Hall, L. H., Kier, L. B., Oloff, S., and Tropsha, A. QSAR modeling of human serum protein binding with several modeling techniques utilizing structure-information representation. *J. Med. Chem.* 2006, *49*, 7169–7181.

343. Jung, E., Kim, J., Kim, M., Jung, D. H., Rhee, H., Shin, J. M., Choi, K., Kang, S. K., Kim, M. K., Yun, C. H., Choi, Y. J., and Choi, S. H. Artificial neural network models for prediction of intestinal permeability of oligopeptides. *BMC Bioinformatics* 2007, *8*, 245.

344. Polley, M. J., Burden, F. R., and Winkler, D. A. Predictive human intestinal absorption—QSAR models using Bayesian regularized neural networks. *Aust. J. Chem.* 2005, *58*, 859–863.

345. Bazeley, P. S., Prithivi, S., Struble, C. A., Povinelli, R. J., and Sem, D. S. Synergistic use of compound properties and docking scores in neural network modeling of CYP2D6 binding: predicting affinity and conformational sampling. *J. Chem. Inf. Model* 2006, *46*, 2698–2708.

346. Molnar, L. and Keseru, G. M. A neural network based virtual screening of cytochrome P450 3A4 inhibitors. *Bioorg. Med. Chem. Lett.* 2002, *12*, 419–421.

347. Wang, Y. H., Li, Y., Li, Y. H., Yang, S. L., and Yang, L. Modeling *K*(m) values using electrotopological state: substrates for cytochrome P450 3A4-mediated metabolism. *Bioorg. Med. Chem. Lett.* 2005, *15*, 4076–4084.

348. Sadowski, J. Database Profiling by Neural Networks, In *Virtual Screening for Bioactive Molecules*, Wiley, New York, 2000.

349. Gregori-Puigjane, E. and Mestres, J. Coverage and bias in chemical library design. *Curr. Opin. Chem. Biol.* 2008, *12*, 359–365.

350. Caffrey, C. R., Rohwer, A., Oellien, F., Marhofer, R. J., Braschi, S., Oliveira, G., McKerrow, J. H., and Selzer, P. M. A comparative chemogenomics strategy to predict potential drug targets in the metazoan pathogen, *Schistosoma mansoni. PLoS One* 2009, *4*, e4413.

351. de Wildt, S. N., Ito, S., and Koren, G. Challenges for drug studies in children: CYP3A phenotyping as example. *Drug Discov. Today* 2009, *14*, 6–15.

352. Ince, I., de Wildt, S. N., Tibboel, D., Danhof, M., and Knibbe, C. A. Tailor-made drug treatment for children: creation of an infrastructure for data-sharing and population PK-PD modeling. *Drug Discov. Today* 2009, *14*, 316–320.

353. Hilmer, S. N. ADME-tox issues for the elderly. *Expert Opin. Drug Metab. Toxicol.* 2008, *4*, 1321–1331.

354. Jamei, M., Dickinson, G. L., and Rostami-Hodjegan, A. A framework for assessing inter-individual variability in pharmacokinetics using virtual human populations and integrating general knowledge of physical chemistry, biology, anatomy, physiology and genetics: A tale of 'bottom-up' vs. 'top-down' recognition of covariates. *Drug Metab. Pharmacokinet.* 2009, *24*, 53–75.

355. Jamei, M., Marciniak, S., Feng, K., Barnett, A., Tucker, G., and Rostami-Hodjegan, A. The Simcyp((R)) population-based ADME Simulator. *Expert Opin. Drug Metab. Toxicol.* 2009, *5(2)*, 211–223.

356. Hodge, A. E., Altman, R. B., and Klein, T. E. The PharmGKB: integration, aggregation, and annotation of pharmacogenomic data and knowledge. *Clin. Pharmacol. Ther.* 2007, *81*, 21–24.

357. Weskamp, N., Hullermeier, E., and Klebe, G. Merging chemical and biological space: Structural mapping of enzyme binding pocket space. *Proteins* 2009, *76*, 317–330.

358. Yildirim, M. A., Goh, K. I., Cusick, M. E., Barabasi, A. L., and Vidal, M. Drug-target network. *Nat. Biotechnol.* 2007, *25*, 1119–1126.

359. Campillos, M., Kuhn, M., Gavin, A. C., Jensen, L. J., and Bork, P. Drug target identification using side-effect similarity. *Science* 2008, *321*, 263–266.

360. Scheiber, J., Jenkins, J. L., Sukuru, S. C., Bender, A., Mikhailov, D., Milik, M., Azzaoui, K., Whitebread, S., Hamon, J., Urban, L., Glick, M., and Davies, J. W. Mapping Adverse Drug Reactions in Chemical Space. *J. Med. Chem.* 2009, *52*, 3103–3107.

361. Schimmel, K. J., Richel, D. J., van den Brink, R. B., and Guchelaar, H. J. Cardiotoxicity of cytotoxic drugs. *Cancer Treat. Rev.* 2004, *30*, 181–191.

362. Mirza, A., Desai, R., and Reynisson, J. Known drug space as a metric in exploring the boundaries of drug-like chemical space. *Eur. J. Med. Chem.* 2009, *44(12)*, 5006–5011.

363. Hohman, M., Gregory, K., Chibale, K., Smith, P. J., Ekins, S., and Bunin, B. Novel web-based tools combining chemistry informatics, biology and social networks for drug discovery. *Drug Discov. Today* 2009, *14*, 261–270.

364. Yang, L., Luo, H., Chen, J., Xing, Q., and He, L. SePreSA: a server for the prediction of populations susceptible to serious adverse drug reactions implementing the methodology of a chemical-protein interactome. *Nucleic Acids Res.* 2009, *37*, W406–W412.

3

ABSORPTION AND PHYSICOCHEMICAL PROPERTIES OF THE NCE

JON SELBO AND PO-CHANG CHIANG

3.1. INTRODUCTION

Attrition of drug candidates during the discovery and development process is a serious problem for the pharmaceutical industry. Other than a lack of *in vivo* efficacy or unintended toxicological issues, failures are often associated with inappropriate physicochemical characteristics contributing to poor absorption and poor pharmacokinetics [1–3]. The absorption of any chemical entity reflects a very complex series of actions and efficacy can be affected by factors acting in concert or independently. In human physiology, for example, the physicochemical properties of the active ingredient, active or passive transport, disease state, formulation, and dose are often important for bioavailability. Other factors such as dosing interval, fed or fasted state, age, and gender can each affect the oral bioavailability of a given drug. Due to this complexity, optimizing absorption of a drug or formulation often requires full knowledge of how these variables interact. For a given compound it may take years of research before such comprehensive knowledge can be accumulated. In the absence of such detailed information on a new compound, optimization of a candidate to fit certain physicochemical properties and the corresponding first in human formulation is often based on common considerations of factors that affect absorption.

ADMET for Medicinal Chemists: A Practical Guide, Edited by Katya Tsaioun and Steven A. Kates

3.2. PHYSICOCHEMICAL PROPERTIES

During the 1990s almost 40% of the failure in clinical trails was attributed to poor absorption and poor pharmacokinetics [4–6]. In response, pharmaceutical researchers began to focus on a better understanding of target selectivity, toxicological, and physicochemical (pharmacokinetics related) properties of new chemical entities (NCEs) [7, 8]. For example, approaches such as "property-based design" [8], a method for understanding how medicinal chemists could manipulate critical combinations of physical and structural properties that contribute to "drug-like properties," were adopted. The outcome was profound and within a decade, candidate attrition for poor absorption and poor pharmacokinetics properties was reduced to less than 10% of the total failures [4–6].

There have been numerous attempts to predict the properties that are the most desirable for a good drug candidate. Analysis of the structures of orally administered drugs, and of drug candidates, headed by Lipinski and his colleagues [9] led to the establishment of the Lipinski rule of five. The rule states that an orally active drug should have as little violations of these guidelines as possible:

- molecular weight less than 500,
- log P (octanol/water partition coefficient) less than 5,
- no more than five hydrogen bond donors,
- no more than 10 hydrogen bond acceptors.

Other parameters such as polar surface area (PSA) and molecular rigidity as indicated by the number of rotatable bonds (NRB) [10] have also been associated with drugability of NCEs.

More recently, PSA and molecular flexibility (measured as NRB) have been demonstrated to be important predictors of good oral bioavailability [11]. After analyzing more than 1100 drug candidates in rats, Veber et al. found that increasing molecular rigidity had a positive impact on bioavailability while increasing the polar surface area lowered bioavailability. They suggested that compounds with 10 or fewer rotatable bonds and a polar surface area below 140 $Å^2$ would have a higher chance of being orally bioavailable. Molecular weight, independent of NRB, did not appear to correlate with oral bioavailability. At first glance, this result appears to be inconsistent with Lipinski's molecular weight rule. However, given that the major contributors to the PSA are hydrogen-bond donors or acceptors and NRB count frequently increases with MW, these findings are still fairly consistent. PSA has also been reported to correlate with transporter activities within a given molecular scaffold that can be useful in building structure–activities relationships (SAR) [12].

It is worth mentioning that statistical analyses of over 1000 marketed drugs and clinical candidates indicate that lower MW, balanced log P, and greater rigidity remain important features of oral drug molecules [12–15]. Authors of those articles tracked the changes of computed property profiles (MW, Clog P, PSA, etc.) relative to the stage of clinical development candidates. By examining a large database of compounds in clinical development, the authors found that as the stage of development progresses (preclinical, Phase 1, Phase 2, Phase 3, and launch), compounds that are advanced further have lower molecular weight, Clog *P*, and polar surface area [16]. Compounds with excessive molecular weight (>500) or high lipophilicity (Clog $P > 5$), tended to be highly disfavored in clinical development [14, 16]. This suggests that physicochemical properties are intimately linked to physiological control.

Vieth et al. [17, 18] compiled a database of physicochemical properties of marketed drugs, compounds in clinical development, and related molecules known to have biological activity, but not moving forward for clinical development. They distinguished between oral and other routes of administration for the known drugs. Their goal was to establish the optimal physicochemical parameters associated with compounds with good pharmacokinetic properties versus those with poor pharmacokinetic properties [16]. Over 1700 compounds were used in their study. It was not surprising that they found that when compared with oral drugs, injectable drugs have significantly higher MW, number of H-bond acceptors/donors, rotatable bonds, aromatic rings, and much lower Clog *P*. Differences were also distinguished for absorbent and topical compounds compared with oral, although these differences were not as large as those found with injectable drugs. The authors also reported that the average property distributions of oral drugs remains fairly constant over time, suggesting that the properties of successful drug candidates are in a narrowly defined property space, which is in agreement with simple rules such as Lipinski's, NRB, and PSA correlations.

Physicochemical properties have also been correlated with the *in vivo* performance of drug candidates. For example, lipophilicity plays an important role in metabolism by Cytochrome P450 enzymes. Theses enzymes, which mediate the clearance of more than 50% of marketed drugs, have lipophilic active sites that accommodate and metabolize drug molecules. In general, drug clearance increases with the increase of lipophilicity. Common examples include the barbituric acid series [19, 20], β-adrenoceptor antagonists and calcium channel blockers [21], and the diverse structures of CYP3A4 substrates [20]. Other investigations correlating plasma protein binding with physicochemical properties have been reported as well [22, 23].

Compounds may fail for a number of reasons in clinical development. Factors such as no or low efficacy, toxicity, or exposure [16, 24] are likely causes. However, certain physical properties are favored for clinical development of human therapeutic agents. In order to ensure the integration of these drug-like properties into the drug design strategy, a strong emphasis on drug "developability" has been raised within the pharmaceutical industry [25–28]. Empirical rules such as the rule-of-five are now widely applied by many pharmaceutical companies as a first *in silico* filter that flags compounds with potential issues for further development.

3.3. STABILITY

Another important property that impacts bioavailability is the chemical and physical (especially gastrointestinal (GI)) stability of a drug candidate. Chemical stability is discussed here and physical form stability in Section 3.5. For an oral drug to have good bioavailability it needs to be stable *in vivo* and in its formulation so that the performance is consistent over the desired dosing interval. For drugs that are ionizable or contain pH-sensitive functional groups, it is important to measure the pH-stability profile so that the impact of stability on absorption and formulation development can be assessed. The major chemical reactions that lead to degradation of the drug in the GI include hydrolysis, oxidations, and reductions [17, 29]. These processes are often catalyzed by pH, and/or enzymes in the small intestine, and the bacterial flora of the lower intestinal tract. Stewart and Tucker have listed some common classes of drugs that are subject to hydrolysis. The list includes esters, thiol esters, amides, sulfonamides, imides, lactams, lactones, and halogenated aliphatics [18, 30–32]. Intestinal (including colonic) stability is an important factor to consider for compounds that need controlled release profiles. Some examples of drugs that are biotransformed in the large intestine include atropine, digoxin, indomethacin, phenacetin, and sulfinpyrazone [18, 33].

Stability assessment in common cosolvents is an important consideration because solubilizing agents are often used to increase solubility in formulations. This is especially true for poorly soluble compounds, where high percentages of organics are used. Other types of stability such as photo, hygroscopicity, and heat sensitivity need to be monitored as well. These can play an important role on the final product development (dosage form), shelf life, and packaging.

3.4. DISSOLUTION AND SOLUBILITY

3.4.1. Dissolution Rate, Particle Size, and Solubility

For oral drug delivery, the availability of a drug to be absorbed depends on its ability to dissolve in GI fluids during the transit time through areas of the GI track where it can be absorbed. If the rate of dissolution (not to be confused with its equilibrium solubility) is the rate-limiting step in drug absorption, any feature affecting the dissolution rate will have an impact on bioavailability. The dissolution rate can be expressed by the well-known diffusion-layer model, modified Noyes–Whitney equation [34–37]:

$$\frac{dc}{dt} = \frac{DA}{hv}(C_s - C)$$

where the dissolution rate is given by dc/dt, D is the diffusion coefficient, h is the diffusion layer thickness, A is the surface area of drug exposed to the dissolution media, v is the volume of the dissolution media, C_s is the saturated solubility of the drug in the dissolution medium at the experimental temperature, and C is the concentration of drug in solution at time t.

A common practice to increase the apparent dissolution rate and subsequently the bioavailability for compounds, where the oral absorption is limited, is to decrease the particle size of the drug. Reducing the particle size increases the surface area available to the dissolution media and increases the overall apparent dissolution rate. The use of nanoparticles for the delivery of poorly water-soluble drugs has been increasingly used [36, 38–46]. In addition to dissolution improvements, nanolized particles offer advantages such as GI retention [51], and solubility improvements. There are various patents and publications describing nanoparticulate drug preparations and applications [47–57].

Particle size reduction is accomplished by two general approaches. These are (1) dissolving the drug and reconstructing particles from their molecular state, such as fast precipitation or rapid expansion; or (2) by breaking large particles, such as by milling. The approach of producing and maintaining a stable particle size reduced system is not free of problems. Challenges such as solid form changes, physicochemical stability, and well-characterized formulations must be addressed. Furthermore, if a wet milling/suspension system is used, the effect on changing particle size in an aqueous environment needs to be understood. The potential for particle agglomeration has been examined by researchers and summarized in detail [36, 47, 48]. In theory, the new surface area generated by either approach requires an energy cost. The energy increase due to the increase in surface area by either procedure will create a less stable system. Such a system will have a tendency to offset the increase in surface area and thereby reduce energy by agglomeration. This phenomenon can be controlled by introducing surfactants and controlling temperature. The addition of surfactants can provide stabilization at longer times due to an increased energy barrier and, along with lowering temperature, prevents particles from coming close enough to cause agglomeration [36, 48].

Despite the advantages of increasing the dissolution rate through particle size reduction, the solubility of the drug plays the most pivotal role in the absorption process. Solubility is one of the most important properties impacting bioavailability because of its role in dissolution and absorption. Solubility and permeability are the two main factors defining the biopharmaceutics classification system (BCS) used by the FDA as a guide for predicting intestinal drug absorption (Figure 3.1) [58].

Although some materials such as glucose and L-amino acids are absorbed by active transport across the intestinal barrier, absorption by passive diffusion is far more common [59]. For a drug administrated orally to enter the circulation system, it must dissolve in the solution phase first and then diffuse into and across the wall of the intestinal lumen. Improving the solubility of the drug is a major approach to absorption enhancement for oral drug delivery. In preclinical and clinical development, various methods and vehicles are used to enhance the solubility of drug candidates. Vehicles such as cosolvents, emulsions, and cyclodextrins are commonly used to improve drug solubility. Despite the success of using these tools, a solid understanding of factors affecting solubility is crucial in addressing deficiencies in formulation caused by poor solubility.

Solubility of a given compound in aqueous media is governed by the intermolecular forces between the solvent and the solute and the entropy changes associated with that interaction. A full treatment of solubility as applied to pharmaceutics is well beyond this text [60–62]. However, it should be understood that factors such as

Permeability

High ↓ Low

Class 1 HS/HP High solubility High permeability	**Class 2** LS/HP Low solubility High permeability
Class 3 HS/LP High solubility Low permeability	**Class 4** LS/LP Low solubility Low permeability

Solubility

High ⟶ Low

Figure 3.1 Biopharmaceutics classification system.

temperature (Van't Hoff equation), pressure, pH (Section 3.4.2), the ionic strength of the aqueous media, and the solid form (Section 3.5) used will affect the balance of these interactions and change the overall solubility.

Increasing solubility and supersaturation in GI fluid are important attributes that can affect drug absorption. Supersaturation is particularly important for compounds with poor intrinsic solubility and is the limiting factor for absorption. Creating or maintaining supersaturation in the GI fluid is a must to enhance absorption of these compounds. Formulations with cosolvents, the use of excipients for solubilization, inclusion, or suspension, and the use of pH adjustment or salts have been used for this purpose.

3.4.2. pH and Salts

In practical terms, the medicinal chemist is often asked to find efficacious candidates within a series that have better solubility and in many cases pharmaceutical scientists are required to formulate low solubility materials to properly assess efficacy and toxicity during exposure. Adding ionizable groups that have a pK_a in a physiologically useful range can provide options for formulators and materials scientists to solve solubility and dissolution rate issues [64]. For ionizable drugs, the intrinsic solubility is defined by the unionized form. However, the solubility profile will be pH sensitive and optimizing solubility in the formulation may be achieved by altering the pH of the solution/suspension or by dosing a soluble salt.

The solubility of an ionizable compound can be calculated from its pH-solubility profile as given by the Henderson–Hasselbalch equation. For example, for a slightly soluble weak acidic electrolyte with single pK_a, the solubility and pH can be expressed as follows:

$$HA_{(\text{solid})} \rightarrow HA_{(\text{sol})}$$

$$HA_{(\text{solid})} \rightarrow A^{-} + H^{+}$$

$$K_a = \frac{[A^-][H^+]}{[HA]_{(sol)}}$$

$$pK_a = \log\frac{[A^-][H^+]}{[HA]_{(sol)}} = \log[H^+] + \log\frac{[A^-]}{[HA]_{(sol)}}$$

$$pH = pK_a + \log\frac{[A^-]}{[HA]_{(sol)}} \quad \text{(Henderson–Hasselbalch equation)}$$

$$\text{Sol}_{(total)} = [HA]_{(sol)} + [A^-], \text{ where } [HA]_{(sol)} = \text{intrinsic solubility} = S_0$$

$$\text{Sol}_{(total)} = S_0\left(1 + \frac{K_a}{[H^+]}\right)$$

$$\begin{aligned}\text{Sol}_{(total)} &= S_0\left(1 + 10^{(pH - pK_a)}\right)_{(Acid)} = S_0\left(1 + 10^{(pK_a - pH)}\right)_{(Base)} \\ &= S_0\left(1 + 10^{(pK_a - pH)} + 10^{(pH - pK_a)}\right)_{(Ampholyte)}\end{aligned}$$

For a simple acid base titration, the above relationship holds only at equilibrium, where the product of the ionized species and counter ion is below its solubility product (K_{sp}). The K_{sp} of a salt is defined as the equilibrium constant for the aqueous disassociation into its ionic species as in the example below:

$$A_xB_{y(S)} = xA^{y+}{}_{(aq)} + yB^{x-}{}_{(aq)}$$

$$K_{sp} = [A^{y+}]^x[B^{x-}]^y$$

This equilibrium region is typically referred to as $pH < pH_{max}$, where pH_{max} is defined as the pH where the solution is saturated with respect to both the free and salt forms. Once the pH drops below pH_{max} and the salt forms, the solubility is governed by the K_{sp} [63–65]. This phenomenon is illustrated in Figure 3.2. The quadratic equation for expressing the pH_{max} of a base is

$$pH_{max} = pK_a + \log\frac{S_0}{\sqrt{K_{sp}}}$$

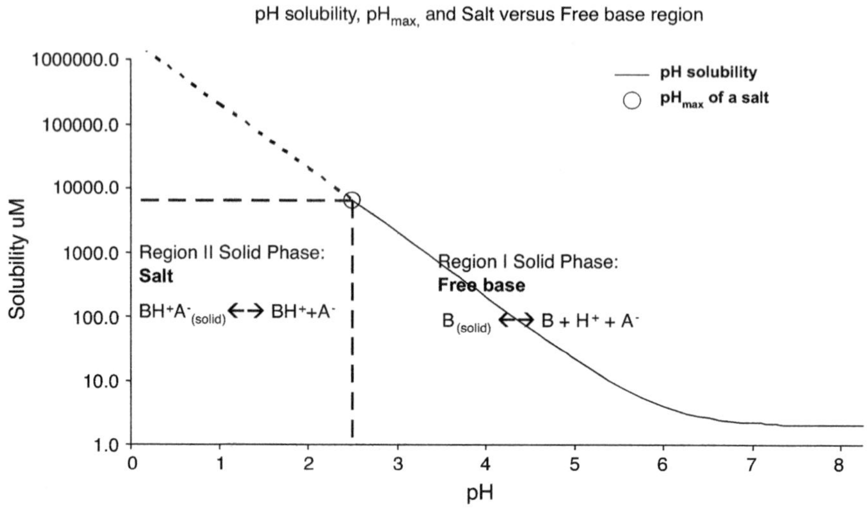

Figure 3.2 pH solubility curve for a basic drug.

However, enhanced salt solubility may not guarantee better *in vivo* absorption [66–68]. When a salt or pH-adjusted formulation is used, the degree of bioavailability improvement may be largely dependent on the degree of supersaturation with respect to the equilibrium solubility in GI tract [69, 70]. The effect of better solubility on bioavailability may be neutralized in the gastric or intestinal environment when changes in the pH decrease the solubility and cause the ionized species to precipitate as the free form. Table 3.1 lists reported pH changes during transit in the GI tract of a fasted and fed human [71, 72]:

For a weak base, when the pH rises above the pK_a, the degree of supersaturation becomes a kinetically controlled phenomenon and the improvement in bioavailability due to supersaturation is dependent on the rate of free form precipitation. Regardless of the pH of the system, the pH change induced by the salt at the dissolution layer may facilitate dissolution and retard free form precipitation. The salt acts as its own buffer once in the solvated state and the dynamics of precipitation and absorption may result in a net enhancement of amount dissolved and absorbed. The kinetic nature of the process often leads to higher exposure variability *in vivo*. The inclusion, if feasible, of

TABLE 3.1 Gastrointestinal pHs for Human Subjects

Site	pH Fasted	pH Fed
Stomach	1.4–2.1	3.0–7.0
Jejunum	4.4–6.6	5.2–6.2
Ileum	6.8–8.0	6.8–8.0
Colon	5.0–8.0	5.0–8.0

basic or acidic functional groups in drug candidates with pK_a's where the molecule will be fully ionized within the desired physiologic relevant pH range will mitigate this issue.

The selection of a suitable counter ion can be important for a salt approach [69, 70]. Supersaturation and precipitation phenomenon can be expressed as the change in Gibbs free energy for transitioning from a supersaturated solution to equilibrium:

$$\Delta G = -R_g T \ln S_x$$

where R_g is the gas constant, T is the absolute temperature, and S_x is the supersaturation ratio which is concentration dependent. As the change in free energy increases, the driving force for precipitation increases. Thus, the salt with the highest solubility may quickly precipitate and may not necessarily provide the highest *in vivo* exposure.

Classically for many drugs hydrochlorides were often the first and sometimes the only salts considered when searching for a more soluble form. However, the presence of chloride ions in gastric acid may well depress solubility *in vivo* compared to other salt forms because of common ion effects [73–76]. It is a particular concern in the stomach, where the acidic pH and high concentration of the chloride ion can be problematic for many basic compounds. Conversion in the stomach to a hydrochloride salt is a problem if the hydrochloride salt is poorly soluble or oppositely if the hydrochloride salt is highly soluble in the stomach but precipitates in the small intestine due to unwanted physicochemical changes (i.e., a salt or particle size change). The conversion to a hydrochloride salt can be avoided by use of enteric coating techniques [18, 77].

In the intestine, the presence of bile salts and other components such as lipids usually improve the intrinsic solubility of the free base and shift pH_{max} to higher values [18]. The potential for absorption enhancement by salts are typically explored via *in vivo* studies in small animals prior to administration to humans. Animal studies provide useful rank ordering for different salts, but are not necessarily linearly predictive of human absorption. Caution should be taken that these preclinical formulations should contain excipients compatible with human administration and it should be understood that they may not encompass all possible human physiological conditions [70].

3.4.3. *In Vivo* Solubilization

Drug solubility can be enhanced by food and natural bile production in the stomach and intestine. Components such as bile salts, lecithin, and monooleins help solubilize drugs. However, depending on the physicochemical properties of the drug, the degree of solubilization may vary. Log *P*, MW, and specific interactions between drugs and bile salts have different degrees of impact on bile–lecithin micelle solubility [78, 79]. There is growing evidence that bile salt–lecithin mixed micelles are good solvents for lipophilic drugs [79–81]. For drugs that fall into this category, the total solubility of the drug is proportional to the bile salt concentration and there is an increase in

TABLE 3.2 Composition of Two Simulated Intestinal Fluid Media Used for *In Vitro* Testing of Drug Solubility

FaSSIF[a]	FeSSIF[b]
Sodium taurocholate 3 mM	Sodium taurocholate 15 mM
Lecithin 0.75 mM	Lecithin 3.75 mM
NaOH (pellets) 0.174 g	NaOH (pellets) 4.04 g
$NaH_2PO_4.H_2O$ 1.977 g	Glacial acetic acid 8.65 g
NaCl 3.093 g	NaCl 11.874 g
Purified water qs. 500 mL	Purified water qs. 1000 mL

[a] FaSSIF media has a pH of 6.50 and an osmolality of about 270 mOsmol/kg.
[b] FeSSIF media has a pH of 5.00 and an osmolality of about 670 mOsmol/kg.

solubilization with an increase in log P [78, 82–85]. Thus, for drugs that are lipophilic, solubility measurements in physiologically relevant media are highly recommended.

Two physiologically relevant media developed by Dressman et al. based on literature and experimental data in dogs and humans have been used extensively in the pharmaceutical industry and academic research. They are the fasted-state simulated intestinal fluid (FaSSIF) and fed-state simulated intestinal fluid (FeSSIF) [86, 87]. The compositions of FaSSIF and FeSSIF are listed in Table 3.2.

3.5. SOLID STATE

The three classical states of matter are solids, liquids, and gases. The most common physical state targeted for storage and formulation of an active pharmaceutical ingredient (API) is a solid because of its relative stability and reproducibility. Even in the case of liquid formulations, the API is typically harvested as a solid and later incorporated with solvents and excipients. An API may precipitate in a number of different solid-state forms. These are commonly classified as amorphous, partially crystalline (crystalline with some degree of disorder), and crystalline. Crystalline materials can further be classified into their polymorphic forms or in the case of solvent inclusion, solvates (desolvated or partially desolvated solvates).

Amorphous materials such as plastics or glasses are solids that are made up of a random arrangement of their constituent parts (atoms or molecules). Figure 3.3 shows a representation of amorphous and crystalline solids. The purely amorphous form is the highest energy (ΔG) solid form available and is thermodynamically unstable with respect to its crystalline counterparts. As a result, if a nucleus of crystalline material was to form and there was enough motility in the system to allow the molecules to rearrange, the amorphous material will change form and crystallize. Materials that become kinetically "stuck" between crystalline and amorphous phases are referred to as partially amorphous, partially crystalline, or crystalline with disorder. This can include mesophases with liquid crystalline behavior [88]. There may be an infinite number of different amorphous and partially crystalline states depending on the

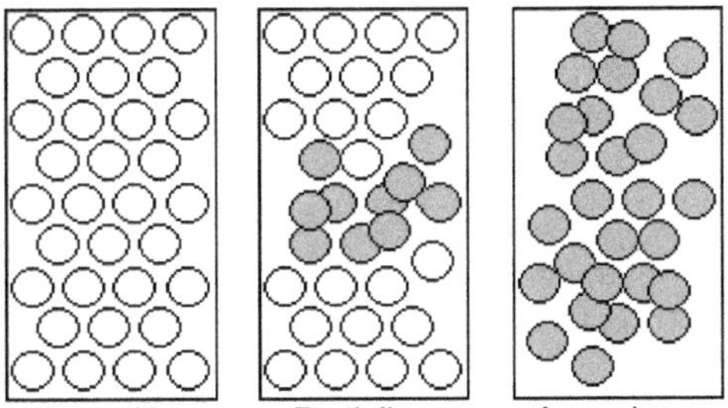

Figure 3.3 A simple two-dimensional example representing a crystalline to amorphous system.

orientation of the molecules in the amorphous material and the degree of crystallinity that is incorporated.

Crystalline materials are well-ordered solids, whose constituent parts are arranged to produce a repeating pattern throughout the solid lattice. The minimum arrangement of parts (molecules) that can be translated throughout the solid is defined as the unit cell. It serves as a building block for the solid and is unique to the molecule in that particular molecular arrangement. However, for a given system, a molecule may crystallize into more than one type of unit cell. These different configurations are defined as polymorphic forms and have different physical properties such as melting points and solubility [89, 90]. Also, there may exist related forms such as hydrates (water) or other solvates, where a solvent molecule is incorporated into the lattice to produce a new form. The most common analytical tool used to identify the form of a drug candidate is powder x-ray diffraction. Figure 3.4 shows powder x-ray diffraction data for an amorphous form, a hydrate, and two polymorphic forms of the same candidate.

Ostwald's rule of stages and Gay-Lussac's observations predict that the progression of discovered forms for a particular molecule over time will be from the highest energy form to the lowest [91]. For the medicinal chemist this often means that an amorphous form is first isolated by quick stripping of the solvent or by lyophilization and then a more stable crystalline form will appear as conditions allow. The most stable form at room temperature will eventually be discovered and the system will be at equilibrium (assuming no solvates). However, in reality this is not necessarily true. The likelihood for crystallization to occur within a given system is completely dependent on the formation of a stable nucleus of a crystalline form and the ability of that nucleus to grow. Given that the most stable form at a particular temperature is thermodynamically favored in any solvent except when a solvate of that solvent exists, only kinetic processes will prevent the transformation from occurring. Factors that affect the rate of polymorphic or solvate transformation can include solvent solubility, impurities that impact nucleation or growth, the energy difference between the two states, and the temperature of the entire system [92–94].

Another important concept is the relationship of polymorphs with respect to temperature at a given pressure. Figure 3.5 shows a general example of the differences

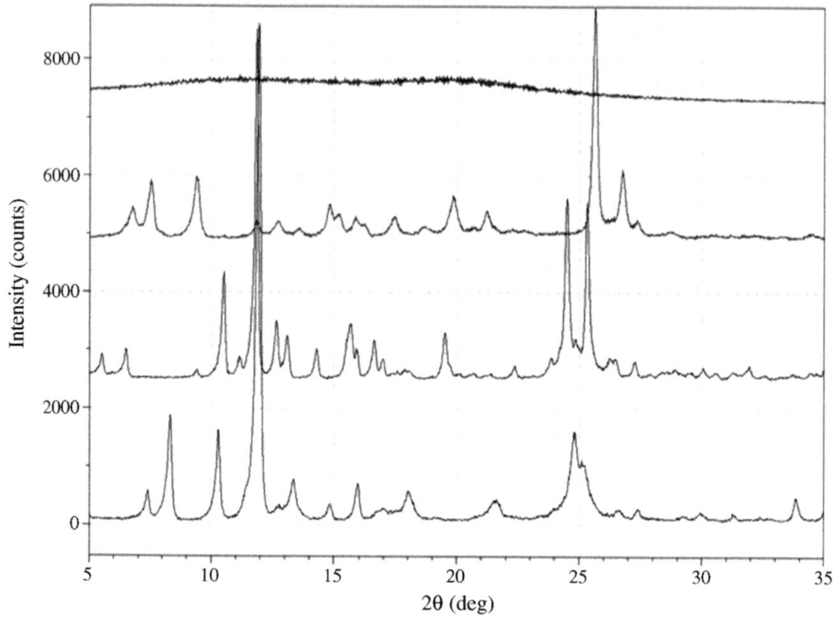

Figure 3.4 Powder X-ray diffraction data showing different forms of the same molecule.

in energy for two types of polymorphic systems with respect to temperature. In each graph, the Gibbs free energy curve for Forms 1 (dashed line) and 2 (solid line) are shown as a function of temperature. The melting points (T_{m1} and T_{m2}) are defined by intersection of the liquidus line (above which the material would be a liquid) with the energy curve for the specific form. T_c is the crossover temperature between Forms 1 and 2.

The energy temperature diagram on the left depicts a monotropic system where Form 1 is metastable (higher energy) with respect to Form 2 at all temperatures below

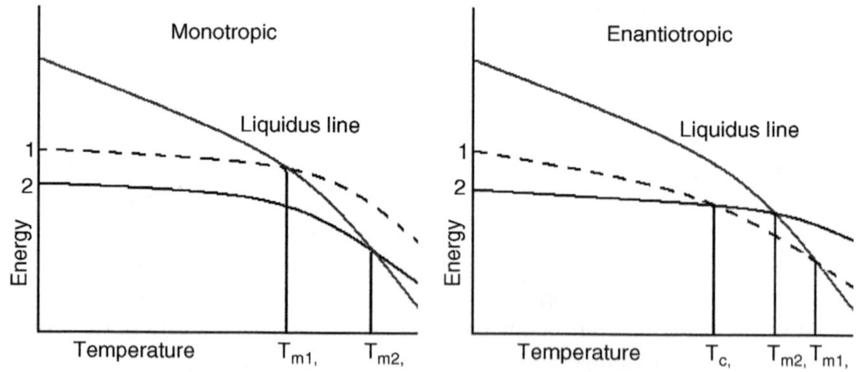

Figure 3.5 Energy diagrams showing an example of the thermodynamic relationships between two polymorphs.

its melt. The diagram on the right shows an example of an enantiotropic system where there is a crossover at some temperature (T_c) prior to the melting onset. For the enantiotropic system, Form 1 becomes more stable (lower energy) above the crossover temperature. Thermodynamically, crystallizations will favor the most stable form at the temperature of the crystallization. However, kinetic conditions and the effect of the microenvironment may cause the nucleation and growth of the unstable form.

For either system if the metastable form is harvested, it may or may not be physically stable depending on the appropriate conditions for the nucleation and growth of the more stable form. Solids may spontaneously undergo a solid-to-solid form conversion without the presence of solvent mediation. However, in most cases the more stable form can be achieved by recrystallization (at a temperature below T_c for the enantiotropic system) with seeding of the stable form or by slurry in a solvent that provides enough solubility to allow for the transfer of material from one form to another. If these techniques are not successful, it is often the role of impurities that may act as nucleation or growth inhibitors [94].

A good method to determine the unknown stable form at a given temperature is to slurry clean material in a panel of solvents of good solubility. Anecdotal evidence suggests that for reasonable slurry times (~1–2 weeks) a solubility of 8 mmol or higher should be targeted [94]. In practice, a number of solvents with varying chemical properties should be used in stable form screening to provide the best chance for solubilization of the API and to minimize/change impurity profiles.

Why do crystallinity, polymorphism, or solvates matter to a discussion of ADME properties? The physical form of a material affects a multitude of physical properties that can impact the bioavailability and development of a drug candidate [89, 95]. Some examples of these include:

- solubility and dissolution rate;
- physical and chemical stability;
- melting point, hygroscopicity, and solvent retention;
- particle size, morphology, hardness, and bulk density;
- purity.

A change in the form of a substance will affect the physical properties. However, the impact of the form on solubility and dissolution rate is the most important consideration for patient safety. If a drug candidate's exposure is dissolution rate-limited (i.e., permeability is high enough that a change in solubility will impact the amount of API being absorbed and the clearance is low enough that the drug becomes systemic), any change that results in the crystallization of a more stable form will cause a loss of exposure and the possibility that the drug may become subtherapeutic. Alternatively, if a higher energy form is used, exposures may become greater due to higher absorption, and toxicity may occur. This may have a deleterious affect on a project at any stage and is the reason that control of the physical form or proof of bioequivalence is required by the FDA [96].

Early in the discovery process there are typically not enough resources, or compound to conduct full solid-state characterization. Frequently hit-to-lead and lead optimization as well as early preclinical development are performed with amorphous or metastable forms of API. Only in late lead optimization or lead profiling stages an assessment of the physical properties of the known forms is commenced. Typical assessed properties include crystallinity (most often by PXRD), melting point, weight loss on heating, moisture sorption, and chemical and physical stability (e.g., formation of a hydrate). The stable form at room temperature should be assessed by a stable form screen and the risks to changes in the form addressed, especially if the stable form was not used during preclinical testing. It is important to remember that the most stable form is thermodynamically favored and any metastable forms will convert given the right conditions. If this occurs in a formulation or even *in vivo*, the result may be a loss of bioavailability causing a significant project setback or even failure. Formation of a hydrate can lead to a multifold loss in solubility. Given the aqueous nature of the gastric process, it can be difficult to dose the API in such a way as to avoid form conversions [70]. Later in development, other factors affected by the solid state, such as formulation stability, tableting characteristics, flow, resistance to deformation on grinding, and intellectual property become important.

Hitherto it has been assumed that the best crystalline form is the most stable form at room temperature, if exposure is not an issue. However, there are a number of formulation-stabilized metastable forms that may provide higher exposures *in vivo*. In the short-term, high-energy amorphous forms may be stabilized so that the delivery of an amorphous API is feasible [97–99]. Examples of stabilization techniques include hot-melt extrusion, freeze drying, and spray drying.

Spray-dried dispersions (SDDs) of low-solubility drugs using hydroxypropyl methylcellulose acetate succinate (HPMCAS) have been prepared. It has been reported that SDDs containing HPMCAS provide supersaturation *in vitro* dissolution determinations and large bioavailability increases *in vivo* [98]. These SDDs provided amorphous drug/polymer colloids and an increased concentration of free drug and drug in micelles relative to crystalline or amorphous drug. A melting temperature (T_m)/glass-transition temperature (T_g) (K/K) versus log P map for 139 compounds formulated as SDDs gave a perspective on an appropriate formulation strategy for low-solubility drugs with various physical properties was also reported [98].

To realistically estimate the impact of solubility on absorption, solubility and the degree of supersaturation in more physiologically relevant media should be determined. Even if an SDD can be prepared and is physically and chemically stable for use, depending on the dose and percent loading of the polymer it may not be useful for attaining project goals. This is especially true for regulatory toxicity studies where the dose required to achieve a desired exposure is often much higher. If the amorphous state of an API becomes important to its development, further characterization should be conducted to determine important solid characteristics that may be used for intellectual property claims.

Although the physical form of a candidate may not be well characterized prior to its selection for advancement into regulatory toxicity studies and clinical development, it can impact *in vitro* and *in vivo* testing. Comparison of exposure results from dissimilar forms may lead to interpretation issues that can complicate candidate comparison or selection. More consistent and reliable *in vitro* and *in vivo* results will be obtained, the earlier in discovery that a stable crystalline form is achieved. The benefit for the medicinal chemist is that data underpinning structure–activity relationships will be more useful for the selection and advancement of a good candidate. As with any endeavor, a balance must be achieved between the amount of work done versus the risk to the success of the project. Given the importance of understanding the physical form, early analysis of the intrinsic physical properties is essential for a well-designed testing funnel.

REFERENCES

1. Hodgson, J. ADMET—turning chemicals into drugs. *Nat. Biotechnol.* 2001, *19*, 722–726.
2. Avdeef, A. High throughput measurements of solubility profiles. In *Pharmacokinetic Optimization in Drug Research; Biological, Physicochemical, and Computational Strategies*, Testa, B. et al. (eds.), Verlag Helvitica Chimica Acta, Zurich, 2001, pp. 305–326.
3. Curatolo, W. Physicochemical properties of oral drug candidates in the discovery and exploratory development settings. *Pharm. Sci. Technol. Today* 1998, *1*, 387–393.
4. Kola, I. and Landis, J. Can the pharmaceutical industry reduce attrition rates? *Nat. Rev. Drug Discov.* 2004, *3*, 711–715.
5. Boyd, R. A. and Lalonde, R. L. Nontraditional approaches to first-in-human studies to increase efficiency of drug development: will microdose studies make a significant impact? *Clin. Pharmacol. Ther.* 2007, *81*, 24–26.
6. Innovation or Stagnation?: Challenge and Opportunity on the Critical Path to New Medical Products. U.S. Department of Health and Human Services, Food and Drug Administration, 2004. Available at http://www.fda.gov/oc/initiatives/criticalpath/whitepaper.pdf.
7. Baxter, A. D. and Lockey, P. M. 'Hit' to 'lead' and 'lead' to 'candidate' optimization using multi-parametric principles. *Drug Discov. World* 2001, *3*, 9–15.
8. Van de Waterbeemd, H., et al. Property-based design: optimisation of drug absorption and pharmacokinetics. *J. Med. Chem.* 2001, *44*, 1313–1333.
9. Lipinski, C. A., Lombardo, F., Dominy, B. W., and Feeney, P. J. Experimental and computational approaches to estimate solubility and permeability in drug discovery and development settings. *Adv. Drug Deliv. Rev.* 1997, *23*, 3–25.
10. Veber, D. F., Johnson, S. R., Cheng, H. Y., Smith, B. R., Ward, K. W., and Kopple, K. D. Molecular properties that influence the oral bioavailability of drug candidates. *J. Med. Chem.* 2002, *45*, 2615–2623.
11. Veber, D. F., Johnson, S. R., Cheng, H.-Y., Smith, B. R., Ward, K. W., and Kopple, K. D. Molecular properties that influence the oral bioavailability of drug candidates. *J. Med. Chem.* 2002, *45*, 2615–2623.
12. Fernandes, J. and Gattass, C. R. Topological polar surface area defines substrate transport by multidrug resistance associated protein 1 (MRP1/ABCC1). *J. Med. Chem.* 2009, *52*, 1214–1218.
13. Wenlock, M. C., Austin, R. P., Barton, P., Davis, A. M., and Leeson P. D. A comparison of physicochemical property profiles of development and marketed oral drugs. *J. Med. Chem.* 2003, *46*, 1250–1256.

14. Blake, J. F. Examination of the computed molecular properties of compounds selected for clinical development. *BioTechniques* 2003, *34*, S16–S20.
15. Oprea, T. I. Current trends in lead discovery: are we looking for the appropriate properties? *J. Comput. Aided Mol. Des.* 2002, *16*, 325–334.
16. Blake, J. F. Integrating cheminformatic analysis in combinatorial chemistry. *Curr. Opin. Chem. Biol.* 2004, *8(4)*, 407–411.
17. Vieth, M., Siegel, M. G., Higgs, R. E., Watson, I. A., Robertson, D. H., Savin, K. A., Durst, G. L., and Hipskind P. A. Characteristic physical properties and structural fragments of marketed oral drugs. *J. Med. Chem.* 2004, *47*, 224–232.
18. Tong, W.-Q. Molecular and Physicochemical Properties Impacting Oral Absorption of Drugs. In *Biopharmaceutics Applications in Drug Development*, Krishna, R. and Yu, L. (eds.), Springer, US, 2008, pp. 26–46.
19. Smith, D. A., Jones, B. C., and Walker, D. K. Design of drugs involving the concepts and theories of drug metabolism and pharmacokinetics. *Med. Res. Rev.* 1996, *16(3)*, 243–266.
20. Davis, A. M., Webborn, P. J. H., and Salt, D. W. Robust assessment of statistical significance in the use of unbound/intrinsic pharmacokinetic parameters in quantitative structure–pharmacokinetic relationships with lipophilicity. *Drug Metab. Dis.* 2000, *28(2)*, 103–106.
21. Van de Waterbeemd, H., Smith, D. A., and Jones, B. C. Lipophilicity in PK Design: Methyl, Ethyl, Futile. *J. Comput. Aided Mol. Des.* 2001, *15*, 273–286.
22. Lobell, M. and Sivarajah V. *In silico* prediction of aqueous solubility, human plasma protein binding and volume of distribution of compounds from calculated pK_a and *A* log*P*98 values. *Mol. Divers.* 2003, *7*, 69–87.
23. Yamazaki, K. and Kanaoka, M. Computational prediction of the plasma protein-binding percent of diverse pharmaceutical compounds. *J. Pharm. Sci.* 2004, *93(6)*, 1480–1494.
24. Venkatesh, S. and Lipper, R. A. Role of the development scientist in compound lead selection and optimization. *J. Pharm. Sci.* 2000, *89*, 145–154.
25. Huang, L. F. and Tong, W. Q. Impact of solid state properties on developability assessment of drug candidates. *Adv. Drug Deliv. Rev.* 2004, *56*, 321–334.
26. Kerns, E. H. and Di, L. Pharmaceutical profiling in drug discovery. *Drug Discov. Today* 2003, *8(7)*, 316–323.
27. Proudfoot, R. Drugs, leads, and drug-likeness: an analysis of some recently launched drugs. *Bioorg. Med. Chem. Lett.* 2002, *12*, 1647–1650.
28. Borchardt, R. T., Kerns, H., Hageman, M. J., Thakker, D. R., and Stevens J. L. *Optimizing the "Drug-Like" Properties of Leads in Drug Discovery*, AAPS Press, Arlington, VA, 2006.
29. Walker, S. E. and Hardy B. G. Alteration in apparent bioequivalency of ibuprofen based on isomer analysis. *J. Clin. Pharmacol.* 1992, *32*, 915–957.
30. Van den Mooter, G. Colon drug delivery. *Expert Opin. Drug Deliv.* 2006, *3(1)*, 111–125.
31. Gibson, M. *Pharmaceutical Preformulation and Formulation: A Practical Guide from Candidate Drug Selection to Commercial Dosage Form*, Interpharm/CRC, Boca Raton, FL, 2004.
32. Stewart, P. J. and Tucker, I. G. Prediction of drug stability—Part 2: hydrolysis. *Aust. J. Hosp. Pharm.* 1985, *15*, 11–16.

33. Sarfaraz, N. *Handbook of Preformulation: Chemical, Biological, and Botanical Drugs*, CRC Press, Boca Raton, FL, 2006.
34. Dressman, J. B. Dissolution Testing of Immediate-Release Products and its Application to Forcasting *In Vivo* Performance. In *Oral Drug Absorption, Prediction and Assessment*, Dressman, J. B. and Lennernas, H. (eds.), Marcel Dekker, New York, 2000, pp. 155–181.
35. Lai, Y., Chiang, P. C., Blom, J. D., Li, N., Shevlin, K., Brayman, T. G., Hu, Y., Selbo, J. G., and Hu, L. Comparison of *in vitro* nanoparticles uptake in various cell lines and *in vivo* pulmonary cellular transport in intratracheally dosed rat model. *Nanoscale Res. Lett.* 2008, *3*, 321–329.
36. Chiang, P.-C., Wahlstrom, J. L., Selbo, J. G., et al. 1,3-Dicyclohexyl urea nanosuspension for intravenous steady-state delivery in rats. *J. Exp. Nanosci.* 2007, *2*, 239–250.
37. Sinko, P. J. (ed.). *Martin's Physical Pharmacy*, 4th Edition, Williams & Wilkins, Baltimore, MD, 1993.
38. Akers, M. J., Fites, A. L., and Robison, R. L. Formulation design and development of parenteral suspensions. *J. Parenter. Sci. Tech.* 1987, *41*, 88–96.
39. Liversidge, G. and Gundy, K. Particle size reduction for improvement of oral bioavailability of hydrophobic drugs: absolute oral bioavailability of nanocrystalline danazol in beagle dogs. *Int. J. Pharm.* 1995, *125*, 91–97.
40. Liversidge, G. and Conzention, P. Drug particle size reduction for decreasing gastric irritancy and enhancing absorption of naproxen in rats. *Int. J. Pharm.* 1995, *125*, 309–313.
41. Viernstein, J. and Stumpf, C. Similar central actions of intravenous methohexitone suspension and solution in the rabbit. *J. Pharm. Pharmacol.* 1992, *44*, 66–68.
42. Boedeker, B. H., Lojeski, E. W., Kline, M. D., and Haynes, D. H. Ultra-long-duration local anesthesia produced by injection of lecithin-coated tetracaine microcrystals. *J. Clin. Pharmacol.* 1994, *34*, 699–702.
43. Moghimi, S. M., Hunter, A. C., and Murray, J. C. Long-circulating and target-specific nanoparticles: theory to practice. *Pharmacol. Rev.* 2001, *53*, 283–318.
44. Lamprecht, A., Schäfer, U., and Lehr, C.-M. Size-dependent bioadhesion of micro- and nanoparticulate carriers to the inflamed colonic mucosa. *Pharm. Res.* 2001, *18*, 788–794.
45. Grau, M. J., Kayser, O., and Muller, R. H. Nanosuspensions of poorly soluble drugs-reproducibility of small scale production. *Int. J. Pharm.* 2000, *196(2)*, 155–159.
46. Sajeesh, S. and Sharma, C. P. Cyclodextrin–insulin complex encapsulated polymethacrylic acid based nanoparticles for oral insulin delivery. *Int. J. Pharm.* 2006, *25*, 147–154.
47. Ziller, K. H. and Rupprecht, H. H. Control of crystal growth in drug suspensions. Part 2. Influence of polymers on dissolution and crystallization during temperature cycling. *Pharm. Ind.* 1990, *52*, 1017–1022.
48. Rabinow, B. E. Nanosuspensions in drug delivery. *Nat. Rev. Drug Discov.* 2004, *3*, 785–796.
49. Merisko-Liversidge, E. Formulation and antitumor activity evaluation of nanocrystalline suspensions of poorly soluble anticancer drugs. *Pharm. Res.* 1996, *13*, 272–278.
50. Garavilla, L., Peltier, N., and Merisko-Liversidge, E. Controlling the acute hemodynamic effects associated with IV administration of particulate drug dispersion in dogs. *Drug Dev. Res.* 1996, *37*, 86–96.

51. Borchard, G. and Kreuter, J. Interaction of serum components with poly (methyl methacrylate) nanoparticles and the resulting body distribution after intravenous injection in rats. *J. Drug Target.* 1993, *1*, 15–19.
52. Peter, K., Leitzke, S., Diederichs, J. E., Borner, K., Hahn, H., Müller, R. H., and Ehklers, S. Preparation of clofazimine nanosuspension for intravenous use and evaluation of its therapeutic efficacy in murine *Mycobacterium avium* infection. *J. Anti. Chemo.* 2000, *45*, 77–83.
53. Clement, M. A., Pugh, W., and Parikh, I. Tissue distribution and plasma clearance of a novel microcrystal encapsulated flurbiprofen formulation. *The Pharmacologist* 1992, *34*, 204.
54. Kipp, J. E. The role of solid nanoparticle technology in the parenteral delivery of poorly water-soluble drugs. *Int. J. Pharm.* 2004, *284*, 109–122.
55. Kattan, J., Dorz, J.-P., Couvreur, P., Marino, J.-P., Boutan-Laroze, A., Rougier, P., Brault, P., Vranckx, H., Grognet, J.-M., Morge, X., and Sancho-Garnier, H. Phase 1 clinical trial and pharmacokinetic evaluation of doxorubicin carried by polyisohexylcyanoacrylate nanoparticles. *Inv. New Drugs.* 1992, *10*, 1991–1999.
56. Haskell, R. J.United States Patent, *Patent No.*: US 6,814,319 B2, 2004.
57. Pannuti, F., Camaggie, C. M., Strocchi, E., and Comparsi, R. Metroxyprogesterone acetate plasma pharmacokinetics after intravenous administration in rabbits. *Cancer Chemo. Pharmacol.* 1987, *19*, 311–314.
58. Amidon, G. L., Lennernas, H., Shah, V. P., and Crison, J. R. A theoretical basis for a biopharmaceutic drug classification: the correlation of *in vitro* drug product dissolution and *in vivo* bioavailability. *Pharm. Res.* 1995, *12(3)*, 413–420.
59. Kararli, T. T. Gastrointestinal absorption of drugs. *Crit. Rev. Ther. Drug Carrier Syst.* 1989, *6(1)*, 39–86.
60. Grant, D. J. W. and Highuchi, T. *Solubility Behavior of Organic Compounds*, Wiley, New York, 1990.
61. Jain, N. and Yalkowsky, S. H. Estimation of the aqueous solubility I: application to organic non-electrolytes. *J. Pharm. Sci.* 2000, *90*, 234–252.
62. Yalkowski, S. H. *Solubility and Solubilization in Aqueous Media*, Oxford University Press, New York, 1999.
63. Stahl, P. H. and Wermuth, G. G. *Handbook of Pharmaceutical Salts Property, Selection, and Use*, Wiley-VCH, Weinheim, Germany, 2002.
64. Li, S., Wong, S., Sethia, S., Almoazen, H., Joshi, Y. M., and Serajuddin, A. T. M. Investigation of solubility and dissolution of a free base and two different salt forms as a function of pH. *Pharm. Res.* 2005, *22(4)*, 628–635.
65. Parshad, H., Frydenvang, K., Liljefors, T., Cornett, C., and Larsen, C. Assessment of drug salt release from solutions, suspensions and *in situ* suspensions using a rotating dialysis cell. *Eur. J. Pharm. Sci.* 2003, *19*, 263–272.
66. Lipinski, C. A., Lombardo, F., Dominy, B. W., and Feeney, P. J. Experimental and computational approaches to estimate solubility and permeability in drug discovery and development settings. *Adv. Drug Deliv. Rev.* 2001, *46*, 3–26.
67. Lin, S. L., et al. Preformulation investigation I. Relation of salt forms and biological activity of a novel antihypertensive. *J. Pharm. Sci.* 1972, *61(9)*, 1418–1422.
68. Walmsley, L. M., et al. Plasma concentrations and relative bioavailability of naftidrofuryl from different salt forms. *Biopharm. Drug Dispos.* 1986, *7(4)*, 327–334.

69. Nikos, S. and Koutsoukos, P. G. Kinetics of precipitation of calcium carbonate in alkaline pH at constant supersaturation. Spontaneous and seeded growth. *J. Phys. Chem. B* 1998, *102*, 6679–6684.

70. Chiang, P. C., South, S. A., Daniels, J. S., Anderson, D. R., Wene, S. P., Albin, L. A., Mourey, R. J., and Selbo, J. G. Aqueous vs. non-aqueous salt delivery strategies to enhance oral bioavailability of a mitogen activated protein kinase activated protein kinase (MK-2) inhibitor in rats. *J. Pharm Sci.* 2009, *98(1)*, 248–256.

71. Dressman, J. B., Amidon, G. L., Reppas, C., and Shah, V. P. Dissolution testing as a prognostic tool for oral drug absorption: immediate release dosage forms. *Pharm. Res.* 1998, *15(1)*, 11–22.

72. Kerns, E. H. and Di, L. *Drug-Like Properties: Concepts, Structure Design and Methods from ADME to Toxicity Optimization*, Academic Press, Boston, 2008, p. 68.

73. Martini, L. G. and Crowley P. J. Physicochemical approaches to enhancing oral absorption. *Pharm. Technol. Europe* 2004, Sept. 1. (See reference at this link: http://www.ptemag.com/pharmtecheurope/issue/issueDetail.jsp?id=4535).

74. Miyazaki, S., Oshiba, M., and Nadi, T. *J. Pharm. Sci.* 1981, *70(6)*, 594–595.

75. Thomas, E. and Rubino, J. Solubility, melting point and salting–out relationships in a group of secondary amine hydrochloride salts. *Int. J. Pharm.* 1996, *130(2)*, 179–183.

76. Engel, G. L., et al. Salt form selection and characterization of LY333531 mesylate monohydrate. *Int. J. Pharm.* 2000, *198(2)*, 239–247.

77. Horter, D. and Dressman, J. B. Influence of physicochemical properties on dissolution of drugs in the gastrointestinal tract. *Adv. Drug Deliv. Rev.* 1997, *25*, 3–14.

78. Mithani, S. D., Bakatselou, V., TenHoor, C. N., and Dressman, J. B. Estimation of the increase in solubility as a function of bile salt concentration. *Pharm. Res.* 1996, *13*, 163–167.

79. Carey, M. C. and Small, D. M. Micelle formation by bile salts. Physical–chemical and thermodynamic considerations. *Arch. Intern. Med.* 1972, *130*, 506–527.

80. Tso, P. Gastrointestinal digestion and absorption of lipid. *Adv. Lipid Res.* 1985, *21*, 143–186.

81. O'Connor, C. J. and Wallace, R. G. Physical–chemical behavior of bile salts. *Adv. Coll. Interface Sci.* 1985, *22*, 1–111.

82. Bakatselou, V., Oppenheim, R., and Dressman, J. Solubilization and wetting effects of bile salts on the dissolution of steroids. *Pharm. Res.* 1991, *8*, 1461–1469.

83. Naylor, L. J., Bakatselou, V., Rodriguez-Homedo, N., Weiner, N. D., and Dressman, J. D. Dissolution of steroids in bile salt solutions is modified by the presence of lecithin. *Eur. J. Pharm. Biopharm.* 1995, *41*, 346–353.

84. Li, C.-Y., Zimmerman, C. L., and Wiedmann, T. S. Solubilization of retinoids by bile salt/phospholipid aggregates, *Pharm. Res.* 1996, *13*, 907–913.

85. Solomon, L. J., Embleton, J. K., and Pouton, C. W. Solubilization of Steroidal Compounds by Mixed Bile Salt/Lecithin Micelles. In *Formulation of Poorly Available Drugs for Oral Administration*, In: Couvreur, P., Duchene, D.,and Kalles, I. (eds.), Editions de Sante, Paris, 1996, pp. 219–220.

86. Kostwicz, E. S., Brauns, U., Becker, R., and Dressman, J. B. Forecasting the oral absorption behavior of poorly soluble weak bases using solubility and dissolution studies in biorelevant media. *Pharm. Res.* 2002, *19(3)*, 345–349.

87. Dressman, J. B. and Reppas, C. *In vitro–in vivo* correlations for lipophilic, poorly water-soluble drugs. *B.T. Gattefosse* 2000, *93*, 91–100.

88. Hartshorne, N. *The Microscopy Series: The Microscopy of Liquid Crystals*, Microscope Publications Ltd., London, 1974.

89. Brittain, H. G., *Polymorphism in Pharmaceutical Solids. Drugs and the Pharmaceutical Sciences*, Vol. 95, Marcel Dekker, New York, 1999.

90. Bernstein, J. *Polymorphism in Molecular Crystals. IUCr Monographs on Crystallography*, Vol. 14, Clarendon Press, Oxford, 2006.

91. Ostwald, W. Studies concerning the formation and transformation of solid bodies. I Discussion: supersaturation and supercooling. *Z. Phys. Chem. Stoechiom. Verwandtschaftsl* 1896, *22*, 289–330.

92. Cardew, P. T. and Davey, R. J. The Kinetics of Solvent-Mediated Phase Transformations. *Proceedings of the Royal Society of London. Series A, Mathematical and Physical Sciences* 1985, *398, 1815*, pp. 415–428.

93. Gu, C.-H., Young, V. Jr., and Grant, D. J. W. Polymorph screening: influence of solvents on the rate of solvent-mediated polymorphic transformation. *J. Pharm. Sci.* 2001, *90(11)*, 1878–1890.

94. Gong, Y., Collman, B., Mehrens, S., Lu, E., Miller, J., Blackburn, A., and Grant, D. J. W. Stable-form screening: overcoming trace impurities that inhibit solution-mediated phase transformation to the stable polymorph of sulfamerazine. *J. Pharm. Sci.* 2008, *97(6)*, 2130–2144.

95. Byrn, S. R., Pfeiffer, R. R., and Stowell, J. G. *Solid-State Chemistry of Drugs*, SSCI, Inc., West Lafayette, IN, 1999.

96. Byrn, S., Pfeiffer, R., Ganey, M., Hoiberg, C., and Poochikian, G. Pharmaceutical solids: a strategic approach to regulatory considerations. *Pharm. Res.* 1995, *12*, 945–954.

97. Gao, P. Amorphous pharmaceutical solids: characterization, stabilization and development of marketable formulations of poorly soluble drugs with improved oral absorption. *Mol. Pharm.* 2008, *5(6)*, 903–904.

98. Friesen, D. T., Shanker, R., Crew, M., Smithey, D. T., Curatolo, W. J., and Nightingale, J. A. Hydroxypropyl methylcellulose acetate succinate-based spray-dried dispersions: an overview. *Mol. Pharm.* 2008, *5(6)*, 1003–1019.

99. Hancock, B. C. and Parks, M. What is the true solubility advantage for amorphous pharmaceuticals? *Pharm. Res.* 2000, *17(4)*, 397–404.

4

ADME

MARTIN E. DOWTY, DEAN M. MESSING, YURONG LAI, AND
LEONID (LEO) KIRKOVSKY

4.1 INTRODUCTION

The term ADME denotes the *a*bsorption, *d*istribution, *m*etabolism, and *e*xcretion of drugs and drug candidates upon administration to animals or humans. The ADME processes occurring after oral administration of drugs are depicted (Figure 4.1).

The purpose of this chapter is to discuss (1) the interplay of physiological phenomena and the properties of drug candidates in biological systems, and (2) the various preclinical tools that may be used to predict human performance. ADME information is critically important from the early drug design stage of discovery to the ultimate clinical development of the most promising candidates. The process of drug discovery requires the prediction of human ADME characteristics through the judicious preclinical use of various *in silico*, *in vitro*, and *in vivo* tools (Figure 4.2). Furthermore, targeted ADME properties need to be integrated into the overall desired potency and efficacy as well as safety requirements of a drug candidate.

Optimizing the use of ADME requires an understanding of the bioavailability of the drug candidate from the route of administration to the ultimate site of activity for the required duration of time in order to elicit the intended pharmacology with an adequate safety margin. The vast majority of drug candidates are intended for oral absorption, requiring an appreciation of drug dissolution and solubility within the gastrointestinal lumen, luminal behavior, enterocyte permeability, and intestinal and liver metabolism. Upon reaching the systemic circulation, it is important to characterize drug distribution to the intended site of activity and the barriers that may influence this delivery. Plasma pharmacokinetics typically dictates the intended

ADMET for Medicinal Chemists: A Practical Guide, Edited by Katya Tsaioun and Steven A. Kates

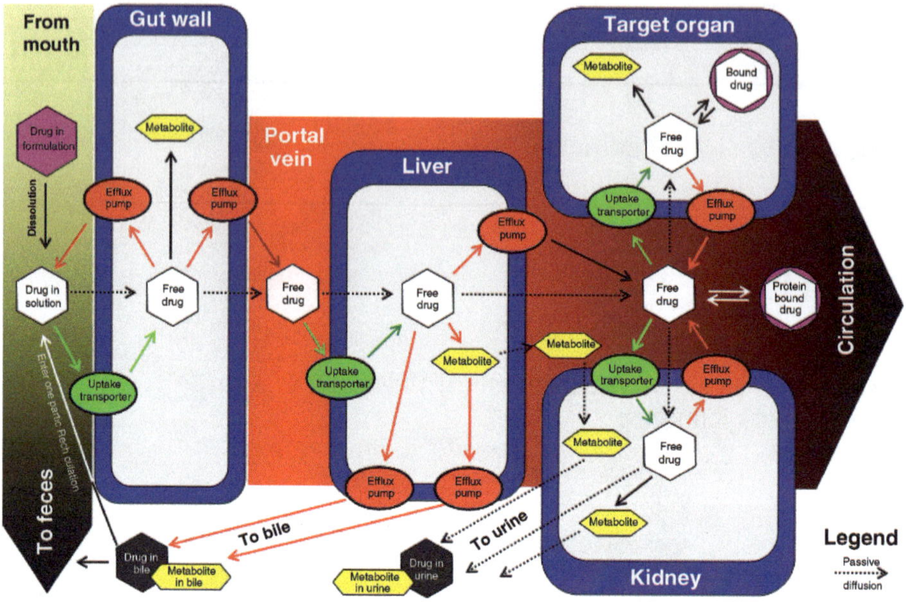

Figure 4.1 The processes during the absorption, distribution, metabolism, and excretion of drugs.

pharmacodynamics as well as unintended toxic effects. The duration of drug activity can be significantly influenced by drug metabolism and elimination. Understanding drug clearance and its influence on elimination pathways are necessary to better understand the potential for concomitant drug interactions. Other factors that may influence the ADME properties of a drug include genetic variability, health or disease state, environment, age, gender, and race/ethnicity. The key to optimal drug design is to understand ADME characteristics that are on the critical path as early as possible in drug discovery while there is adequate time to make appropriate alterations in chemical structure. Consequently, understanding the ADME properties of potential drug candidates is an important goal of the medicinal chemist.

4.2 ABSORPTION

Absorption of a drug is the first process a molecule must navigate in order to reach the systemic circulation. The properties of both the drug and the route of administration will influence the overall bioavailability of the compound. Much of the emphasis of this section will be on the oral route, which is typically the preferred one for patients and is the major focus of the pharmaceutical industry.

4.2.1 Route of Administration

Therapeutics can be delivered into the systemic circulation via a number of different routes. Generally, these include the oral and parenteral (intravenous, intramuscular,

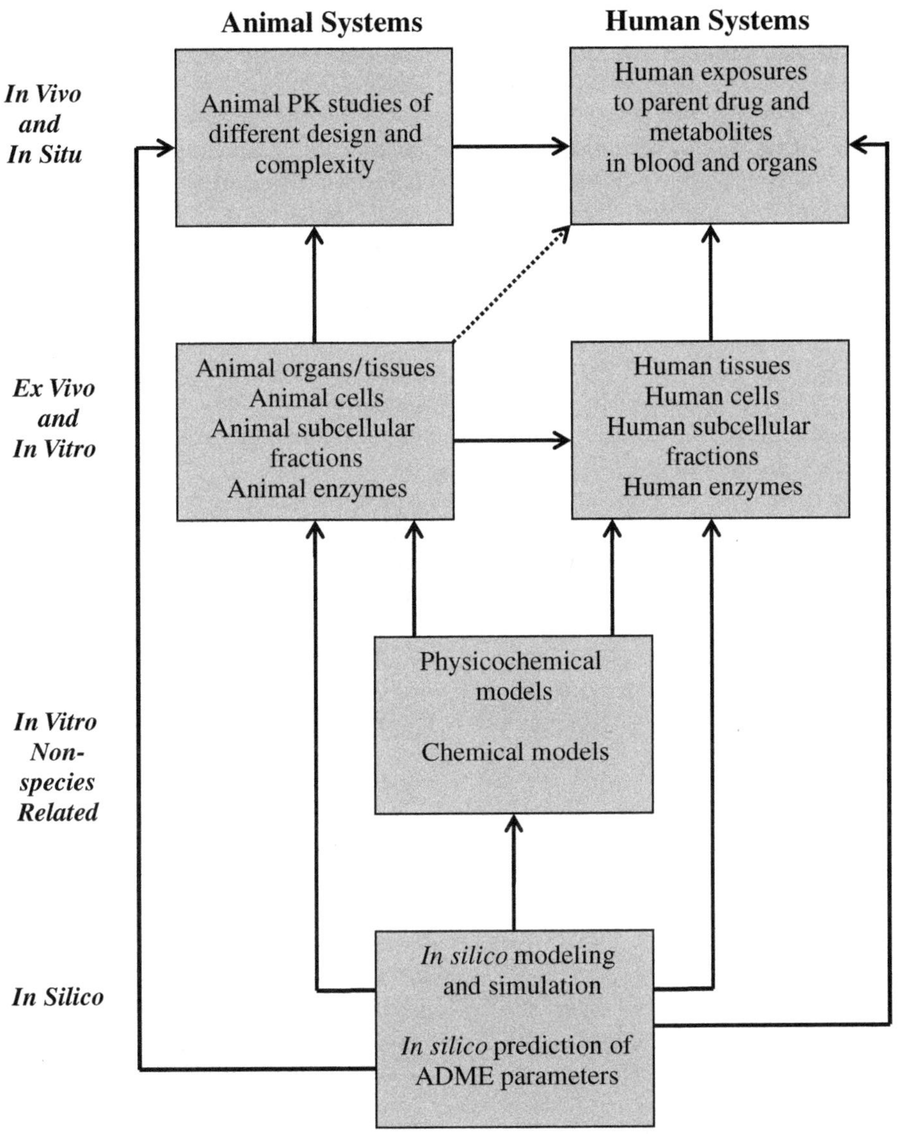

Figure 4.2 The network of preclinical tools used to predict human ADME behavior of new drug candidates.

intraperitoneal, and subcutaneous) routes of delivery. For various reasons including the need for local therapy or the infeasibility of the oral route, drugs can also be administered through other routes such as topically to the eyes (ocular), dermally or transdermally, nasally, rectally or intratracheally (inhalation). The drug administration route should be judiciously evaluated in the drug discovery phase, based on the target of delivery (systemic versus local treatment), therapeutic indication and the properties of both the drug and the route of administration [1]. The characteristics of a drug that make it an ideal candidate for one route of administration do not necessarily allow it to be effectively delivered via an alternative route.

4.2.1.1 ***Oral Administration*** As oral administration is the most convenient, safest, and least expensive way to deliver a drug, it is the route most often used. Following drug dissolution, the drug initially must pass intact through the oral cavity, esophagus, stomach, and finally intestinal epithelium into the portal vein system, and subsequently through the liver before it is transported via the bloodstream to its systemic target site (Figure 4.1). Because of the large surface area created in the small intestine by the presence of villi and microvilli, the majority of drug absorption occurs in this region [1]. In addition to the absorption surface area, several factors such as pH stability, intestinal blood flow, the physical state of the drug (solution/solid dosage form), solubility and dissolution of drug, and the luminal drug concentration also influence oral absorption.

While the drug travels from the gastrointestinal tract to the systemic circulation, the intestine and the liver can metabolize many drugs, decreasing the amount of drug reaching the bloodstream (referred to as first-pass or presystemic clearance) [2, 3]. In this regard, both the drug properties and the physiology of the gastrointestinal tract determine overall drug oral absorption. Good oral bioavailability of a drug essentially implies that the drug is able to reach the systemic circulation if administered by mouth. The absorption of drugs via the oral route is a subject of intense and continuous investigation in drug discovery and will be an important component of further discussion here.

4.2.1.2 ***Parenteral Administration*** The parenteral route includes a number of administration routes other than through the gastrointestinal tract [4] such as intravenous, subcutaneous, intraperitoneal, and intramuscular, which have little in common except that they require a hypodermic needle for delivery. These routes bypass a number of physiologic barriers present with the oral route and can be particularly useful for the delivery of biotherapeutic drugs, but may also provide rapid systemic access when studying the biological effects of small molecules. The intravenous and subcutaneous routes of administration are discussed here.

Intravenous Injection The intravenous (IV) route is a well-controlled and optimal way to deliver a precise dose quickly into the body, not possible by other administration routes. IV administration requires delivery of a solution containing the drug directly into the vein as a single dose through a needle puncture. The drug can also be continuously infused by gravity or by an infusion pump through a catheter inserted into a vein for greater control of drug concentrations. IV delivery can be used for more irritating solutions, which might otherwise cause pain and damage to tissues if given by the subcutaneous or intramuscular routes. There are both advantages and disadvantages to the use of IV administration. An advantage is that drug injected directly into the bloodstream can take effect more quickly than by any other route of administration. A disadvantage is that a high concentration of drug may be attained rapidly, which may result in an unfavorable reaction or undesired side effects related to the maximal plasma concentration.

Subcutaneous Injection A solution-containing drug can be administered by a needle inserted into tissues just beneath the skin surface, where the drug diffuses into small blood vessels and capillaries and then is carried away by the bloodstream or reaches the bloodstream through the lymphatic vessels. The subcutaneous injection (SC) route has been used for many biotherapeutics, such as protein drugs or vaccines, because such drugs are not stable in digestive fluid and SC administration avoids degradation of drug in the gastrointestinal tract. Biotherapeutics like insulin are large in size and usually reach the bloodstream slowly through the lymphatic vessels, thus prolonging absorption. Through SC injection, a drug can be prepared for controlled release delivery in order to prolong drug absorption from the injection site for hours, days, or longer. Certain drugs such as progestin for birth control may be given subcutaneously by inserting plastic capsules under the skin for very long duration of activity [5].

4.2.1.3 Other Routes of Administration Alternatively, drugs can be delivered through various other routes of administration including pulmonary, nasal, sublingual, ocular, rectal, vaginal, and transdermal [1, 6]. These routes may be used when a drug is needed, for example, to produce rapid absorption (e.g., sublingual for nitroglycerin delivery) or for a local therapeutic effect (e.g., antiasthmatic drugs). Each of these routes can require vastly different physicochemical drug properties for optimal delivery.

4.2.2 Factors Determining Oral Bioavailability

Bioavailability is a term used to indicate the fractional extent of a dose of drug reaching the systemic circulation. Oral bioavailability is the result of both absorption and clearance processes. The important factors determining oral bioavailability include drug solubility and dissolution, chemical and enzymatic stability in the intestinal lumen, interacting luminal contents (food), gastrointestinal transit time, enterocyte permeability, and intestinal and hepatic metabolism (Figure 4.1).

The bioavailability (F) of a compound is defined by the equation

$$F = f_a(1 - E_g)\,(1 - E_h)$$

where f_a is the fraction absorbed representing all processes from dissolution of the solid dosage form to the intestinal transport of the drug; and E_g and E_h are the first pass metabolic extraction/removal from the gut and the liver, respectively.

While the permeability, solubility, and metabolic stability of the compound may be important individually, the interrelationship of these properties will determine the overall *in vivo* bioavailability of a drug. A drug with very low solubility may be problematic for a high dose compound but acceptable for one with a low dose. The maximum absorbable dose (MAD) model has shown some value in relating aqueous solubility and intestinal permeability to absorption potential [7, 8]:

$$\mathrm{MAD} = SK_{\mathrm{a}} \times \mathrm{SIV} \times \mathrm{SIT}$$

where S is maximal solubility, K_{a} is a rate constant of absorption, SIV is the small intestinal volume, and SIT is transit time of the small intestine.

Overall PO bioavailability can be evaluated *in vivo* by comparing the dose-normalized area under the concentration (AUC) time curve following PO and IV administration. A first assessment of PO bioavailability comes from animal models. It is important to appreciate the potential differences between preclinical animal models and human in order to understand approaches to best predict human performance.

As drug solubility and dissolution have been thoroughly discussed in Chapter 3, this subject will not be reviewed in detail here. The following sections will primarily discuss the aspects of the intestinal permeability of drugs. As metabolism, in general, is covered in Section 4.4, the following discussion will only include some highlights of intestinal metabolism.

4.2.2.1 Mechanism of Drug Absorption A drug can cross the intestinal mucosa via a number of different pathways. The mechanisms involved in the passage of drug across the enterocyte into the portal system include: (1) passive diffusion (paracellular and transcellular); (2) active transport including facilitated uptake as well as active efflux, and (3) receptor-mediated endocytosis [9, 10]. The absorption mechanisms are not independent from each other, and will take place in parallel for susceptible molecules. Figure 4.3 illustrates the mechanisms of intestinal absorption.

For typical drug design, the important mechanisms of absorption to consider are passive permeability and carrier-mediated transport.

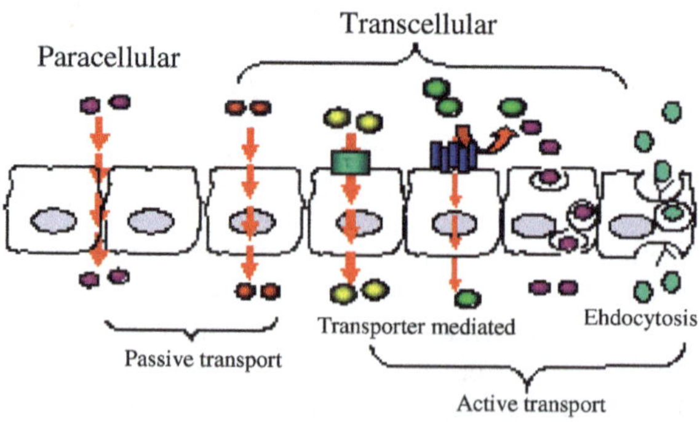

Figure 4.3 Mechanisms of absorption in the gastrointestinal tract.

4.2.2.2 Passive Permeability Permeability is the velocity of drug traveling across a biological membrane. It is a kinetic parameter related to lipophilicity, which in turn is related to the partition and distribution coefficients. Physicochemical profiling of drug molecules is important in assessing the potential for good oral absorption [11, 12]. At the same time, physicochemical properties are not independent of each other, and effective use is in the collective assessment of these parameters. Lipinski's guidelines have been useful in this regard, stating that good oral absorption is more probable for molecules that have MW < 500, clog $P < 5$, hydrogen-bond donors <5, and hydrogen-bond acceptors <10 [13]. Polar surface area (PSA) is another parameter that can correlate with the permeability of drug candidates [14], with low PSA values corresponding to high permeability.

Passive diffusion is not a saturable process and so cannot be inhibited by other drugs unless the physical properties of the drug or membrane are affected in some way. The process of crossing the gastrointestinal tract follows the solubility–diffusion model, which is defined by the following equation derived from Fick's law:

$$\text{Flux rate} = [D \times A \times K \times \Delta C]/X$$

where D represents the diffusion constant, which is inversely proportional to the molecular weight of the drug; A represents the area of the membrane available for permeability; K represents the membrane partition coefficient, which is represented by lipid solubility and is the most important determinant of the speed of transfer across the membrane; ΔC is the concentration gradient across the membrane; and X is the thickness of membrane. The permeability coefficient, a useful parameter for comparing drugs, is defined as $[D \times K]/X$.

The luminal surface of the gastrointestinal tract is lined with a monolayer of epithelial cells tethered together through apical tight junctions. There are two passive permeability pathways available for drug molecules: transcellular and paracellular diffusion. Transcellular diffusion involves the movement of drug through the epithelial cells by passing directly through the cell membrane. In contrast, paracellular transport is defined as drug movement into bloodstream *between* epithelial cells by simple diffusion [15, 16]. The small paracellular pore size limits the permeation of hydrophilic compounds [17], where increasing molecular size decreases the rate of paracellular penetration. Paracellular permeability is both size and charge dependent [18]. Generally, paracellular permeability is relevant for smaller drugs with molecular weights of less than about 300 Da. Paracellular transport is preferred for drugs with a positive charge and log $D < 0$.

The transcellular passive mechanism is the preferred pathway for drugs that are in the 500 Da range or less, are moderately lipophilic (log $D > 0$), and uncharged. As the majority of drugs are relatively lipophilic in nature, the transcellular route is thought to be the major mechanism of permeability for most marketed drugs [19, 20].

4.2.2.3 Tools to Assess Passive Permeability A number of tools are available to assess the passive permeability of molecules and are discussed below.

In Vivo Models for Assessing Permeability The extent of the drug absorption from the gastrointestinal tract can be evaluated by comparing the PO dose plasma AUC with the AUC of the compound in samples collected from a hepatic portal vein cannulated animal [21, 22].

In Situ and Ex Vivo Models for Assessing Passive Permeability Absorption processes can be assessed *in situ* and *ex vivo* through perfusion of a drug solution through an isolated intestinal segment [23–25]. Two ends of an intestinal segment are cannulated, setting up a closed circulation loop through which a buffered drug solution is circulated. Drug absorption is assumed from a measurement of drug disappearance from the circulating solution, which may not always be the case.

The permeation of a drug across intestinal mucosa can also be studied *ex vivo* in an using chamber, which consists of two sampling chambers with a section of intestinal mucosa mounted between the chambers [21, 26]. The Using chamber provides a physiological system to measure the transport of ions, nutrients, and drugs across various epithelial tissues [27].

Another *ex vivo* technique used for studying drug absorption is the inverted gut sac [28]. It is prepared by removing the small intestine from the animal, inverting it over a glass rod and dividing it into segments. Sacs (mucosal side out) are then submerged in culture medium containing the drug, and accumulation within the inner compartment is measured. Under optimal conditions, sacs remain viable for up to 120 min [21].

Cell Culture Systems for Assessing Passive Permeability A major method of permeability assessment is the use of various cell culture systems such as Caco-2, MDCK, HT29, and LLCK-1 cell lines. In this method, the immortalized cells are grown on a semipermeable filter, generating a cell monolayer with tight junctions. Theoretically, any cell line that could form a cell monolayer with tight junctions may be applied in the permeability assessment.

Among the cell lines, Caco-2 has received the greatest attention and characterization. These cells are of human colon adenocarcinoma origin and develop microvillus that mimic the morphology of intestinal epithelial cells as well as the expression of some drug transporters [29]. However, the long time needed for cell differentiation (18–21 days in culture) hinders its high-throughput use in the pharmaceutical industry. A 5 day Caco-2 system has been developed for permeability assessment, however, its transporter expression and functionality are not optimal [30].

Recently, the use of MDCK cells has increased in popularity due to ease of handling and shorter differentiation times (4–5 days). MDCK cells are of canine origin and kidney phenotype. Since these cells lack human P-glycoprotein expression, they are useful as a good background model for over-expression of human transporters such as P-glycoprotein [31]. With any of the cell culture systems, it is important to understand potential sources for variation [32]. Transport and metabolic properties of cultured cells can vary due to culture conditions, seeding density, passage number, confluency, filter support, monolayer age, and stage of differentiation. Therefore, permeability assays typically include various positive and negative controls to allow for facilitated comparison between studies and laboratories.

The distinction between paracellular and transcellular permeability is commonly made with the use of *in vitro* epithelial monolayer cell lines. Any cell line, such as Caco-2 and MDCK, which form tight junctions can be used for this purpose. The paracellular pathway is investigated by opening it with the use of EDTA to chelate calcium, which is important for tight junctional integrity [33–35]. The tight junctions can also be disrupted by cytochalasin D [36]. The disruption of tight junctions increases the space for paracellular compounds to penetrate while leaving the integrity of transcellular permeability intact. During testing, mannitol (paracellular probe) and propranolol (transcellular probe) are commonly used as a positive and negative controls, respectively [37].

Noncell Systems for Assessing Passive Permeability Two common cell membrane mimetic systems include immobilized artificial membrane (IAM) HPLC columns [38, 39] and the parallel artificial membrane permeability assay (PAMPA) [40, 41]. IAM columns contain covalently bound phosphatidylcholine analogs that serve as a surface for drug membrane interactions and are highly amenable to high-throughput screening [42]. The PAMPA system uses a hexadecane or other lipid-filled membrane as a lipophilic barrier and has been shown to correlate to cell culture and human jejunum permeability [43, 44]. Both of these systems are used as a measure of passive permeability only and not for assessment of potential active transport (see below). Highly lipophilic compounds can be difficult to assess with these systems because of issues with high retention to lipophilic matrix.

In Silico Tools for Assessing Passive Permeability Computational methods for the prediction of drug permeability are increasing [45]. Numerous commercial software programs are available for the prediction of intestinal absorption. *In silico* prediction models are especially useful tools for virtual screening, when a medicinal chemist investigates the permeability effects of various substitutions before actually synthesizing compounds. However, the prediction capability of software varies and the user should avoid over-interpreting the results. The computational models are most useful when the *in silico* predictions can be validated against *in vitro* permeability data from a testing set of compounds (see Chapter 2 for a comprehensive discussion).

4.2.2.4 Transporter-Mediated Permeability A number of membrane transporters within the intestinal tract can influence drug disposition [46]. They are responsible for two major permeability mechanisms: active uptake and efflux. Figure 4.4 illustrates the distribution of drug transporters in epithelial cells of the intestine.

Epithelial cells in the intestine contain several uptake and ATP-dependent efflux transporters in the luminal membrane including the organic transporting polypeptide family (OATP/SLCO), oligopeptide transporter (PEPT/SLC15A), monocarboxylic acid transporter (MCT/SLC16A), apical sodium-bile acid co-transporter (ASBT/ALC10A2), P-glycoprotein (MDR1/ABCB1), multidrug resistance protein 2 (MRP2/ABCC2), and breast cancer resistance protein (BCRP/ABCG2). On the basolateral membrane, the transport systems include the organic cation transporter 1 (OCT1;

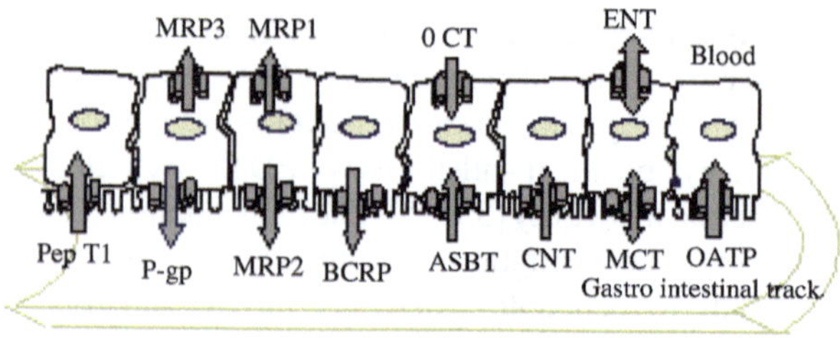

Figure 4.4 The distribution of drug transporters in epithelial cell of the intestine.

SLC22A1), heteromeric organic solute transporter (OSTα-OSTβ), and multidrug resistance protein 3 (MRP3; ABCC3). Some drugs utilize these transporters for systemic availability. For example, the PEPT system is a proton coupled transporter that plays a critical role in the oral absorption of β-lactam antibiotics, anticancer drugs, and dopamine receptor antagonists [46].

The utility of these uptake transporters as a platform delivery vehicle provides new knowledge for strategies to enhance intestinal absorption of drugs [47]. In contrast to the uptake transporters, ATP-dependent efflux pumps may serve as a barrier to oral absorption [48–50]. Transporter-mediated drug absorption is saturable and affected by competitive inhibitors [51]. Therefore, drug–drug interactions (DDI) may be more of a concern for efflux transporters [52, 53]. Drug transporter research is still a relatively young area of investigation, but is rapidly progressing in terms of transporter function, substrate specificity, spectrum, and kinetics, and overall implications for drug discovery and development. Based on the current understanding of transporter molecular biology and the role of transporters in pharmacokinetics, guidelines for drug transporter interaction studies have been proposed [54].

4.2.2.5 Tools to Assess Transport-Mediated Permeability A number of tools are available to assess the transport-mediated permeability of molecules and are discussed below.

In Vivo Systems for Assessing Transport-Mediated Permeability Confirming *in vitro* findings in *in vivo* dynamic living system can provide greater confidence and understanding of the interaction with the transporters. Genetic knockout or naturally occurring transporter-deficient animal models and chemical knockout models are popular assays used in drug discovery and development to characterize transporter effects. Numerous transporter gene knockout mice have been characterized in recent years and are commercially available [55]. For example, the Mdr-1 gene knock out model has been used in assessing the impact of P-glycoprotein on ADME in drug discovery and development [22, 56].

Extrapolation of preclinical transport findings to the clinic remains challenging because of species differences in transporter expression, substrate affinity, physiological function, the interplay between transporters and enzymes, and occasionally unpredicted differential regulation of transporters between genetically modified and wild-type animals [57]. Recently, humanized transporter animal models and stem cell derived cell lines have been introduced as promising tools that may prove to be useful in the near future to study discovery compounds and transporter interactions [58].

In Vitro Systems for Assessing Transport-Mediated Permeability Cell-based assay systems include gene transfected cell lines and polarized cell lines. Caco-2 cells are known to express many of the drug transporters existing in epithelial cell of the gastrointestinal tract [59]. Polarized transport in bidirectional transport studies is useful as a first indication of transporter involvement. Chemical knockdown experiments using the co-administration of a transporter-specific inhibitor with test compound identify the involvement of specific transporters. Transporter cDNA stably or transiently expressed in various cell lines can also be used to characterize drug transporter interactions. Recently, several laboratories have developed polarized cells that express both an uptake transporter in their basolateral membrane and an efflux transporter in their apical membrane to mimic *in vivo* vectoral transport [60–62]. However, whether these doubly transfected cells represent the true *in vivo* situation is still under discussion [63].

Cell membrane preparations from transporter gene over-expressed insect cells are commercially available for characterizing drug interactions with transporters. For ATP-dependent efflux pump assessments, substrate-dependent ATP hydrolysis methods have been developed. The simplicity of these assays is an advantage in high-throughput applications [64]. However, as the assay only monitors ATPase activity and not substrate transport, a high incidence of false positives might occur. Recently, inverted cell membrane vesicle preparation have been employed primarily to study efflux transporter-mediated uptake activity [65]. The advantage of this type of assay is to enable detailed substrate and inhibitor kinetic measurements for SAR analyses. In addition, the assays are readily automated for high-throughput screening.

In Silico Tools for Assessing Transport-Mediated Permeability Compared to the general prediction tools for intestinal absorption, commercial models for predicting specific transporter interactions are still limited. With the increasing availability of higher quality data sets, the application of computational modeling algorithms to assess transporter substrate/inhibitor interactions has advanced [66–70].

4.2.2.6 Solubility and Permeability The Biopharmaceutics Classification System (BCS) (Figure 4.5) has commonly been used in pharmaceutics to classify discovery compounds in terms of their permeability and solubility and is adapted by the FDA to rationalize the critical components related to oral absorption (http://www.fda.gov/AboutFDA/CentersOffices/CDER/ucm128219.htm).

The classification system allows pharmaceutical companies to bypass clinical bioequivalence studies if their drug product meets the specifications detailed in the guidance [11, 71]. The BCS is a simplification of Fick's first law. The diffusion equation reduces simply to a product of permeability and solubility, which can be characterized *in vitro* based on certain assumptions. The scientific rationale in the BCS is that if the highest dose of a drug candidate is readily soluble in the fluid

	High solubility	Low solubility
High permeability	Class I	Class II
Low permeability	Class III	Class V

Figure 4.5 Biopharmaceutics classification system.

volume of the gastrointestinal tract (250 mL in human) and the drug is more than 90% absorbed, then the *in vitro* drug product dissolution profiles should allow assessment of equivalence of different drug formulations. In principle, the BCS classification system can be applied to clinical development as well as to postapproval changes in drug manufacturing. Therefore, early investments in optimizing the permeability and solubility of a drug candidate in discovery research can provide significant savings in future development costs.

4.2.2.7 ***First Pass Drug Metabolism*** Oral bioavailability can be affected by chemical reactions in the gastrointestinal tract, which includes the potential formation of a drug complex, hydrolysis by gastric acid or digestive enzymes in the intestinal lumen, and intestinal and liver metabolism (Phase I and II metabolism). The enterocytes express most of the metabolic enzymes that exist in intestine, including UDP-glucuronyltransferases, sulfotransferases, esterases, and cytochromes P450s (3A4 major). Therefore, drugs that interact with liver metabolic enzymes may also be chemically removed during passage through the gut wall [72] (see also Section 4.4).

The distribution of metabolizing enzymes and transporters is uneven along the intestinal tract. The metabolic activity of Phase I and II metabolism is higher in the duodenum and jejunum than in the ileum and colon in both rat and human [23]. Conversely, P-glycoprotein mRNA levels increase longitudinally along the intestine, with the lowest levels in the stomach and highest in the colon [22]. There may also be an interplay between substrates for both P-glycoprotein and CYP3A4 substrates where efflux cycling can increase the time that a drug interacts with CYP3A4 within the enterocyte [73].

Tools to Assess First Pass Metabolism From *in vivo* pharmacokinetic studies, it is difficult to clearly identify the first pass extraction contribution from the intestine and liver. However, transgenic mouse models with selective organ expression of CYP3A4 offer the opportunity to investigate the first-pass metabolism of the anticancer agent docetaxel by the gut wall, and not the liver [74]. The study helped explain the major cause of low oral bioavailability in humans and interpatient differences in efficacy and safety following oral therapy with CYP3A4 substrates.

The extent of first pass drug metabolism by the liver can be evaluated by comparing the plasma AUC of the compound dosed PO with the AUC of the compound administered into the portal vein of hepatic portal vein cannulated animals, bypassing the process of oral absorption (see Section 4.4).

4.3 DISTRIBUTION

The fate of a drug following absorption begins with an understanding of its distribution. The factors that determine its ultimate delivery to the intended target site must be appreciated and are discussed in the following sections.

4.3.1 Drug Distribution

The distribution of drug refers to the reversible movement of the compound from one compartment to another within the body (Figure 4.6). Following drug absorption into blood, the rate and extent of distribution between the blood and various tissues will depend both on the physicochemical properties of the drug and the biological properties of tissue compartments. Useful information as to the rate and extent of drug distribution can be derived from an assessment of drug concentrations in blood or plasma.

Movement of drug from the intravascular to the extravascular space is typically rapid as the mean aqueous pore diameter in capillary membranes is of the order of 50–100 Å (Figure 4.6). Therefore, most drugs have ready access to cell surface

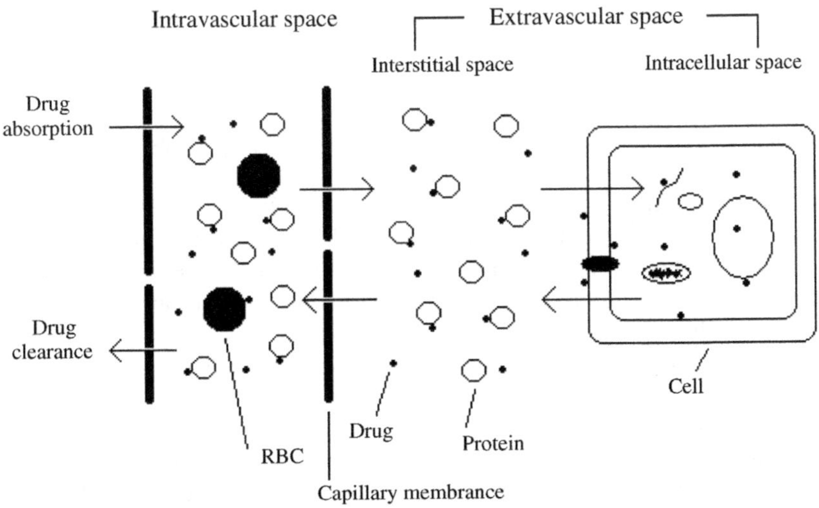

Figure 4.6 Schematic representation of drug distribution between the intravascular and extravascular spaces [75]. Drug available for distribution is influenced by both drug absorption and clearance. The free drug hypothesis suggests that only unbound drug moves between compartments and is at relatively equal concentrations at steady state.

targets. One exception is the capillary bed of the central nervous system (CNS), which possesses a system of circumferential tight junctions that limit paracellular entry of compounds. In this case, the ability of drugs to readily diffuse across the phospholipid cell membrane is important for entry into the CNS as well as to other intracellular target sites. At the same time, both absorptive (e.g., OATP in the liver) and exsorptive (e.g., MDR1 in the CNS) transporters within the cell membrane can influence the efficiency with which drugs can cross various cell barriers.

4.3.2 Volume of Distribution

The apparent volume of distribution is simply a proportionality factor between the total amount of drug present in the body and drug concentration in a reference fluid (typically plasma) at a given time. It is a theoretical value that reflects in part tissue affinity. The volume of distribution at steady state (V_{ss}) describes the extent of drug distribution from the plasma pool into tissues in the body as

$$V_{ss} = V_p + K_p V_t$$

where V_p is the volume of plasma, V_t is the volume of the extravascular space plus the erythrocyte volume into which drug distributes, and K_p is the steady-state tissue-to-plasma drug concentration ratio.

For a drug that is confined to the blood, the apparent volume of distribution would be about 0.08 L/kg (i.e., total blood volume). Similarly, a drug that distributes only into total body water would have an apparent volume of distribution of about 0.6 L/kg. Beyond these values, the volume of distribution only has mathematical significance. For example, a volume of 4 L/kg means that about 2% of the drug is in circulation. The rest of the drug may be moderately distributed to many tissues or concentrated in only a few. Ions such as bromide do not readily pass through cell membranes but distribute rapidly throughout extracellular water volume, having a volume of distribution of about 0.4 L/kg [76]. On the other hand, neutral lipid-soluble drugs, such as antipyrine [77], readily diffuse through cell membranes and easily distribute throughout extra- and intracellular water volume and can have a volume of distribution of about 0.6 L/kg (i.e., total body water). Compounds such as basic drugs, like amlodipine, have a higher affinity for tissue than for plasma proteins, and can easily have volumes of distribution greater than 10 L/kg [78]. This observation can, in part, be attributed to the ion pairing that occurs between the positive charge of basic compounds and the net negative charge of cell membrane constituents such as phospholipids, sialic acid residues on glycolipids, and the carbohydrate-rich glycocalyx.

Table 4.1 summarizes some generalizations regarding acidic, neutral, and basic compounds. A general comparison between acidic, neutral, and basic compounds and volume of distribution is shown in Figure 4.7, with reference to lipophilicity [79]. Since half-life ($t_{1/2}$) is determined by both the volume of distribution (V_β) and clearance (CL), $t_{1/2} = \ln 2(V_\beta/\mathrm{CL})$, manipulation of the volume of distribution (with a concomitant understanding of changes in clearance) can be used to change the drug half-life and, potentially, the duration of effect.

TABLE 4.1 General Volume of Distribution Trends for Acidic, Neutral, and Basic Drugs

Compound Type	Volume of Distribution (L/kg)	Binding Behavior	Distribution Characteristics
Acidic	<0.4	Plasma > tissue	Drug mainly confined to plasma with limited tissue distribution
Neutral	0.4–1.0	Plasma ~ tissue	Drug uniformly distributes between plasma and tissue
Basic	>1.0	Tissue > plasma	Drug may be more concentrated in particular tissues

If a drug gradually diffuses from the plasma to various tissue compartments, the volume of distribution actually increases with time. This is exemplified when a plasma concentration–time profile exhibits a biexponential (two-compartment model) decline following IV administration. Three different volumes of distribution apply in this case: the early apparent volume of distribution of the central compartment (V_c), the apparent volume of distribution at steady state (V_{SS}) or distributional equilibrium between plasma and tissue compartments, and the later maximal apparent

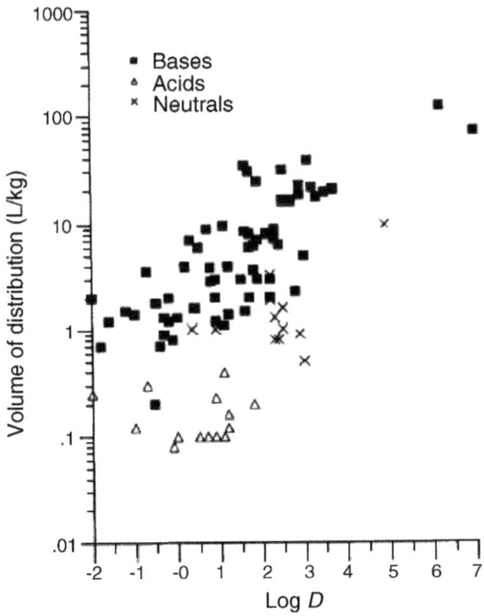

Figure 4.7 Illustration of differences in volume of distribution between acidic, neutral, and basic compounds, as well as the relationship of volume of distribution to lipophilicity (log *D*) [79].

volume of distribution at pseudodistribution equilibrium (V_β). In the case of a monoexponential concentration–time profile, the body behaves like a single compartment, and the three volume of distribution terms, V_c, V_{ss}, and V_β become the same and are independent of time.

4.3.2.1 ***In Vivo Tools to Assess Drug Distribution*** Whole animals can be used to assess the volumes of distribution following IV administration (see Chapter 5), although this value does not provide information about drug distribution to specific organs or tissues. Specific tissue distribution may be assessed by collecting various tissues and assessing total drug concentration with time following bolus or infusion (steady state) administration.

A spatial tissue distribution of drug candidates can also be obtained using the technique quantitative whole body autoradiography (QWBA), which quantifies the total radioactivity of tissues in thin sliced sections of the animal after the administration of a radiolabeled drug candidate. This technique does not distinguish between intact drug and radiolabeled metabolites. Newer techniques such as matrix-assisted laser desorption/ionization (MALDI) mass spectrometric imaging can simultaneously measure compound and metabolites distributed in whole-body tissue sections, using nonradiolabeled compounds [80].

The comparison of the tissue distribution data with and without the use of chemical transport inhibitors [81] or knock-out animals may also provide valuable information about the mechanism of distribution.

4.3.3 Free Drug Concentration

Within blood, drug can bind to various components including red blood cells and plasma proteins. As a consequence of binding, the concentration of total drug in whole blood and plasma, and unbound drug in blood and plasma, can vary significantly. Examples of plasma proteins in human blood are listed in Table 4.2. The two most important proteins are albumin and α_1-acid glycoprotein, which have a preference for acidic and basic drugs, respectively, although basic drugs can bind to albumin as well.

TABLE 4.2 Representative Plasma Proteins in Human

Plasma Protein	Molecular Weight (kDa)	Concentration (μM)	Preference in Binding
Albumin	67	500–700	Acidic drugs
α_1-acid glycoprotein	42	9–23	Basic drugs
Lipoproteins	200–2400	Variable	Lipophilic and basic drugs, triglycerides, phospholipids, and cholesterol
Cortisol-binding globulin (transcortin)	53	0.6–1.4	Steroids

Source: From Ref. 83.

Approximately 40% of the total albumin in the body is in the plasma, with the remaining located mainly in interstitial fluid (Figure 4.6). Binding of drug to plasma proteins is typically reversible, occurs with rapid equilibrium, and is saturable. Lipophilicity is one, but not the only general descriptor influencing plasma protein binding [82].

Characterization of drug protein binding is important in the understanding of the overall pharmacokinetic and pharmacodynamic properties of the drug. According to occupancy theory of drug response, receptor activation is assumed to be directly proportional to the number of receptors occupied by a given drug ligand. It is generally assumed that only free drug can exert pharmacological activity and that unbound drug is free to move across cell membranes. Because the intended site of activity may not be directly sampled, the pharmacodynamic relationship is typically investigated when drug concentrations at the site of activity are in equilibrium with those compartments that are accessible such as plasma or blood. Two important aspects are important when correlating plasma concentrations with those at the active site:

1. Drug has the appropriate physicochemical properties that allow it to diffuse freely across tissue compartments and cell membranes and it is not subject to transporter and/or metabolic activity.
2. Unbound drug has direct access to the receptor.

In addition to the importance of free drug and pharmacologic activity, it is also generally assumed that only unbound drug is subject to processes of hepatic and renal clearance. The relationship between the free fraction of drug in blood (f_u^b) and hepatic clearance (CL_h) is illustrated by considering the well-stirred hepatic clearance model [84]:

$$CL_h = [Q_h f_u^b\ (CL_{int}/f_u^{mic}]/[Q_h + f_u^b(CL_{int}/f_u^{mic})]$$

where Q_h is the hepatic blood flow (20 mL/min/kg in human), CL_{int} is the intrinsic hepatic clearance of the drug, and f_u^{mic} is the fraction of drug not associated with microsomes. The free drug concentration in red blood cells is related to free plasma concentration as follows:

$$f_u^b C^b = f_u^p C^p$$

where C^b and C^p are the total concentration in blood and plasma, respectively, and f_u^p is the free fraction of drug in plasma. It is generally assumed that free drug concentration in red blood cells is the same as that in plasma, but drug can preferentially partition into red blood cells and impact the interpretation of organ clearance [85]. The well-stirred hepatic clearance model would suggest that greater binding in blood or plasma would reduce free drug concentrations within hepatocytes. Whether a change in blood or plasma binding of a drug impacts overall hepatic clearance also depends on its intrinsic hepatic clearance and microsomal association.

Protein binding is also important in the renal clearance (CL_r) of drug

$$CL_r = f_u^b[GFR + (Q_r\, CL_{int}^s)/(Q_r + f_u^b\, CL_{int}^s)][1 - F_r]$$

where GFR is the glomerular filtration rate, Q_r is the renal blood flow, CL_{int}^s is the intrinsic clearance for active renal tubular secretion, and F_r is the fraction of drug reabsorbed from urine back into blood. Renal clearance generally trends lower with increasing lipophilicity [86].

4.3.3.1 Tools to Assess Free (Unbound) Drug Concentrations Microdialysis can be used to assess free drug concentrations in various organs or blood circulation *in vivo* [87]. There are also a number of *in vitro* methods available to assess unbound drug concentrations in plasma, blood, or tissue homogenate including human albumin-immobilized chromatographic columns, ultrafiltration, and equilibrium dialysis [88–90]. Among them, equilibrium dialysis is considered the preferred standard method and has more recently become amenable to higher throughput [91]. The technique is based on the establishment of an equilibrium between two chambers separated by a semipermeable membrane; one chamber containing plasma, blood, or tissue homogenate and the other only buffer. Drug is added to the buffer chamber and its equilibrium allowed to be established between the two chambers (steady state should be validated). Both temperature and pH during the experiment are critical in order to accurately assess binding.

4.3.4 CNS Penetration

The blood–brain barrier (BBB) is the most important barrier for drug entry into the central nervous system [92–96].

The brain capillaries form a continuous layer of endothelial cells joined together by circumferential tight junctions, which highly restricts paracellular diffusion of molecules. Drug penetration across the BBB is essential for centrally active compounds; however, the BBB can also be exploited to minimize potential central side effects [97].

Good brain penetration requires that a compound has good passive permeability. Lipophilic physicochemical properties have been shown to be particularly important for CNS active drugs [98] (Table 4.3). Good brain penetration also requires avoidance of P-glycoprotein (MDR1) susceptibility [94, 99, 100]. While other transporters have been identified at the BBB [101], P-glycoprotein has been currently shown to have the greatest clinical relevance [100]. P-glycoprotein is located at the luminal capillary surface of the BBB and possesses a highly promiscuous substrate specificity. Greater molecular weight, log P, polar surface area, and H-bonding increase the probability of P-glycoprotein interaction [102, 103].

In addition to permeability across the BBB, brain distribution and, in particular, unbound brain concentration are important for overall drug delivery to the brain [104–108]. It is generally assumed that free brain concentration will be the primary driver of physiological response. Consistent with this argument, central dopamine D_2 receptor

TABLE 4.3 Calculated Physicochemical Properties of CNS Drugs [98]

Property	Mean	Range
MW	319	151–655
cLog *P*	3.43	0.16–6.59
cLog *D*	2.08	− 1.34–6.57
Polar surface area (Å)	40.5	4.63–108
H-bond donors	0.67	0–3
H-bond acceptors	1.85	0–7
Positive charges	1.19	0–3
Negative charges	0	0

occupancy has been shown to significantly correlate to free brain concentrations for a number of antipsychotics, whereas total brain to plasma ratios were less useful [109]. In fact, simply considering total brain to plasma ratios has not generally been a useful correlation to pharmacological action [106, 110]. Large amounts of drug in the brain may be reflective of extensive binding to brain tissue rather than free drug available for interaction with its target receptor.

The relationship between free plasma, free brain, and total cerebrospinal fluid (CSF) concentrations can be described by a three compartment model [106] (Figure 4.8). It is important to understand that this equilibrium is only relevant for freely diffusing drugs that are not subject to active transport (e.g., P-glycoprotein) or metabolism between compartments [109, 111]. Under these circumstances, drug concentration at the central target site can be predicted simply by measuring free plasma or CSF concentration at steady state [112, 113].

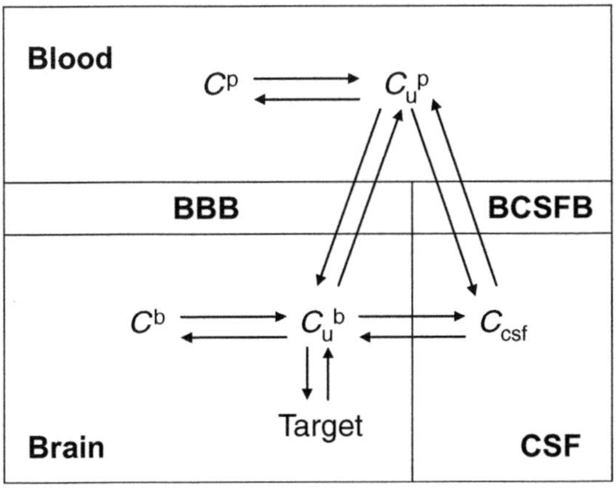

Figure 4.8 Relationship between drug concentration in plasma, brain, and CSF compartments for a freely diffusing molecule. Key: C^p, C^b, and C_{csf} are total plasma, brain, and CSF concentrations, respectively; C_u^p and C_u^b are unbound plasma and brain concentrations, respectively; BBB, blood–brain barrier; BCSFB, blood–CSF barrier.

4.3.4.1 Tools to Assess CNS Delivery of Drugs In terms of experimental tools in drug discovery, at a minimum, the three most important aspects of assessing compounds for CNS delivery are as follows:

- passive transcellular permeability,
- human P-glycoprotein substrate susceptibility.
- free brain concentrations.

The first two parameters will characterize the rate of BBB penetration, while the last parameter relates to the extent of brain distribution.

Tools to Assess Passive Transcellular Permeability into CNS There are a number of *in vitro* transwell cell permeability models available to assess passive permeability, where Caco-2 and Madin–Darby canine kidney (MDCK) cells are the most common for industrial use. The major criterion for any *in vitro* BBB permeability model is that it possesses a restrictive paracellular pathway [114]. Much work has been done to characterize *in vitro* brain endothelial cell lines for this purpose, but these tend to be limited by high paracellular permeability or lack high-throughput capacity [100, 115]. Noncell-based *in vitro* models such as PAMPA methodology have shown some value in assessing passive permeability of potential drug candidates as well [116].

Tools to Assess P-Glycoprotein Substrate Susceptibility Assessment of P-glycoprotein substrate specificity is typically performed in the cell types discussed above, where the stably transfected human MDR1-MDCK cell line has received significant attention [117, 118]. The P-glycoprotein knockout mouse is also a valuable tool and has shown widespread use in assessing the *in vivo* function of the efflux transporter in drug disposition [119, 120]. There have been reports of species differences in the brain uptake of P-glycoprotein substrates [121] and some breeds of dog, such as Collie, actually lack functional P-glycoprotein [122]. In general, compounds found to be substrates in rodent models are also likely to be substrates in higher species [100, 118, 122]. It is important to appreciate that the majority of marketed CNS active drugs have weak to no human P-glycoprotein interaction [100].

Tools to Assess Free Brain Concentrations of Drugs Techniques used to assess free brain concentrations include *in vivo* microdialysis and *in vitro* binding to brain tissue homogenate or slices [106, 123]. While microdialysis is a direct measure of free *in vivo* brain concentrations, there are challenges of nonspecific drug binding and the methodology is quite labor intensive and low throughput. Greater use is being made of indirectly estimating free brain concentrations by combining *in vivo* assessments of total brain to plasma concentration ratios and estimates of *in vitro* brain binding [104, 105, 107, 108]. Total brain to plasma ratios are successfully assessed by either measurement of total brain and plasma AUC values following a single PO dose or with terminal brain, plasma, and CSF concentrations following a steady-state IV infusion. Care should be taken initially with single point plasma and brain measurements following single PO doses without an understanding of potential differences in peripheral and central absorption and clearance rates. When using *in vitro* brain homogenate binding techniques, consideration should be given to the ability of a compound to move freely between intracellular and extracellular compartments, where brain slices retain greater cellular integrity [123].

4.4 ELIMINATION

Elimination is the process by which a drug is irreversibly removed from the systemic circulation by metabolism and/or excretion. Metabolism, also referred to as biotransformation, is the chemical alteration of a drug or substance in the body by the action of enzymes. Metabolites occasionally can be converted back to parent compound; thus metabolism is an elimination process only if the metabolite is excreted or lost from the body irreversibly. Excretion is the irreversible removal of unchanged drug and/or metabolites from the body by all possible routes [124]. Quantitatively, renal excretion and hepatic biliary secretion are the two most important excretion mechanisms, although drugs and metabolites can also be excreted from lung, sweat, tears, and other bodily fluids.

4.4.1 Elimination Versus Clearance

The terms elimination and clearance are often used interchangeably, particularly with respect to the mechanism of clearance, including in this chapter. However, elimination refers to the physiological process of removing drug from the systemic circulation, while clearance is a pharmacokinetic parameter defined as the quantitative measure of the rate at which a substance is removed from the blood, and is usually derived from blood or plasma concentration data.

4.4.2 Metabolism Versus Excretion

In a pharmaceutical discovery setting, *in vivo* pharmacokinetic studies in preclinical animal species are used to elucidate the elimination pathways in animals and predict the principal elimination pathways of drug candidates in humans. As a first step, compound is dosed intravenously and the parent compound concentrations are determined in plasma (or blood) and urine. The contribution of renal excretion can be determined from the urine concentrations, and the remainder of the elimination is likely to be hepatic, especially for lipophilic compounds. Hepatic elimination occurs via metabolism or biliary secretion, or a combination of the two mechanisms. The contribution of biliary secretion to elimination can be assessed by dosing the compound intravenously in a bile-duct cannulated animal, such as a rat, and determining the amount of parent compound secreted into bile. When a parent compound is initially metabolized, the elimination mechanism is metabolism, even though the metabolites may be subsequently excreted in urine and feces (via bile).

4.4.3 Drug-Free Fraction and Clearance

An important assumption in clearance is that only the free compound is available to be cleared from systemic circulation whether by biotransformation or excretion. The compound must be unbound to plasma proteins or other cellular or tissue components in order to be eliminated because protein-bound compounds cannot be readily metabolized or transported across membranes by hepatic or renal transporters (see earlier discussion in Section 4.3.3).

4.4.4 Lipophilicity and Clearance

Lipophilicity is the major determinant of clearance for neutral drugs and drug-like compounds. In general, lipophilic drugs are most often eliminated by hepatic metabolism, whereas hydrophilic drugs tend to be eliminated renally. A relationship between log $D_{7.4}$ and clearance has been established (Figure 4.9). For drugs with log $D_{7.4}$ below 0, excretion is predominantly renal, and renal excretion decreases as log $D_{7.4}$ becomes more lipophilic, while metabolic clearance increases as log $D_{7.4}$ becomes more lipophilic [79].

4.4.5 Transporters and Clearance

In addition to lipophilicity, another key determinant of clearance is affinity for transporter proteins in the liver and kidney, especially for charged molecules and compounds containing both lipophilic and hydrophilic functionalities.

4.4.5.1 Hepatic Uptake Transporters In the liver, drugs enter hepatocytes by either passive diffusion through the cellular membrane or by hepatic uptake transport

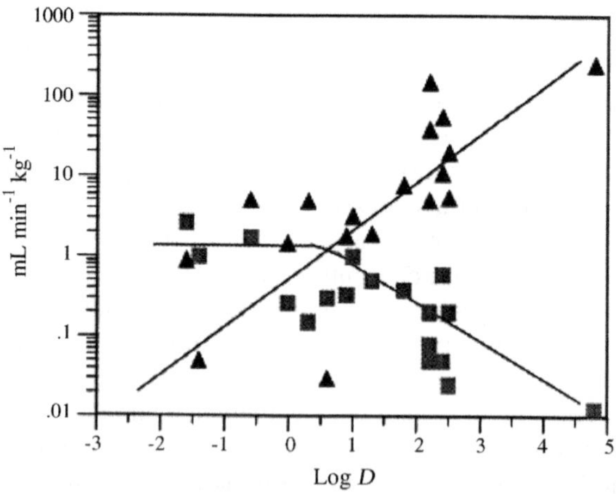

Figure 4.9 Relationship between lipophilicity and unbound renal (squares) and metabolic clearance (triangles) for a range of neutral drugs in man [79].

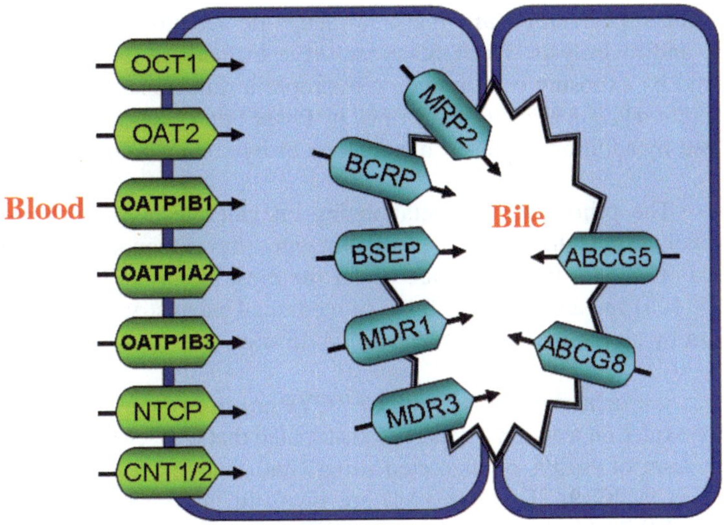

Figure 4.10 Hepatic uptake and biliary secretion transporters.

proteins, or by a combination of these two mechanisms. Hepatic uptake transporters are especially important for anionic or cationic compounds of molecular weight >400. For ionizable compounds of molecular weight >500, hepatic uptake may even serve as the rate-limiting step in clearance [125]. Important hepatic uptake transporters are shown in Figure 4.10.

4.4.5.2 Biliary Transporters and Secretion While lipophilic, low-molecular weight compounds can easily diffuse out of hepatocytes through the cellular membrane, hepatic efflux transporters are required for secretion of ionizable and higher molecular weight compounds into the bile. Important biliary transporters are shown in Figure 4.10.

4.4.5.3 Renal Transporters Renal transport mechanisms are important for the excretion of drugs that are positively or negatively charged at physiological pH and are discussed below in Section 4.4.7.1.

4.4.6 Metabolism

Metabolism by biotransformation enzymes is the primary mechanism of elimination for many drugs and other xenobiotic substances, especially for lipophilic compounds. Drug metabolism and biotransformation are often used interchangeably and refer to the structural modification of a chemical by enzymes in the body. The drug or xenobiotic compound can be metabolized by direct modification, referred to as a Phase I reaction, and by the addition of a conjugate functionality, which is termed a Phase II reaction.

4.4.6.1 Phase I Metabolism Phase I metabolic reactions include oxidation, reduction, and hydrolysis. These reactions serve to increase the hydrophilicity of a compound by exposing or introducing hydrophilic functional groups, thus facilitating excretion [126]. Metabolites formed by Phase I processes may be sequentially metabolized by additional Phase I metabolism or by conjugation reactions.

Oxidation The principal drug-metabolizing enzymes responsible for oxidation reactions include cytochrome P450 (CYP) enzymes, flavin monooxygenases (FMO) and several others. CYP enzymes are by far the most important for metabolism of drugs [127, 128] and are the major focus of medicinal chemistry strategies to reduce metabolism by alteration of metabolically labile sites.

CYP ENZYMES AND THEIR CLINICAL IMPORTANCE CYP enzymes are capable of catalyzing a variety of oxidation reactions. It has been estimated that CYP enzymes contribute to the metabolism of ~75% of marketed drugs, and that five major CYP isoforms (CYP1A2, 2C9, 2C19, 2D6, and 3A4) are involved in 95% of all Phase I reactions [129]. CYP3A4 is the most important CYP isoform for the metabolism of drugs and is involved as a major or minor drug-metabolizing enzyme in more than half of all drugs [130]. The human CYP isoforms most often involved in the metabolism of drugs along with characteristics of typical substrates are listed in Table 4.4. In general, the

TABLE 4.4 Characteristics of Human CYP Isoforms and their Substrates[a]

CYP	% Total Hepatic CYP[b]	Substrate Range of log *P*	Substrate Average log *P*	Substrate Molecular Characteristics	Typical Substrate
1A2	12	0.08–3.61	2.01	Poly(hetero)aromatic amines and amides	MeIQ[c]
2A6	4	0.07–2.79	1.44	Relatively small neutral molecules	Losigamone
2B6	1	0.23–4.89	2.54	Basic (unionized) compounds	Bupropion
2C8	[d]	0.06–6.98	3.38	Acidic (ionized) compounds	Rosiglitazone
2C9	[d]	0.89–5.18	3.20	Acidic (unionized) compounds	Naproxen
2C19	[d]	1.49–4.42	2.56	Amides and amines	Proguanil
2D6	4	0.75–5.04	3.08	Basic (ionized) compounds	Propranolol
2E1	6	−1.35 to 3.63	2.07	Small neutral molecules	4-Nitrophenol
3A4	30	0.97–7.54	3.10	Large neutral molecules	Nifedipine

[a]Adapted from Ref. 131.
[b]Adapted from Ref. 132.
[c]MeIQ = 2-amino-3,4-dimethylimidazo[4,5-*f*]quinoline.
[d]Total CYP2C is approximately 20%; quantification of individual isoforms is limited by antibody cross-reactivtiy.

binding affinity of a substrate to CYP enzymes is determined by the log *P* and the number of hydrogen bond donor and acceptor atoms [131]. Additional factors affecting which CYP isoforms are likely to contribute to the metabolism of a compound include molecular weight, planarity, and acidity/basicity. Because of overlapping substrate specificity, compounds can be substrates of multiple CYP enzymes, and the site of metabolism may be the same or can vary.

CYP1A2 CYP1A2 tends to oxidize small, planar lipophilic compounds such as caffeine and phenacetin and is often a minor or secondary contributor to the metabolism of a drug. It is additionally important because it plays a role in the metabolic activation of some carcinogens.

CYP2C8 CYP2C8 has a larger active site than the other CYP2C enzymes and tends to metabolize medium to large molecular weight acidic and lipophilic compounds. CYP2C8 has substrate affinity that overlaps somewhat with CYP3A. Paclitaxel, amiodarone, and rosiglitazone are examples of CYP2C8 substrates.

CYP2C9 CYP2C9 preferentially metabolizes compounds that are hydrophobic and weakly acidic, including drugs such as phenytoin, (*S*)-warfarin, and numerous nonsteroidal anti-inflammatory drugs.

CYP2C19 CYP2C19 tends to metabolize medium to large molecular weight lipophilic amine and amide compounds such as (*S*)-mephenytoin and omeprazole and has substrate affinity that overlaps somewhat with CYP3A.

CYP2D6 CYP2D6 preferentially metabolizes ionized basic compounds and often oxidizes metabolizable sites 7 or 9 Å from a basic nitrogen. Many drugs are metabolized by CYP2D6 including most beta andrenergic blocking drugs and a wide variety of psychotherapeutic agents.

CYP3A4/5 CYP3A4 is the most abundant human CYP isoform and is the most important human drug-metabolizing enzyme due to its relative abundance combined with its large active site and broad substrate specificity for metabolizing lipophilic molecules. The closely related CYP3A5 has similar metabolic properties, although it is only expressed in approximately one-fourth of humans. In those humans possessing this isoform, expression levels are typically only one-third as high as for CYP3A4.

CYP2A6, CYP2B6, AND CYP2E1 These are minor CYP isoforms that can contribute to the metabolism of drugs but are not usually identified as the major contributor. CYP2E1 is important for the metabolism of many low molecular weight compounds, including organic solvents and some inhalable anesthetics.

FLAVIN MONOOXYGENASE FMO enzymes catalyze the oxidation of nucleophilic nitrogen, sulfur, and phosphorous heteroatoms present in a variety of drugs [133]. The most important FMO reactions are the oxidation of tertiary amines to *N*-oxides, the oxidation of secondary amines to hydroxylamines, and the oxidation of thiols, thiones, and thioethers to *S*-oxides. Many oxidation reactions catalyzed by FMO can also be catalyzed by CYP, and experimental procedures have been developed to determine the contribution of FMO compared to CYP enzymes for a specific reaction.

OTHER ENZYMES PREFORMING OXIDATION REACTIONS Other important enzymes that are capable of performing oxidation reactions of drugs include alcohol dehydrogenase, aldehyde dehydrogenase, aldehyde oxidase, xanthine oxidase, monoamine oxidase, and diamine oxidase [126].

Reduction Reduction reactions include azo, nitro, carbonyl, disulfide, sulfoxide, quinone reductions, and also reductive dehalogenation reactions. The drug-metabolizing enzymes responsible for these reduction reactions vary with the type of reduction. Azo- and nitro-group reductions can be performed by intestinal microflora, CYP enzymes, and NAD(P)H-quinone oxidoreductase. Carbonyl group reductions can be catalyzed by alcohol dehydrogenase and a family of carbonyl reductases. Disulfides can be reduced in a reaction involving glutathione-*S*-transferase, sulfoxide, and *N*-oxide reductions can be catalyzed by CYP. Quinone reductions are catalyzed by NAD(P)H-quinone oxidoreductase, and reductive dehalogenation reactions are catalyzed by CYP.

Hydrolysis The main enzymes responsible for hydrolysis reactions are carboxylesterases, peptidases, and epoxide hydrolases. Hydrolysis reactions are especially important for the metabolism of prodrugs and can occur in blood, intestine, or liver.

4.4.6.2 Species Differences in Phase I Metabolism The differences in homology and expression levels of Phase I metabolizing enzymes between humans and preclinical animal species are great enough that cross-species metabolism is not predictable. This is especially true of CYP enzyme in which it has been shown experimentally using site-directed mutagenesis studies that a single amino acid substitution in the active site of an enzyme can change the catalytic specificity such that a different oxidation product is formed. Therefore, human *in vitro* drug-metabolizing systems are considered to be the most relevant predictor of human metabolism, and likewise, *in vitro* systems for other preclinical animal species should be used to predict their respective *in vivo* metabolic rates and/or profiles. Species differences in Phase I metabolism are reviewed elsewhere [134, 135].

4.4.6.3 Phase II Metabolism (Conjugation) Phase II metabolic reactions add conjugate functionalities that result in a large increase in hydrophilicity, usually greater than that achieved by Phase I reactions [126]. Compounds do not need to undergo Phase I metabolism prior to Phase II. Metabolites formed by Phase II processes are often vastly more amenable to excretion than the parent compound, but still may be sequentially metabolized by additional Phase I or II reactions.

Glucuronidation Glucuronidation represents a major biotransformation pathway for drugs, as well as steroid, bile acids, bilirubin, and other dietary components [136, 137]. Uridine-diphoshphate glucuronosyltransferase (UGT) enzymes utilize uridine-diphoshphate (UDP) glucuronic acid as a cofactor, which can be conjugated with compounds containing an electron-rich heteroatom such as O, S, or N. Hydroxyl and carboxyl functionalities are most often subject to glucuronidation. Glucuronidation of carboxylic acids can result in acyl migration of the glucuronide and may lead to the formation of reactive metabolites.

Sulfation Many of the same substrates that undergo *O*-glucuronidation can also be metabolized to sulfate conjugates by sulfotranserases using 3′-phosphoadenosine-5′-phosphosulfate (PAPS) as the cofactor. The conjugation reaction is carried out by the transfer of SO_3^- from PAPS to the drug compound.

Glutathione Conjugation Conjugation with glutathione by glutathione-*S*-transferase represents a major detoxification mechanism by reducing reactive metabolite concentrations in circulation.

Other Phase II Processes Other important Phase II reactions include amino acid conjugation, acylation, and methylation.

Species Differences in Phase II Metabolism As with Phase I metabolic reactions, numerous species differences exist between Phase II metabolism reactions in humans and preclinical animal species [138]. Some species differences are mainly quantitative, in which differing amounts of the same conjugate metabolite are formed, for example, guinea pigs have an unusually high capacity for methylation compared to human. Others species differences involve a complete inability to catalyze a specific metabolic reaction, for example, dogs cannot acetylate aromatic amines and pigs cannot catalyze sulfate conjugations [135]. In some cases these species differences in metabolism can lead to differences in toxicity or carcinogenicity.

4.4.6.4 Extrahepatic Metabolism Although liver is the major site of metabolism for drugs and is the organ most thoroughly studied, other organs and tissues can also contribute to the metabolism of drugs [139]. Small intestine, kidney, and lung contain significant amounts of drug-metabolizing enzymes, although, in terms of functional enzyme capacity, these organs are one to two orders of magnitude lower compared to the liver. In particular, CYP enzymes are known to be distributed throughout the body and are found in most tissues, including brain and skin, albeit often at low levels of expression.

4.4.7 Excretion

Excretion of unchanged compound is the primary mechanism of elimination for many drugs and other xenobiotic substances, especially for hydrophilic compounds and those that are charged at physiological pH. Quantitatively, excretion into urine and feces (via secretion into bile) comprises the majority of drug and metabolite removal from the body, except for some low molecular weight compounds, such as inhalable anesthetics, which can be excreted by exhalation from the lungs.

4.4.7.1 Renal Excretion Drugs that have polar functionality and molecular weight <500 are water soluble and predominantly excreted in the kidney. Recently, an analysis of human renal clearance data for a set of 391 compounds showed that renal clearance contributes to >50% of total body clearance for 31% of the compounds [140]. The excretory functional unit of the kidney is the nephron, which is composed of the glomerulus, proximal tubule, loop of Henle, distal tubule, and the collecting tubule. The three mechanisms involved in drug excretion through the kidney are glomerular filtration, tubular reabsorption, and active secretion. The renal transporters that are important for active secretion are shown in Figure 4.11.

Glomerular Filtration Glomerular filtration is the nonselective passive process by which many drugs and small molecules are filtered through the glomerulus of the nephron. This process is driven by hydrostatic pressure formed in the capillaries.

Tubular Reabsorption Tubular reabsorption takes place after glomerular filtration and occurs all along the renal tubule. Lipophilic drugs undergo extensive reabsorption, while hydrophilic drugs and compounds are not reabsorbed and are more readily excreted in the urine.

Active Tubular Secretion For acidic and basic compounds ionized at physiological pH, active tubular secretion is the most important excretion process. The active

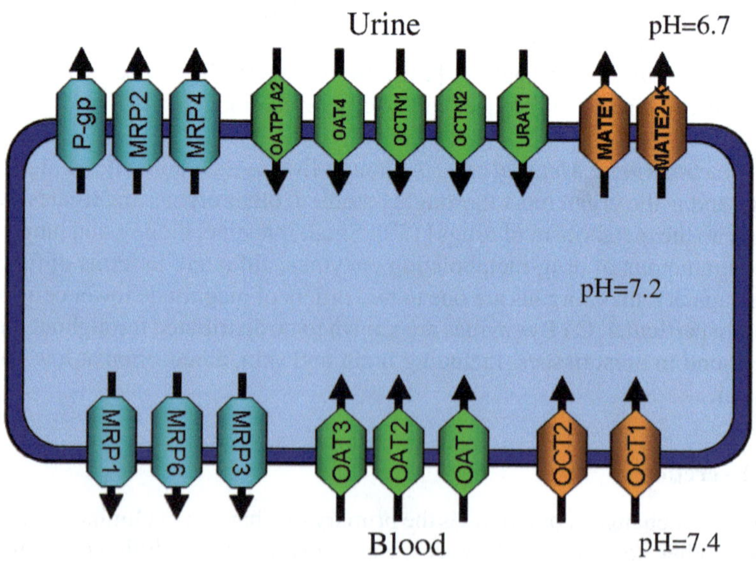

Figure 4.11 Renal transporters.

secretion is performed by transport proteins in the proximal tubule, with different sets of transporters existing for acids and bases.

The Role of Lipophilicity in Renal Excretion The extent of reabsorption of drug in the kidney depends on both the lipophilicity and ionization of the drug. If a drug has sufficient lipophilicity, the drug is reabsorbed by passive diffusion and concentrated as the kidney reabsorbs water. For neutral compounds, reabsorption only occurs at log $D_{7.4}$ values >0 and excretion into urine is more likely as log $D_{7.4}$ decreases [79].

The Role of Charge in Renal Excretion Because tubular pH (6.5) is often more acidic than plasma pH (7.4), the renal clearance of acidic drugs may be higher than their log $D_{7.4}$ might suggest, and conversely, the renal clearance of basic drugs may be lower than their log $D_{7.4}$ might suggest. Particularly for lipophilic charged compounds, the renal excretion can be very high due to interactions with active tubular secretion transporters [79].

4.4.7.2 Biliary Excretion In addition to renal excretion, the other major route is hepatic excretion into the bile, which is produced in the liver and flows into the intestinal tract. As opposed to the kidney, the liver cannot passively filter chemicals but can actively secrete chemicals into bile and eventually eliminate them via excretion of feces. Biliary secretion of a chemical may not result in the immediate elimination of chemical from the body because of hepatobiliary recirculation, which is discussed in more detail in the section "Enterohepatic Recirculation of Drugs".

Bile Composition The production and recirculation of bile is the main excretory function of the liver. Bile is composed primarily of bile salts and smaller amounts of cholesterol, phospholipids, bilirubin, protein, and other components [141]. The bile salts function as detergents that dissolve dietary fat and also solubilize lipophilic drugs.

Compound Properties Leading to Biliary Excretion Anions, cations, and neutral compounds containing both hydrophilic and lipophilic groups can be secreted into bile. Generally, the molecular weight must be >300 for biliary secretion to occur because lower molecular weight compounds are generally reabsorbed before being secreted into the bile duct. In humans, the threshold for preferential excretion of compounds into bile is a MW in the 500–600 Da range [142]. This threshold varies across species and is as low as approximately 235 Da in rats.

The Role of Transporters in the Biliary Secretion of Drugs For drugs that cannot exit hepatocytes by simple passive diffusion into the plasma, a number of transport proteins exists that actively secrete the drugs and/or their metabolites into the bile [125].

Enterohepatic Recirculation of Drugs An issue that can affect both drugs and metabolites, particularly glucuronide conjugates, is enterohepatic (or hepatobiliary) recycling (EHR, see Section 5.2.1.5). After a drug is conjugated with glucuronic acid to form a glucuronide metabolite, the metabolite can be secreted into bile, which flows to the gall bladder and is released into the small intestine. In the intestine, the glucuronide conjugate can be hydrolyzed back to the parent compound by β-glucuronidases present in intestinal bacteria. The parent compound can then be reabsorbed and returned to circulating blood and the liver where it can be metabolized and the cycle repeats [143].

4.5 DRUG INTERACTIONS

Adverse drug reactions are undesirable and can result in the clinical failure of drug candidates and can also lead to alteration of the dosing regimen of approved products and even withdrawal from the market. Although individual drugs can cause adverse drug reactions, many adverse reactions result from DDI due to concomitant administration of multiple medicinal products. The two main categories of DDI are pharmacological and pharmacokinetic. Pharmacological DDI occurs when one or more drugs alters the pharmacological effect of another. Examples of this type of DDI include the synergistic and additive effect of multiple central nervous system depressants, resulting in severe respiratory depression; and the inhibition of platelet aggregation by nonsteroidal anti-inflammatory drugs, leading to increased bleeding when anticoagulants are co-administered. Reviews of pharmacological DDI are provided elsewhere [144].

Pharmacokinetic DDI affect the disposition of a drug and can occur when any ADME process is interfered with, including absorption, distribution, metabolism, and/or excretion.

4.5.1 Absorption-Driven DDI

Absorption can be affected by the chemical interaction of drugs that complex or chelate with each other, by drugs that change the rate of gastric emptying, drugs that alter the pH of gastrointestinal fluids, and drugs that alter the composition of intestinal microflora, for example, antibiotics. In addition, drugs and excipients can interact in the gastrointestinal tract and affect drug absorption. Most clinically important drug–excipient interactions have been shown to affect disintegration and/or dissolution processes [145].

4.5.2 Distribution-Driven DDI

Distribution processes are typically only affected when drugs displace each other from plasma protein binding sites [146]. This type of drug interaction only results in significant consequences in very limited situations and is not a major source of clinical DDI.

4.5.3 Excretion-Driven DDI

Excretion of drugs can be inhibited due to interactions with renal or biliary transporters. Renal excretion of ionizable compounds can be either reduced or increased by concomitant administration of drugs that affect the pH of urine.

4.5.4 Metabolism-Driven DDI

Metabolic DDI due to perturbations of drug metabolism are by far the major cause of pharmacokinetic DDI and have lead to the withdrawal of numerous marketed products [147]. Metabolic DDI are discussed in detail below, and are a main focus of medicinal chemistry strategies to reduce compound attrition in Pharmaceutical Discovery and Development.

4.5.4.1 DDI via Inhibition of Drug-Metabolizing Enzymes Metabolic DDI occurs when a drug causes either an increase or decrease of systemic exposures of other drugs due to alterations of drug metabolism, or is susceptible to an increase or decrease of its own systemic exposures due to effects on its metabolism by other concomitantly administered drugs. Multiple strategies are used to screen drug candidates for metabolic DDI potential and are tailored to the discovery or development stage. The FDA has issued a Guidance to Industry that provides suggestions for approaches to studying the potential for metabolic DDI using *in vitro* techniques [148, 149] (www.fda.gov/downloads/Drugs/GuidanceComplianceRegulatory-Information/Guidances/ucm072101.pdf).

Perpetrator DDI The most clinically significant type of DDI occurs when a drug is a potent inhibitor (perpetrator) of one or more CYP enzymes. The consequence of this inhibition can result in a severe reduction of drug-metabolizing capacity and the loss of the major elimination mechanism for many other drugs that are metabolized by the same enzymes, which can lead to toxic or even lethal increases in circulating blood concentrations. This is especially the case for potent inhibitors of CYP3A4, such as antifungal drugs and some antiviral agents.

Although metabolic DDI can be caused by inhibition of drug-metabolizing enzymes other than CYPs, clinically relevant examples are rare. Glucuronidation is an elimination mechanism for approximately one in ten of the most highly prescribed drugs, yet the likelihood of metabolic DDI is low for drugs cleared by glucuronidation [150].

Victim DDI Drugs that are eliminated via metabolism by a single drug-metabolizing enzyme can greatly increase circulating blood concentrations if that metabolic pathway is inhibited significantly. This type of drug is often referred to as the "victim" of a metabolic DDI such as the interaction between ketoconazole and terfenadine. Ketoconazole is a potent inhibitor of CYP3A4, and terfenadine is dependent on CYP3A4 metabolism as its sole route of elimination. Terfenadine is thus the victim of the ketoconazole inhibition, and this clinically significant DDI eventually resulted in the withdrawal of terfenadine from the market.

4.5.4.2 Metabolism by Polymorphic CYPs Another type of undesirable metabolic drug interaction occurs when a drug is eliminated primarily via metabolism of a polymorphically expressed human CYP isoform; most notably CYP2C19 and CYP2D6. For each of these two CYP isoforms a significant fraction of the population exhibits a poor metabolizer phenotype. The result of a drug relying on one of these enzymes for its elimination can lead to greatly increased circulating blood concentrations in those subjects who completely lack or possess significantly reduced drug-metabolizing capacity for that enzyme. In this case the increased risk of toxicity is not caused by an interaction between two drugs, but rather the drug and its mechanism of elimination.

4.5.4.3 DDI via Induction of Drug-Metabolizing Enzymes Induction occurs when drug metabolism capacity is increased due to an increase in intracellular metabolizing enzymes occurring primarily in the liver, but also in the lung, small intestine, kidney, and other tissues. Unlike inhibition of drug-metabolizing enzymes that can happen immediately, induction takes longer (several days) to achieve a higher steady-state level of enzyme activity. The most important clinical example of induction is the effect of the potent CYP3A4 inducer rifampicin on reducing the systemic exposure of the tissue rejection drugs cyclosporine and tacrolimus, which have a very narrow therapeutic index [151]. Rifampicin causes an increase in CYP3A4 activity that reduces blood concentrations of these immunosuppressant drugs and can lead to tissue rejection. In the pharmaceutical industry, induction of CYP3A4 is the greatest concern for DDI and drug candidates are often compared to rifampicin to ascertain their potential to cause a clinically relevant CYP3A4 induction.

Cause of Induction and Sequence of Events CYP induction is caused by a sequence of events starting with the binding of a drug or dietary component to a nuclear receptor such as PXR or CAR, followed by an increase in gene transcription, protein translation, and finally, an increase in the level of functional drug-metabolizing enzyme [152]. The induction process takes several days to occur and usually is not maximal in humans until 10–14 days.

Assessment of Potential for CYP Induction Strategies for assessment of CYP induction are employed at every step of the sequence. The highest throughput method is to assess binding of compound to the pregnane-X receptor (PXR), the human nuclear receptor most responsible for upregulation of CYP3A4, using a reporter gene assay. The definitive and most predictive assay uses cultured primary human hepatocytes. Compounds of interest are incubated with hepatocytes and the increases in CYP3A4 mRNA and protein are measured. Increases in functional drug-metabolizing capacity are assessed by incubating the induced cells with a CYP3A4 probe substrate and measuring the formation of marker metabolites.

Issues with Prediction of CYP Induction Assessment of CYP induction potential often results in low confidence in the quantitative prediction of induction, even when using human *in vitro* systems, because of the high variability of induction response in the human population. The ability to form structure–activity relationships with PXR is challenging due to the wide variety of chemical structures that are able to bind to the receptor. In addition, induction of CYP3A4 has been shown to be a species specific process due to species differences in the ligand binding domain of PXR [153]. For example, rifampicin is known to be a potent inducer of CYP3A in human but not in rat. Conversely, pregnenolone 16α-carbonitrile is a very potent inducer of CYP3A in rat but not in human. Prediction of human induction potential from preclinical animal *in vivo* exposure data may not be predictive.

4.5.5 Tools for Studying Drug Metabolism

A variety of tools can be utilized to investigate drug metabolism in the various stages of drug discovery and development:

- *In vivo* studies
- *In situ* perfused organs
- Liver slices
- *In vitro* cell-based systems (hepatocyte suspensions)
- *In vitro* subcellular fractions (microsomes, S9, cytosol)
- *In vitro* recombinant drug-metabolizing enzymes
- *In silico* tools.

Usually these tools are used in combination to address different aspects of drug metabolism. Understanding of the advantages and disadvantages of certain tools as well as their best application to the projects of different stages is critical for medicinal chemists and their ADME partners.

Most of the tools are derived from liver tissue because the liver is the major site of drug metabolism, although preparations from other tissues such as kidney, intestine, or lung may also be used in order to elucidate the contribution of metabolism in those tissues.

4.5.5.1 In Vivo Studies in Animals Pharmacokinetic clearance data from intravenously dosed preclinical animals can be used to assess the rate of hepatic metabolism, provided it can be determined that hepatic metabolism is the major route of elimination and excretion is minor. For screening a large number of compounds, rat is the species utilized most often, however the preclinical species most relevant to human should be used if possible. Animal pharmacokinetic studies are also used as a source of *in vivo* metabolites, which can be isolated from plasma, urine, bile, feces, and other fluids or tissues. Profiling parent and metabolites in plasma and excreta using radiolabeled drug in an *in vivo* mass balance study is considered more definitive because it does not require prior knowledge of expected metabolites.

The extent of first-pass metabolism by the liver may be evaluated *in vivo* by comparing the plasma AUC of the drug-dosed PO with that following direct infusion into the portal vein system. The use of various chemical inhibitors such as 1-aminobenzotriazole, a potent, nonspecific inhibitor of CYP enzymes, can be used to assess CYP contributions to metabolism, although care should be taken in understanding the specificity of inhibition [154].

Knock-out or humanized animals may also be used to assess specific metabolism clearance mechanisms [155].

4.5.5.2 In Situ Perfused Organs Isolated perfused organs have been used to investigate drug metabolism in numerous preclinical animal species. Isolated liver models in the rat have been used most extensively and the procedure is described elsewhere [23, 156–158]. The *in situ* perfusion of liver has several advantages including intact tissue architecture, cell polarity, and bile flow. This model is able to perform both metabolism and hepatic uptake and biliary secretion, and thus can be used to determine the overall hepatic elimination.

4.5.5.3 Liver Slices Liver slices are prepared from liver by using a razor blade or a precision-cutting device to cut small sections of liver tissue to a thickness of 200–500 μm [159]. The slices can then be incubated in buffer or cell culture medium and used for drug metabolism experiments. As drug metabolism tools, liver slices contain intact cells and have some of the same advantages as hepatocytes [160].

4.5.5.4 In Vitro Cell-Based Systems Hepatocyte suspension is a very popular system for studying drug metabolism. Hepatocytes are intact cells and thus are capable of performing both Phase I and Phase II metabolic reactions and also sequential biotransformation reactions.

Hepatocytes are prepared from intact liver by perfusing the liver with collagenase to isolate the hepatocytes from the extracellular matrix. The isolated hepatocytes can be incubated immediately with test compound in cell culture medium in an oxygenated atmosphere, or can be cryopreserved for future use.

4.5.5.5 In Vivo Subcellular Fractions Subcellular fractions isolated from animal or human liver such as microsomes, S9 fraction, and cytosolic fraction are widely used in drug discovery to study the rate of metabolism, reaction phenotyping, and predicting metabolic profiles of drug candidates, and their potential DDI. Microsomes preparations are the system most frequently used for high-throughput metabolic screening as well as for more mechanistic drug metabolism studies *in vitro*.

Liver Microsomes Liver microsomes are prepared by further centrifuging liver S9 in an ultracentrifuge at 100,000 × *g* or greater. This procedure compresses the endoplasmic reticulum, which contains membrane-bound drug-metabolizing enzymes, into vesicles called microsomes, which can be resuspended in buffer and stored frozen. The microsomes contain the important CYP, FMO, and UDP-GT enzymes, among others.

MICROSOMES VERSUS HEPATOCYTES Microsomes and hepatocytes can both be used for determination of metabolic stability and intrinsic clearance. Each system has advantages and disadvantages. Microsomes that are subcellular fractions lack cell membranes and provide ready access of the test compound to the metabolizing enzymes. They are used mostly for determining metabolism by CYP enzymes, which represent a viable screening strategy since CYP metabolism has the greatest overall impact on metabolic stability. Microsomes can also be used to determine the metabolic rates of other membrane-bound drug-metabolizing enzymes. However, the addition of exogenous cofactors may be required, for example, UPD-glucuronic acid fortified systems are used to facilitate formation of glucuronide conjugates by UDP-GT enzymes. Hepatocyte incubations, by comparison, use cultured intact cells, and thus have the advantage of structurally intact membrane-bound and cytosolic enzymes. They are capable of catalyzing the entire complement of hepatic drug-metabolizing functions, and may thus provide a more relevant prediction of *in vivo* metabolism. Hepatocyte systems sometimes yield artifactual low rates of metabolism particularly for highly lipophilic compounds often encountered in early discovery because of either poor solubility of test compound in the cell culture medium or inability to enter the hepatocytes to gain access to the drug-metabolizing enzymes. For lipophilic compounds, especially in screening mode, microsomal incubations tend to provide higher rates of metabolism and are more useful for decision making and rank ordering of compounds.

Liver S9 Fractions Liver S9 is a subcellular fraction prepared by homogenizing liver, centrifuging at 9000 $\times$ *g* and saving the postmitochondrial supernatant, which can be stored frozen and used as a crude source of drug-metabolizing enzymes. An advantage of liver S9 fraction is that it contains both cytosolic and membrane-bound drug-metabolizing enzymes.

Liver Cytosolic Fractions Liver cytosolic fraction is prepared from the liver S9 fraction during the preparation of microsomes (see section "Liver Microsomes"). During the final centrifugation step, the microsomes form the pellet and the supernatant comprises the cytosolic fraction, which contains soluble drug-metabolizing enzymes, as opposed to the membrane-bound enzymes in the microsomes. The cytosolic fraction is an excellent source of numerous Phase I drug-metabolizing enzymes, including epoxide hydrolase, several reductases, alcohol dehydrogenase, aldehyde oxidase, xanthine oxidase, and also Phase II enzymes capable of conjugating drugs with sulfate, glutathione, and methyl and acyl groups.

4.5.5.6 In Vivo Recombinant Drug-Metabolizing Enzymes Recombinant cDNA-expressed human drug-metabolizing enzymes are metabolism tools that are now commercially available from numerous sources. A specific human drug-metabolizing enzyme mRNA is used as the source for generation of a cDNA, which is recombined with an expression vector and introduced into a cell culture system suitable for production of a large quantity of human enzyme. The cells can be homogenized and centrifuged to prepare microsomes or the enzymes can be further purified and reconstituted.

4.5.5.7 In Silico Tools *In silico* models have been developed to predict drug metabolism properties [161]. The simplest models are used for screening and utilize physicochemical properties to predict metabolic stability. More sophisticated models have been developed for predicting hepatic clearance, metabolite formation, the potential for metabolic DDI, and other metabolism properties [20, 162].

4.5.6 Applications of Drug Metabolism Tools

A variety of tools are available to investigate the role of metabolism in the overall disposition of a test compound or drug candidate. The main uses of metabolism tools are for the prediction of human exposure and safety, and generally fall into the following four categories:

1. metabolic stability and the intrinsic clearance;
2. reaction phenotyping (identification of enzymes contributing to the metabolism of a particular chemical entity);
3. metabolic profiling; and
4. prediction of potential metabolic DDI.

4.5.6.1 Metabolic Stability and Intrinsic Clearance The determination of metabolic stability of the newly synthesized compounds is usually done at a very early stage of the drug discovery projects in a high-throughput screening mode aiming to determine basic metabolic liabilities of the compounds, estimate their intrinsic metabolic clearance, and establish so-called *in vitro–in vivo* correlations (IVIVC).

Metabolic Stability Liver microsomes and S9 fraction are the tools of choice for determining metabolic stability, and fully automated, high-throughput systems for these are applied at early stages of drug discovery. Test compounds are incubated *in vitro* with the enzyme preparation and an NADPH regenerating system to supply electrons for the CYP reactions. Consumption of parent compound from the incubation mixture is measured either at a fixed time point or using a time course to determine the *in vitro* metabolic disappearance half-life. The resulting information is used to advance compounds for further testing based on a pass/fail criterion or to determine the rank order of a series of drug candidates.

Drugs that are eliminated principally by metabolism require a rate of metabolism that is appropriate for the desired pharmacokinetic profile: short elimination half-life for fast acting drugs, longer half-life suitable for BID or QD dosing regimen for most chronically administered drugs. For drug candidates intended for chronic administration, rapid metabolism is often a key factor in poor pharmacokinetics. Several tools and techniques are used at various discovery stages to screen out compounds demonstrating undesirable high rates of metabolism.

Intrinsic Clearance Metabolic stability assays that measure an *in vitro* half-life are used to determine intrinsic clearance, which essentially represents the fraction of hepatic clearance driven by metabolism. The *in vitro* half-life is converted to an *in vitro* intrinsic clearance value, and then physiological scaling factors are applied. The scaled value is incorporated into a calculation of *in vivo* hepatic clearance, such as the well-stirred model (described previously in Section 4.3.3). The *in vivo* hepatic clearance can be used for elucidation of the metabolic contribution to clearance and also can be incorporated into the prediction of the *in vivo* elimination half-life [84].

In Vitro–In Vivo Clearance Correlation An important technique in the investigation of the rate of drug metabolism is the determination of the correlation of *in vitro* predicted hepatic clearance to that of *in vivo* hepatic clearance from animal pharmacokinetic studies. A lack of correlation such that the *in vivo* clearance is significantly higher than the *in vitro* predicted value usually indicates that the *in vitro* system represents only a part of the overall clearance mechanism. In the case of underpredicted clearance using microsomes, either an S9 system fortified with cofactors or a hepatocyte incubation system may provide the missing metabolic contribution and a more accurate prediction. If metabolic intrinsic clearance still underpredicts *in vivo* clearance, the results may indicate that either biliary secretion or extrahepatic metabolism are significant factors in the elimination of the compound.

4.5.6.2 Reaction Phenotyping An important discovery stage activity is the determination of which drug-metabolizing enzymes are responsible for the elimination of a drug candidate. This knowledge is used to predict if the drug candidate will be eliminated by a single metabolic pathway, resulting in a potential metabolic DDI risk (especially for CYP3A4). It is also implemented to predict whether the drug candidate will be metabolized by an enzyme that is polymorphically expressed in human and could lead to high variability of drug exposures, which could result in clinical safety issues [163]. The polymorphically expressed human drug-metabolizing enzymes of most concern are CYP2D6 and CYP2C19 [164]. Depending on which enzymes and how many enzymes contribute to metabolism, different techniques are employed.

In vitro incubation with different subcellular liver fractions can be used to assess the location of the enzyme (microsomal membrane-bound or cytosolic fraction). Addition or subtraction of required cofactors and/or specific chemical inhibitors to *in vitro* incubations can be used to assess the type of enzyme (CYP, UDP-GT, etc.). For CYP enzymes, the battery of assays used to determine the fraction of metabolism catalyzed by the various CYPs is referred to as reaction phenotyping [163] and utilizes pooled human liver microsome incubations in combination with isoform-selective inhibitors and additional experiments with recombinant human CYP enzymes.

4.5.6.3 Metabolic Profiling The aim of the metabolic profiling of drug candidates at early stages of the discovery projects is to determine the structural elements of the molecules causing high metabolic instability of the compounds. Those functional groups ("soft spots") can then be modified or replaced with different functional groups in order to reduce the rate of the metabolism of the drug candidates.

At later stages of discovery projects, metabolic profiling is typically used to compare the metabolites formed in the preclinical animal species with those that can be formed in the humans to ensure the safety of human subjects in clinical trials.

Identification of Metabolites and Metabolic "Soft Spots" Metabolic soft spot identification is utilized in early discovery to identify metabolically labile sites that cause unacceptably high rates of metabolism. For a compound of interest or a few compounds in a chemical series, major metabolites are putatively identified using LC–MS/MS (liquid chromatography–electrospray tandem mass). The metabolic profiles are examined to determine whether a single site can be blocked or if multiple metabolic routes exist and thus metabolism will be more difficult to reduce by strategic modifications. Liver microsome, S9 or hepatocyte incubations, as well as animal plasma and urine can all be used as the source of metabolites for assessment of highly labile sites, although in early discovery screening, microsomes are the tool used most often.

In vitro metabolizing systems, particularly liver microsomes, are used as a source of metabolites for the assessment of active metabolites in early discovery pharmacology screens. Test compounds are incubated *in vitro* with liver microsomes to generate metabolites. The incubations are then subjected to a simple purification procedure and the resulting supernatants or resuspended extracts are tested for *in vitro* potency. In later stages of discovery, major metabolites (>10% in circulation compared to parent compound) may be purified or synthesized and submitted to pharmacology testing to more accurately evaluate the contribution of the metabolite to the overall *in vivo* pharmacological activity.

Animal and Human Metabolites in Safety Testing Prediction of the human metabolic profile is required in order to predict the elimination mechanisms in humans and to understand the likely role of metabolism in human clearance. An additional important consideration is that all predicted human metabolites should be adequately represented in preclinical animal species during safety studies. The only relevant tools for prediction of the human metabolic profile in the discovery stages are human *in vitro* systems, due to species differences in metabolism, most significantly for CYP enzymes.

Hepatocyte incubations are preferred as they provide the best overall picture of metabolism. For low turnover compounds, liver microsomes and occasionally recombinant expressed human CYP enzymes may be used to generate and identify putative human metabolites. In the development stage, when human plasma and urine become available from clinical Phase I studies, metabolite scouting can be performed, while definitive human metabolite identification is typically performed later in development using radiolabeled compound.

Cross-species metabolite identification is performed in the late discovery stage to determine if the predicted human metabolite profile is qualitatively similar to the metabolic profiles in the preclinical animal species (usually rat and dog or monkey) used for toxicology testing. Identification of the formation of a metabolite that is unique to human represents a drug development risk because the metabolite cannot be generated by the toxicity species and thus cannot be evaluated prior to clinical trials. Also, predicted human major metabolites may be subject to required preclinical toxicity assessment in addition to the testing required for the parent compound as described in the FDA Guidance for Industry called MIST (Metabolites in Safety

Testing) [165]. Cross-species metabolite identification is performed, minimally, by incubating the test compound *in vitro* with hepatocytes from human and all relevant toxicity species, and then determining and comparing the metabolic profiles. Additional profiling of *in vivo* plasma and/or urine from the toxicity species can help to understand the relevance of the *in vitro* metabolite profile to the *in vivo* situation and strengthen the human prediction.

4.5.6.4 Prediction of Metabolic Drug–Drug Interactions A variety of human *in vitro* systems are used for the prediction of a potential metabolic DDI due to the inhibition or the induction of the CYP enzymes.

CYP Inhibition and Potential DDI CYP inhibition studies are conducted to assess the potential for new chemical entities or drug candidates to potently inhibit any of the major human CYP isoforms, typically CYP1A2, CYP2C9, CYP2C19, CYP2D6, and CYP3A4. Different techniques are used in different stages of discovery but most assays use pooled human liver microsomes as the CYP enzyme source and either a single concentration or varying concentrations of test compounds to generate IC_{50} values.

Early stage discovery assessment of CYP inhibition employs high-throughput assays to screen large numbers of compounds and facilitate building structure–inhibitor relationships that can be used for lead compound design [147].

In later stages of discovery, emphasis shifts to the determination of K_i values and investigation of possible atypical kinetics and determination of the type of inhibition, especially nonreversible time-dependent inhibition [166]. In addition, rigorous, validated assays have been developed for the definitive determination of CYP inhibition during development [167]. Understanding of the potency and type of CYP inhibition, combined with knowledge of the fraction metabolized by individual CYP isoforms, can be used effectively to predict the potential for human metabolic DDI using commercially available prediction software.

CYP Induction and Potential DDI Several *in vitro* models can be utilized to predict the likelihood of a metabolic DDI due to induction. The main focus of these models is to assess the potential for induction of CYP3A4 via binding to the nuclear receptor PXR, which is the mechanism for most of the important examples of clinical metabolic DDI caused by induction.

In early discovery, a CYP3A4 reporter gene assay can be used to screen a large number of compounds. The cell line most often used is the HepG2 cell line [168]. In this assay, compounds can be rank-ordered and compared to known clinical inducers to categorize them as potential inducers. For definitive assessment of induction potential, either the immortalized hepatocyte cell line Fa2N-4 can be used, or preferably, primary cultured human hepatocytes. In either system, CYP3A4 induction can be measured by increases in CYP3A4 mRNA, CYP3A4 protein, and CYP3A4 functional enzyme activity using a probe substrate. These increases can be compared to established potent inducers such as rifampicin. The Fa2N-4 system has the advantage of cell availability and batch-to-batch reproducibility, but has disadvantages such as low expression of some hepatic uptake transporters.

Cultured human hepatocytes have been proposed as the preferred system for definitive *in vitro* determination of human induction potential [149] (http://www.fda.gov/downloads/Drugs/GuidanceComplianceRegulatoryInformation/Guidances/ucm072101.pdf) and is considered to be most predictive. However, this system has the disadvantage of limited availability and batch to batch variability of induction response [169].

4.5.7 Tools for Studying Drug Excretion

Tools for determining the role of excretion in the elimination of a drug candidate can be employed at various stages of the drug discovery process and include *in vivo* pharmacokinetic studies, *in situ* models, and cell-based or membrane vesicle transporter systems.

As opposed to the myriad of tools for assessing drug metabolism, excretion tools are more limited and in many cases utilized only after it has been determined that metabolism is not the major mechanism of elimination.

4.5.7.1 In Vivo Animal Studies Due to the complexity of the excretion process that often involves a combination of passive and active transport processes, *in vivo* animal models are useful tools for investigating the role of excretion in drug elimination.

Renal Excretion In Vivo Pharmacokinetic studies in preclinical animal species can be used to determine the renal clearance of test compounds from urine concentration data (Section 5.2.4.1). For compounds that are hydrophilic or charged at physiological pH, renal excretion may represent the main route of elimination. Renal clearance in human is generally well predicted by preclinical animal species [170, 171], especially for passive glomerular filtration. Renal clearance data from pharmacokinetics studies can be effectively used to screen discovery compounds.

Biliary Excretion In Vivo The most useful tool for evaluating the contribution of biliary secretion to drug elimination is the bile-duct cannulated animal model, and rat is the species most widely used for this purpose. In this model, animals are surgically cannulated so that bile can be continuously collected from the bile ducts in the liver. Following intravenous administration of compound, a time course of bile samples can be collected, concentrations determined, and biliary secretion calculated. Knowledge of the rate of biliary secretion can also be used to investigate the role of hepatobiliary recirculation in the disposition of compound.

In Situ and Ex Vivo Animal Models The use of the *in situ* excretion models is fairly limited and is not very frequently used in the discovery settings.

Renal Excretion In Situ The isolated perfused kidney (IPK) model can be used to study specific aspects of renal excretion [172, 173], and the effect of drug on various renal functions can be determined by adding the drug to the recirculating perfusion medium. In addition to excretion, kidney metabolism and toxicity may also be investigated using this model. The renal clearance of drug candidates may also be estimated by measuring drug uptake in kidney slices [174].

Renal Excretion Ex Vivo The renal clearance of drug candidates can be estimated by measuring the drug uptake by using kidney slices [174].

4.5.7.2 In Vitro Cell-Based Excretion Models The use of the *in vitro* cell-based systems for studying drug excretion is a rapidly growing area of science and technology driven by the need to assess the mechanism of the excretion processes mediated by a broad variety of the transporters.

Cell-based transporter systems can be utilized to provide information pertaining to the involvement of individual transporters in the excretion process. Specific transporters can be transfected into cells with low background activity. The transporters are expressed in the cell membrane and the transport of compound into the cell can be measured quantitatively. The most important application of this technology is to determine if transport is likely to be saturable, which represents a safety liability.

Primary Cell Cultures Primary cell systems can be used to investigate transporters that are important for renal or biliary excretion. An advantage of primary cell systems is that they express the full complement of transporters and may best represent the *in vivo* situation. A disadvantage is that these systems exhibit limited cell viability and are also limited by the availability of tissue.

Sandwich-cultured rat and human hepatocytes have been developed and used as tools to evaluate the *in vivo* biliary clearance of drugs [175]. The sandwich-cultured cells are able to form intact bile canalicular networks and maintain functional expression levels of uptake and efflux transporters for several days. This system may be useful for predicting the human biliary secretion of drug candidates.

Immortalized Cells Immortalized cell systems are capable of expressing high levels of specific transporters and can be grown in large quantities. However, expression of some normal transport systems may be lacking, and transporter expression and activity may become unstable in culture over time.

Transfected Cell Lines Numerous heterologous expression (transfected) systems have been developed to investigate the function of renal and biliary excretion transporters. Transfected cell lines can express specific transporters of interest. Although the transporters are expressed in a nonnative cell background, which may affect the transport kinetics, these systems are especially useful tools for screening because large quantities can be easily produced.

Membrane Vesicle Transporter Systems For polar or charged compounds that cannot enter cells via passive permeability, membrane vesicle systems can be used to study efflux transport. Membrane vesicles are prepared from cells resulting in an inverted transporter configuration, such that the test compound has access to the transporter, and uptake of the compound into the vesicle indicates functional efflux transport.

4.6 STRATEGIES FOR ASSESSING ADME PROPERTIES

Designing the right ADME properties into a molecule starts with an understanding of the pharmacokinetic properties needed to deliver the targeted pharmacodynamics (PK–PD). Biomarker identification as an efficacy surrogate is also becoming more important for the success of discovery programs. As nonclinical models are used to predict efficacy in human disease, attention to the consistency of biology system drivers in preclinical models is paramount. Otherwise, predicting efficacious human doses may be quite difficult. Designing in the correct ADME properties can be easier for precedented targets and mechanisms, where benchmark compounds are likely available for comparison. However, unprecedented targets provide more significant challenges to the discovery scientist. The tools applied in the assessment of ADME properties within a screening paradigm will vary by stage of a program and can vary with time as greater knowledge is gained. In general, the logic of applying ADME tools starts with an understanding of the defined *in vivo* targets and using the appropriate *in silico* (presynthesis) and *in vitro* (postsynthesis) tools to predict the desired *in vivo* behavior. The judicious use and cross-validation of *in silico*, *in vitro*, and *in vivo* tools, with an appreciation for their limitations, should provide a framework for efficient drug design. The primary focus of screening should be on early identification of rate-limiting ADME properties and subsequent optimization. This is the topic of further discussion in Section 4.6.1.

4.6.1 Assessing ADME Attributes at Different Stages of Discovery Projects

A typical discovery project involves four major stage gates: Target Identification, Lead Selection, Lead Optimization, and Preclinical Development (Figure 4.12). An example of a similar process can be found in the literature [176, 177].

4.6.1.1 Target Identification The Target Identification stage focuses primarily on the biology of a selected target. In addition, an initial assessment is made of the ADME space to which the chemical space of interest belongs. This can provide an early read of the deliverability of targeted molecules.

Animal testing, primarily in rodents, may be utilized for preliminary evaluation of PK properties of screening hits and/or benchmark compounds described in the literature. It is also used for selecting an appropriate dose and route of administration to deliver sufficient exposures in the animal efficacy models to build confidence in the rationale of the biology of the target.

4.6.1.2 Lead Selection The primary purpose of the Lead Selection stage of the discovery project is to (1) identify the spectrum of ADME properties of several chemical templates (series) and (2) determine the drivers of efficacy (and biomarkers)

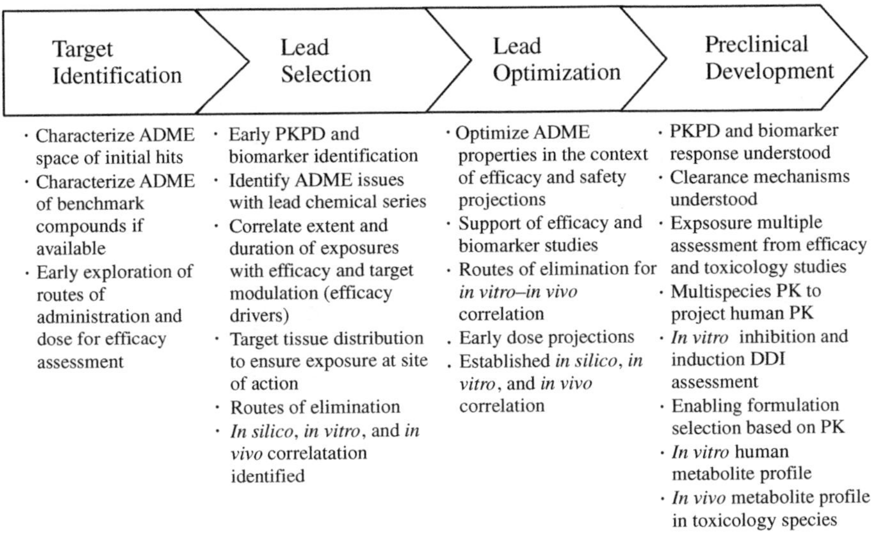

Figure 4.12 The stages of the discovery process and primary purposes of ADME studies.

by analyzing the relationships between the extent and the duration of *in vivo* exposure, efficacy and target modulation. Certain tissue distribution studies (e.g., brain penetration) and receptor occupancy assessments may provide valuable information as to target site availability. Initial screening PK is used at this stage to assess clearance mechanisms and IVIVC. Initial *in vivo* mechanistic studies aimed at evaluating the primary routes of elimination may be conducted, and may include bile-duct cannulated (BDC) rats or even dogs. Another important goal at this stage is to begin setting up *in silico*, *in vitro*, and *in vivo* relationships so that these tools can be appropriately incorporated into the screening paradigm paying particular attention to model interrelationships. The Lead Selection stage of the project is particularly important in establishing the program as the working chemical space is narrowed significantly.

4.6.1.3 Lead Optimization Selection of the lead series is a significant milestone for the discovery project, which now moves to the Lead Optimization stage. At this point, much effort is applied to specifically fixing any revealed ADME problems and to identify the best compounds for further advancement. *In vitro* and *in silico* tools for ADME assessment are widely used at this stage of the project. In particular, predictive *in silico* tools provide an effective way to rationally design and enrich the pool of compounds that likely will possess the proper *in vivo* ADME properties.

4.6.1.4 Preclinical Development In the Preclinical Development stage, typically a front running candidate is chosen from a handful of leads for eventual clinical development. More *definitive* ADME-related studies are typically conducted *in vitro* and *in vivo* to revise early assessments from *screening* studies. More extensive safety evaluations are run to assess exposure multiples between projected human doses and

TABLE 4.5 ADME Phenomena and the Tools for their Evaluation

Tool	Absorption	Distribution	Metabolism	Renal Excretion	Biliary Excretion
In vivo	• PO administration • ID administration • Portal vein sampling • Formulation • Food effect • KO animals • Humanized animals • Chemical inhibitors • *In situ* intestinal perfusion	• Tissue distribution • QWBA • MALDI • Microdialysis • KO mice • Chemical inhibitors	• Mass balance • Portal vein dosing • KO animals • Humanized animals • Chemical inhibitors • Allometric scaling	• Mass balance • Urine collection • Transgenic/ humanized mice	• Mass balance • Bile cannulated animals
In situ *Ex vivo* and *in vitro*—species specific	• Isolated intestinal • Intestinal sections • Inverted intestinal sacs • Cell monolayers • Hepatocytes • Transfected cells • Membrane vesicles • Artificial membranes	• Isolated organ • Tissue/plasma protein binding • BBB/tissue permeability models	• Isolated liver • Intestinal sections • Liver slices • Hepatocytes • Sandwiched hepatocytes • Microsomes • S9	• Isolated kidney • Kidney slices • Transfected cells	• Isolated liver • Sandwiched hepatocytes • Transfected cells

In vitro—nonspecies specific		• Albumin-immobilized columns	• Recombinant enzymes	• Physicochemical properties	• Physicochemical properties
	• Physicochemical properties • Dissolution/solubility	• Artificial membranes • Physicochemical properties	• Physicochemical properties		
In silico	• Physicochemical properties	• Volume	• Clearance	• Renal clearance	• Biliary clearance
	• Permeability • Solubility • Absorption profile • MAD • Transporter SAR	• Protein binding • PK profile • Transporter SAR • BBB uptake • MDR1	• Sites of metabolism • Half-life • Inhibition/induction • Transporter SAR • Allometric scaling		

preclinical safety findings usually in multiple day *in vivo* toxicology screens in both rodent and nonrodent species. Plasma protein binding data should be available in efficacy models, safety species, and human so that unbound drug concentrations and multiples can be compared. A more detailed ADME evaluation of selected final dosage form of the compound that is expected to be used for initial regulated toxicology studies and human dosing is conducted in several animal species including rodents and nonrodents.

As part of an early risk assessment, some mechanistic DDI studies may be conducted in human cell systems *in vitro*. Early comparisons of the metabolism of drug candidates in both *in vitro* human systems and *in vitro* and *in vivo* animal models are conducted to ensure the absence of unique human metabolites not present in animal species used for safety evaluation.

A significant number of additional studies are usually performed to support further development of a drug candidate and include more definitive radiolabeled ADME studies to assess metabolite profiles in humans and toxicology species, a broader safety evaluation of the drug candidate (e.g., longer term toxicology, reproductive toxicology, carcinogenicity, and juvenile toxicology), and special studies to address some specific issue of clinical development (e.g., metabolite safety, mechanistic understanding of an unexpected clinical finding).

4.7 TOOL SUMMARY FOR ASSESSING ADME PROPERTIES

The various ADME tools discussed in this chapter are provided as a quick reference (Table 4.5).

REFERENCES

1. Washington, N., Washington, C., and Wilson, C. *Physiological Pharmaceutics: Barriers to Drug Absorption*, 2nd Edition, Taylor & Francis Series in Pharmaceutical Sciences, CRC, Boca Raton, FL, 2001, p. 328.
2. Ueda, C. T., Williamson, B. J., and Dzindzio, B. S. Absolute quinidine bioavailability. *Clin. Pharmacol. Ther.* 1976, *20(3)*, 260–265.
3. Paine, M. F., et al. First-pass metabolism of midazolam by the human intestine. *Clin. Pharmacol. Ther.* 1996, *60(1)*, 14–24.
4. Stegman, J. K. *Stedman's Medical Dictionary*, 28th Edition, Lippincott Williams & Wilkins, Baltimore, MD, 2006, p. 2100.
5. Mishell, D. R., Jr., Pharmacokinetics of depot medroxyprogesterone acetate contraception. *J. Reprod. Med.* 1996, *41(5)*, 381–390.
6. Brunton, L., Lazo, J., and Parker, K. *Goodman & Gilman's The Pharmacological Basis of Therapeutics*, 11th Edition, McGraw-Hill Professional, New York, 2006.
7. Johnson, K. C. and Swindell, A. C. Guidance in the setting of drug particle size specifications to minimize variability in absorption. *Pharm. Res.* 1996, *13(12)*, 1795–1798.

8. Hilgers, A. R., et al. Predicting oral absorption of drugs: a case study with a novel class of antimicrobial agents. *Pharm. Res.* 2003, *20(8)*, 1149–1155.
9. Amidon, G. L., et al. A theoretical basis for a biopharmaceutic drug classification: the correlation of *in vitro* drug product dissolution and *in vivo* bioavailability. *Pharm. Res.* 1995, *12(3)*, 413–420.
10. Lennernas, H. Human intestinal permeability. *J. Pharm. Sci.* 1998, *87(4)*, 403–410.
11. Avdeef, A. Physicochemical profiling (solubility, permeability and charge state). *Curr. Top Med. Chem.* 2001, *1(4)*, 277–351.
12. Hartmann, T., et al. ADME related profiling in 96 and 384 well plate format—a novel and robust HT-assay for the determination of lipophilicity and serum albumin binding. *Curr. Drug. Deliv.* 2006, *3(2)*, 181–192.
13. Lipinski, C. A., et al. Experimental and computational approaches to estimate solubility and permeability in drug discovery and development settings. *Adv. Drug Deliv. Rev.* 1997, *23, 3–25.*
14. Lennernas, H. Modeling gastrointestinal drug absorption requires more *in vivo* biopharmaceutical data: experience from *in vivo* dissolution and permeability studies in humans. *Curr. Drug Metab.* 2007, *8(7)*, 645–657.
15. Ishizawa, T., Hayashi, M., and Awazu, S. Paracellular and transcellular permeabilities of fosfomycin across small intestinal membrane of rat and rabbit by voltage-clamp method. *J. Pharmacobiodyn.* 1991, *14(10)*, 583–589.
16. Hayashi, M., Tomita, M., and Awazu, S. Transcellular and paracellular contribution to transport processes in the colorectal route. *Adv. Drug Deliv. Rev.* 1997, *28, 191–204.*
17. Grass, G. M. and Robinson, J. R. Mechanisms of corneal drug penetration. II: ultrastructural analysis of potential pathways for drug movement. *J. Pharm. Sci.* 1988, *77(1)*, 15–23.
18. Artursson, P., Ungell, A. L., and Lofroth, J. E. Selective paracellular permeability in two models of intestinal absorption: cultured monolayers of human intestinal epithelial cells and rat intestinal segments. *Pharm. Res.* 1993, *10(8)*, 1123–1129.
19. Mandagere, A. K., Thompson, T. N., and Hwang, K. K. Graphical model for estimating oral bioavailability of drugs in humans and other species from their Caco-2 permeability and *in vitro* liver enzyme metabolic stability rates. *J. Med. Chem.* 2002, *45 (2)*, 304–311.
20. van de Waterbeemd, H., Lennernäs, H., and Artursson, P. Drug Bioavailability: Estimation of Solubility, Permeability, Absorption and Bioavailability. In *Methods and Principles in Medicinal Chemistry*, Mannhold, R., Kubinyi, H.,and Folkers, G. (eds.), Wiley-VCH Verlag GmbH, Weinheim, 2003, xxiv, p. 579.
21. Bohets, H., et al. Strategies for absorption screening in drug discovery and development. *Curr. Top Med. Chem.* 2001, *1(5)*, 367–383.
22. Zhang, Y. and Benet, L. Z. The gut as a barrier to drug absorption: combined role of cytochrome P450 3A and P-glycoprotein. *Clin. Pharmacokinet.* 2001, *40(3)*, 159–168.
23. van de Kerkhof, E. G., de Graaf, I. A., and Groothuis, G. M. *In vitro* methods to study intestinal drug metabolism. *Curr. Drug Metab.* 2007, *8(7)*, 658–675.
24. Cummins, C. L., et al. *In vivo* modulation of intestinal CYP3A metabolism by P-glycoprotein: studies using the rat single-pass intestinal perfusion model. *J. Pharmacol. Exp. Ther.* 2003, *305(1)*, 306–314.

25. Fisher, R. B. and Parsons, D. S. A preparation of surviving rat small intestine for the study of absorption. *J. Physiol.* 1949, *110(1–2)*, 36–46.
26. Dowty, M. E. and Dietsch, C. R. Improved prediction of *in vivo* peroral absorption from *in vitro* intestinal permeability using an internal standard to control for intra- and inter-rat variability. *Pharm. Res.* 1997, *14(12)*, 1792–1797.
27. Clarke, L. L. A guide to using chamber studies of mouse intestine. *Am. J. Physiol. Gastrointest. Liver Physiol.* 2009, *296(6)*, G1151–G1166.
28. Wilson, T. H. and Wiseman, G. The use of sacs of everted small intestine for the study of the transference of substances from the mucosal to the serosal surface. *J. Physiol.* 1954, *123(1)*, 116–125.
29. Artursson, P., Palm, K., and Luthman, K. Caco-2 monolayers in experimental and theoretical predictions of drug transport. *Adv. Drug Deliv. Rev.* 2001, *46(1–3)*, 27–43.
30. Zhu, C., et al. A comparative study of artificial membrane permeability assay for high throughput profiling of drug absorption potential. *Eur. J. Med. Chem.* 2002, *37(5)*, 399–407.
31. Tang, F., Horie, K., and Borchardt, R. T. Are MDCK cells transfected with the human *MRP2* gene a good model of the human intestinal mucosa? *Pharm. Res.* 2002, *19(6)*, 773–779.
32. Volpe, D. A. Variability in Caco-2 and MDCK cell-based intestinal permeability assays. *J. Pharm. Sci.* 2008, *97(2)*, 712–725.
33. Wielinga, P. R., et al. *In vitro* transepithelial drug transport by on-line measurement: cellular control of paracellular and transcellular transport. *J. Pharm. Sci.* 1999, *88(12)*, 1340–1347.
34. Artursson, P. and Magnusson, C. Epithelial transport of drugs in cell culture. II: effect of extracellular calcium concentration on the paracellular transport of drugs of different lipophilicities across monolayers of intestinal epithelial (Caco-2) cells. *J. Pharm. Sci.* 1990, *79(7)*, 595–600.
35. Knipp, G. T., et al. Paracellular diffusion in Caco-2 cell monolayers: effect of perturbation on the transport of hydrophilic compounds that vary in charge and size. *J. Pharm. Sci.* 1997, *86(10)*, 1105–1110.
36. Stevenson, B. R., et al. Tight junction structure and ZO-1 content are identical in two strains of Madin–Darby canine kidney cells which differ in transepithelial resistance. *J. Cell. Biol.* 1988, *107(6 Pt 1)*, 2401–2408.
37. Lazorova, L., et al. Quantification and imaging of mannitol transport through Caco-2 cell monolayers using a positron-emitting tracer. *Pharm. Res.* 1998, *15(7)*, 1141–1144.
38. Pidgeon, C. and Venkataram, U. V. Immobilized artificial membrane chromatography: supports composed of membrane lipids. *Anal. Biochem.* 1989, *176(1)*, 36–47.
39. Alvarez, F. M., et al. Immobilized Artificial Membrane Chromatography: Prediction of Drug Transport Across Biological Barriers. In *Molecular Interactions in Bioseparations*, In: Ngo, T. T. (ed.), Plenum Press, New York, 1993, pp. 151–167.
40. Kansy, M., Senner, F., and Gubernator, K. Physicochemical high throughput screening: parallel artificial membrane permeation assay in the description of passive absorption processes. *J. Med. Chem.* 1998, *41(7)*, 1007–1010.
41. Wohnsland, F. and Faller, B. High-throughput permeability pH profile and high-throughput alkane/water log *P* with artificial membranes. *J. Med. Chem.* 2001, *44(6)*, 923–930.

42. Valko, K., et al. Rapid-gradient HPLC method for measuring drug interactions with immobilized artificial membrane: comparison with other lipophilicity measures. *J. Pharm. Sci.* 2000, *89(8)*, 1085–1096.

43. Avdeef, A. High-Throughput Measurement of Permeability Profiles. In *Drug Bioavailability: Estimation of Solubility, Permeability, Absorption and Bioavailability*, van de Waterbeemd, H., Lennernäs, H.,and Artursson, P. (eds.), Wiley-VCH Verlag GmbH, Weinheim, 2003, pp. 46–71.

44. Kerns, E. H., et al. Combined application of parallel artificial membrane permeability assay and Caco-2 permeability assays in drug discovery. *J. Pharm. Sci.* 2004, *93(6)*, 1440–1453.

45. Stenberg, P., et al. Experimental and computational screening models for the prediction of intestinal drug absorption. *J. Med. Chem.* 2001, *44(12)*, 1927–1937.

46. Kerns, E.and Di, L. (eds.). *Drug-Like Properties: Concepts, Structure Design and Methods: From ADME to Toxicity Optimization*, Academic Press, New York, 2008, p. 552.

47. Tsuji, A. and Tamai, I. Carrier-mediated intestinal transport of drugs. *Pharm. Res.* 1996, *13(7)*, 963–977.

48. Terao, T., et al. Active secretion of drugs from the small intestinal epithelium in rats by P-glycoprotein functioning as an absorption barrier. *J. Pharm. Pharmacol.* 1996, *48(10)*, 1083–1089.

49. Chan, L. M., Lowes, S., and Hirst, B. H. The ABCs of drug transport in intestine and liver: efflux proteins limiting drug absorption and bioavailability. *Eur. J. Pharm. Sci.* 2004, *21 (1)*, 25–51.

50. Kim, H. R., et al. Comparative gene expression profiles of intestinal transporters in mice, rats and humans. *Pharmacol. Res.* 2007, *56(3)*, 224–236.

51. Cao, J., et al. Role of P-glycoprotein in the intestinal absorption of glabridin, an active flavonoid from the root of *Glycyrrhiza glabra*. *Drug Metab. Dispos.* 2007, *35(4)*, 539–553.

52. Takano, M., Yumoto, R., and Murakami, T. Expression and function of efflux drug transporters in the intestine. *Pharmacol. Ther.* 2006, *109(1–2)*, 137–161.

53. Zhang, L., et al. A regulatory viewpoint on transporter-based drug interactions. *Xenobiotica* 2008, *38(7–8)*, 709–724.

54. Giacomini, K. M., et al. Membrane transporters in drug development: report from the FDA Critical Path Initiative Sponsored Workshop. *Nat. Rev. Drug Discov.* 2010, *9(3)*, 215–236.

55. Klaassen, C. D. and Lu, H. Xenobiotic transporters: ascribing function from gene knockout and mutation studies. *Toxicol. Sci.* 2008, *101(2)*, 186–196.

56. Chen, C., Liu, X., and Smith, B. J. Utility of Mdr1-gene deficient mice in assessing the impact of P-glycoprotein on pharmacokinetics and pharmacodynamics in drug discovery and development. *Curr. Drug Metab.* 2003, *4(4)*, 272–291.

57. Vlaming, M. L., et al. Carcinogen and anticancer drug transport by Mrp2 *in vivo*: studies using Mrp2 (Abcc2) knockout mice. *J. Pharmacol. Exp. Ther.* 2006, *318(1)*, 319–327.

58. van de Steeg, E., et al. Methotrexate pharmacokinetics in transgenic mice with liver-specific expression of human organic anion-transporting polypeptide 1B1 (SLCO1B1). *Drug Metab. Dispos.* 2009, *37(2)*, 277–281.

59. Maubon, N., et al. Analysis of drug transporter expression in human intestinal Caco-2 cells by real-time PCR. *Fundam. Clin. Pharmacol.* 2007, *21(6)*, 659–663.

60. Keppler, D. Uptake and efflux transporters for conjugates in human hepatocytes. *Methods Enzymol.* 2005, *400, 531–542.*

61. Sasaki, M., et al. Prediction of *in vivo* biliary clearance from the *in vitro* transcellular transport of organic anions across a double-transfected Madin–Darby canine kidney II monolayer expressing both rat organic anion transporting polypeptide 4 and multidrug resistance associated protein 2. *Mol. Pharmacol.* 2004, *66(3)*, 450–459.

62. Cui, Y., Konig, J., and Keppler, D. Vectorial transport by double-transfected cells expressing the human uptake transporter SLC21A8 and the apical export pump ABCC2. *Mol. Pharmacol.* 2001, *60(5)*, 934–943.

63. Bartholome, K., et al. Data-based mathematical modeling of vectorial transport across double-transfected polarized cells. *Drug Metab. Dispos.* 2007, *35(9)*, 1476–1481.

64. Ishikawa, T., et al. High-speed screening of human ATP-binding cassette transporter function and genetic polymorphisms: new strategies in pharmacogenomics. *Methods Enzymol.* 2005, *400, 485–510.*

65. Xia, C. Q., Milton, M. N., and Gan, L. S. Evaluation of drug-transporter interactions using *in vitro* and *in vivo* models. *Curr. Drug Metab.* 2007, *8(4)*, 341–363.

66. Crivori, P., et al. Computational models for identifying potential P-glycoprotein substrates and inhibitors. *Mol. Pharm.* 2006, *3(1)*, 33–44.

67. Lai, Y., et al. Structure–activity relationships for interaction with multidrug resistance protein 2 (ABCC2/MRP2): the role of torsion angle for a series of biphenyl-substituted heterocycles. *Drug Metab. Dispos.* 2007, *35(6)*, 937–945.

68. Chang, C., et al. Pharmacophore-based discovery of ligands for drug transporters. *Adv. Drug Deliv. Rev.* 2006, *58(12–13)*, 1431–1450.

69. Ha, S. N., Hochman, J., and Sheridan, R. P. Mini review on molecular modeling of P-glycoprotein (P-gp). *Curr. Top. Med. Chem.* 2007, *7(15)*, 1525–1529.

70. Ekins, S., et al. *In vitro* and pharmacophore-based discovery of novel hPEPT1 inhibitors. *Pharm. Res.* 2005, *22(4)*, 512–517.

71. Polli, J. E., et al. Summary workshop report: bioequivalence, biopharmaceutics classification system, and beyond. *AAPS J.* 2008, *10(2)*, 373–379.

72. Thummel, K. E., et al. Oral first-pass elimination of midazolam involves both gastrointestinal and hepatic CYP3A-mediated metabolism. *Clin. Pharmacol. Ther.* 1996, *59(5)*, 491–502.

73. Wu, C. Y. and Benet, L. Z. Predicting drug disposition via application of BCS: transport/absorption/elimination interplay and development of a biopharmaceutics drug disposition classification system. *Pharm. Res.* 2005, *22(1)*, 11–23.

74. van Herwaarden, A. E., et al. Knockout of cytochrome P450 3A yields new mouse models for understanding xenobiotic metabolism. *J. Clin. Invest.* 2007, *117(11)*, 3583–3592.

75. Kwon, Y. *Handbook of Essential Pharmacokinetics, Pharmacodynamics and Drug Metabolism for Industrial Scientists.* Kluwer Academic/Plenum Publishers, New York, NY, 2001.

76. Wong, W. W., et al. Measurement of extracellular water volume by bromide ion chromatography. *Am. J. Clin. Nutr.* 1989, *50(6)*, 1290–1294.

77. Brans, Y. W., et al. Simultaneous estimation of neonatal total body water by antipyrine and $H_2^{(18)}O$ dilution. *Biol. Neonate* 1990, *58(3)*, 137–144.

78. Stopher, D. A., et al. The metabolism and pharmacokinetics of amlodipine in humans and animals. *J. Cardiovasc. Pharmacol.* 1988, *12(7)*, S55–S59.

79. Smith, D. A., Waterbeemd, H.v.d., and Walker, D. K. Pharmacokinetics and Metabolism in Drug Design. In *Methods and Principles in Medicinal Chemistry*, Vol. *13, Mannhold, R., Kubinyi, H.,and Timmerman H. (eds.)*, Wiley-VCH Verlag GmbH, Weinheim, 2001, xi, p. 64.

80. Stoeckli, M., Staab, D., and Schweitzer, A. Compound and metabolite distribution measured by MALDI mass spectrometric imaging in whole-body tissue sections. *Int. J. Mass Spectrom.* 2007, *260, 195–202.*

81. Turk, D. and Szakacs, G. Relevance of multidrug resistance in the age of targeted therapy. *Curr. Opin. Drug Discov. Devel.* 2009, *12(2)*, 246–252.

82. Kratochwil, N. A., et al. Predicting plasma protein binding of drugs: a new approach. *Biochem. Pharmacol.* 2002, *64(9)*, 1355–1374.

83. Rowland, M. and Tozer, T. N. *Clinical Pharmacokinetics: Concepts and Applications*, 2nd Edition, Lea & Febiger, Philadelphia, PA, 1989.

84. Obach, R. S. Prediction of human clearance of twenty-nine drugs from hepatic microsomal intrinsic clearance data: an examination of *in vitro* half-life approach and nonspecific binding to microsomes. *Drug Metab. Dispos.* 1999, *27(11)*, 1350–1359.

85. Hinderling, P. H. Red blood cells: a neglected compartment in pharmacokinetics and pharmacodynamics. *Pharmacol. Rev.* 1997, *49(3)*, 279–295.

86. Smith, D. A., Jones, B. C., and Walker, D. K. Design of drugs involving the concepts and theories of drug metabolism and pharmacokinetics. *Med. Res. Rev.* 1996, *16(3)*, 243–266.

87. Bertera, F. M., et al. Comparison of different pharmacodynamic models for PK-PD modeling of verapamil in renovascular hypertension. *J. Pharmacol. Toxicol. Methods* 2008, *57(3)*, 212–219.

88. Pacifici, G. M. and Viani, A. Methods of determining plasma and tissue binding of drugs. Pharmacokinetic consequences. *Clin. Pharmacokinet.* 1992, *23(6)*, 449–468.

89. Oravcova, J., Boehs, B., and Lindner, W. Drug-protein binding studies. New trends in analytical and experimental methodology. *J. Chromatogr. B* 1996, *677(1)*, 1–28.

90. Cohen, L. Plasma Protein-Binding Methods in Drug Discovery. In *Optimization in Drug Discovery: In Vitro* Methods, Yan Z.and Caldwell, G. (eds.), Humana Press, Totowa, NJ, 2004, pp. 111–122.

91. Banker, M. J., Clark, T. H., and Williams, J. A. Development and validation of a 96-well equilibrium dialysis apparatus for measuring plasma protein binding. *J. Pharm. Sci.* 2003, *92(5)*, 967–974.

92. Pardridge, W. M. *Introduction to the Blood–Brain Barrier: Methodology, Biology, and Pathology*, Cambridge University Press, Cambridge, UK, 1998, xiv, p. 486.

93. Cornford, E. M. and Hyman, S. Blood–brain barrier permeability to small and large molecules. *Adv. Drug Deliv. Rev.* 1999, *36(2–3)*, 145–163.

94. Hitchcock, S. A. and Pennington, L. D. Structure–brain exposure relationships. *J. Med. Chem.* 2006, *49(26)*, 7559–7583.

95. Pardridge, W. M. Blood–brain barrier delivery. *Drug Discov. Today*, 2007, *12(1–2)*, 54–61.

96. Hammarlund-Udenaes, M., et al. On the rate and extent of drug delivery to the brain. *Pharm. Res.* 2008, *25(8)*, 1737–1750.

97. Chen, C., et al. P-glycoprotein limits the brain penetration of nonsedating but not sedating H1-antagonists. *Drug Metab. Dispos.* 2003, *31(3)*, 312–318.

98. Mahar Doan, K. M., et al. Passive permeability and P-glycoprotein-mediated efflux differentiate central nervous system (CNS) and non-CNS marketed drugs. *J. Pharmacol. Exp. Ther.* 2002, *303(3)*, 1029–1037.

99. Schinkel, A. H. P-Glycoprotein, a gatekeeper in the blood–brain barrier. *Adv. Drug Deliv. Rev.* 1999, *36(2–3)*, 179–194.

100. Liu, X., Chen, C., and Smith, B. J. Progress in brain penetration evaluation in drug discovery and development. *J. Pharmacol. Exp. Ther.* 2008, *325(2)*, 349–356.

101. Begley, D. J. ABC transporters and the blood–brain barrier. *Curr. Pharm. Des.* 2004, *10 (12)*, 1295–1312.

102. Pajeva, I. K. and Wiese, M. Pharmacophore model of drugs involved in P-glycoprotein multidrug resistance: explanation of structural variety (hypothesis). *J. Med. Chem.* 2002, *45(26)*, 5671–5686.

103. Varma, M. V. and Panchagnula, R. Prediction of *in vivo* intestinal absorption enhancement on P-glycoprotein inhibition, from rat *in situ* permeability. *J. Pharm. Sci.* 2005, *94(8)*, 1694–1704.

104. Kalvass, J. C. and Maurer, T. S. Influence of nonspecific brain and plasma binding on CNS exposure: implications for rational drug discovery. *Biopharm. Drug Dispos.* 2002, *23(8)*, 327–338.

105. Kalvass, J. C., Maurer, T. S., and Pollack, G. M. Use of plasma and brain unbound fractions to assess the extent of brain distribution of 34 drugs: comparison of unbound concentration ratios to *in vivo* P-glycoprotein efflux ratios. *Drug Metab. Dispos.* 2007, *35 (4)*, 660–666.

106. Liu, X. and Chen, C. Strategies to optimize brain penetration in drug discovery. *Curr. Opin. Drug Discov. Devel.* 2005, *8(4)*, 505–512.

107. Maurer, T. S., et al. Relationship between exposure and nonspecific binding of thirty-three central nervous system drugs in mice. *Drug Metab. Dispos.* 2005, *33(1)*, 175–181.

108. Summerfield, S. G., et al. Toward an improved prediction of human *in vivo* brain penetration. *Xenobiotica* 2008, *38(12)*, 1518–1535.

109. Watson, J., et al. Receptor occupancy and brain free fraction. *Drug Metab. Dispos.* 2009, *37(4)*, 753–760.

110. Martin, I. Prediction of blood–brain barrier penetration: are we missing the point? *Drug Discov. Today* 2004, *9(4)*, 161–162.

111. Ohe, T., et al. Effect of P-glycoprotein-mediated efflux on cerebrospinal fluid/plasma concentration ratio. *Drug Metab. Dispos.* 2003, *31(10)*, 1251–1254.

112. Liu, X., et al. Evaluation of cerebrospinal fluid concentration and plasma free concentration as a surrogate measurement for brain free concentration. *Drug Metab. Dispos.* 2006, *34(9)*, 1443–1447.

113. Liu, X., et al. Unbound drug concentration in brain homogenate and cerebral spinal fluid at steady state as a surrogate for unbound concentration in brain interstitial fluid. *Drug Metab. Dispos.* 2009, *37(4)*, 787–793.

114. Garberg, P., et al. *In vitro* models for the blood–brain barrier. *Toxicol. In Vitro* 2005, *19 (3)*, 299–334.

115. Johnson, M. D. and Anderson, B. D. *In vitro* models of the blood–brain barrier to polar permeants: comparison of transmonolayer flux measurements and cell uptake kinetics using cultured cerebral capillary endothelial cells. *J. Pharm. Sci.* 1999, *88(6)*, 620–625.

116. Vastag, M. and Keseru, G. M. Current *in vitro* and *in silico* models of blood–brain barrier penetration: a practical view. *Curr. Opin. Drug Discov. Devel.* 2009, *12(1)*, 115–124.

117. Wang, Q., et al. Evaluation of the MDR-MDCK cell line as a permeability screen for the blood–brain barrier. *Int. J. Pharm.* 2005, *288(2)*, 349–359.

118. Feng, B., et al. *In vitro* P-glycoprotein assays to predict the *in vivo* interactions of P-glycoprotein with drugs in the central nervous system. *Drug Metab. Dispos.* 2008, *36 (2)*, 268–275.

119. Schinkel, A. H., et al. P-glycoprotein in the blood–brain barrier of mice influences the brain penetration and pharmacological activity of many drugs. *J. Clin. Invest.* 1996, *97 (11)*, 2517–2524.

120. Doran, A., et al. The impact of P-glycoprotein on the disposition of drugs targeted for indications of the central nervous system: evaluation using the MDR1A/1B knockout mouse model. *Drug Metab. Dispos.* 2005, *33(1)*, 165–174.

121. Syvanen, S., et al. Species differences in blood–brain barrier transport of three positron emission tomography radioligands with emphasis on P-glycoprotein transport. *Drug Metab. Dispos.* 2009, *37(3)*, 635–643.

122. Roulet, A., et al. MDR1-deficient genotype in Collie dogs hypersensitive to the P-glycoprotein substrate ivermectin. *Eur. J. Pharmacol.* 2003, *460(2–3)*, 85–91.

123. Friden, M., et al. *In vitro* methods for estimating unbound drug concentrations in the brain interstitial and intracellular fluids. *Drug Metab. Dispos.* 2007, *35(9)*, 1711–1719.

124. Rowland, M. and Tozer, T. N. *Clinical Pharmacokinetics: Concepts and Applications*, 3rd Edition, Williams & Wilkins, Baltimore, MD, 1995, xiv, p. 601.

125. Shitara, Y., Horie, T., and Sugiyama, Y. Transporters as a determinant of drug clearance and tissue distribution. *Eur. J. Pharm. Sci.* 2006, *27(5)*, 425–446.

126. Parkinson, A. Biotransformation of Xenobiotics. In *Casarett & Doull's Toxicology: The Basic Science of Poisons*, Klaassen, C. D. (ed.), McGraw-Hill Professional, New York, 2001, pp. 133–224.

127. Furge, L. L. and Guengerich, F. P. Cytochrome P450 enzymes in drug metabolism and chemical toxicology. *Biochem. Mol. Biol. Educ.* 2006, *32(2)*, 66–74.

128. Rendic, S. Summary of information on human CYP enzymes: human P450 metabolism data. *Drug Metab. Rev.* 2002, *34(1–2)*, 83–448.

129. Guengerich, F. P. Cytochrome p450 and chemical toxicology. *Chem. Res. Toxicol.* 2008, *21(1)*, 70–83.

130. Gibbs, M. A. and Hosea, N. A. Factors affecting the clinical development of cytochrome p450 3A substrates. *Clin. Pharmacokinet.* 2003, *42(11)*, 969–984.

131. Lewis, D. F. and Ito, Y. Human P450s involved in drug metabolism and the use of structural modelling for understanding substrate selectivity and binding affinity. *Xenobiotica* 2009, *39(8)*, 625–635.

132. Anzenbacher, P. and Anzenbacherova, E. Cytochromes P450 and metabolism of xenobiotics. *Cell. Mol. Life Sci.* 2001, *58(5–6)*, 737–747.

133. Cashman, J. R. Role of flavin-containing monooxygenase in drug development. *Expert Opin. Drug Metab. Toxicol.* 2008, *4(12)*, 1507–1521.

134. Martignoni, M., Groothuis, G. M., and de Kanter, R. Species differences between mouse, rat, dog, monkey and human CYP-mediated drug metabolism, inhibition and induction. *Expert Opin. Drug Metab. Toxicol.* 2006, *2(6)*, 875–894.

135. Caldwell, J. The current status of attempts to predict species differences in drug metabolism. *Drug Metab. Re.v* 1981, *12(2)*, 221–237.

136. Tukey, R. H. and Strassburg, C. P. Human UDP-glucuronosyltransferases: metabolism, expression, and disease. *Ann. Rev. Pharmacol. Toxicol.* 2000, *40, 581–616.*

137. Miners, J. O., et al. Predicting human drug glucuronidation parameters: application of *in vitro* and *in silico* modeling approaches. *Ann. Rev. Pharmacol. Toxicol.* 2004, *44, 1–25.*

138. Williams, R. Species variations in the pathways of drug metabolism. *Environ. Health Perspect.* 1978, *22, 133–138.*

139. Krishna, D. R. and Klotz, U. Extrahepatic metabolism of drugs in humans. *Clin. Pharmacokinet.* 1994, *26(2)*, 144–160.

140. Varma, M. V., et al. Physicochemical determinants of human renal clearance. *J. Med. Chem.* 2009, *52(15)*, 4844–4852.

141. Monte, M. J., et al. Bile acids: chemistry, physiology, and pathophysiology. *World J. Gastroenterol.* 2009, *15(7)*, 804–816.

142. Ghibellini, G., Leslie, E. M., and Brouwer, K. L. Methods to evaluate biliary excretion of drugs in humans: an updated review. *Mol. Pharm.* 2006, *3(3)*, 198–211.

143. Stenner, R. D., et al. Enterohepatic recirculation of trichloroethanol glucuronide as a significant source of trichloroacetic acid. Metabolites of trichloroethylene. *Drug Metab. Dispos.* 1997, *25(5)*, 529–535.

144. Edwards, I. R. and Aronson, J. K. Adverse drug reactions: definitions, diagnosis, and management. *Lancet* 2000, *356(9237)*, 1255–1259.

145. Jackson, K., Young, D., and Pant, S. Drug–excipient interactions and their affect on absorption. *Pharm. Sci. Technol. Today* 2000, *3(10)*, 336–345.

146. Kedderis, G. L. *Pharmacokinetisc of Drug Interactions.* In *Drug–Drug Interactions: Scientific and Regulatory Perspectives,* Li, A. P. (ed.), Academic Press, New York, 1997, pp. 189–204.

147. Hutzler, M., Messing, D. M., and Wienkers, L. C. Predicting drug–drug interactions in drug discovery: where are we now and where are we going? *Curr. Opin. Drug Discov. Devel.* 2005, *8(1)*, 51–58.

148. FDA, Guidance for Industry. *Drug Metabolism/Drug Interaction Studies in the Drug Development Process: Studies In Vitro*, 1997.

149. FDA, Guidance for Industry. *Drug Interaction Studies—Study Design, Data Analysis, and Implications for Dosing and Labeling. Graft Guidance*, 2006.

150. Williams, J. A., et al. Drug–drug interactions for UDP-glucuronosyltransferase substrates: a pharmacokinetic explanation for typically observed low exposure (AUCi/AUC) ratios. *Drug Metab. Dispos.* 2004, *32(11)*, 1201–1208.

151. Armstrong, S. C., Cozza, K. L., and Pimentel, E. A. Immunosuppressants. *Psychosomatics* 2002, *43(5)*, 424–427.

152. Lin, J. H. CYP induction-mediated drug interactions: *in vitro* assessment and clinical implications. *Pharm. Res.* 2006, *23(6)*, 1089–1116.

153. LeCluyse, E. L. Pregnane X receptor: molecular basis for species differences in CYP3A induction by xenobiotics. *Chem. Biol. Interact.* 2001, *134(3)*, 283–289.

154. Linder, C. D., Renaud, N. A., and Hutzler, J. M. Is 1-aminobenzotriazole an appropriate *in vitro* tool as a nonspecific cytochrome P450 inactivator? *Drug Metab. Dispos.* 2009, *37(1)*, 10–13.

155. Botre, F. Humanized animal models to study drug metabolism: no longer a "chimera"? *Clin. Chem.* 2009, *55(10)*, 1763–1764.

156. Kukan, M. The Isolated Perfused Liver as a Tool in Drug Metabolism. In *Handbook of Drug Metabolism*, Woolf, T. F. (ed.), Marcel Dekker, New York, Basel, 1999, p. 596.

157. Lau, Y. Y., et al. *Ex situ* inhibition of hepatic uptake and efflux significantly changes metabolism: hepatic enzyme-transporter interplay. *J. Pharmacol. Exp. Ther.* 2004, *308(3)*, 1040–1045.

158. Wu, C. Y. and Benet, L. Z. Disposition of tacrolimus in isolated perfused rat liver: influence of troleandomycin, cyclosporine, and gg918. *Drug Metab. Dispos.* 2003, *31(11)*, 1292–1295.

159. Lerche-Langrand, C. and Toutain, H. J. Precision-cut liver slices: characteristics and use for *in vitro* pharmaco-toxicology. *Toxicology*, 2000, *153(1–3)*, 221–253.

160. Ekins, S., et al. Xenobiotic metabolism in rat, dog, and human precision-cut liver slices, freshly isolated hepatocytes, and vitrified precision-cut liver slices. *Drug Metab. Dispos.* 1996, *24(9)*, 990–995.

161. Wishart, D. S. Improving early drug discovery through ADME modelling: an overview. *Drugs R D* 2007, *8(6)*, 349–362.

162. Gombar, V. K., Silver, I. S., and Zhao, Z. Role of ADME characteristics in drug discovery and their *in silico* evaluation: *in silico* screening of chemicals for their metabolic stability. *Curr. Top. Med. Chem.* 2003, *3(11)*, 1205–1225.

163. Zhang, H., et al. Cytochrome P450 reaction-phenotyping: an industrial perspective. *Expert Opin. Drug Metab. Toxicol.* 2007, *3(5)*, 667–687.

164. Kirchheiner, J., et al. CYP2D6 and CYP2C19 genotype-based dose recommendations for antidepressants: a first step towards subpopulation-specific dosages. *Acta Psychiatr. Scand.* 2001, *104(3)*, 173–192.

165. US FDA. *Guidance for Industry: Safety Testing of Drug Metabolites*, 2008, pp. 1–11.

166. Grimm, S. W., et al. The conduct of *in vitro* studies to address time-dependent inhibition of drug-metabolizing enzymes: a perspective of the pharmaceutical research and manufacturers of America. *Drug Metab. Dispos.* 2009, *37(7)*, 1355–1370.

167. Walsky, R. L. and Obach, R. S. Validated assays for human cytochrome P450 activities. *Drug Metab. Dispos.* 2004, *32(6)*, 647–660.

168. Sinz, M., et al. Evaluation of 170 xenobiotics as transactivators of human pregnane X receptor (hPXR) and correlation to known CYP3A4 drug interactions. *Curr. Drug Metab.* 2006, *7(4)*, 375–388.

169. Fahmi, O. A., et al. Prediction of drug–drug interactions from *in vitro* induction data: application of the relative induction score approach using cryopreserved human hepatocytes. *Drug Metab. Dispos.* 2008, *36(9)*, 1971–1974.

170. Mahmood, I. (ed.). *Interspecies Pharmacokinetic Scaling: Principles and Application of Allometric Scaling*, Pine House Publishers, Rockville, MD, 2005, p. 393.

171. Mahmood, I. Application of allometric principles for the prediction of pharmacokinetics in human and veterinary drug development. *Adv. Drug Deliv. Rev.* 2007, *59(11)*, 1177–1192.

172. Nakatani-Freshwater, T. and Taft, D. R. Renal excretion of emtricitabine II. Effect of trimethoprim on emtricitabine excretion: *in vitro* and *in vivo* studies. *J. Pharm. Sci.* 2008, *97(12)*, 5411–5420.

173. Sweeney, K. R., et al. Renal disposition and drug interaction screening of (−)-2′-deoxy-3′-thiacytidine (3TC) in the isolated perfused rat kidney. *Pharm. Res.* 1995, *12(12)*, 1958–1963.

174. Watanabe, T., et al. Prediction of the hepatic and renal clearance of transporter substrates in rats using *in vitro* uptake experiments. *Drug Metab. Dispos.* 2009, *37(7)*, 1471–1479.

175. Abe, K., Bridges, A. S., and Brouwer, K. L. Use of sandwich-cultured human hepatocytes to predict biliary clearance of angiotensin II receptor blockers and HMG-CoA reductase inhibitors. *Drug Metab. Dispos.* 2009, *37(3)*, 447–452.

176. Tabrizi, M. A., et al. Translational strategies for development of monoclonal antibodies from discovery to the clinic. *Drug Discov. Today* 2009, *14(5–6)*, 298–305.

177. Gan, L.-S., et al. Case Study—Use of ADME Studies for Optimization of Drug Candidates, In *Optimizing the 'Drug-Like' Properties of Leads in Drug Discovery*, Borchardt, R. T., et al. (eds.), American Association of Pharmaceutical Scientists, New York, NY, 2006, pp. 81–101.

5

PHARMACOKINETICS FOR MEDICINAL CHEMISTS

LEONID (LEO) KIRKOVSKY AND ANUP ZUTSHI

5.1 INTRODUCTION

The purpose of this chapter is to give medicinal chemists a brief overview of the theory of pharmacokinetics followed by some practical considerations that need to be taken into account for planning PK studies and interpreting and troubleshooting PK data. The primary focus of the chapter is using PK studies in discovery settings because this stage of the drug invention and advancement is most relevant to medicinal chemists. This chapter will not provide a comprehensive overview of PK theory and practices but rather give junior medicinal chemists and other scientists with less experience with PK a flavor of the challenges and considerations in using animal PK data.

5.1.1 History of Pharmacokinetics as Science

The term *pharmacokinetics* (from the Greek "pharmacon" meaning drug and "kinetikos" meaning putting in motion) is a branch of pharmacology that involves the rates of movement (disposition) of a drug (or any other substance) when administered to a living organism. Specifically, pharmacokinetics is the study of the rates of absorption, distribution, metabolism, and excretion of a drug (ADME) once it is administered to a living organism.

Pharmacokinetics (PK) describes what the body does to the drug and is dependent on the dose administered, site of administration, and physiological state of the organism. A typical PK study involves administering a fixed amount of the drug (the dose) to the subject (human or animal) and at various times postdose, samples of

ADMET for Medicinal Chemists: A Practical Guide, Edited by Katya Tsaioun and Steven A. Kates

an easily accessible tissue (usually blood/plasma) are drawn and collected for analysis of the drug and its metabolite(s) concentrations. These concentration values are plotted against the sampled times and the data mathematically analyzed to yield parameters that are associated with the disposition of the drug.

Toxicokinetics (TK) is pharmacokinetics applied to high doses used in toxicity testing of drugs. Sometimes such high doses result in a saturation of kinetic (mass transfer) pathways, which can affect the PK profile.

Clinical pharmacokinetics is pharmacokinetics applied to clinical situations and the therapeutic management of patients.

Population pharmacokinetics is the study of the sources and correlates variability in drug concentrations among individual patients (inter- and intraindividual variability) such that, if necessary, dose adjustments can be made to offset the variability and maximize therapeutic benefit.

The term *pharmacokinetics* was first coined by F.H. Dost in 1953 and presented on page 244 of his now famous treatise Der Blutspiegel (Blood Levels)—Kinetic der Knozentrationsablaufe in der Kreislauffussigkeit [1]. The concepts of PK, however, were known almost a 100 years prior to Dost's definition. Table 5.1 assimilates a historical record of the discipline.

5.2 ADME

As described earlier, the acronym ADME is absorption, distribution, metabolism, and excretion and is used to describe the various physiological processes in sequence that the drug substance encounters from its initial input (dosing) to its final removal from the body. The "E" in the acronym is excretion and not, as sometimes mistakenly presented, elimination. In fact, metabolism and excretion together are elimination and many texts may refer to the process as ADE where the "E" is elimination.

5.2.1 Absorption

Absorption is the process of movement of a drug from an extravascular site of administration (such as the GI tract for PO, subcutaneous site [SC], intramuscular [IM], rectal, inhalation [INH], etc.) into the systemic circulation (blood). Although, there are great similarities between biomembranes in the GI tract and other tissues, the absorption behavior of drugs from each of these sites can be very different.

5.2.1.1 Parenteral Routes of Administration (IM, SC) Absorption by the intramuscular route is very consistent and predictable and relatively fast. In cases where drug cannot be administered by an IV route, however, a rapid delivery into the systemic circulation is desired, IM is the preferred route.

In subcutaneous administration, the drug is injected into the tissue just under the skin. Typically a larger volume of drug (10 mL/kg [3]) can be administered in the SC space and sometimes if necessary, multiple SC injections can be made at different sites in the body to increase availability. Typically, the absorption from the SC site is

TABLE 5.1 The Historical Milestones in Pharmacokinetics

Year	Author	Achievement
1847	Buchanan	Showed that the anesthetic effect (depth of narcosis) of ether was related to its brain concentration, which in turn depended on the arterial concentration and the strength of the ether in the inhaled mixture
1847–1924	Sollman, Hanzlik, Haggard, and others	Quantitative study of the disposition kinetics of various chemicals in animals
1913	Michaelis and Menton	Mathematical treatment of enzyme kinetics
1924	Widmark and Tandberg	Defined one-compartment model
1924	Haggard	Studied the disposition of diethyl ether
1931	Jolliffe	Introduced the concept of clearance
1932	Hamilton	Mean residence time
1934	Dominguez and Pomerone	Volume of distribution
1937	Teorrell	Multicompartmental PBPK model
1945	Oser	Bioavailability
1948	Boxer	Multiple dosing model
1953	Dost	Introduced the term pharmacokinetics
1960	Perl	Multiexponential curve fitting to PK data
1960	Garrett and Wiegand	Use of an analog computer for curve fitting and simulations
1961–1972	Wagner, Garrett, Levy, Riegelman, Yaffe, Nelson, Ritschel	The growth period of pharmacokinetics when most of the terms and methods were established and concepts defined
1965	Krueger-Thiemer	Multiple dosing therapeutic model
1972	Levy and Gibaldi	Defined clinical pharmacokinetics
1977	Sheiner	Introduced population pharmacokinetics

Source: Adapted from Ref. 2.

slow and usually similar to an orally administered dose. Drugs that are needed for prolonged exposure in the body are preferably dosed via this route as are drugs that have a nonaqueous (less polar) formulation.

5.2.1.2 Inhalation Route of Administration The inhalation route is employed for local delivery of drugs to the lungs (bronchodilation, inflammation) or as a portal for systemic delivery of the drug. Absorption from the lungs is very rapid and sometimes, particularly for small molecular weight compounds (<1000 Da), almost as quick as an IV dose. This is because the lungs are highly perfused, particularly in the alveolar regions and drugs deposited in this region are rapidly absorbed.

5.2.1.3 Topical Route of Administration Drugs administered topically are usually meant for local application and therapy. Thus drugs for opthalmic, nasal, vaginal, ear, and skin have a local effect and utility. The skin has been used to deliver drugs to the systemic circulation (transdermal delivery). Although the transdermal route suffers from more variability in absorption than the other routes of administration, many drug preparations have been developed for delivery through the skin. The transdermal route is a noninvasive route and is suitable for patients that cannot consume a drug through other routes. It also enjoys a higher compliance profile for usage among patients.

5.2.1.4 Oral Route of Administration The oral route of drug delivery is the most common, convenient, and widely used route of administration. Absorption from this route varies with the region of the GI tract as the physicochemical nature of the GI tract is very different in the stomach, duodenum, small intestine, and large intestine.

The pH, surface area, composition of the GI tract membranes, presence and absence of transporters, and presystemic P450s and other metabolizing enzymes, presence and absence of bile, presence and absence of food, and a host of other factors can influence the absorption of the drug.

Once absorbed, the drug is brought to the liver via the hepatic-portal vein and if the drug is susceptible to first pass effects, the drug may be cleared before it reaches the systemic circulation. All the mesenteric blood supply (from the entire GI tract except for a small region close to the anal opening where the drug can directly access the systemic circulation) collects into the hepatic-portal vein, thereby bringing the absorbed drug in direct contact with the liver.

5.2.1.5 Enterohepatic Recycling Drugs and or their metabolites that pass into the bile and are excreted into the intestine have the potential to be reabsorbed into the systemic circulation. This transfer of drug from the body to the intestine and back into the body is called enterohepatic recycling (EHR) [4].

Although all drugs that are excreted through the biliary pathway have the potential to be recycled, the drug or its metabolite must possess certain physicochemical characteristics for EHR to occur. Thus the drug or metabolite must be polar and have a molecular weight greater than 350 Da. Many glucouronide metabolites (morphine, naloxone, etc.) are excreted through the bile and into the intestine. The alkaline environment of the intestine hydrolyzes the glucouronide and the released parent molecule is reabsorbed into the systemic circulation.

5.2.2 Distribution

Distribution is the reversible transfer of drug molecules from one part of the body to the other (Figur 5.1). The blood and to a smaller extent the lymph are the major tissues responsible for distributing the drug molecules from one location of the body to another. The ability of a drug molecule to distribute into tissues depends on the affinity of the drug and its partitioning into the tissues, the strength of binding to the blood components (RBCs, plasma proteins, platelets, etc.), and the physiological volume of the tissue.

The PK parameter that characterizes the distribution of the drug is the volume of distribution (V_d). Although this parameter does not have any true physiological relevance (the volume measure is not related to any body space), it does give a

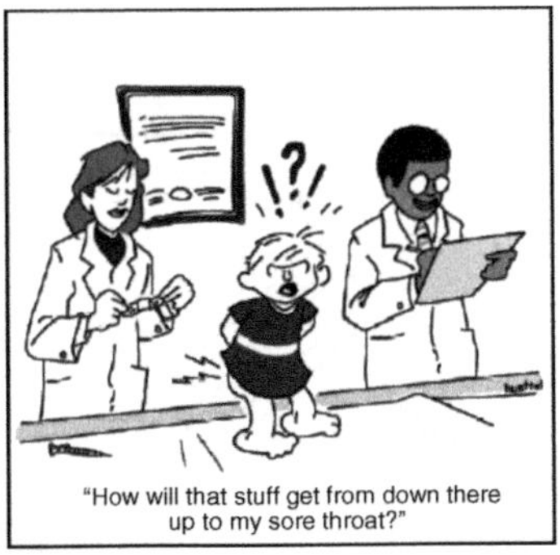
"How will that stuff get from down there
up to my sore throat?"

Figure 5.1 Schematic representation of the pharmacokinetic distribution of drugs (www.stjude.org/SJFile/pharmaco_pharmacokinetics.pdf).

qualitative assessment of the extent of distribution (and the dilution of the dose). Further details are provided in Section 5.4.1.3.

5.2.2.1 Plasma Protein Binding Since the blood is the major tissue that transports drugs from one part of the body to the other, the components of blood can interact with the drug. Plasma proteins comprise a significant fraction of plasma (8%) and drugs usually bind to these proteins in a reversible manner (irreversible binding is considered to lead to toxicity). This reversible binding of the drug to the proteins in plasma is called the plasma protein binding (PPB).

It is acknowledged that drug bound to proteins is not available for interacting with the target of action and is also not available for metabolism (clearance [CL]) and excretion. However, PPB is an equilibrium and like any other equilibria, PPB obeys the law of mass action. If the drug has an affinity for a target over the plasma protein, the drug will partition into the target. Similarly, the drug may be readily cleared even if the PPB is high (Figure 5.2).

Predicting PPB is difficult and hence trying to chemically modify a drug compound to increase or decrease its PPB is a futile exercise. Instead, discovery programs should focus on increasing the affinity of the drug to the target and reducing its CL liabilities rather than trying to manipulate the PPB.

In discovery, the PPB is determined in all the preclinical species being investigated. If the values for PPB are similar between the species, then correcting for free fraction is not necessary as the information gained from using total or free concentrations on the values of parameters is the same. If the values between the species are different, then it is important to convert all concentrations and parameter estimates to the corresponding free estimates for comparisons and decision making.

If it has been determined that the PPB varies in different species (rat, dog, monkey, human, etc.), it appears prudent to measure the PPB in different strains of the same species. If different strains of mice (CD-1, BALB/c, DBA, Swiss-Webster, etc.) or rats (Sprague-Dawley, Wistar, Lewis, etc.) are being used for different studies on a project and the PPB is different in these strains, then PPB should be determined in each strain and the free concentrations or free parameter estimates should be used.

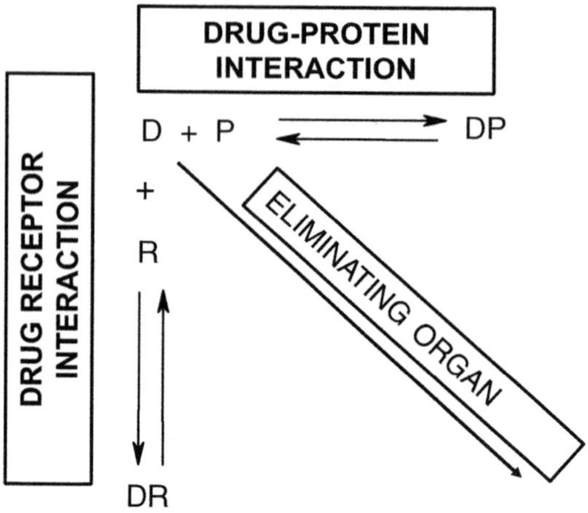

Figure 5.2 Competing equilibria depicting the importance and relevance of PPB.

Additionally, PPB may decrease with the increasing drug concentration in the systemic circulation, particularly if the therapeutic levels of the drug approach the concentrations of the primary binding components in the human plasma, albumin (670 μM), or α1-acid glycoprotein (16 μM) [5]. For the vast majority of drugs binding to albumin, the therapeutic levels are significantly below the albumin concentrations and consequently the PPB remains constant in each subject for a broad range of administered doses. However, if the drug target protein is present in the plasma along with the plasma proteins, the saturation of some high-affinity but low-capacity proteins may occur at therapeutic doses that subsequently can lead to a change in the PK properties of the compounds at high and low doses. This has been reported for the angiotensin-converting enzyme (ACE) inhibitors RU44403 [6] and ramipril [7] and dipeptidyl peptidase 4 inhibitor BI-1356 [8]. Nonetheless, the clinical relevance of the changes in PPB needs to be carefully evaluated [9]. Some additional discussion of the PPB of drugs can be found in the following review articles [10–13].

In cases where data from a PK study is being compared with data from a toxicology study, the concentration ranges may impact the PPB. It is recommended to determine the PPB at various concentrations to help bridge the divide between the low concentrations used in efficacy studies and the high concentrations used in toxicology studies. If there is a PPB difference, the free concentrations should be compared.

5.2.2.2 ***Red Blood Cell Partitioning*** Another major component of blood is the red blood cell (RBC). Many drugs can partition or bind to the RBCs and similar to PPB are considered unavailable to elicit a pharmacodynamic response or for clearance.

RBC distribution has been used as a carrier system for some anticancer drugs. However, for most compounds the impact of RBC partitioning is small. It must be determined for each species and if different, must be used to normalize concentration, efficacy, and toxicology data.

In some instances, the extent of RBC partitioning of the drug is large and rate limiting (hemoglobin modifiers such as the clofibric acids, etc.). This may result in treating the RBCs as a separate kinetic compartment [14].

5.2.3 Metabolism

The irreversible conversion or biotransformation of the compound into a relatively more polar entity (usually) is called metabolism. This biotransformation is affected by a number of enzymes. The major family of enzymes that is involved in metabolism of xenobiotics are called the cytochrome P450s. These enzymes are found in many different organs but the major presence and source of these enzymes is the liver, the largest metabolizing organ in the body. The kidneys and lungs are other organs that express cytochrome P450s as well as other drug-metabolizing enzymes. Other enzymes such as conjugating enzymes (glucouronidase, sulfatase) mono-oxygenating enzymes, such as FMOs, dehydrogenases, etc. can also contribute to the biotransformation of drug substances.

These metabolic processes convert the drug into a more polar entity (in most cases) and prepare it for being excreted and removed from the body.

5.2.4 Excretion

Ultimately the absorbed dose has to be excreted. A fraction of the dose administered orally that never gets absorbed passes unchanged into the feces and is not the subject of this section's discussion.

5.2.4.1 Renal Excretion The kidneys play a significant role in excreting drugs into the urine. Most of this excretion occurs by a passive process through the glomerulus (glomerular filtration [GF]). The proximal and distal tubules are lined with various organic anion and cation transporters that excrete (tubular secretion [TS]) or reabsorb (tubular reabsorption [TR]) drugs from the circulation and urine, respectively (Figure 5.3), by an active energy driven process. These transporters are saturable (leading to nonlinear PK) at high concentrations. For drugs that may compete for the same transporters for excretion, the potential for drug–drug interaction exists, when these drugs are administered concomitantly. Renal excretion requires that the drug be water soluble and have a relatively polar structure.

Analyzing urine data (applies for biliary data also) from a PK data analysis is slightly different than for plasma. First, the urine is considered to be collected in the bladder from which there is no return of drug back into the circulation. Second, the urine samples are collected over an interval, usually in 0–4 h intervals, and during this time the plasma levels are constantly changing. This makes it difficult to assign a specific plasma level to the excreted amount in the urine. Although the urine collecting interval can be shortened (to less than 4-h duration), there is a risk of incomplete bladder emptying which can result in errors in the estimation.

For a drug being cleared unchanged through the kidneys, the amount of drug (concentration of the drug in the urine sample multiplied by the volume of the urine

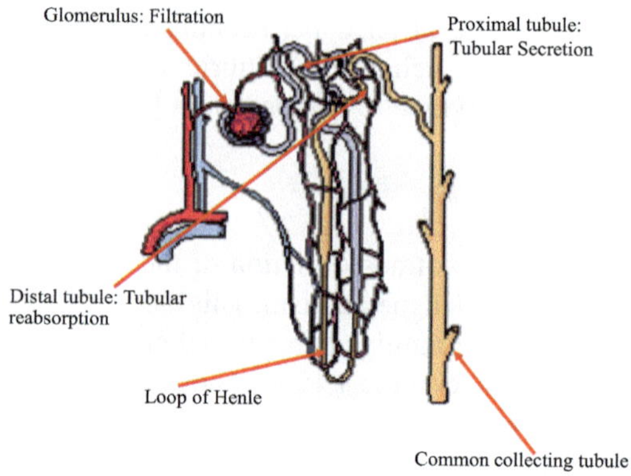

Figure 5.3 Kidney diagram of excretory pathways (www.abbysenior.com/biology/kidney_system.htm).

collected) in each interval is computed and all these amounts are added to help estimate the renal clearance as

$$CL_{\text{ren}} = \frac{\sum U_t}{\text{AUC}} \tag{5.1}$$

where ΣU_t is the cumulative amount of unchanged drug excreted in the urine from all collections and the AUC is the plasma area under curve (AUC) for the duration of the collection.

It is important that times for AUC calculation should match the time duration for which the urine was collected. If one uses the AUC_∞ value in the denominator of Equation 5.1, then the numerator is the value of U_∞, which is the complete excretion of the drug through this pathway (Figure 5.4).

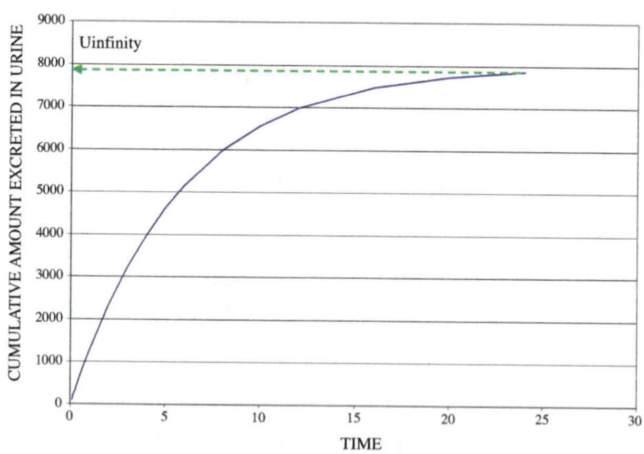

Figure 5.4 The cumulative amount of drug excreted in the urine reaching an asymptote indicating that all drug has been excreted through this pathway.

The fraction of the dose that is excreted through the urinary pathway is shown in Equation 5.2. It is important to collect urine for at least 4–6 half-lives of plasma disposition. The collected urine data will yield a more accurate estimate of renal clearance. It is also important to recognize the relationship, where

$$\frac{U_\infty}{\text{Dose}} = \frac{CL_{\text{ren}}}{CL_{\text{tot}}} = \frac{k_{\text{ren}}}{k_{\text{e}}} \tag{5.2}$$

where k_{ren} is the first-order rate constant for renal elimination (from plasma).

A semimechanistic understanding ([15], pp.169–178) of the value of the unbound renal clearance CL_{ren}/fu (fu = fraction unbound to plasma proteins) is made by comparing it to the glomerular filtration rate (GFR) in an animal [16].

If the $CL_{\text{renal}} = fu \times \text{GFR}$, then it is assumed that the only renal excretory mechanism for the drug is filtration (GF), which is considered a first-order (diffusion-controlled) process or it is filtration with equal amounts of TS and TR such that the latter cancels out.

If the $CL_{\text{renal}} > fu \times \text{GFR}$, then it is assumed that the renal excretory mechanism involves GF as well as TS and perhaps a small amount of TR.

If the $CL_{\text{renal}} < fu \times \text{GFR}$, then the excretory mechanism involves GF with a large TR but perhaps an insignificant TS.

5.2.4.2 Biliary Excretion The biliary process in mammals is responsible for aiding in the saponification, digestion, and absorption of fats. The bile is formed in the canaliculi of the liver and accumulated into the gall bladder (except in rodents who do not have a gall bladder and continuously secrete bile into the intestine). The bile is concentrated in the gall bladder and eventually secreted into the intestine. The biliary excretory system is also controlled by a plethora of transporters similar to the tubules of the kidneys. Some of the major transporters are P-gp, MRP1, and MRP2 (Figure 5.5). These transporters maintain bile physiology and are responsible for excreting toxic chemicals [17]. Many drugs are substrates and are excreted through these transporters. There have been no examples of any uptake transporters that reabsorb drugs back from the bile. It has been observed that typically drugs excreted through the biliary pathway have a molecular weight > 350 Da.

The biliary data is treated very similar to the urine data. Bile is collected in intervals and the cumulative amounts excreted are determined. The complete biliary excretion profile is as shown in Figure 5.6.

Using a similar approach to the data analysis, a biliary clearance value can be calculated from the bile data as

$$\frac{B_\infty}{\text{Dose}} = \frac{CL_{\text{bil}}}{CL_{\text{tot}}} = \frac{k_{\text{bil}}}{k_{\text{e}}} \tag{5.3}$$

where k_{bil} is similar to k_{ren} in Equation 5.2

Noteworthy, the biliary clearance is a part of the hepatic clearance and cannot exceed it (Equation 5.31).

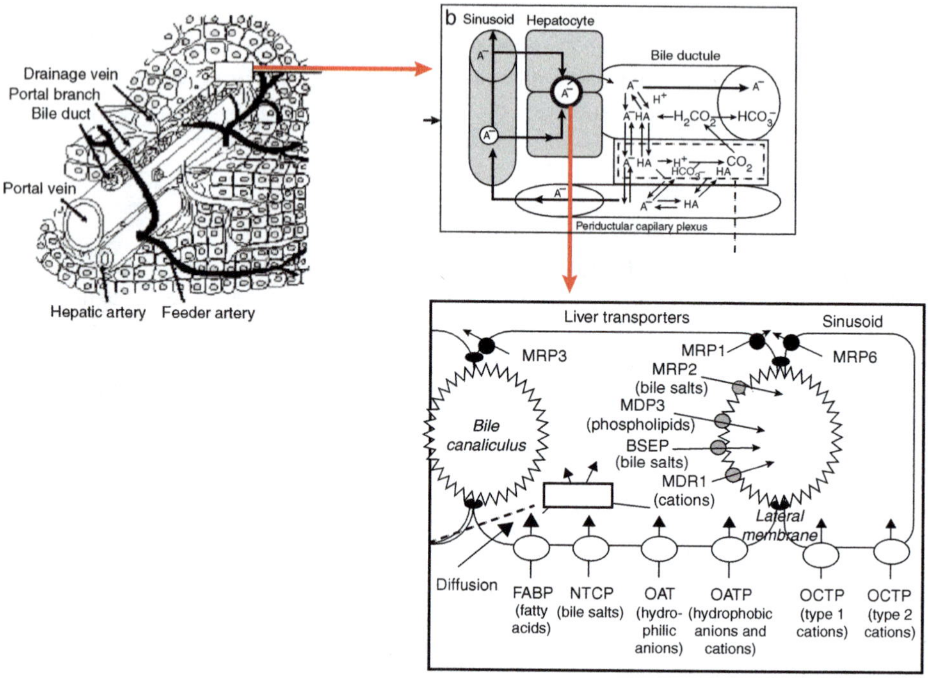

Figure 5.5 The biliary excretion apparatus in the liver.

For all drugs, it is important to have multiple pathways of clearance so that if any one pathway is immobilized due to saturation or a DDI, the other pathways can take over and clear out the drug, thereby reducing the potential for an adverse event to occur. Although the potential for urinary or biliary excretion is difficult to engineer in a drug, the discovery team should consider advancing compounds with multiple pathways of clearance preferably over those that do not possess such properties.

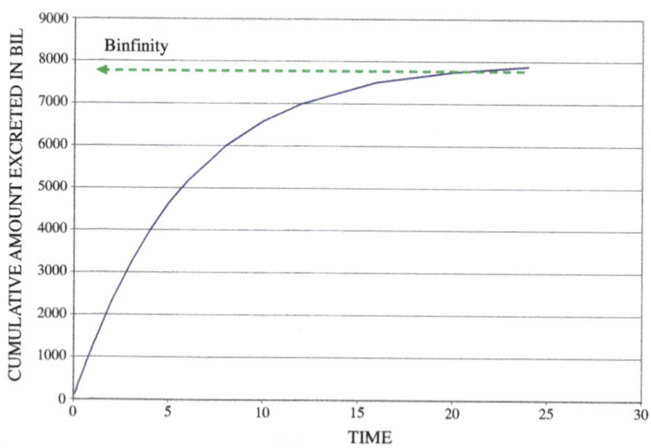

Figure 5.6 Biliary excretion profile.

5.3 THE MATHEMATICS OF PHARMACOKINETICS

The rate of decline of the amount (or concentration) of a drug in the body depends on the amount present at that time. This kinetic first-order process is depicted by a differential equation of the form

$$-\frac{dC}{dt} = k \times C \tag{5.4}$$

where dC/dt is the rate of change of concentration, which is proportional to the first-order of C. The negative sign indicates the declining concentration. The proportionality constant k is a first-order rate constant and is an indication of the rate of the decline.

Separating the variables in Equation 5.4

$$-\frac{dC}{C} = k \times t \tag{5.5}$$

Integrating throughout provides

$$\text{Ln } C|_0^t = k \times t \tag{5.6}$$

which simplifies to

$$C = C_0 \times e^{-kt} \tag{5.7}$$

where C_0 is the concentration at time = 0. Transforming both sides of Equation 5.7 by taking the natural log (log to the base "e") obtains

$$\text{Ln } C = \text{Ln } C_0 - k \times t \tag{5.8}$$

It is for this reason that an exponential equation of the form in Equation 5.7 when plotted on a rectilinear graph gives a curved profile, while the same equation plotted on a semilog paper is a straight line as in Equation 5.8.

Note the semilog plots seen in pharmacokinetic figures are based on the log to the base 10 (abbreviated simply as Log). This form of log transformation is only meant for visualization purposes and no calculations are usually undertaken in this format. However, it is easy to transform the natural log "Ln" to the base log base 10 "Log" as Ln (X) = 2.303 × Log (X).

As long as the pharmacokinetics remains linear (i.e., the rate of change of concentration is proportional to the concentration), the equations in PK are very symmetrical and all PK data can be explained by a sum of exponentials depending on the number of kinetic phases seen in the semilog plots of concentration versus time. Just as the plasma or blood data (when plotted) reflect the route of administration and type of dosing, these equations reflect the curves and hence the route of

TABLE 5.2 Sum of Exponentials Equations Used to Model Typical PK Data

Route/Type	Equation	Exponentials	Compartments
IV/Bolus	$C = C_0 \times e^{-kt}$	1	1
IV/Bolus	$C = A \times e^{-\alpha t} + B \times e^{-\beta t}$	2	2
IV/Bolus	$C = A \times e^{-\alpha t} + B \times e^{-\beta t} + C \times e^{-\gamma t}$	3	3
IV/Infusion	$C = C_0 \times e^{-kt} + C_{ss}(1 - e^{-kt})$	1	1
EV/Bolus	$C = I \times \{e^{-k_e t} - e^{-k_a t}\}$	2	1
EV/Bolus	$C = A \times e^{-\alpha t} + B \times e^{-\beta t} - D \times e^{-k_a t}$	3	2

Note: (1) The number of exponentials (or compartments) is based on the number of distinct parameters associated with the exponent; (2) The negative sign before the exponent indicates absorption or increasing concentrations from an infusion.

administration and type of dosing (Table 5.2). Further, based on the number of exponentials used to describe the plasma data, a number of distinct body spaces (arbitrarily based on blood perfusion concepts—to be discussed later) are assigned to the disposition of the drug.

5.3.1 Compartmental Versus Noncompartmental Analysis

In a discovery setting and particularly at the early stages of lead identification, PK data analysis using simple noncompartmental methods is adequate to help in estimating most of the basic PK parameters. Although, commercially available software packages readily guide through the noncompartmental data analysis process, these analyses can be done in Microsoft Excel or in some cases on a hand-held calculator. Many of the LIMS (laboratory information management systems) used to capture bioanalytical data have built-in PK parameters estimation capability and typically use the noncompartmental methods of estimation.

If PK data is required to understand mechanistic aspects (how many distinct body compartments, movement of drug from each compartment, rates of metabolism, sequential metabolism, multiple excretory pathways, etc.) of the disposition of the drug, then compartmental sums of exponentials modeling is a must. Some of the basic models can be managed using Microsoft Excel or a hand-held calculator, but it is advisable to do the calculations and curve fitting on commercially available software platforms, many of which are tailored for PK data analysis.

A comparison of noncompartmental and compartmental method of PK data analysis is shown in Table 5.3.

5.4 DRUG ADMINISTRATION AND PK OBSERVATIONS

Once the drug has been administered, the blood, urine, bile, feces, and other tissues (depending on the objectives of the study) are sampled and submitted for chemical or biochemical analysis using sensitive, reproducible, and rugged analytical methods.

TABLE 5.3 Comparison of Noncompartmental and Compartmental Method of PK Data Analysis

Noncompartmental	Compartmental
Uses terminal phase data and AUC to derive all other PK parameters	Uses the entire data to obtain the PK parameters
Quick, easy, and high throughput. Ideal for screening/binning compounds	Relatively difficult. Ideal for late-stage compound development
Requires basic knowledge of math/statistics	Requires a more detailed understanding of math/statistics
Not as detailed and provides no mechanistic interpretation of the data	Very robust and can provide mechanistic detail of drug disposition
Not helpful in simulations or for the treatment of PK–PD data analysis	Valuable for future predictions, simulations, and treatment of PK–PD data

The actual time of data (not the nominal protocol specified times) and sample collection is recorded and this time is used for PK calculations. The resultant data is analyzed and interpreted.

Depending on the matrix, each PK data set is treated differently and subsequently plotted to examine the profile depending on the route of administration and the dose.

Blood/Plasma Data Analysis The blood/plasma concentrations are plotted against time on a rectilinear graph and examined for inconsistencies. The data is subsequently plotted on a semilogarithmic graph and checked to identify the number of distinct kinetic phases. Based on this observation, an initial estimate is made on the type of PK model that may be applied to analyze the data.

Excreta Data Analysis Excreta (urine, bile, feces)—The amounts excreted during a collection interval (0–4, 4–8, etc.) are estimated and the cumulative amounts up to the interval are calculated. The cumulative amounts are plotted against time to establish the extent of excretion (fraction of the dose) and estimate clearance parameters through the particular excretion pathway.

Tissue Data Analysis The concentration of the drug in the tissue expressed as concentration of the drug per gram of tissue or per milliliter (if the density is estimated) of tissue matrix is plotted similar to the blood and plasma data. The tissue data can be overlaid on the same graph as the plasma data to assess the kinetics of the drug in the tissue.

5.4.1 Analysis of Intravenous PK Data

The plasma (blood) data following an IV bolus dose if administered correctly always shows a declining profile as time increases (Figure 5.7).

The following parameters can be derived from the plasma (blood) PK profile shown above including the area under the curve, clearance, mean residence time (MRT), and half-life ($t_{1/2}$) of the compound.

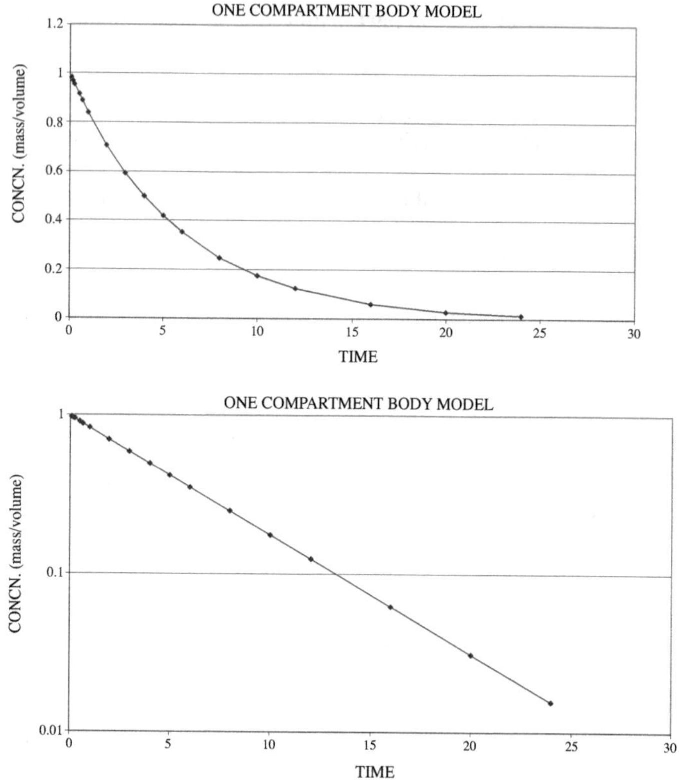

Figure 5.7 Rectilinear (top) and semilogarithmic (bottom) IV PK.

5.4.1.1 Area under the Curve The area under the plasma (blood) concentration versus time curve is a scalar quantity that measures drug exposure. This PK parameter cannot be compared across drugs but for a given drug the AUC values for different doses can be compared. The AUC parameter is useful in toxicology, biopharmaceutics, and pharmacokinetics.

AUC in Toxicology Since AUC is a measure of drug exposure, the AUC values plotted against dose (Figure 5.21) can be evaluated to assess dose linearity. Dose linearity is when AUC is proportional to dose (solid line).

Thus if the AUC values increase more than proportionally to increasing dose (dashed line), then a clearance pathway has been saturated resulting in a systemic nonlinearity. If the AUC values plateau as dose increases (dotted line) then either absorption is saturated or nonlinear protein binding occurred (Figure 5.21).

AUC in Biopharmaceutics The AUC value can be used for a direct comparison of different formulations of the same drug. In bioequivalency testing, the AUC values following administration of a generic product must be within 80–120% of the value of the innovator product administered to the same individuals. In a discovery setting, the AUC values can be used to compare the performance of different formulations or the impact of salt forms, or crystal structure of the same drug administered at the same dose.

AUC in Pharmacokinetics The AUC values can be used to determine other PK parameters such as the total body clearance, fraction bioavailable, and mean residence time.

Estimating AUC The easiest method of calculating the AUC is the linear trapezoidal rule. The trapezoidal rule is a general purpose method of graphically calculating the AUC (can be used for any type of curve) and is independent of the pharmacokinetics associated with the curve.

The technique involves breaking down the curve into individual trapezoids (Figure 5.8) and estimating the area under each trapezoid. Adding all the trapezoids, then gives the area under the entire curve

One can further break down each trapezoid into a triangle (gray) and a rectangle (black) and estimate the area of the triangle as 1/2 × base × height and the area of the rectangle as length multiplied by width (Figure 5.9). Adding these two parts gives the area of the trapezoid as follows.

Once all the trapezoids are summed, the area under the curve up to the last sampled time point is obtained:

$$\mathrm{AUC_{last}} = \sum \frac{C_n + C_{n-1}}{2} \times (t_2 - t_1) \tag{5.9}$$

Since the plasma levels decline exponentially (approach but never get to zero; as $t \rightarrow \infty$, $C \rightarrow 0$), the area under the curve to infinity is a measure of the complete exposure of the drug:

$$\mathrm{AUC_{\infty}} = \mathrm{AUC_{last}} + \frac{C_{\mathrm{last}}}{k_{\mathrm{e}}} \tag{5.10}$$

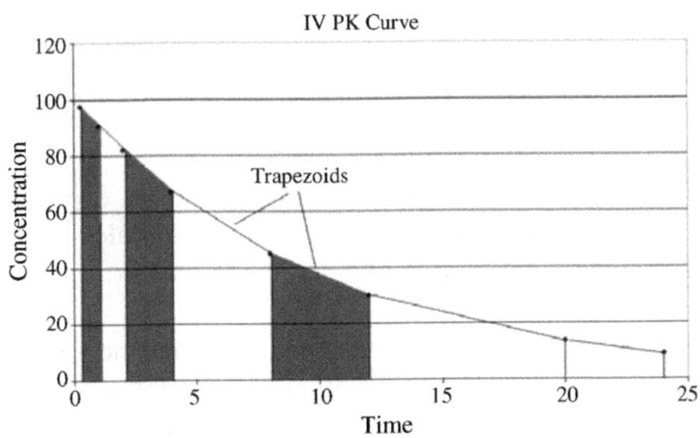

Figure 5.8 A series of trapezoids making up the area under the curve.

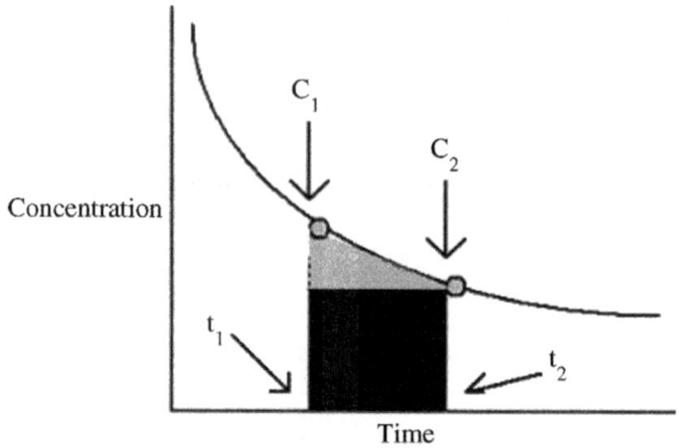

Figure 5.9 An expanded view of the trapezoid to measure the AUC. Area of trapezoid = $\frac{1}{2}(C_1 + C_2) \times (t_2 - t_1)$.

where C_{last} is the last measured time point and k_e is the slope of the terminal phase of the log transformed plasma concentration versus time profile.

If the plasma concentration versus time data has been fit to a sum of exponentials then the AUC_∞ is calculated mathematically using

$$AUC_\infty = \int_0^\infty C\,dt = \sum_1^n \frac{C_{i-1}}{\lambda_i} \tag{5.11}$$

and thus for a monoexponential decline (one-compartment model), the AUC_∞ will be

$$AUC_\infty = \int_0^\infty C\,dt = \int_0^\infty C_0 \times e^{-kt}\,dt = \frac{C_0}{k_e} \tag{5.12}$$

and for a biexponential decline (two-compartment model) the AUC_∞ will be

$$AUC_\infty = \int_0^\infty C\,dt = \int_0^\infty (A \times e^{-\alpha t} + B \times e^{-\beta t})\,dt = \frac{A}{\alpha} + \frac{B}{\beta} \tag{5.13}$$

Similar expressions can be derived for every sum of exponential modeling analysis, and most commercially available software will calculate the AUC value by this method in compartmental analysis.

5.4.1.2 Clearance Every drug is a foreign substance and the body tends to remove it once detected in circulation. In a first-order kinetic domain, this elimination is proportional to the concentration of the drug. The clearance of the drug is the proportionality constant between the rate of elimination and the concentration of the drug (usually measured in plasma, although it can refer to an individual tissue) such that

$$\frac{\mathrm{d}E}{\mathrm{d}t} \propto C \tag{5.14}$$

where $\mathrm{d}E/\mathrm{d}t$ is the rate of elimination and C is the plasma concentration. Solving Equation 5.14 gives

$$\frac{\mathrm{d}E}{\mathrm{d}t} = CL \times C \tag{5.15}$$

where CL is the proportionality constant called "clearance." Solving for clearance (separating the variables and integrating from zero to infinity) gives

$$CL = \frac{\text{Dose}}{\text{AUC}_{\infty}} \tag{5.16}$$

where dose is the dose that is systemically available. The formula in Equation 5.16 is most often used for estimating clearance and although it does not help to define the term, it is easy to note that CL is a volumetric term with units of volume/unit time.

Clearance is defined as that volume of blood, which, when passing through an organ per unit time, is completely cleared of drug. Thus, a CL value of 10 mL/min would indicate that it takes 1 min to remove all traces of drug from 10 mL of blood.

Individual Organ Clearance Although drug clearance can take place from any organ, the liver is the most significant organ for drug clearance and hence has been studied extensively.

The liver is responsible for detoxifying the body of all foreign entities and eliminating them from the body. Most drugs are metabolized by the liver through the cytochrome P450 enzymes that biotransform the drug into more polar metabolites. These polar metabolites are rendered ready for excretion and removed from the body. Other organs that also play a significant role in clearing drugs are the kidneys, lungs, blood, GI tract, skin, and so on.

The clearance estimated from Equation 5.16 is the total body clearance and is the sum of all the individual clearance in the body so

$$CL_{\text{tot}} = CL_{\text{hepatic}} + CL_{\text{renal}} + CL_{\text{other}} \tag{5.17}$$

If the individual organ CL (renal CL as an example) is determined, one can use Equation 5.18 to determine the fractional clearance of each organ as

$$f_e^{\text{renal}} = \frac{CL_{\text{renal}}}{CL_{\text{total}}} \tag{5.18}$$

Of all PK concepts, clearance is one of the most closely associated with the physiology of the body (volume of distribution also has physiological significance). By recognizing that the maximum clearance by an organ will be limited by the blood flow to the organ, a direct comparison is made of the estimated clearance (using Equation 5.16) and the blood flow through the major clearing organs of the body as in Appendix 5.A.5. If the calculated clearance value approaches the hepatic and renal blood flows, the clearance of the compound is considered high.

The liver clears drugs by metabolism and by excretion of the unchanged drug into the bile so

$$CL_{\text{hepatic}} = CL_{\text{metabolic}} + CL_{\text{biliary}} \tag{5.19}$$

The hepatic clearance is dependent on (a) the hepatic blood flow and (b) the extraction efficiency (or ratio) of the liver such that

$$CL_{\text{hepatic}} = Q_{\text{H}} \times E_{\text{H}} \tag{5.20}$$

where Q_{H} is the hepatic blood flow and E_{H} is the extraction efficiency. The E_{H} is dependent on the inherent ability of the liver to clear a drug substance or the intrinsic clearance ($CL_{\text{intrinsic}}$) of the liver for the particular drug such that

$$E_{\text{H}} = \frac{fu_{\text{b}} \times CL_{\text{intrinsic}}}{Q_{\text{H}} + fu_{\text{b}} \times CL_{\text{intrinsic}}} \tag{5.21}$$

where fu_{b} is the fraction of the drug unbound in blood (this is one of the few times that the unbound concentration in blood rather than plasma is important).

From Equation 5.21, the maximum value of the extraction efficiency (a fraction) is 1. When E_{H} approaches unity, the term $fu_{\text{b}} \times CL_{\text{intrinsic}} \gg Q_{\text{H}}$ and hence, the hepatic clearance in Equation 5.20 approaches the hepatic blood flow Q_{H}. This means that the impact of $CL_{\text{intrinsic}}$ is negligible. Chemically manipulating such compounds may not result in affecting the hepatic clearance. Usually, an E_{H} value > 0.7 for a drug is considered a high extraction ratio.

Similarly, if $Q_{\text{H}} \gg fu_{\text{b}} \times CL_{\text{intrinsic}}$, then E_{H} depends on Q_{H}, fu_{b}, and $CL_{\text{intrinsic}}$ and when substituted in Equation 5.20, the CL_{hepatic} depends on fu_{b} and $CL_{\text{intrinsic}}$. Here the hepatic clearance can be manipulated by changing the intrinsic clearance of the drug. Typically an $E_{\text{H}} < 0.3$ is considered a low extraction efficiency for the drug.

The E_{H} range between 0.3 and 0.7 is considered as intermediate. Very few drugs fall into this intermediate range and simple substitutions in Equation 5.21 after assuming $fu_{\text{b}} = 1$ show that only drugs with intrinsic clearance values in the range between $0.43 \times Q_{\text{H}}$ to $2.3 \times Q_{\text{H}}$ will be in the intermediate range.

The fu_{b} must be the fraction unbound in blood and can be substituted for the fraction unbound in plasma provided that the blood-to-plasma ratio ($C_{\text{blood}}/C_{\text{plasma}}$) is ≤ 1.

Notice that no suggestion is made to manipulate the fu_{b} since trying to design a drug with a certain fu_{b} or plasma protein binding is a futile exercise.

Such individual organ clearance can be estimated for other organs such as kidneys in a similar manner as shown for the liver.

Estimating $CL_{intrinsic}$ The intrinsic clearance is estimated by *in vitro* experiments where the drug is incubated with hepatic (or renal) microsomes or hepatocytes and the degradation of the drug is studied at the initial conditions of the Michaelis–Menten kinetic equation

$$\text{Rate of metabolism} = \frac{V_{max} \times C}{K_m + C} \tag{5.22}$$

where V_{max} is the maximum rate of the metabolism (also called the velocity) and K_m is the concentration "C" of the metabolite where the rate is $^1/_2 V_{max}$.

At low concentrations where $K_m \gg C$, the impact of C in the denominator is ignored resulting in

$$\text{Rate of metabolism} = \frac{V_{max} \times C}{K_m} \tag{5.23}$$

which is a first-order equation in concentration. The ratio V_{max}/K_m is called the intrinsic *CL*. Most discovery organizations use this feature to determine the intrinsic *CL* of their chemical series via high-throughput assays (usually 2–4 points) at low concentrations of the drug relative to its K_m.

5.4.1.3 Volume of Distribution Once a drug enters the blood stream, it distributes to various parts and tissues of the body, to a degree dependent on its physicochemical properties. A pseudoequilibrium is established (in reality a drug never experiences a true equilibrium as clearance process begins as soon as the drug is in the systemic circulation) and the concentration in plasma that is achieved is based on the amount (dose) administered or absorbed and the extent of distribution.

The plasma concentration reflects the extent to which the dose was diluted (or distributed). The factor that relates the amount of the drug to its concentration is called the "volume of distribution" (V_d). This extent of dilution could be due to extensive distribution throughout the body or it could be due to binding to specific tissues in the body or in some unusual cases it could reflect the sequestration of the drug to a single tissue. Assessing the true extent of distribution from the V_d could be misleading as many factors contribute to the magnitude of the estimate of V_d. It is for this reason that the term "apparent volume of distribution" is used to describe this factor and hence

$$\text{Apparent volume of distribution} = \frac{\text{Amount (dose)}}{\text{Concentration}} \tag{5.24}$$

The volume of distribution does not reflect true physiological volumes but by definition the value cannot be less than the blood (or plasma) volume of the animal.

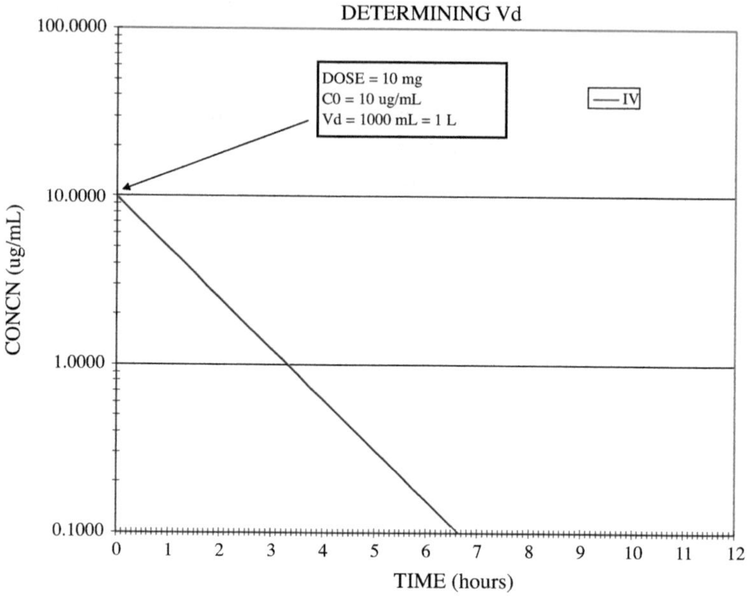

Figure 5.10 The one-compartment (monoexponential) model.

There is no upper limit to the volume of distribution, and it can exceed the total body water of the animal.

Since the volume of distribution characterizes the relationship between the amount of drug and its concentration, the value of the volume of distribution will change as the shape of the pharmacokinetic profile changes. For illustration, a monoexponential (Figure 5.10) and a biexponential PK (Figure 5.11) disposition curve (semilog transformed) are considered.

In Figure 5.10, the entire curve needs a single volume term (V_d) to describe the relationship outlined by Equation 5.24.

In Figure 5.11, the plasma curve following an IV bolus is biphasic and each kinetic phase is explained by a different volume term. This biphasic curve is explained by

$$C = A \times e^{-\alpha t} + B \times e^{-\beta t} \tag{5.25}$$

where A and B are the intercepts of the distribution and elimination phases of the drug, respectively, and α and β are the corresponding distribution and elimination rate constants, respectively. It is important to note that the terminal phase represents elimination and the slope of the line defining this phase is "β" and the intercept on the Y-axis is "B." The preterminal phase, however, is related to distribution and elimination. Once the elimination phase is deconvoluted (subtracted) from the preterminal phase, the resultant curve represents the distribution phase and its slope is "α" and intercept is "A."

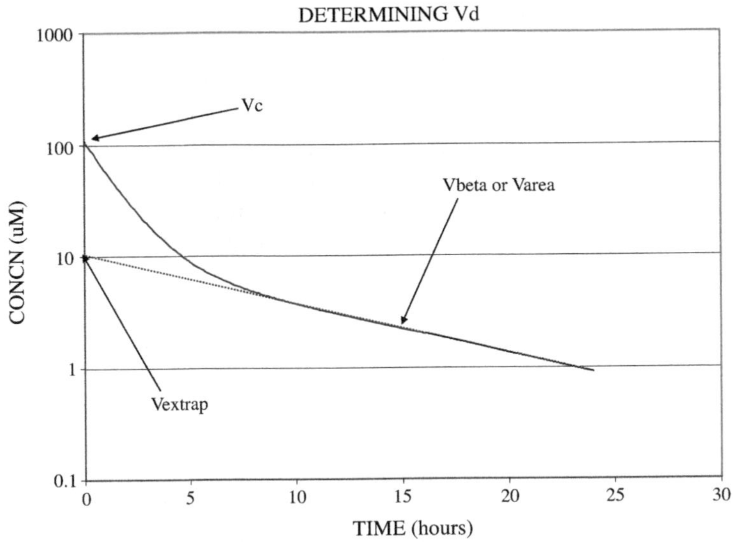

Figure 5.11 The two-compartment (biexponential) model.

Volume of Distribution of the Central Compartment (V_c) This term is estimated by extrapolating the preterminal phase (also called the alpha phase) of the curve to time = 0, (*Y*-axis intercept), and can also be estimated by utilizing Equation 5.25 as

$$V_c = \frac{\text{Dose}}{A + B} \tag{5.26}$$

The V_c cannot be less than the blood volume because the drug, at a minimum, has to equilibrate into the blood and will be diluted to that extent.

Volume of Distribution Extrapolated (V_{extrap}) This term is obtained by dividing the dose with "*B*," the intercept on the ordinate axis that is extrapolated from the terminal phase (Figure 5.11). This term is an overestimate of the volume of distribution and does not have any scientific utility. It was sometimes calculated mainly to inform "budding" pharmacokineticists of the perils of estimating erroneous parameters.

Volume of Distribution of the Beta Phase (V_β or V_{darea}) This term explains the relationship between amount and concentration in the terminal phase or the elimination phase of the disposition. It is estimated from the total body clearance as

$$V_\beta = \frac{CL_{\text{tot}}}{\beta} \tag{5.27}$$

where β is the slope of the terminal phase.

Volume of Distribution at Steady State (V_{ss}) When the elimination of a drug is very rapid as compared to its distribution, the drug does not get an opportunity to distribute to a pseudoequilibrium. Consequently, using Equations 5.26 and 5.27 to estimate the volumes of distribution will result in inflated numbers, rather than the true volume of distribution. In such cases and as applied more generally, the volume of distribution measured at a steady state would give a more accurate value. If one was to infuse a drug to a steady state and measure the volume of distribution, the value would be a true representation of the distribution of the drug. It can be derived that

$$V_{ss} = V_c\left\{1 + \frac{k_{12}}{k_{21}}\right\} = MRT \times CL_{tot} \tag{5.28}$$

where V_c is as described in Equation 5.25. The ratio of k_{12} to k_{21} is the ratio of the intercompartmental rate constants in a two-compartment model. MRT is the mean residence time (Section 5.4.1.4) and CL_{tot} is the total body clearance.

As in the case of clearance, the volume of distribution value can be compared to the volumes of the various body spaces in an animal. Although this comparison does not have absolute physiological significance, it nevertheless gives a sense of the extent of distribution that the drug undergoes. Table 5.9 (Appendix 5.A.3) compares the various body space volumes in a variety of laboratory animal species.

The volume of distribution is a difficult variable to control via chemical manipulations of the structure as opposed to clearance, which can be manipulated by changing chemical structure.

5.4.1.4 Mean Residence Time Mean residence time is defined as the time for 63.2% of the administered drug molecules (dose) to be eliminated from the body.

Statistical Moments The concept of residence times has been adopted into the PK arena from its extensive use in chemical engineering where it is used to describe flow data.

Every time a drug is dosed, a large number of drug molecules are introduced into the body (system). If the body is considered to be a stochastic space (drug molecules do not interact with each other) and these drug molecules distribute in this space, then each molecule spends a finite amount of time residing in the body before it is eliminated. If the residence times of each molecule in the body were plotted, a normal statistical distribution would be obtained. The probability of finding a molecule in this distribution can be considered to be a probability density function [18].

Simple statistical evaluations to this probability density function and estimating parameters that are equivalent to the mean, standard deviation, and so on, of a normal distribution can be applied (Table 5.4). A mathematical description of such probability density functions are called "moments."

TABLE 5.4 Similarities of Statistical Moments and Normal Statistics

Moment (M)	Description	Normal Distribution	Probability Density Function
0	Number	N	AUC
1	Mean	$\bar{X} = \frac{\sum X_i}{N}$	MRT
2	Variance	$\sigma^2 = \frac{\sum (X_i - \bar{X})^2}{N}$	VRT
3	Skewness	$\gamma = \frac{\sum (X_i - \bar{X})^3 / N}{(\sigma^2)^{3/2}}$	SRT

Hence, the plasma (or blood) PK curve can be considered a statistical distribution and the descriptors for this distribution can be calculated as

$$M_r = \int_0^\infty t^r \times C(t)\mathrm{d}t \quad r = 0, 1, 2, 3, \ldots, n \tag{5.29}$$

and for $r = 0$,

$$M_0 = \int_0^\infty t^0 \times C(t)\mathrm{d}t = \text{AUC} \tag{5.30}$$

and for $r = 1$,

$$M_1 = \int_0^\infty t^1 \times C(t)\mathrm{d}t = \text{AUMC} \tag{5.31}$$

and for $r = 3$,

$$M_2 = \int_0^\infty t^2 \times C(t)\mathrm{d}t = \text{VRT} \tag{5.32}$$

These parameters can also be estimated by the trapezoidal rule and typically for most PK analyses, the zero and the first moments are estimated by the trapezoidal rule where AUC is estimated as in Equations 5.29 and 5.30 and

$$M_1 = \text{AUMC} = \sum \frac{C_n t_n + C_{n-1} t_{n-1}}{2} \times (t_2 - t_1) \tag{5.33}$$

$$\text{AUMC}_{\infty} = \text{AUMC}_{\text{last}} + \frac{C_{\text{last}} t_{\text{last}}}{k_{\text{e}}} + \frac{C_{\text{last}}}{k_{\text{e}}^{2}} \tag{5.34}$$

where AUMC is the area under of the first moment curve and terms C_{last}, t_{last}, and k_{e} are as defined before (Equations 5.29 and 5.30).

Calculation of Mean Residence Time The central or the average tendency of this residence distribution of drug molecules is called the mean residence time and is defined as the time for 63.2% of the administered dose to be eliminated ([19], p. 409).

For an IV dose, the MRT is estimated as

$$\text{MRT}_{\text{IV}} = \frac{\text{AUMC}}{\text{AUC}} \tag{5.35}$$

The MRT is related to the half-life of the drug and

$$\text{MRT}_{\text{IV}} = \frac{1}{K} \tag{5.36}$$

where $K = CL_{\text{tot}}/V_{\text{ss}} = 0.693/t_{1/2}$ or the elimination rate constant following IV dosing.

Sometimes for a drug with a multiexponential decline, it is more important to estimate an effective half-life to understand the "meaningful" rate of elimination and this is estimated as

$$t_{1/2}^{\text{eff}} = 0.693 \times \text{MRT}_{\text{IV}} \tag{5.37}$$

A similar approach can be taken for a PO (or EV) dosed system, except the drug is administered into a separate compartment (GI tract, SC site, etc.) before it enters the systemic circulation. In order to account for the time the drug spends in this dosed compartment, the equation for PO or EV dosing is

$$\text{MRT}_{\text{PO}} = \text{MRT}_{\text{IV}} + \text{MAT} \tag{5.38}$$

where MAT is the mean absorption time and is similar to considering the average time the drug molecules spend in the absorption compartment waiting to be absorbed. Similar to Equation 5.36, the MAT can be used to determine an absorption rate constant (k_{a})

$$\text{MAT} = \frac{1}{k_{\text{a}}} \tag{5.39}$$

This value of k_{a} is useful when a dose curve is to be predicted in humans following extrapolations from preclinical data.

The MRT can also be used to estimate the volume of distribution at steady state (V_{ss}) as per Equation 5.28 where $V_{\text{ss}} = \text{MRT} \times CL_{\text{tot}}$.

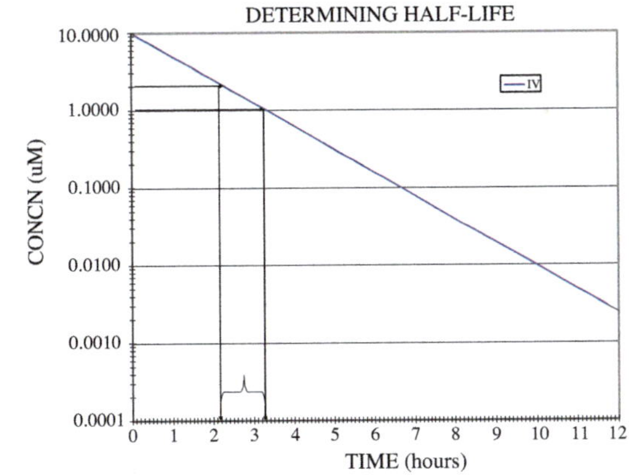

Figure 5.12 Determining half-life; concentration drop from 2 units to 1 unit is a half-life.

5.4.1.5 Half-Life ($t_{1/2}$) The time for the drug concentration to fall to half of its (initial) maximum value is the half-life. This PK parameter is the most often used and easiest to understand for the nonkineticist but is the most misinterpreted as well.

In a first-order process, the half-life is estimated as

$$t_{1/2} = \frac{\text{Ln } 2}{k} = \frac{0.693}{k} \tag{5.40}$$

where k is any first-order rate constant.

The half-life is simple and easy to understand when describing a monoexponential decline because a single half-life explains the entire disposition (Figure 5.12).

For a drug undergoing a multiexponential decline, there are many half-lives that can be determined for each of the kinetic phases (Figure 5.13). The α-phase and β-phase have different estimates. Which one is relevant? It could be argued that the terminal phase represents the true elimination phase of the drug and the half-life associated with that phase is more relevant. However, there are many instances where

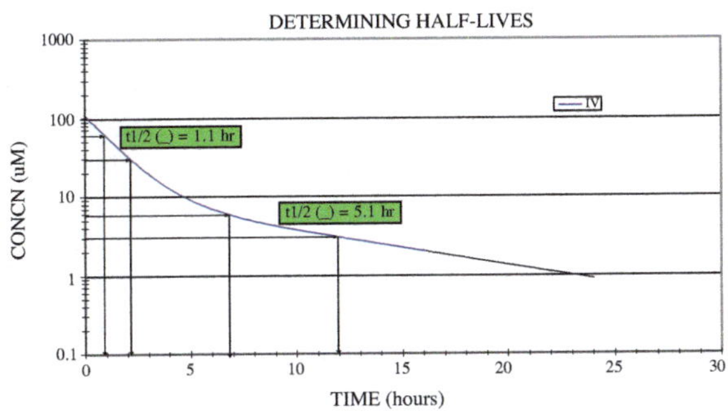

Figure 5.13 A biphasic PK profile with different half-lives for each phase.

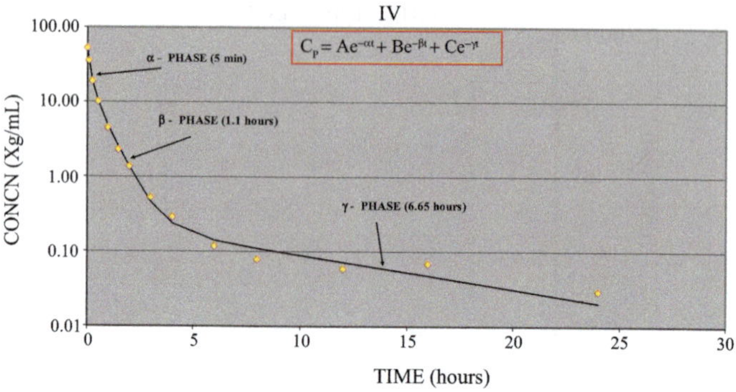

Figure 5.14 IV profile showing a three-exponential decline with a rapid α- and β-phases and a slower γ-phase. The γ-phase contributes to less than 10% of the total AUC.

the terminal phase does not contribute to the overall disposition of the compound and can be misleading in its interpretation (Figure 5.14).

In Figure 5.14, the drug has undergone three log orders of concentration change by the time the terminal phase is realized. The terminal phase contributes to less than 10% of the total AUC of the disposition. If the half-life of the terminal phase is used (~7 h in this example) as a guide, then a once a day (QD) or twice a day (BID) profile would suffice to achieve a steady state (it takes ~6 $t_{1/2}$ to achieve a steady state). In reality, either of these dosing regimens would not reach a steady state because the kinetic phase with the 7 h half-life has an insignificant impact on the accumulation to steady state. In fact the "meaningful" half-life is associated with the phase immediately prior to the terminal phase ($\sim t_{1/2} = 1.1$ h in this example) and it would be impractical to dose such a drug to a steady state unless one was using an IV infusion.

This suggests that the half-life can be a confusing parameter. Further, this parameter is not an independent PK parameter. It in fact depends on two physiologically based PK parameters CL_{tot} and V_{d} (V_{ss} in a multiexponential decline) as

$$t_{1/2} = 0.693 \times \frac{V_{\mathrm{ss}}}{CL_{\mathrm{tot}}} \tag{5.41}$$

One can clearly appreciate the association between Equations 5.28, 5.37 and 5.40 in defining the relationships between half-life, effective half-life, and MRT.

In practice, it is important to compare the terminal half-life value with the MRT estimate to check if the half-life being considered is meaningful (the MRT value and the half-life value should be similar); otherwise it may be more appropriate to use the effective half-life (Equation 5.37).

Further, it is difficult or next to impossible for chemists to conduct SAR around half-life because it requires controlling both the volume of distribution and the clearance. The latter can be manipulated by structural modifications of metabolic "soft" spots on the molecule but the former (V_{d}) is very difficult to control and predict.

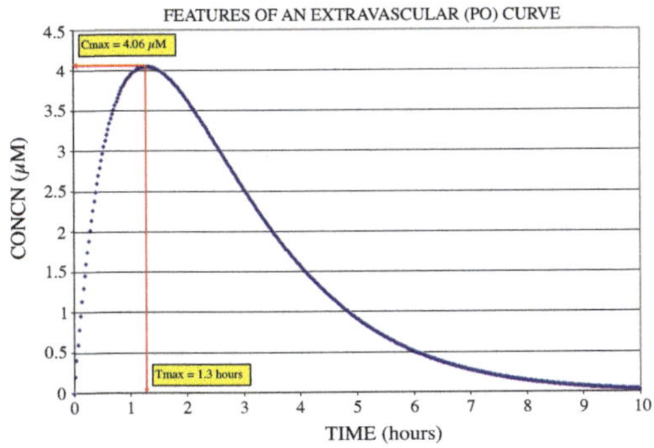

Figure 5.15 A typical plasma PK profile observed following EV administration.

5.4.2 Analysis of Extravascular PK Data

A drug delivered into an extravascular space such as an oral, subcutaneous, intramuscular, inhalation, transdermal, etc. formulation, will result in a growth curve in the plasma profile, reaching a maximum (C_{max}) followed by a decline in plasma levels. Drug delivered to any body compartment, where the drug has to traverse biomembranes before it can enter the blood/plasma circulation, will show a profile similar to that shown in Figure 5.15.

The structure of the plasma or blood level curve following extravascular administration is characterized by C_{max}, T_{max}, absorption rate (for the absorption phase), and the post absorption phase.

5.4.2.1 Maximum Concentration The maximum observed plasma (or blood) level following EV dosing is the C_{max}. It is obvious that since this is an observed value, there should be adequate sampling postdose to be able to accurately identify and estimate the C_{max} of the drug. The C_{max} of the drug is also dependent on the formulation and a change in the formulation can cause a change in the C_{max}.

In toxicokinetics, the C_{max} value is used to establish "safety margins" in multiples above some NOAEL (no observed adverse effect level) and hence it needs to be determined accurately. In toxicokinetic studies, as the dose is increased, it is quite possible that the absorption of the drug becomes saturated or dissolution-limited (solubility is usually the major contributing factor to a slower dissolution). As the overall rate of absorption slows, the plasma kinetics tends to reflect a "flip–flop" kinetic pattern (see Section 5.4.2.5) and the profile acquires a flattened shape with a C_{max} that is shifted to a higher time value. Such a "right" shift in the C_{max} along the time axis (higher T_{max}) is indicative of a saturable absorption or dissolution-limited absorption. It is therefore important to interpret the C_{max} value cautiously in a dose escalation protocol.

In bioequivalence studies, the FDA requires that the C_{max} observed for the generic product must be within 80–120% of the innovator compound.

5.4.2.2 Time to Maximum Concentration The time to obtain maximum plasma concentration (C_{max}) is T_{max} and the challenges faced in determining the accuracy of

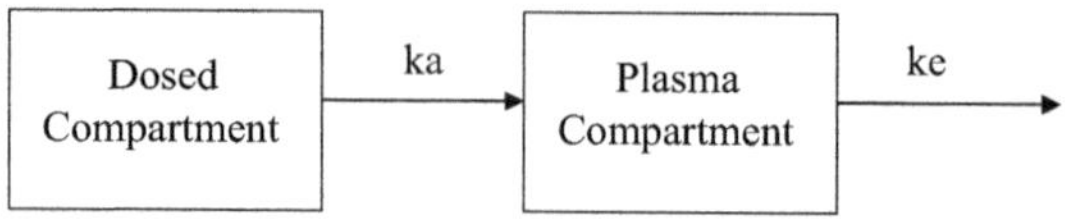

Figure 5.16 A one-compartment model with first-order absorption and first-order elimination.

C_{max} are the same as for determining T_{max}. This parameter can be used qualitatively to understand the mechanism of absorption and the associated kinetics (see discussion in C_{max} Section 5.4.2.1).

5.4.2.3 Absorption Rate The absorption rate constant (k_a) is a first-order rate constant that defines the absorption of the drug from the dosed compartment into the systemic circulation as shown in the simplified Figure 5.16.

In most cases, the absorption rate constant $k_a > k_e$ (rapid absorption) such that the plasma level curves show a C_{max} and the terminal phase (post-C_{max}) reflects the elimination phase with the elimination rate constant k_e.

5.4.2.4 Bioavailability The probability of having the entire dose absorbed from the dosing compartment is usually low. Moreover, the net dose that is available into the systemic circulation is low with drugs having a low solubility or high clearance.

The fraction of the dose administered that enters the systemic circulation unchanged is the fraction bioavailable.

By definition, the bioavailability is the rate and extent of absorption of a drug from the dosing compartment.

The rate is determined by the time to C_{max}, (T_{max}) and also the absorption rate constant (K_a).

The extent is determined by estimating the fraction bioavailable (F) from

$$F = \frac{\text{AUC}_{\text{EV}}}{\text{AUC}_{\text{IV}}} \times \frac{\text{Dose}_{\text{IV}}}{\text{Dose}_{\text{EV}}} \tag{5.42}$$

This equation assumes that the CL for both the IV and EV doses remains a constant. It is important to recognize that if the EV dose is very high (such as in a toxicokinetics study) and if there is a potential for this high dose to be in the nonlinear range, this equation cannot be applied to calculate the fraction bioavailable.

When the AUC for EV is compared against the drug dosed as an IV, the bioavailabilty is "absolute." If the AUC for EV is compared against another EV formulation (Equation 5.42), then the bioavailability is "relative."

The bioavailability from an EV site can never exceed 100%. However, in many instances the calculated value for the bioavailability shows an apparent value that exceeds 100%. There are many reasons for this to occur and are to some degree an error or misinterpretation of the data. Some instances when the percent bioavailability exceeds 100% are as follows:

1. Measuring plasma concentrations with a nonspecific assay for the parent drug and its metabolites. This can create an additive effect of the AUC values (AUC of parent + AUC of metabolite(s)) for the EV data as opposed to the IV data particularly if the EV administration is a PO dose.
2. Estimating the bioavailability when the EV dose is much higher than the IV dose, thereby resulting in a nonlinear kinetic profile for the EV dose and a linear kinetic profile for the IV dose. This requires that the EV dose be similar to the IV dose for comparisons.
3. Estimating the bioavailability of a prodrug by analytically measuring the drug content released by hydrolysis of the prodrug. When such a prodrug is administered via the PO route, it is almost completely converted to the drug during the first pass through the liver, but the same prodrug injected into the vein will take multiple cycles through the liver before it is completely converted. The AUC (of the drug) from the PO route is inflated as compared to the corresponding AUC from the IV route and the bioavailability is inflated.
4. In flip–flop kinetics (Section 5.4.2.5), the estimate of the AUC extrapolated to infinity following IV administration may be smaller than when the same extrapolation is done for the EV route. This may add on a large fraction of area to the AUC following EV administration, thereby inflating the bioavailability calculations. Typically, the AUC values up to a time point (post-T_{max}) that is shared by both routes of administration should be compared.

5.4.2.5 Flip–Flop Kinetics In some cases, the absorption is slower than the elimination ($k_a <<< k_e$) and the terminal phase represents the absorption. This is "flip–flop kinetics" and simplest to confirm by dosing the drug via the IV route and comparing the terminal phase of the IV curve with the terminal phase of the extravascular curve. Typically in flip–flop kinetics, the curve acquires a "flatter"

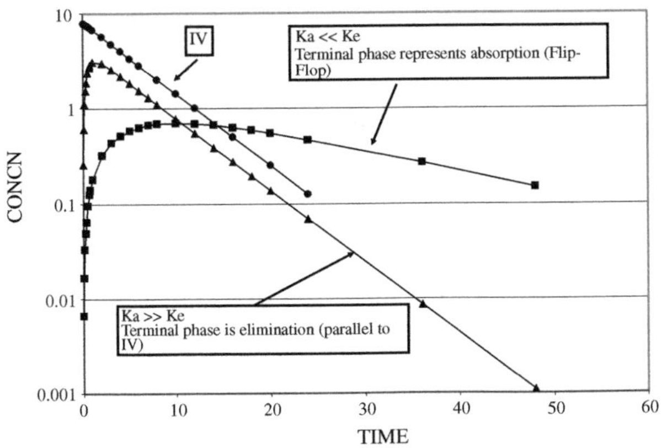

Figure 5.17 Absorption plots showing rapid absorption and flip–flop kinetics or slow absorption.

shape and the C_{max} is lower and T_{max} is right-shifted (Figure 5.17). In many instances (such as in toxicokinetic studies), the low doses will reflect the standard absorption kinetics, while at higher doses a flip–flop kinetic situation might arise.

It is important for discovery teams to realize that the terminal phase observed via EV dosing does not *a priori* reflect an elimination phase until the phase can be confirmed by an IV formulation or another EV formulation that has a faster (or slower) absorption profile.

5.4.2.6 ***First-Pass Effect*** Most drugs are designed for oral administration (PO) and are meant to be absorbed into the systemic circulation from the membranes of the GI tract. Following absorption, the drug has to pass through the hepatic-portal vein through the liver and into the systemic circulation. If a drug is susceptible to metabolism, it may not be able to enter the systemic circulation because it would be metabolized in the GI tract or in the enterocytes or be completely destroyed by the liver. The degradation of a drug as it passes through clearing organs for the first time en-route to the systemic circulation is called the "first pass effect."

The only way to protect the drug molecule from the first-pass effect is to modify the metabolic "soft spots" on the molecule and if this is not feasible, the route of administration should be changed (perhaps to an SC or IM, etc.) to bypass the first-pass metabolizing organ.

5.4.3 Analysis of Intravenous Infusion Data

In many instances, the drug cannot be delivered for some reason (e.g., poor solubility) through an IV bolus. If dosing the drug to a steady-state level is desired, then an IV infusion is optioned. Typically, the drug is infused into the vein for a fixed duration of time using an infusion pump. Depending on the pharmacokinetic half-life of the drug, a steady state is achieved, if the duration of the infusion is greater than 4–6 half-lives of the drug (see Table 5.5 and Figure 5.18).

5.4.3.1 ***Steady State for Infusion*** As the drug is delivered into the body via a continuous infusion, the plasma (or blood) levels of the drug rise. Correspondingly,

TABLE 5.5 Half-Life and Disposition of the Drug

No. of Half-Lives Elapsed	Percentage of Initial Concentration Eliminated	Percentage of Initial Concentration Remaining
0	0	100
1	50	50
2	75	25
3	87.5	12.5
4	93.75	6.25
5	96.875	3.125
6	98.4375	1.5625
7	99.21875	0.78125

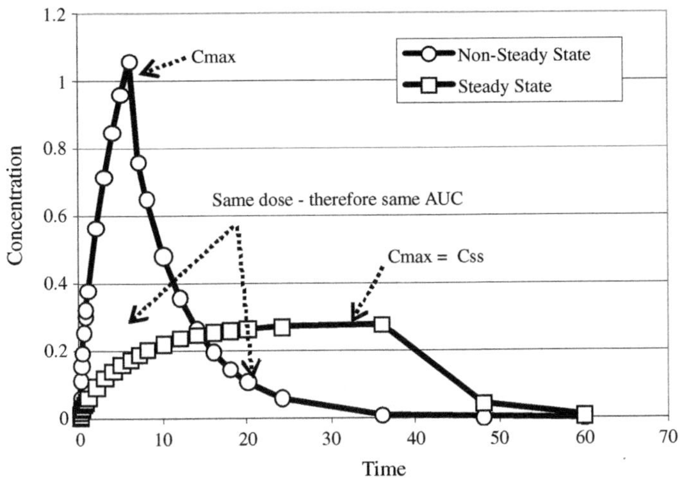

Figure 5.18 A plasma PK profile after an IV infusion to a steady-state or a nonsteady-state outcome.

as would be expected in a first-order process, the rate of elimination also increases. When the rate of input (from the infusion) and the rate of elimination are the same, then the resultant plasma levels remain unchanged as long as the infusion continues at the same rate. Changing the rate of infusion will result in a new steady state to be established (Figure 5.19).

Since kinetic processes are first order, the time to steady state is approximately six half-lives (Table 5.5). By six half-lives, the drug has reached almost 99% of the true steady state (the time to steady state is independent of any other criterion).

It takes approximately six half-lives to achieve ~99% of steady state (Table 5.5), and this time to steady state is independent of any other criterion. The steady-state levels (C_{ss}) depend on the rate of delivery and the CL of the compound such that

$$k_0 = C_{ss} \times CL_{tot} \tag{5.43}$$

where k_0 is the drug input rate (zero order, like an infusion) and C_{ss} is the steady-state level.

If steady state is lost due to a missed dose or an overdose, it will take ~6 $t_{1/2}$ to reestablish the same steady state.

5.4.4 Analysis of PK Data after Multiple Dose Administrations

Most drugs are used for chronic therapy and hence are typically dosed at multiple times during the day for many days (and sometimes are used for the lifetime of the patient). Multiple dosing is most convenient for drugs that are administered via noninvasive methods such as PO, INH, and TD.

Depending on the dosing frequency and the half-life of the drug, multiple dosing usually is tailored to achieve an SS. By design, each dose administration results in

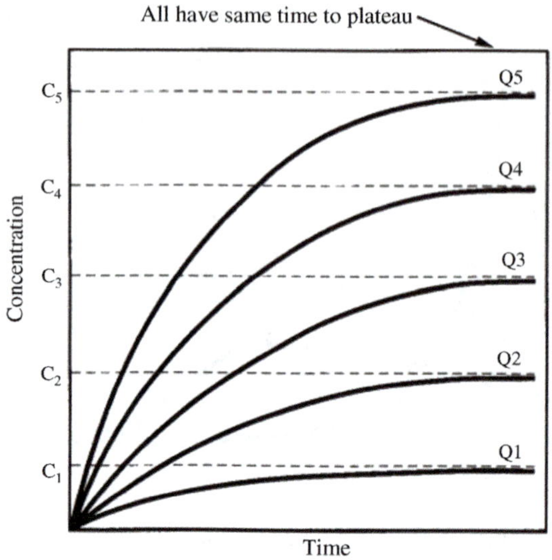

Figure 5.19 Time to steady state is six half-lives. The different steady-state levels are because the infusion rate is different [20].

an absorption followed by an elimination such that blood levels fluctuate in an oscillatory manner. The impact of the frequency of dosing on the steady-state levels as well as the fluctuation of the maximum and minimum response is shown in Figure 5.20. As one doses closer to the half-life of a drug, the fluctuations (C_{max} to C_{min}) reduce. It is for discovery teams to evaluate the right dosing frequency required for maximum therapeutic benefit.

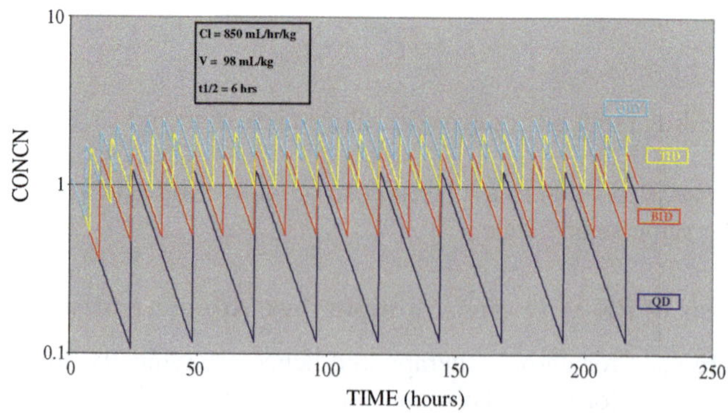

Figure 5.20 Simulated plasma levels showing impact of various dosing frequency on the C_{ss} and the degree of fluctuations for a drug with $t_{1/2} = 6$ h. Blue = QD (once a day); red = BID (twice a day); yellow = TID (three times a day), and aqua = QID (four times a day). See insert for color representation of this figure.

For any dosing scenario, an average steady-state concentration can be predicted by

$$\bar{C}_{ss} = \frac{AUC}{\tau} \tag{5.44}$$

where the AUC is after a single dose and the "τ" is the dosing interval (24 h for QD, 12 h for BID, and so on).

5.4.5 Analysis of PK Data after Escalating Dose Administrations

In all the above discussions, the PK of the drugs were assumed to be linear, that is, the relationship between dose and AUC (as a measure of exposure) is proportional. This means that if the dose is doubled, then the AUC must double and so on. In many cases, and particularly at higher doses, this relationship fails and increasing dose results in more than or less than proportional changes in AUC. This lack of proportionality results in "nonlinear PK."

Nonlinearity is considered a "problem' situation in PK because the ability to extrapolate and predict is lost. Since the PK now depends on the dose and the plasma levels, PK parameters such as CL and V_d are no longer constant and independent of dose. Consequently, achieving a SS is difficult and the potential of increasing plasma levels rapidly and in an uncontrolled and unpredictable manner can lead to severe adverse events.

An initial discussion about recognizing nonlinearity was made in section "AUC in Toxicology" and shown in Figure 5.21. Comparing AUCs at different doses to check for proportionality will help to identify the nonlinearity.

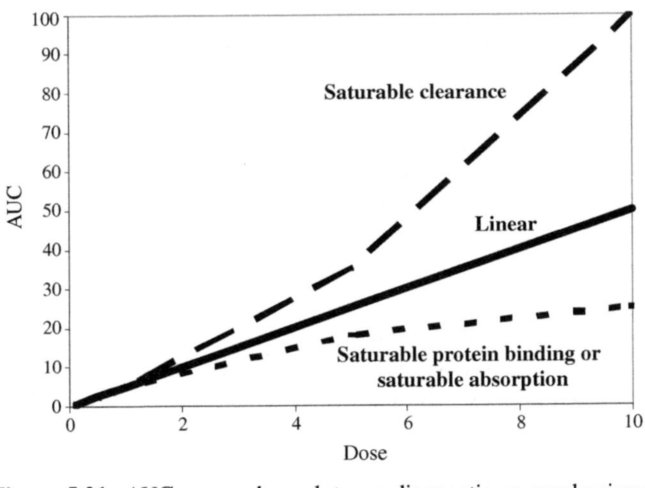

Figure 5.21 AUC versus dose plots are diagnostic on mechanisms.

5.4.5.1 Nonlinearity A linear first-order system demands that the concentrations should change proportionally to the dose. If the dose is doubled, then the concentrations should double and so on. As long as this condition holds, extrapolations and interpolations between such linear doses can be readily made as the PK parameters such as CL and V_d do not change as the dose changes. This linear assessment is best made by comparing the AUC to the given dose or recognizing that in a linear system the dose/AUC $= CL =$ a constant.

When this condition is not met, the PK system is nonlinear and extrapolations cannot be made. Depending on the type of nonlinearity, there could be a safety issue if drug concentrations following multiple administrations increase unbridled due to a systemic nonlinearity.

Presystemic Absorption Nonlinearity If the AUC at higher doses increases in a less than proportional manner, then absorption has become rate-limiting (Figure 5.21). This rate-limited absorption could be due to a saturation of the absorption through the biomembranes of the GI tract or for compounds with poor solubility, resulting in a dissolution rate limit. Increasing the dose does not achieve a higher plasma level. A possible approach to rectifying this problem may be to change the formulation (salt form, dosage form, etc.).

Nonlinear Protein Binding Sometimes at higher plasma levels, all the binding sites for the drug are saturated and the unbound fraction of the drug increases. Higher concentrations of free drug are present resulting in an increase in the rate of CL. In effect, the AUC decreases, as the dose and the corresponding plasma levels increase, result in the plateau effect seen in Figure 5.21. In a nonlinear protein-binding case, all concentrations should be converted to the free levels, and the free plasma concentrations should be used for any further PK calculations.

Nonlinearity due to Saturable Clearance When the AUC increases more than proportionally (see Figure 5.21), a CL pathway has become saturated. Typically, for drugs that are metabolized by the cytochrome P450 enzymes, higher plasma levels can result in concentrations in the liver that may saturate the capacity of the enzyme to metabolize the drug. In this case, drug starts to accumulate in the system and if unchecked, can increase alarmingly to levels that can cause toxicities. Some drugs have the ability to inhibit or interact with the metabolizing enzyme or a transporter, thereby making the enzyme unavailable for metabolism and CL. This can also be a cause for the nonlinearity. If such a nonlinearity (green curve) is observed at very low plasma levels, the only recourse is to change the molecule or increase potency to the target and reduce the dose.

A nonlinearity can be caused if the drug induces an enzyme that is responsible for the drug's own metabolism (autoinduction). This type of nonlinearity is not observed after a single dose and it usually requires multiple doses of the drug to induce the expression and synthesis of the enzyme. The blood levels measured (and the corresponding AUCs) after multiple dosing for a week (usually) are much lower (red curve) than expected despite the PK properties of the drug (adequate $t_{1/2}$ to

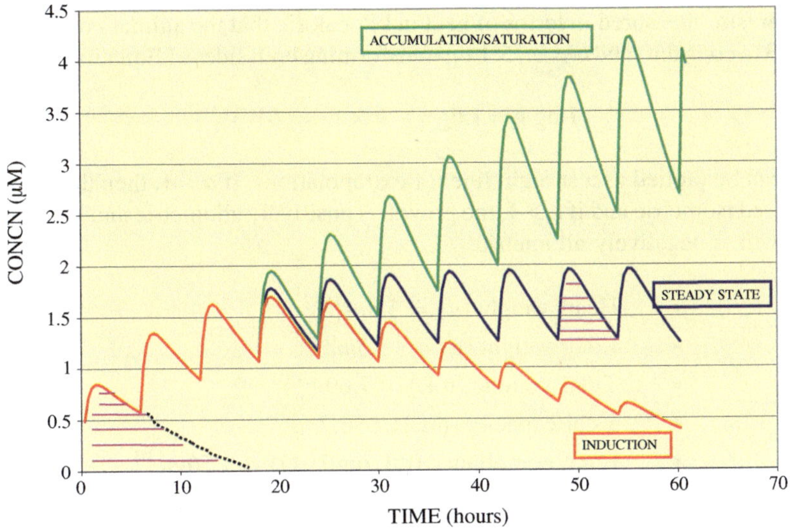

Figure 5.22 The impact of nonlinearities on the steady-state exposures of a hypothetical drug undergoing saturable *CL* (green) and autoinduction (red). See insert for color representation of this figure.

expect accumulation and an increase in SS). This induction can be overcome by adjusting the dose to a higher level.

5.5 HUMAN PK PROJECTION

The primary focus of accomplishing the PK studies in various laboratory animal species is to have the ability to predict the human PK for the compound. Various methods have been used to establish correlations of the PK properties between animals and man; however, even if successful, these correlations work within a series but do not translate across all compounds. There are two primary approaches in scaling animal PK properties to humans, namely, allometric scaling and physiologically based pharmacokinetic (PBPK).

5.5.1 Allometric Scaling

Allometry is the study of the differential growth rates of different parts of the organism's growth or behavior. In 1947, Max Kleiber [21] demonstrated that the basal metabolic rate of an organism was related to the body weight in a power function. This was quantified in an equation of the form

$$y = a \times (BW)^b \tag{5.45}$$

where a = allometric coefficient and is different for different relationships studied and b = power function. Kleiber described $y = P_{\text{met}}$, which is the basal metabolic rate of the organism (measured in terms of heat in kilocalorie that the animal produces) and $a = 73.3$ (a constant) and $b = 0.75$. Log transforming both sides of Equation 5.45 gives

$$\text{Log}\, y = \text{Log}\, a + b \times \text{Log}\,(BW) \tag{5.46}$$

which can be plotted as a straight line for extrapolations. If $a = 1$, then the growth is considered isometric and if $a > 1$, the growth is positively allometric and if $a < 1$ then the growth is negatively allometric.

- Heart weight (g) $= 5.8m_b^{0.98}$
- Long weight (g) $= 11.3m_b^{0.98}$
- Tidal volume (mL) $= 7.69m_b^{1.04}$
- Vital capacity (mL) $= 56.7m_b^{1.03}$
- Lung compliance (mL/cmH_2O) $= 1.56m_b^{1.04}$
- Blood volume (mL) $= 65.6m_b^{1.02}$
- Muscle mass $= 0.40m_b^{1.00}$
- Skeletal mass $= 0.0608m_b^{1.08}$

Using the above concept and applying it to pharmacokinetics the *CL* of a compound measured in various animal species could be scaled and extrapolated to humans (Figure 5.23).

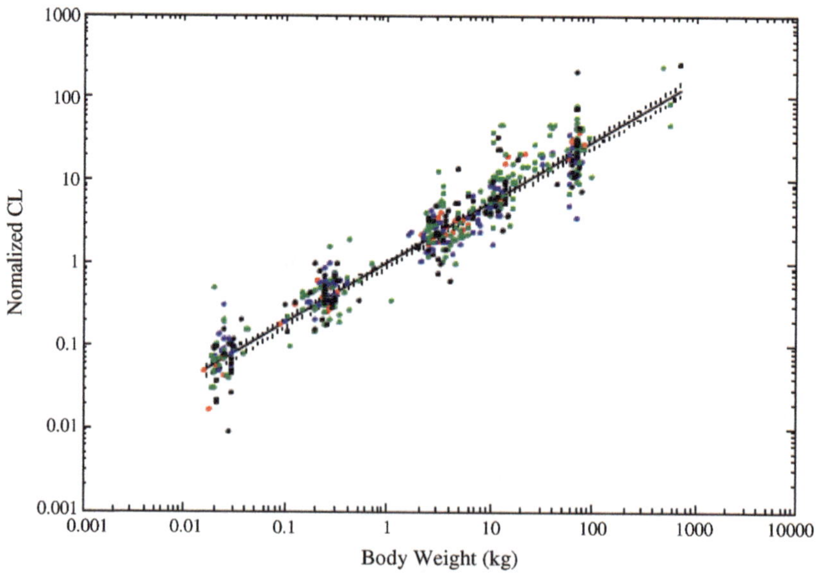

Figure 5.23 Allometric scaling of 91 xenobiotics (red, proteins; green, drugs eliminated by metabolism; blue, drugs eliminated by renal excretion; and black, drugs eliminated by both renal excretion and metabolism [22]. See insert for color representation of this figure.

The important PK parameters that are scaled are the CL, V_d, and by extension the half-life. As mentioned before, the CL scales according to the following equation:

$$CL = a \times (BW)^{0.75} \tag{5.47}$$

and the V_d scales isometrically as

$$V_d = a \times (BW) \tag{5.48}$$

and recognizing that the half-life depends on both the CL and the V_d (Equation 5.41), it scales as

$$t_{1/2} = a \times (BW)^{0.25} \tag{5.49}$$

where a is a constant (a is not the same constant for each relation).

Typically, these PK parameters are determined in three to four different laboratory animal species such as mouse, rat, rabbit, dog, monkey, pig, and so on, and use the allometric relationships mentioned above to scale the PK parameters to humans.

Many investigators have acknowledged that better correlations are obtained when the CL of a compound are normalized to brain weight or *in vitro* intrinsic clearance, or other physiological variables [23, 24]. These correlations are not based on any scientific concepts but for a given compound can result in better estimates. The practitioner is encouraged to try various approaches to establish a correlation and use it for predictions to man.

5.5.1.1 Single-Species Scaling Recently, it has been shown that the rat alone scales to human with an accuracy which is within ±twofold of the actual CL observed in the clinic [25]. This level of accuracy is considered adequate by many clinicians who cautiously study the PK of the investigational compound in first in human studies. Taking the ratio of Equation 5.47 gives

$$\frac{CL_{\text{human}}}{CL_{\text{rat}}} = \left(\frac{BW_{\text{human}}}{BW_{\text{rat}}}\right)^{0.75} \tag{5.50}$$

where the BW_{human} is usually assumed to be 70 kg and the BW_{rat} is usually around 0.25 kg. The CL value used in Equation 5.50 is expressed in absolute units of volume per time (e.g., mL/min or L/h, etc.).

Correspondingly, the volume of distribution scales linearly such that on an mL/kg (or a L/kg) basis the value between species will remain the same.

5.5.2 Scaling by Physiologically Based Pharmacokinetic Modeling

Many investigators have suggested that a better method of scaling the pharmacokinetic parameters is based upon physiological processes, which in turn scale via allometric equations such as shown before for various organ weights, volumes, blood

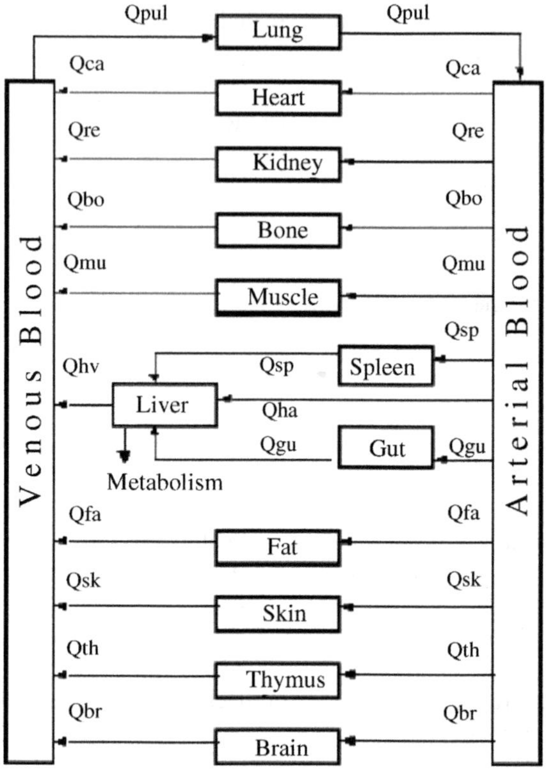

Figure 5.24 The physiological representation of the body for PBPK modeling [26].

flows, etc. The body is considered to be a series of compartments (usually associated with each of the organs; see also Figure 5.24) and relating CL and V_d of a drug in the rat to the physiology of the rat allows one to apply the same physiological rational to humans to predict the properties of the drug in human.

A series of differential equations is written to account for the movement of the drug from the arterial to the venous side taking into account the role of the clearing organs. Fitting these differential equations to the data collected from each tissue is accomplished (Figure 5.25) and using various organ- and tissue-specific scaling factors the corresponding profiles for the drug in human tissues can be simulated.

Many commercially available software packages assist with scaling using the PBPK approach such as Gastroplus®. In this software, distribution characteristics of a drug into various tissues have been extrapolated from the basic physicochemical properties of the drug, thereby requiring minimum experimentation. Using this approach, De Buck et al. [28] compared the predictions of 26 clinically tested drugs with projections from Gastroplus®. They reported a 65–74% success in predicting various PK and PD parameters within twofold of the actual data. Although the concepts used in PBPK modeling are scientifically the most relevant, the only way an accurate model can be constructed is if each tissue in the animal body is taken and

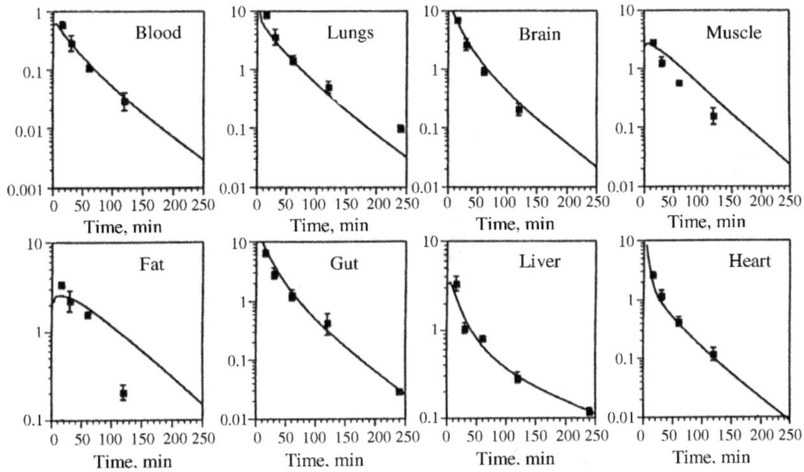

Figure 5.25 PBPK modeling of cocaine in the rat [27].

the drug content measured as a function of time. Since this is very tedious in a discovery setting, it has found minimum favor among PK practitioners for the purpose of scaling.

5.5.3 *In Vitro–In Vivo* Correlations

In discovery, there are many examples as well as published papers that have used *in vitro* results as a guide to better predict and project *in vivo* data. A majority of these methods have been developed to improve the ability to scale the *CL* of the compound. Scaling the *CL* using the *in vitro* intrinsic *CL* values estimated using the well-stirred, parallel tube, and dispersion models predicted that the scaling factors ($CL_{\text{intrinsic } in\ vivo}/CL_{\text{intrinsic } in\ vitro}$) in humans were very varied. Using the *in vitro* human *CL* intrinsic values along with the human scaling factors, the predictions were poor; incorporating the animals scaling factors improved the predictions [29].

Other investigators have used sandwich-cultured human hepatocytes to predict human biliary clearance [30] and *in vitro* expressed UDP-glucuronosyltransferase to predict the Phase II glucuronidation [31] of compounds. Judicious decisions should be made by project teams in deploying such techniques and methods to benefit the various stages of discovery and development continuum.

5.6 PK PRACTICES

The following section is dedicated to describing practical considerations that should be taken into account when designing and executing PK studies and when analyzing and interpreting PK data. Because of the limited size of this chapter, only a brief outline of the key issues will be given below. More relevant information can be found in the references provided.

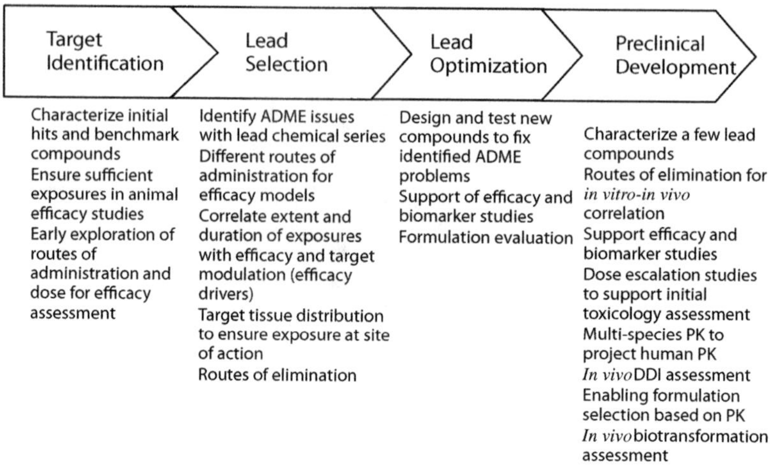

Figure 5.26 The stages of the discovery process and primary purposes of animal PK studies.

5.6.1 PK Studies for Different Stages of Discovery Projects

Animal PK testing is widely used in pharmaceutical discovery. Although different companies may utilize somewhat different approaches and processes in discovering new drugs, the key stages of the discovery projects are fairly similar. A typical discovery project involves four major stage gates: target identification, lead selection, lead optimization, and preclinical development (Figure 5.26). An example of a similar process can be found in the literature [32]. A similar discovery assay by stage (DABS) approach is described by the group of the scientists from Millenium Pharmaceuticals [33] who broke the discovery process into four stages: (1) high-throughput screening (HTS), hit-to-lead (HTL), lead optimization (LO), and development candidate (DC).

5.6.1.1 Target Identification The target identification stage focuses primarily on the biology of a selected target. Animal testing, primarily in rodents, is utilized for preliminary evaluation of PK properties of screening hits and/or benchmark compounds described in the literature. At this stage, animal PK data can be used to select an appropriate dosage and route of administration that would deliver sufficient exposures in the animal efficacy models to build confidence in the rationale of the biology of the target.

5.6.1.2 Lead Selection The primary purposes of the lead selection stage of the discovery project are to (1) identify the spectrum of ADME properties of several chemical templates (series) and (2) identify the drivers of efficacy by analyzing the relationships between the extent and the duration of the *in vivo* exposures, efficacy, and target modulation.

In this case, certain tissue distribution studies (e.g., brain penetration) may provide valuable information. Some initial screening PK is used at this stage to quickly assess *in vitro–in vivo* correlation (IVIVC) and identify the reason for their absence. Some initial *in vivo* mechanistic studies aimed at evaluation of the primary routes of elimination may be conducted in bile-duct cannulated (BDC) rats or even dogs. The lead selection stage of the project is probably the most critical for the success of the entire program because it narrows down the chemical space in which the program will operate and limits the opportunity to modulate and correct any critical pharmaceutical properties (ADME, potency and efficacy, etc.).

5.6.1.3 Lead Optimization Selection of the lead series is a very significant milestone for the discovery project, which now moves to the lead optimization stage. At this stage, the primary efforts of animal testing are to fix any identified ADME problems and to identify the best compounds for further advancement. Screening PK studies aimed at driving the design of new compounds with better properties are conducted and PK data continues to be used to support efficacy and biomarker studies as well as find reasonable formulations for early safety assessments. A small number of the most promising compounds are identified prior to moving to the next stage.

5.6.1.4 Preclinical Development In the preclinical development stage, research is carried out to prepare for the first-in-human (FIH) dosing of the selected front-running drug candidate. Animal studies may be conducted in a "definitive" rather than a "screening" format because they are used to predict human PK and project an FIH dose. A more detailed evaluation of PK/PD relationships is done in different animal species using biomarkers and efficacy readouts. Usually a fair number of animal studies are done to develop a formulation that will be used in investigational toxicology (IVT) evaluations in rodent (usually rats) and nonrodent (usually dogs but occasionally monkeys) species. As part of a risk assessment, some mechanistic drug–drug interaction (DDI), *in vivo* biotransformation and metabolite identification studies may be conducted in different animal species and compared to human *in vitro* DDI studies. Such comparisons help properly select toxicology species.

Once the preclinical package is ready for filing in an investigational new drug (IND) application, preclinical development may be considered complete. Nonetheless, a significant number of animal studies are usually performed to support further development of the drug candidate. The goal of these studies may be to support a broader safety evaluation of the drug candidate (e.g., reproductive toxicology, carcinogenicity, etc.) or address some specific issues of clinical development (e.g., biotransformation).

5.6.2 Key Parameters of PK Studies

There are several key parameters that have to be taken into account when planning for an animal PK study:

- compound
- formulation
- animal species and strain

- dosing route and frequency
- sample collection
- bioanalysis
- data analysis and reporting.

Those parameters are discussed in the subsequent sections.

5.6.2.1 Compounds There are several critical properties of the compound (sometimes referred to as "test compound" or "test article" or "test material") that need to be discussed and agreed upon between medicinal chemists and the ADME scientists when planning and performing an animal PK study:

- metabolic stability in expected biological matrices
- properties related to formulations
- purity
- supply
- physical form.

Compound Metabolic Stability in Expected Biological Matrices Compound stability in the biological matrices planned to be collected and analyzed is a property that may either prevent conducting the study or correctly interpreting the PK data. The metabolic stability of a newly synthesized compound can be measured *in vitro* in metabolizing organs' subcellular fractions (such as microsomes or S9 fractions) or whole cells (such as hepatocytes). This stability may be estimated based upon information obtained for closely related structural analogs or on general knowledge of the metabolism of similar classes of compounds. Ester prodrugs and peptide drug candidates are two well-known examples of compounds whose metabolic stability in biological media needs to be evaluated prior to animal dosing. Although challenging, PK studies of some metabolically unstable compounds can be conducted if some special sample collection techniques are used. For example, exposure to ester prodrugs can be assessed in animal blood or plasma samples if plasma esterases are inhibited immediately upon sample collection by using esterase inhibitors such as paraoxon [34], phenylmethylsulfonyl fluoride (PMSF), sodium fluoride or others [35], or by mixing the blood or plasma samples with water-miscible quenching agents (acetonitrile, methanol, acids, etc.). These agents coagulate proteins and destroy enzymatic activity. However, there is a potential risk of re-esterification of the prodrugs if alcohols are used as the blood- or plasma-quenching agents. While technically feasible, such techniques need to be considered in the context of drug development program, and a team should consider whether a molecule with such metabolic liabilities is an appropriate clinical candidate.

Metabolic instability of test compounds in biological media may lead to an overestimated total clearance of the compound, which may be higher than the total hepatic blood flow in the animal species. When a new series of chemical compounds is chosen for evaluation in the lead selection stage of the project, metabolic instability may become a deselecting criterion for the entire series or individual molecules.

In vitro metabolic stability in animal plasma is typically evaluated as the first parameter for new compounds. The assay is fairly straightforward and may be performed by spiking a stock solution of the compound into animal plasma to produce an incubation mixture maintained at 37°C and monitoring the disappearance of the parent molecule or appearance of some known or expected metabolites usually using liquid chromatography mass spectrometry (LC/MS) quantitation.

The use of at least one positive control (a compound with a known and accurately measurable metabolic half-life) is highly recommended for these experiments since enzymatic activity of the plasma may be reduced upon its storage and handling.

Also, some organic solvents (e.g., DMSO) used for preparation of the stock solution may inhibit plasma enzymes responsible for biotransformation of the compounds. As a rule of thumb, the maximum concentration of DMSO in the incubation mixture should not exceed 0.1%. Higher percentages of organic solvents can potentially be used for low-solubility compounds if a positive control with a similar mechanism of metabolism is used as a reference.

Another potential source of data variability or error is evaporation from the incubation mixture. This can happen if the mixture is sampled multiple times to determine metabolic stability of the compounds at multiple time points. A better assay format may utilize preparing a "bulk" amount of the incubation mixture sufficient for generating multiple individual incubation samples in the tubes with caps or on the plate with tight lids. These individual samples can be quenched at different time points to establish a metabolic stability time course.

If the compound needs to be quantified in the animal's organs and tissues, it may be necessary to generate some data for metabolic stability in those tissues, homogenates, or subcellular fractions.

Usually the PK matrix metabolic stability experiments are performed in a "quick and dirty" format with a relative rather then absolute LC/MS quantitation. The analyte peak area is used for quantification and ranking of compounds (see Section 5.6.2.7).

Compound Properties Related to Formulations The solubility and the chemical and physical stability of the test compounds are critical for preparing a suitable formulation for *in vivo* administration.

SOLUBILITY Sufficient solubility of the compound is especially important for intravenous formulations that require true solutions with no microparticles. Another limitation for IV formulation is that the dose volumes are more restricted and typically should not exceed 5 mL/kg. If the maximum solubility of a compound in a particular IV formulation is 1 mg/mL, the maximum IV dose that can be achieved in the animal study is 5 mg/kg.

CHEMICAL STABILITY Chemical stability of the compound may be experimentally evaluated prior to preparing an appropriate formulation. Typically, acid- or base-catalyzed degradation of the compound may lead to its limited stability in solution or solid form. The stability of the compound in solution typically can be assessed at pH 1–2 (representing gastric pH of human and some animal species) and pH 6–9 (representing intestinal pH of different sections of the intestine from duodenum to colon). The duration of the stability experiments depends on the expected time between the formulation preparation and animal dosing, which may range from several minutes to 12–24 h.

If the compound is prepared as a salt of a strong acid (e.g., HCl or TFA) for PK, it is recommended to assess its stability at least at room temperature with a typical ambient humidity. It is strongly advised to conduct this stability if the salt form is hygroscopic.

Another source of compound instability is photodegradation due to light exposure. In this case, the compound can be maintained in amber glass vials and handled in the labs equipped with yellow lamps.

Oxidation by atmospheric oxygen may make handling the compound challenging and reduce the probability for commercialization.

HYGROSCOPICITY Hygroscopicity of the compound may lead to higher instability in solid form as well as to the absorption of atmospheric moisture that may change the correction factor for the content of the parent compound content in the material used for animal studies.

CRYSTALLINITY A crystalline form of the compound does not impact true solution formulations but may have a profound effect on suspension formulations used for oral dosing.

Usually, in the early stages of a project, a new compound is purified using liquid chromatography followed by lyophilization of the collected fractions. Frequently this process leads to an amorphous form of the compound with a lower melting point and higher solubility. Higher solubility of the amorphous compound may facilitate its dissolution in oral dosing suspensions which, in turn, may lead to a higher fraction absorbed and higher oral bioavailability of the amorphous compound compared to its crystalline form. If the compound may exist in different crystalline forms (polymorphs), different polymorphs may exhibit different PK properties such as ritonavir [36, 37].

ELECTROSTATICS If the compound is amorphous (frequently fluffy), it may be electrostatic and require special handling to avoid loss of material when transferring to a vial. When possible, transfer of the material should be minimized or avoided. A potential good practice may be to determine the weight of the empty vials used for lyophilization so the weight of the solid material can be accurately determined and used for formulation work without material transfer. If transfer of solid material is still required, certain devices reducing static electricity can be used to reduce the risk of losing compound.

Compound Purity There are several aspects of compound purity that may impact PK studies. The test compound must be pure enough for safe administration in animals. Even if the impurities do not cause animal death, animal health and physiology can be impacted, which, in turn, may affect ADME properties of the compound. Both the absolute content of the desired compound in the material prepared for animal dosing as well as the quantity and spectrum of potential biological/toxicological properties of undesired impurities must be well understood.

Typically, the total purity of the compound intended for animal administration in preclinical PK is expected to be not less than 95%. Lower content of the test compound may be scientifically justified if the impurities are represented by known and fairly safe components (water, certain salts). Conversely, greater than 95% purity of the test compound may not be sufficient for animal PK if the impurities are highly toxic components of chemical synthesis or purification of the compounds (reagents, catalysts, side products).

The total content of the test compound (purity) needs to be taken into account in calculating the total amount of the material required for animal dosing. Total content of the test compound may change due to sample storage and handling. For example, if the acid in the salt form of the compound is not strongly associated with the parent molecule, there is a possibility for the acid to be fully or partially released from the test material leading to increased formal purity of the material. If the compound is hygroscopic, it may absorb atmospheric moisture and reduce the percentage of the test compound in the material leading to a reduced formal purity of the test material. It is critical for medicinal chemists to clearly communicate to their ADME colleagues the best practices in compound storage and handling.

Residual solvent in the amorphous samples of the compound needs to be calculated to determine the purity of the compound. Proton or ^{13}C-NMR may provide qualitative and in some cases quantitative information about the residual solvent content.

Amount of Compound Required for Rat PK Studies The amount of compound required for a particular PK study can be calculated using the following equation:

$$CR = \frac{DL \times BW \times GS \times NA}{P} \text{Overage} \qquad (5.51)$$

where *CR* is the amount of the compound required for the study (mg), *DL* is a dose level (mg/kg), *BW* is the animal body weight (kg), *GS* is an animal group size (the number of animals on study), *NA* is the number of administrations (in case of a multidose experiments), *P* is the purity of the test material.

Typical animal weights can be found in Appendix 5.A.1. However, it may be a good practice to consult with ADME scientists on the actual weight of the animals for a particular study especially if less typical animal strains or younger or older animals are used.

Additional material may be needed to be reserved for the formulation work if the compound is new and a suitable formulation is not yet developed.

Some material needs to be reserved for preparation of the calibration standards and quality control samples for bioanalysis of the PK samples. Usually this amount is relatively low compared to the test material required for animal dosing. It is a good practice to reserve a small quantity (at least several milligrams) of the most pure material as an analytical standard for bioanalysis.

The number of administrations depends on the duration of the study and the frequency of daily administration. Early PK studies typically utilize a single once-daily (QD) administration of the compound. However, some efficacy or toxicology studies may require multiday and more than once-daily administration.

Overage of the compound is needed due to the inevitable loss of material during sample transfer, formulation preparation, and administration of the compound especially in the case of oral gavage of suspensions. Studies with smaller animals may require higher overage due to higher loss of material in the formulation vessels, syringes, etc. Studies with different animals may require different overages typically ranging from 1.1 to 1.5 with an average of about 1.2.

Example: The total amount of a 95% pure material for a single dose 1 mg/kg PK study with two rats on study can be estimated based on a 0.3-kg rat weight as

$$CR\,(\text{mg}) = \frac{1\ \text{mg/kg} \times 0.3\text{kg/rat} \times 2\ \text{rats} \times 1\ \text{administration}}{0.95}\,1.2 \qquad (5.52)$$

In this example, the minimum amount not including the material for the formulation development and bioanalysis is 0.75 mg.

Physical Form of Compounds The compound for animal dosing can be delivered to ADME scientists in several forms such as solids, solutions, or oils.

SOLIDS Solid materials are perhaps most frequently used as a source of animal dosing. Advantages of solid materials include ready transferability from one container to another (assuming they are not electrostatic) and the stability may potentially be higher than a solution form. It is common in the pharmaceutical industry to maintain the samples of small molecule drug candidates as a solid material in dry and oxygen-free conditions. The disadvantage of solid material for animal dosing is that more material is usually lost due to transfer between containers.

Careful consideration is required when several different batches of the compound are combined in order to create a single batch for animal dosing. The advantage of combining several batches is that the final batch has uniform purity and crystallinity if the batches are dissolved together and recrystallized. When supplying compound to the ADME scientist for animal dosing, avoid delivering several batches in separate vials. This forces either the scientist preparing the dose or the analyst to determine the percentage of parent compound out of a variety of salt forms and/or purities and can lead to mathematical or dosing errors.

SOLUTIONS Dissolving a newly synthesized compound in certain organic solvents (typically DMSO) to prepare a concentrated stock solution for initial testing is a common practice in the pharmaceutical industry. The advantage of using a solubilized form of the compound is that it is easy to transfer the solution from container to container (e.g., from a master 96-well plate to secondary plates) with minimal loss.

This process can be highly automated to increase efficiency and human error. The disadvantage of using a solution of the compound is that different compounds may require individualized selection of the best solvents for solubilization, which is difficult to achieve in the modern industrialized pharmaceutical setting. Incomplete solubility of the compounds in standard solvents (e.g., DMSO or acetonitrile) may lead to erroneous initial concentrations of the stock solutions. Even if the compound is initially fully soluble in the stock solution, it may absorb atmospheric moisture or fall out of solution.

Incomplete solubility of the compound in the solution or its falling out of solution upon storage may cause inconsistency of the PK data. A potential solution to incomplete solubility of the compound may be to spin down the stock solution and use the supernatant as a source for formulation work and as the stock solution for preparing calibration curves in bioanalysis.

A compound may not be completely chemically stable in a solvent. Although frequently used as a solvent, DMSO may chemically react with certain compounds (e.g., thiol- or isothiocyanate-containing molecules).

Another potential disadvantage of using solutions as a source of animal testing is that the formulation of the compound will contain the solvent that may not be acceptable or preferred as a component of the formulation vehicle.

OILS Some compounds may exist in an oil form due to a low melting point (lower than the ambient temperature) or due to the presence of some residual solvents used for the synthesis or purification. Transferring and weighing oily compounds may be a challenging task for ADME scientists especially if the oils are very viscous. Another problem is that the oily compounds may contain a significant and/or not well-defined amount of the residual solvents. Thus, it is difficult to calculate the purity of the compound and the actual concentration in the dosing solution.

5.6.2.2 Formulations A very brief overview of formulation development for animal dosing, some examples of the excipients and formulation recipes, and practical suggestions for formulating discovery compounds are presented. The area of drug formulations is large and more information can be found in the following publications [38–46]. Additionally, medicinal chemists should consult with their pharmaceutical science colleagues on the best approaches in formulation development.

Developing a suitable formulation of a compound for animal dosing is one of the major limitations for early PK studies because the current information about the solubility and chemical and physical stability of the compound may be very limited. Evaluation of potential formulations may require a fairly substantial amount of the test material and experimentation. Thus medicinal chemists should collect as much *in vitro* ADME, solubility, and chemical and metabolic stability for the compound series. Even incomplete information or "educated guesses" may be valuable for initial solubilization of the compound that can then be diluted in some standard formulation vehicle.

Additional techniques can be used to solubilize the compound. Prolonged and vigorous vortexing may be helpful if the dissolution kinetics is slow. Sonication and heating may help dissolve the compound, although there is a risk of thermal degradation of the compound. Any information or observations noted during the synthesis or purification of the compound may be very valuable for formulating the compound.

Described below are some typical formulation vehicles that can be used as a starting point when the information about the newly synthesized compound is limited.

Some strategies for selecting appropriate formulations are described in these publications [43, 44].

IV Formulations The formulations used for IV administration may vary significantly between labs and researchers. An ideal formulation for IV administration should contain only water and water-soluble components (salts, buffers). The aqueous solubility of some compounds can be increased by using an appropriate buffer to make the molecule more polar by ionizing its functional groups such as amines, heterocycles, acids, and others [43]. The acceptable pH range for IV formulations may vary from 2 to 12 [44]. The acceptable range of pH for the IV formulation may be expanded with the use of a lower dosing volume but must be balanced with the *in vivo* tolerability requirements [47].

The majority of newly synthesized drug candidates possess low aqueous solubility and may require the use of acceptable organic cosolvents such as dimethylacetamide (DMA), propylene glycol (PG), ethanol, or polyethylene glycol 400 (PEG400) (DMA), *N*-methyl-2-pyrrolidone (NMP; pharmasolve), dimethylsulfoxide (DMSO), and others [44] in order to achieve a desired concentration of the compound in the IV formulation. These solvents are fully miscible with water and aqueous solutions (e.g., PBS, phosphate buffered saline). Although the use of undiluted (straight) organic solvents as the only or the major excipient in the formulations for animal dosing is documented in the literature, there is a potential impact on the oral bioavailability, the rate and the mechanism of absorption, and other PK properties of the test compound. The use of the cosolvents may be combined with pH adjustment. A detailed evaluation of organic solvents in formulations is described in a series of publications by Yalkowski et al. [48–53].

The formulation of a compound for IV administration must be a true solution and may need to be filtered before administration to animals. Although visual inspection of the IV formulation for apparent absence of particles may be sufficient in many cases, there are examples when some insoluble microparticles may cause significantly erroneous PK profiles.

The requirements for single-dose studies are less stringent than for multiple-dose studies. In the case of a single-dose IV administration, a higher concentration of organic cosolvents or other excipients can be used.

PO Formulations Oral administration of animals can be done via oral gavage, oral administration of capsules, or adding the test compound to animal food or drinking water (dietary admixtures).

ORAL GAVAGE Oral gavage is the most typical form of administration in discovery settings. In this case, a solution or a suspension formulation can be used to administer the compound directly into the animal's stomach via a plastic or a metal gavage needle attached to a syringe. Usually, oral gavage is followed by some washing step to rinse the remaining formulation from the syringe and administered to the animals.

SOLUTION FORMULATIONS FOR ORAL GAVAGE A solution formulation of a compound typically provides the "best case scenario" for achieving the highest possible exposure and oral bioavailability after PO administration. Compounds in solution do not have to change from a solid form and are essentially ready for absorption after administration. If the compound is formulated using a relatively high amount of an organic cosolvent, there is a possibility for the compound to precipitate from the solution in the stomach after dosing. The formulation may become diluted with gastric fluid and the reduced concentration of the organic cosolvent may not be sufficient to maintain the compound in solution. The dilution phenomenon should be remembered when comparing the PK data after administration of poorly soluble compounds in solution and suspension formulations. If this occurs, the PK profile may show some animal-to-animal and study-to-study variability depending on the rate of oral gavage, the fed/fasted state of the animals, and other parameters.

An ideal PO formulation should contain only aqueous buffers, which may be achieved in certain cases by adjusting the pH of the formulation to ionize certain functional group of the compound similar to the IV formulation. The range of the acceptable pHs for oral formulations is typically broader: from 2 to 10 [44].

If pH adjustment is not sufficient to achieve a target concentration of the compound in the PO formulation, certain water-miscible cosolvents may help solubilize the compound at a higher concentration in PO formulations. Some of the water-miscible organics that can be used are polyethylene glycol 400, ethanol, propylene glycol, and glycerin along with many water-soluble nonionic surfactants [44].

An alternative strategy for PO formulations of highly water-insoluble compounds may be to use nonwater-miscible organic media such as peanut oil, corn oil, and others [44].

In addition to using organic cosolvents, an oral solution may be developed using some pharmaceutically acceptable surfactants such as Cremophor EL, polysorbate 80 (Tween 80), and many others [44]. Although surfactants are widely used even for human formulations, it is important to consider that some of the surfactants (e.g., Cremophor EL) may serve as the inhibitor of the intestinal P-gp efflux pumps [54] and increase oral bioavailability of some drugs like saquinavir in a dose-dependent manner [55].

SUSPENSION FORMULATIONS FOR ORAL GAVAGE Suspension formulations are widely used for oral administration of newly synthesized compounds in discovery settings to conduct PK, efficacy, or toxicology studies.

Suspension formulations have several advantages over solution formulations for oral dosing:

- Multiple standard or well-established recipes are available in the literature.
- The compound is less likely to degrade chemically in a suspension formulation because only the surface of the solid material is in contact with the solution.

- A suspension formulation may provide more realistic assessment of oral bioavailability that may be easier to translate to a tablet formulation.
- In toxicology studies, suspension formulations allow avoidance of organic cosolvents, surfactants, or other excipients, which may exhibit toxicity by themselves or exacerbate the toxicity of the test compound causing difficult interpretation of toxicology results.

At the same time, suspension formulations may have some disadvantages compared to solution formulations for oral gavage:

- Their PK properties may strongly depend on the particle size and size distribution, which may be difficult to reproduce in discovery settings (especially for early stage projects when the amount of the material is limited).
- Their PK properties may strongly depend on the crystalline or amorphous form of the material and on a polymorphic composition, which may be challenging to reproduce for discovery compounds.
- The loss of material in the preparation of a suspension formulation may be much higher compared to the solution formulation.
- It may be more challenging to maintain homogeneity of a suspension formulation prior to in-life administration. Some suspensions may tend to sediment on the bottom or the edges of the formulation vessel, which may lead to inconsistent filling of the gavage syringe, and as a result, an inconsistent dosing of the animals.
- Reproducible administration of suspension formulations may be more challenging even for highly trained animal technicians, which may lead to higher variability of PK data. Special attention is required to wash the gavage syringe.
- Smaller animals such as mice may require a very fine suspension formulation due to the small gauge of the gavage needle. The needle may clog leading to inconsistent dosing of animals.

ADMINISTRATION OF CAPSULES Small-sized capsules can be used to administer compound to larger animals such as dogs or monkeys and even rats although this technique is not frequently used in discovery studies.

DIETARY ADMIXTURES Adding compound to animal food or drinking water may be a reasonable formulation option for long-term efficacy studies. The advantage of this formulation is in minimal animal handling (essentially, the compound is self-administered), which reduces animal stress and the risk of dosing error compared to oral gavage. However, this type of formulation may provide variable PK profiles in animals.

Other Formulations The use of formulations other than IV and PO for PK studies in discovery settings is less common. Less common PK studies typically aim to provide data to support animal efficacy and toxicology studies and occasionally FIH dose projection.

5.6.2.3 Animal Species Used for PK Studies The selection of an animal species for a discovery PK study may depend on the stage of the project and the purpose of the PK study. If the study is conducted to compare a new compound with a known benchmark compound, then the same species and ideally the same strain should be used for PK assessment. If the PK study is conducted in support of efficacy studies, the species and strain selection may be driven by the type of animals used for efficacy measurement [33]. For the preparation of safety studies, the toxicology species selection is likely to drive the decision. Unfortunately, there is no single species that can be used for all the above and additional purposes.

Described below are the animal species and strains most frequently used for PK discovery studies. These include mice, rats, dogs, and monkeys, and with lesser frequency guinea pigs, hamsters, and rabbits. Since animals have been used in pharmaceutical development for decades, a significant amount of literature exists describing a broad spectrum of applications of animals for discovery and development purposes [3, 56–58].

Gender Male animal species are used much more frequently than female species in discovery studies except for the studies in preparation for reproductive toxicology assessment. In this case, female rats and rabbits are generally the rodent and nonrodent species for embryo–fetal development studies. It is important to evaluate PK properties of new drug candidates in both males and females due to some obvious difference in their hormonal status as well as less appreciated differences in brain and neurochemical processes, which may be critical for CNS targeting drugs [59].

There are certain drug-metabolizing enzymes that are gender-specific. For example, the carbonyl reductase is expressed only in male rats. This enzyme reduces the carbonyl group of acetohexamide, an oral antidiabetic drug [60].

It is a good scientific practice to match the gender of the animal species used for PK assessment and respective efficacy studies especially if a particular gender is more prone to developing a certain disease. Since female nonobese diabetic (NOD) mice have higher propensity of spontaneously developing diabetes [61], it is more rational to evaluate drug candidates for the treatment of diabetes in this gender.

Animal Age The difference in the age of the animals may lead to a noticeable difference in PK parameters of the compounds. Some PK parameters of ibuprofen in older Fischer rats were different than in young adults due to decreases in albumin concentration, the number of albumin-binding sites and reduction in metabolic activity in aged animals [62].

Genetically Modified Animals Although some genetically modified rat models are presently available, the mouse is the most widely used genetically modified animal model for research in integrative biology, toxicology, and pharmacokinetics [63].

A significant number of genetically modified mice (GeMMs) have been developed since the introduction of the techniques in the 1980s and their use in PK studies is well documented in the literature [64, 65]. Some of the mouse models allow for the evaluation of the ADME properties. Transporter null mice may provide information about role of transporters in drug PK [66]. The chimeric mice with humanized liver can be used for the advanced prediction of human pharmacokinetics and toxicity [67–70]. In spite of their advantages, there are limitations of genetically modified mouse models [63].

Rats Rats are frequently used for discovery PK and other studies because of the significant historical data set that can be used to compare a newly synthesized compound with its benchmark compounds. There are three main classes of rats used in research—outbred stocks (e.g., Sprague-Dawley [SD], Wistar), inbred strains (e.g., Fischer), and mutants (including transgenic stocks) [71]. The outbred stock animals contain the maximum amount of genetic differences [72], while the inbred animals are more genetically homogeneous [73]. Selecting the most appropriate rat strain may depend on the stage of the project and the purpose of the PK study. For early stage projects, some standard rat strains are more practical because they are commercially available on a regular basis in cannulated and noncannulated form, less expensive, and have a significant amount of historical reference data for other compounds. For some later stage projects, there may be a need to switch to a different rat strain to match with the strain used for efficacy or biomarker studies or to prepare PK data for toxicology evaluations. There is no "ideal" rat strain that fits all the needs of pharmaceutical discovery. The choice of rat can be complicated, especially when over 200 different strains of rat are known to exist [71].

The variation of the ADME-related properties between the different strains of rats is well documented in the literature. They need to be taken into account when selecting a particular rat strain for specific PK experiments. For example, the activity of aldehyde oxidase may vary between SD and Wistar rats as well as the different SD and Wistar substrains [74, 75]. These differences lead to a marked strain differences in the *in vivo* metabolism of methotrexate [74]. The difference in the activation of brain zones in different rat strains may perhaps be important for selecting the most appropriate model for the drugs targeting CNS [76].

SPRAGUE-DAWLEY SD, an outbred rat strain (CRL strain SAS SD #400, HSD:Sprague Dawley SD), has been widely used historically in discovery settings. A large amount of well-documented information about SD rats exists in the literature. SD rats are a general multipurpose model most frequently implemented for safety and efficacy testing. SD rats tend to be heavier than WH rats of the same age and gain weight faster than WH rats. The typical age and weight of male SD rats used for PK studies is in the range of 10–13 weeks and 300–325 g, respectively.

WISTAR HAN Wistar Han (CRL:WI(Han) strain #273, HSD:RccHan:WIST) is an outbred multipurpose rat strain. The typical age and weight of male WH rats used for PK studies is in the range of 10–13 weeks and 300–325 g, respectively.

OTHER RAT STRAINS Lewis (CRL strain #004) rats are inbred. They are commonly used in efficacy studies, in particular in induced arthritis/inflammation animal models. Other commonly used rat strains are Fischer (inbred), Long-Evans (inbred or outbred), Lister-Hooded (outbred), Brown Norway (inbred), and spontaneously hypertensive rats (SHR) (inbred).

The differences between rat strains and substrains are important because laboratory animals are bred by different breeders. Despite having a similar name, these animals may have different genetic and physiological characterizations that can alter the ADME-related data. For example, Zucker Diabetic Fatty (ZDF) inbred rat (CRL strain #370) is a mutant version of Zucker rat and listed separately from Zucker obese rats (CRL strain #185) on the CRL website (www.criver.com).

Mice Mice are frequently used for early stage discovery PK studies aiming to support efficacy results as well as selection of doses and formulations during efficacy evaluation. There are three main classes of mice used in research—outbred stocks (e.g., Swiss-Webster, CF1, ICR (CD-1)), inbred strains (e.g., C57BL, DBA/2, C3H, and BALB/c), and mutants (including transgenic animals) [73]. Hybrids which consist of crossing two strains of mice are also available (B6C3F1). Transgenic and genetically modified models are also available. Choice of strain and type of mouse used for studies is dependent of study purpose and disease model being considered. Certain strains of mice may be more susceptible to a certain disease than others. More information about the mouse strains can be found on the websites of the common US vendors including Charles River Laboratories (www.criver.com), Harlan (www.harlan.com), Taconic (www.taconic.com), and Jackson Labs (www.jax.org).

The advantage of using mice for PK is their small weight ranging from 15 to 30 g, which allows for conducting studies with less amount of compound. Typically, several mice (frequently $N = 3$) are sacrificed after dosing at predetermined time points to collect blood or tissue samples for PK assessment.

The compound savings in mouse PK studies may become less significant if a mouse study protocol calls for collecting 10 or more time points per administration. In this case, the amount of the compound may become comparable to or even higher than a similar rat study (e.g., $N = 3$ rats per study).

There is a widespread perception that the clearance of the drugs in mice is higher than in rats [77, 78] and other species. The difference is attributed to the higher blood flow in the mouse compared to other species such as the clearance becomes very similar once normalized to a heartbeat rate as shown on Figure 5.27 [79]. There are examples of drugs whose clearance is very similar in rats and mice such as ciclesonide [80].

Dogs As a nonrodent species, dogs are often used in safety and/or pharmacology testing. Purposely bred, beagle dogs are often the breed of choice ([3], p. 567). Desirable features in the beagle are its medium size, moderate hair coat, and even temperament. The body weight of dogs is dependent on the gender and the age of the animals. An average weight of 15 kg can be safely used for calculation of the amount of the compound needed for dog studies.

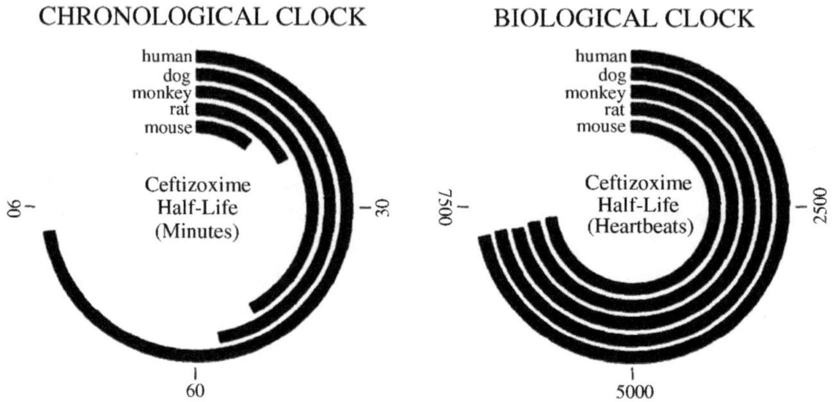

Figure 5.27 Perceived differences in the half-life of ceftizoxime in various mammals depend on the references system used to denote time: (a) half-life is reported in minutes, the smaller mammals eliminate 50% of the drug more rapidly than the larger species. (b) When half-lives are reported in heartbeats, all mammals eliminate 50% of the drug in the equivalent time. Adapted from Refs. [79, 81].

Dogs are a United States Department of Agriculture (USDA) regulated species and animal facilities using dogs are required to follow stringent requirements of the regulatory authorities [82]. The total number of dogs used for research purposes in the United States was about 72,000 in 2007, which was an increase from about 67,000 used in 2005 [83].

Dogs used for PK studies are often used for multiple studies following a washout period, unlike mice or rats that typically are used for a single study. Dogs along with cynomolgus monkeys are the most commonly used nonrodent species for toxicology studies. An estimated 140,000 dogs are used worldwide in research and testing every year primarily in the United States (~50%) and Japan [82].

Nonhuman Primates The use of nonhuman primates (NHP) in animal testing for new drug discovery and development has a long history but also associated with significant ethical, legal, and scientific challenges and controversy. Although there is a strong desire to replace NHPs in pharmaceutical animal testing, a significant and a rising number of primates are used in the United States (around 70,000 in 2007 compare to about 58,000 in 2005) [83].

Monkeys are used in discovery PK studies perhaps least frequently compared to rodents and dogs. This is because of ethical considerations as well as the cost and availability of the animals. In some cases, monkeys rather than dogs may be used for toxicology studies if, for example, monkeys show a metabolic profile more consistent with that in human. Although there is a widespread perception that monkeys may predict human PK better than rats or dogs [84, 86], there is no consensus regarding better translation of monkey PK data to human PK. Some recent analyses showed that a single animal species scaling to human may produce similarly acceptable results based on either rat, dog, or monkey data [25].

RHESUS AND CYNOMOLGUS MONKEY The rhesus and cynomolgus macaques are the species of choice for the studies in nonhuman primates [87, 88]. The studies in monkeys are usually conducted in preparation to toxicology studies in those species if the dog model is found less predictive of the human safety outcome.

CHIMPANZEES Although the studies in chimpanzee played a crucial role in the development of the vaccine for hepatitis B [89], the use of chimpanzees for pharmaceutical research causes much discussion in the scientific community [90–94].

Others Species Other animal species used for discovery PK are rabbits, mini-pigs, guinea pigs, and hamsters. Rabbit PK studies are usually conducted in preparation for a reproductive toxicology studies or in some specialized areas such as ophthalmic PK and efficacy.

Genetically Modified Animals Genetically modified animals, primarily mice, have become more and more commercially available. Certain genetically modified mice can provide valuable information about the route of elimination of compound and can be used for better prediction of human clearance. Humanized mice can be used for better prediction of human clearance. For example, the elimination of the glucuronides can be studied in the UGT1A1 × 28/ugt1–/– humanized mice [95]. Some information about genetically modified animals can be found at http://www.srtp.org.uk/srtga014.htm.

Animal Physiology in Comparison with Human Physiology Information about laboratory animal physiology and anatomy can be found in the literature [16, 96]. A summary of selected PK relevant physiological parameters of laboratory animals and humans can be found in Section 5.8 (Appendices).

5.6.2.4 Animal Dosing There are multiple publications describing most commonly acceptable animal dosing and sample techniques [3, 97].

Potential routes of administration of compounds to the body and potential routes of biological sample collection for PK evaluation are shown in Figure 5.28. Compounds can be injected into a vein or portal vein representing systemic or presystemic circulation, respectively. Alternatively, compound can be administered extravascularly (EV), that is, external to the circulation. The most frequently used EV routes of administration are oral (PO), intraperitoneal (IP), subcutaneous (under the skin), and intramuscular administrations. There are several routes of administration of a compound directly into different sections of the digestive tract such as intraduodenal (ID, into the duodenum of the small intestine) or intragastric (IG, into the stomach).

Additionally, compound can be introduced into the body in a very short period of time via a so-called bolus administration or it can be infused into the body via an infusion mechanism typically by using infusion pumps. Depending on the purpose of a PK study, it may require using different combinations of routes of administration and routes for sample collection.

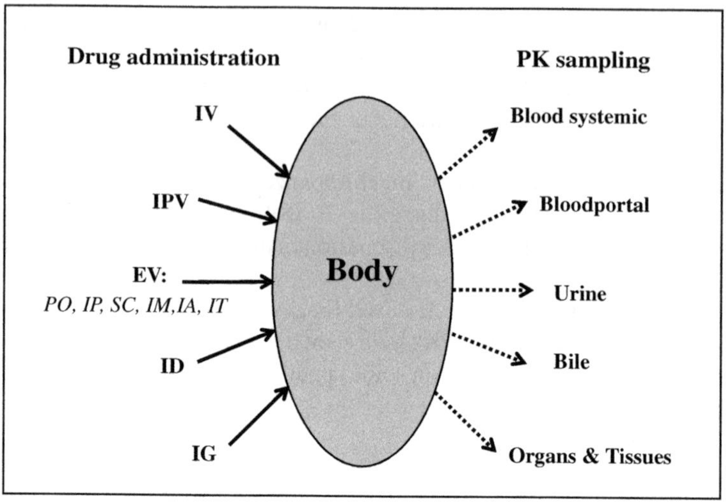

Figure 5.28 Potential routes of administration of the compounds and the sampling routes.

If a PK study is conducted to support an efficacy study in an experimental animal model, then the route of administration is dictated by the efficacy study design. If a PK study is conducted in preparation to a toxicology study, then the route of administration has to be the same as the intended route of administration in FIH study.

The most frequently used methods of compound administration are described below. Intravenous (IV) and oral (PO) routes of administration by far are the most frequently used in discovery settings.

Single-Dose Bolus Administration

SINGLE-DOSE INTRAVENOUS ADMINISTRATION Intravenous administration allows for the direct presentation of compound to the body with no loss of material. The disadvantage of IV administration is that it is invasive and may be more stressful for animals. IV administration is usually used to determine some primary PK parameters of the compound such as AUC, total clearance, the volumes of distribution, terminal half-life, and others. The plasma AUC of the compound is frequently used as a reference (the highest possible) value to determine bioavailability of the compound after oral or other routes of administration.

The major limitation associated with IV administration is that the maximum dose volume typically should not exceed 5 mL/kg. Due to this limitation, the maximum IV dose that can be administered to animals depends on the compound solubility in suitable vehicles. For example, if the solubility of the compound in a selected formulation is 2 mg/mL, the maximum dose that can be achieved in a PK study is going to be 10 mg/kg.

It is critical for an IV study to select the most optimal time points for sample collection, especially early time points, for compounds with a fast distribution phase.

SINGLE-DOSE ORAL ADMINISTRATION Single oral dose (usually via oral gavage) introduces the compound directly into the animal's stomach using a gavage needle attached to a syringe. This administration is usually used to evaluate oral bioavailability of newly synthesized compounds or compare different formulations of the same compound.

The dose volume for oral gavage is as large as 20 mL/kg, and the selection of the formulation suitable for dosing is much wider than for IV administration. Both solution and suspension formulations can be used for PO dosing. It is very important to evaluate the potential effect of the components of the formulation on the physiology of the intestine in order to correctly estimate PK parameters.

INTRAPERITONEAL ADMINISTRATION An IP administration may provide an efficient delivery for some compounds with low oral bioavailability. Most frequently, PK studies with IP dosing are conducted in support of efficacy studies with the same route of administration. The dose volume for IP administration usually should not exceed 20 mL/kg in the mouse and 10 mL/kg in the rat [97].

SC AND IM ADMINISTRATION Subcutaneous (under the skin) or intramuscular (into the muscles) routes of administration are less frequently used in discovery settings and primarily conducted to support efficacy studies with the same route of administration.

IM administration is limited by the dose volume that can be delivered (1 mL/kg [3]), the local irritation at the injection site, and is dependent on the excipients in the formulation. Care should be taken with larger volumes and if necessary should be administered in divided doses.

INTRATHECAL ADMINISTRATION A lumbar intrathecal (IT) injection is a method to deliver compound into the cerebrospinal fluid (CSF), which may be a useful route of administration for CNS-active compounds.

INTRA-ARTICULAR ADMINISTRATION The intra-articular (IA) route of administration is a direct injection of compound into a joint. This type of dosing is used for some rheumatoid arthritis studies.

OTHERS ROUTES OF ADMINISTRATION There are some less frequently used routes of administration for PK studies such as hepatic-portal vein (HPV or IPV), oral gastric, and intraduodenal dosing. Those routes of administration are usually used to troubleshoot low oral bioavailability of the compounds.

IG ADMINISTRATION Intragastric catheterization offers the advantage of an oral dose without the stress and handling involved with conventional PO administration via gavage needle or feeding tube.

HEPATIC-PORTAL VEIN ADMINISTRATION Hepatic-portal vein, sometimes called IPV (intraportal vein) dosing is similar to IV dosing. The difference is that compound is delivered directly to the liver by introduction into the portal vein as opposed to the systemic circulation. Typically, the hepatic-portal vein of the animal has to be cannulated in order to conduct this type of dosing.

PK studies with HPV administration may provide valuable information about first-pass metabolism of the compound and may be used as a diagnostic tool to determine if low oral bioavailability is driven by low permeability or fast metabolism.

The choice of formulation and maximum dose volume is similar between HPV and IV administration.

INTRADUODENAL ADMINISTRATION A direct intraduodenal administration of compound may help estimate first-pass metabolism across the gastrointestinal mucosa [98].

Continuous Administration The most commonly used continuous administration of a compound is IV infusion.

SINGLE-DOSE IV INFUSION Single-dose IV infusion of a compound is typically done via an infusion pump attached to a cannula inserted into a jugular vein. This type of dosing allows for achieving a steady-state concentration of compound in both the systemic circulation and the organs into which the compound distributes. IV infusion can provide a more accurate estimation of clearance of compounds with low solubility. Analysis of compound in the organs and tissues collected shortly after the termination of the IV infusion provides the steady-state distribution of the compound in those organs. This information may be valuable for better understanding of PK/PD and exposure–toxicity relationships.

Escalated Single-Dose Administrations PK studies with escalating dose are typically conducted in preparation for animal efficacy or safety studies.

The purpose of pre-efficacy escalating dose studies is usually to identify a dose range that provides exposures that are sufficient for achieving target *in vivo* concentrations that are close to or above an expected efficacious compound concentration. Ideally the dose escalation study should be performed in the same animal strain with the same health status as will be used in the efficacy study. Certain diseases may impact the physiology of the animals and, as a result, the PK properties of the compound.

The purpose of pretoxicology dose escalation studies is to determine the maximum dose for subsequent toxicology studies and thus referred to as dose-range finding (DRF) studies. The maximum dose in DRF studies may be based upon either toxicology observations at higher doses or the leveling of the exposures at higher administered doses. Most frequently, the DRF studies are conducted in rodents (usually rats) and nonrodent species (usually dogs and less frequently monkeys) to match the species that are expected to be used in the subsequent toxicology studies.

Multiple Administrations via Different Routes (Crossover) The crossover studies are conducted by the PO administration of a compound followed by an IV administration after a washout period (typically 24 h but may be longer for the compounds with a long terminal half-life). In order to ensure that the compound is cleared from the body between the first and the second administration, the PO dose is usually initially administered. This is because the PO dose typically generates lower exposures due to less than 100% oral bioavailability compared to the IV administration.

The purpose of the crossover study design is to decrease the impact of animal-to-animal variability on PK data by using each animal as its own control between the two routes of administration. An additional benefit of the crossover design is that it reduces the number of animals especially larger animals that are typically nonterminal (dogs, monkeys, etc.).

Multiple Administrations via the Same Route PK studies with multiple doses administered sequentially with frequencies such as daily (QD or SID), twice daily (BID), three times a day (TID), four times a day (QID), or with some other dosing regimen, aim to achieve a steady-state concentration to mimic exposure to compound in chronic efficacy or toxicology studies. The frequency and duration of the administration required to achieve steady state is described in Section 5.4.4.

Cassette Versus Singleton Dosing If an animal PK model is used in compound screening, throughput may become a bottleneck in the discovery project. A potential solution to this problem is to combine several compounds in a cassette and dose them together. The biggest challenge of the cassette PK studies is data interpretation due to a potential drug–drug interaction. To mitigate the risk of DDI, the dose levels of individual compounds in the cassette are reduced to compare typical singleton studies. The number of individual compounds in a cassette does not usually exceed 10 with 4 or 5 being more reasonable from a practical and a scientific standpoint. This may present analytical challenges for compounds with poor mass spectrometer source ionization properties. Additionally, compounds with the same exact mass (isobaric) should not be used in the cassette studies because their quantitation in biological samples may be challenging unless these compounds can be separated by using chromatography or some capabilities of triple-quadrupole mass spectroscopy (Section 5.6.2.7).

5.6.2.5 Sampling Collecting biological samples from the animal after administration of a compound is a critical step in evaluation of PK parameters of the compound. Figure 5.28 shows some typical routes of sample collection.

The most important parameters of the sample collection step of a PK study are the type of collected biological matrix, collection frequency, sample handling, and storage.

Biological Matrices Collected for PK Purposes Typical biological samples collected in a PK experiment are blood (or derived plasma or serum), urine, bile, feces, and tissues. Each of these matrices has its unique properties and has to be understood and considered during sample collection and storage.

There are some additional biological matrices (cerebrospinal fluid and synovial fluid) that can be collected for more specialized purposes.

BLOOD Blood can be collected from multiple points representing a systemic circulation or in certain cases from the hepatic-portal vein representing presystemic circulation. The blood samples collected from the systemic circulation represent a central PK compartment. This route of sampling is by far the most frequently used for the majority of PK studies. Blood sampling from the portal vein is typically used to evaluate the level of first-pass metabolism and the fraction absorbed after PO administration.

COLLECTING BLOOD FROM RATS Rats can be bled manually from jugular, saphenous, submandibular, and tail veins. These sampling procedures may or may not require using anesthesia depending upon the comfort and competence of the ADME scientist. Blood samples can be collected via retro-orbital (RO) bleeding but requires anesthesia.

Blood can be collected from rats either manually or via a cannula (catheter) implanted into a certain vessel usually jugular or carotid. Cannulation of rats facilitates blood sample collection and provides less stress on the animals. Cannulation requires a surgical modification of the animal, which may not be successful in 100% of the cases. The cannula may not be patent (stay intact) over a prolonged period of time and rats should be used for PK studies within 2 weeks of cannulation.

Manual bleeding of rats is typically used in toxicology studies especially in longer term studies for which the cannulas most likely will not remain patent. Another reason for using manual blood collection in toxicology studies is a desire to minimally impact the physiology of the animals due to surgical intervention.

The total blood volume that can be collected from rats within 2 weeks is limited to approximately 1% of the total body weight. Approximately 3 mL of blood can be collected from a 300 g rat. Different animal use protocols (AUP) may permit slightly different maximum allowed blood volumes. The terminal blood volume is usually collected via cardiac puncture and provides a larger sample (~2 mL) suitable for additional analyses (e.g., safety measures such as hematology and clinical pathology as well as biomarker or metabolite ID work).

COLLECTING BLOOD FROM MICE Most frequently each individual mouse provides a single blood sample collected by cardiac puncture or from the posterior vena cava upon termination of an animal. Approximately 0.25–1 mL of blood is collected, depending on the body weight of the animal.

There are some procedures for collecting more than one sample from an individual mouse. Blood samples can be collected via tail or saphenous veins, or by submandibular or retro-orbital bleeding. Multiple sample collection (serial bleeding) from mice may provide serial PK data instead of "population" (composite) PK and PD profiles similar to larger animals. Serial bleeding from mice can be done manually or via a cannula inserted in the jugular vein or carotid artery similar to cannulated rats. Cannulation of mice is much less common than cannulation of larger animals such as rats. This technique requires more specialized surgical skills and improper placement of the catheter may lead to frequent failure of the surgery and less catheter patency.

Manual mouse bleeding via jugular vein or carotid artery does not require the use of anesthesia as opposed to retro-orbital bleeding.

The maximum blood volume that is allowed for the collection from each mouse is typically limited to ~1% of the total body weight for a 2 week period but may be as large as ~1.8% for certain AUPs. Approximately 0.3 mL of blood can be collected from a 30 g mouse.

If multiple (serial) blood samples are collected from each mouse, the size of each sample is much smaller than the size of samples collected from, for example, rats. The quantitation of drug in mouse samples may require using more sensitive bioanalytical methods.

COLLECTING BLOOD FROM DOGS Dogs are usually bled manually from the cephalic or jugular vein. For frequent initial blood collections, a catheter can be placed in the cephalic vein of each dog prior to dosing.

Due to the larger size of dogs (~10–15 kg for an adult male dog), the maximum total blood volume that can be collected from each animal does not usually represent a hurdle for a PK study.

COLLECTING BLOOD FROM MONKEYS Monkeys are usually bled manually from femoral, cephalic, or saphenous veins [97]. This procedure does not require using anesthesia.

Similar to the dog, the larger size of monkeys (~2 kg for young adults and up to ~10 kg for mature adults) allows a greater maximum total blood volume collected from each animal and does not usually represent a hurdle for a PK study.

PLASMA/SERUM Once the whole blood is collected from an animal, it can be centrifuged to deliver plasma (typically with ~40–50% yield). The blood samples have to be collected in tubes containing an anticoagulant to prevent the blood from rapid clotting. Alternatively, the blood can be collected without using an anticoagulant so the blood coagulates with time (usually within ~30 min) to produce the serum. The primary difference between the composition of the plasma and the serum is that the serum lacks the blood-clotting proteins.

The maximum volume of plasma that can be collected from the laboratory animal is determined by the volume of the blood allowed for the collection.

URINE Urine is collected for the evaluation of renal clearance by quantitation of the parent compounds and their metabolites. The urine is usually collected in time intervals using cages equipped with devices for separation of the urine from the feces. The urine samples are usually collected in time intervals unlike the blood samples collected at certain time points. The urine volume collected at different time intervals may significantly vary in volume because the animals urinate voluntarily. It is critical then to measure and record the urine volume collected per time interval. It is also important to record the actual weight of each individual animal in order to calculate urinary recovery and renal clearance. The accuracy of the urine collection is typically lower than the accuracy of the blood collection so the calculated urine clearance may be subject to higher variability.

BILE Bile can be collected for measuring biliary clearance of compound as well for evaluation of Phase II metabolism, especially glucuronide formation and excretion.

PK experiments in bile-duct cannulated rats are usually conducted with quadruple cannulated animals: the jugular vein and carotid artery for IV dose administration and sample collection as well as the bile duct and duodenum for bile collection and bile salt infusion. Typically a solution of bile salts or the natural bile from additional animals should be returned back to the study rats to minimize the potential impact of bile removal on rat physiology.

As with urine collection, bile is collected in time intervals. The bile volumes collected in each interval have to be measured and recorded as does the weight of each animal used for the BDC PK experiment.

FECES Feces may provide some information about the amount of compound not absorbed after PO administration. Some compounds excreted in the bile may be measured in the feces. A potential degradation of compound in the feces due to digestion by intestinal microflora needs to be taken into consideration when planning and interpreting data from the PK experiment.

The collection of the feces is not used very frequently in discovery PK experiments.

ORGANS AND TISSUES The collection of organs and tissues may provide valuable information about compound distribution and organ-specific metabolism. Measuring the actual concentration of the compound in a target organ may be critical for establishing translatable PK/PD relationships.

The collection of organs and tissues is typically done upon termination of the experimental animals at a predetermined time point. Nonterminal sample collection procedures can be used in larger animals (dogs, monkeys, or chimpanzees). In this case, a needle biopsy from the liver can be performed on anesthetized animals although the number of nonterminal sampling is usually limited to 1–2 samples.

The collection of highly perfused organs may require removal of the blood in those organs prior to or immediately after the termination of the animals to differentiate compound located in the organ or blood. If the organs are not perfused upon collection, it is necessary to correct the concentrations of the test compound in the organ homogenate for the amount of the blood in the organ. The values for the blood content in different rat organs are summarized in Appendix 5.A.4. This data should be used with caution since the results were obtained using different techniques from various labs and are not always consistent.

Organs that are typically collected from experimental animals are liver, kidneys, brain, heart, lungs, adrenal glands, testes, and muscles.

Duration and Frequency of PK Sampling The duration and frequency of sample collection may have a significant impact on the quality of the PK data and in certain cases may lead to erroneous or misleading PK data. The frequency of sampling typically represents a compromise between a desire to obtain a more complete PK profile with denser sampling and some practical and regulatory considerations. The latter may be the speed that *in vivo* scientists can collect the first blood sample after IV administration, the availability of animal technicians to collect samples after work hours, the total blood volume that can be collected, etc.

A well-executed PK study will continue to collect samples until 4–5 half-lives of a drug's disposition is complete. This is based on the premise that by 4–5 half-lives, more than 95% of the drug has been eliminated from the body (Table 5.5) and the disposition of the drug is *almost* complete. The use of the word "*almost*" is deliberate because all drugs eventually follow an exponential decline and, as such, concentrations approach zero but never attain it. Drug elimination from the body does not refer to all drug-based entities (metabolites, impurities, etc.) in the body, but to the existence of the drug as a distinct chemical entity only.

It is relatively easy to design a PK study if the disposition of the drug is known, but how does one design a PK study for a new chemical entity that has never been dosed before? In a discovery setting, particularly at a lead development stage, costs and adherence to aggressive timelines and schedules should be adapted to experimental study designs.

FREQUENCY OF PK SAMPLING

IV Bolus Administration The frequency of blood sampling after IV administration has to be sufficient to capture the initial phase of the PK profile especially for compounds with very rapid distribution. In this case, an insufficient frequent sampling may lead to an underestimation of the AUC and initial systemic concentration and cause an overestimated clearance and volume of distribution, respectively.

An insufficient frequent sampling at the terminal elimination phase of the PK profile may provide fairly inaccurate terminal half-life ($t_{1/2}$) of the compound.

Extravascular Bolus Administration The most characteristic PK parameters of a compound after an extra-vascular administration (e.g., PO, IP, SC, or IM) are the C_{max}/T_{max} and the terminal $t_{1/2}$. Insufficient blood sampling around the maximum concentration on the PK curve may lead to inaccurate values for C_{max} and T_{max}. Similarly to IV administration, inadequate frequent sampling at the terminal phase of the PK profile may provide inaccurate values of terminal half-life.

IV Infusion The duration of an IV infusion administration is driven by the time necessary to achieve a steady state of the compound concentration in the blood. For practical purposes, the duration of IV infusion can be estimated as approximately seven terminal half-lives of the compound after IV bolus administration. It is common to collect at least several blood samples during the infusion especially close to the end of the infusion to ensure that at least the last two blood concentrations are close in value. After the termination of the infusion, blood samples can be collected for the period of time and with the frequency similar to the IV bolus administration with the first sample collection being as close as practically possible to the infusion termination time.

Sample Handling and Storage Samples collected from a PK study must be handled appropriately so that the analytes of interest do not degrade during the storage process. Approaches to sample handling and storage may vary depending on the purpose of the

PK study, the type of the collected biological matrix, and the properties of the compound of interest (analyte) that need to be quantified.

BLOOD When collecting blood, hemolysis of the red blood cells should be prevented. Blood collected in tubes should be maintained on wet ice but not frozen until used for further processing.

Blood can be collected and stored in a liquid or dry form. If the total concentration of compound in the blood is a desired PK measure, the compound has to be released from the red blood cells to ensure complete recovery of the analyte. Mixing the blood samples with water is a common method for disrupting the RBC. It may be practical to sonicate the processed blood samples to reduce potential capturing of the analyte by the blood components.

As an alternative to using liquid blood, the blood sample can be placed on a filter paper to form a so-called dried blood spot (DBS) that can be used for subsequent drug bioanalysis [99] similar to clinical DBS analysis [100]. The extent and the rate of the partitioning of the drug to the cellular components of the blood, primarily red blood cells is critical [14].

PLASMA Once separated from red blood cells, the plasma can be frozen and stored at − 20 to − 80°C until processed for analysis. It is important to ensure that there is adequate anticoagulant in the blood collection tubes such that the plasma does not coagulate on storage.

URINE Urine should be collected on ice/dry ice and can be treated and stored similar to plasma.

BILE The handling of the bile samples is similar to urine samples.

FECES After the wet weight of the sample is recorded, a weighed amount of solvent (invariably water or methanol) should be added and the sample homogenized and stored at –20 or –80°C until further analysis.

ORGANS AND TISSUES Collecting different organs and tissues is usually conducted by experienced *in vivo* scientists and may require some additional skills and knowledge. The most common way of preserving tissues and organs is freezing in dry ice or liquid nitrogen.

5.6.2.6 Animal Handling Ethical and scientifically reasonable handling of experimental animals used for preclinical testing is more likely to lead to better quality animal data due to reduced animal stress. This should allow better prediction of human PK, which will reduce the risk of incorrect prediction of human exposures in initial human studies and harm to healthy volunteers in first-in-human studies. In effect, better care of laboratory animals is more likely to lead to better care of human beings.

IACUC It is mandatory in the United States, European Union, and some other countries and federations that animal study protocols (or animal use protocols) be reviewed and approved by the local animal use committee. The group consists of scientists and representatives of the community to ensure ethical treatment of animals used for PK and other animal studies. In the United States, the IACUC (Institutional Animal Care and Use Committee) is a self-regulating entity that, according to US federal law, must be established by institutions that use laboratory animals for research or instructional purposes to oversee and evaluate all aspects of the institution's animal care and use program. Some additional information about IACUC functions and procedures can be found at the American Association for Animal Laboratory Science (AALAS) at their website (www.aalas.org).

It is important for medicinal chemists and other scientists to realize that any new animal study design or changes to an existing study design have to be reviewed and approved by the IACUC before the new study protocol is allowed for execution.

In general, there are well-accepted principles known as the "3Rs" that should be applied to all studies in laboratory animals [101]:

- Refinement of the use of research animals to use less painful or the least invasive procedures whenever possible.
- Reduction of the numbers of animals used in each study to the absolute minimum necessary to obtain valid results.
- Replacement of animal experiments with nonanimal experiments such as mathematical models, computer simulations, and *in vitro* biological systems wherever appropriate.

Fed Versus Fasted Rats are fasted overnight prior to PO dosing and access to food provided at 4 h post dose. Access to water is usually *ad lib*. Animals should be fasted no longer than 24 h without justification.

The animals used for an IV study are usually not fasted before dosing. Animals are typically not fasted during any PK studies with multiday administration of compound.

The quality and quantity of animal feeding and the feeding time may impact the PK profile of certain compounds, especially compounds that are poorly soluble or are substrates of transporters or efflux pumps located in the intestinal mucosa. Food effects are well documented in the literature [102–109].

Dosing Volume The allowed and most commonly used dosing volumes for different routes of administration are described in Section 5.6.2.4.

Total Blood Volume The volume of the blood allowed for collection in different animal species is described in Section 5.6.2.5.

Anesthesia Some sample collection techniques may require using anesthesia because they may be distressful or painful to the animals. Avoiding animal pain is based not only on the ethical consideration for the study but also should be based on a scientific consideration due to a potential impact of the animal pain and stress on the

PK parameters of the study. Retro-orbital bleeding, penile vein dosing, and surgical implanting of catheters and osmotic pump require anesthesia.

The choice of an anesthetic for the study should be carefully evaluated based on the prior knowledge and experience with a particular anesthetic or based on some general principles of animal physiology [110, 111].

Certain types of anesthesia may not be compatible with frequent sample collection. A CO_2/O_2 anesthesia may cause animal dysfunction or even death if applied too frequently.

Animal Stress Animal dosing and sampling may be stressful for animals especially if some invasive procedures are used in the PK study (e.g., manual bleeding). Since stress may modulate the animal's physiology and subsequently PK parameters of a studied compound, it is ethical as well as scientifically rational to minimize animal stress. Methods to reduce stress include using anesthesia when possible, reducing sample frequency, reducing sample size via microsampling (*Microsampling* section), using cannulated animals (*Cannulated Versus Noncannulated Animals* section), and using automated instead of manual blood collection (*Automated and Manual Bleeding* section).

Cannulated Versus Noncannulated Animals The use of cannulated animals may ease the sample collection process, reduce the chances of human error (e.g., missing the vein for dosing or bleeding), and reduce the stress on the animals used for a PK study.

Many animal species and strains are commercially available in a single or a multiple cannulated form. There are different sites that can be used for cannulation such as jugular, carotid, and portal vein. The catheters can be installed to access the stomach or the duodenal section of the small intestine.

The disadvantage of the cannulated animals is commercial availability and when available are more expensive than noncannulated animals. The patency of the cannula may be limited to a fairly short period of time (e.g., couple of weeks in rats).

Automated and Manual Bleeding Automated collection of blood samples from cannulated rats and mice has become possible due to the relatively recent development of new automated blood sampling (ABS [112]) instrumentation such as Culex by BASi (www.basinc.com/products/culex) [113] and AccuSampler by DiLab (www.dilab.com). Each system has its own advantages and disadvantages so the selection of the most appropriate ABS may depend on the specific needs of the studies, familiarity, and prior experience with a particular system, etc.

The use of ABS can greatly reduce the stress involved with serial sampling. Stress can possibly alter the PK resulting in inconsistent and even faulty PK and PK/PD data. ABS greatly reduces the human workload allowing for fewer employees to generate a high-quality and high-throughput PK data. By automating the blood-drawing time course, technicians are not required to be in the vivarium at extreme hours of the night.

Microsampling Collecting less than conventional size blood samples from mice may present the benefit of generating serial PK profiles in each individual animal. There are some examples of serial bleeding from mice described in the literature [114–120].

5.6.2.7 Bioanalysis Some basic concepts of bioanalysis of PK samples using liquid chromatography and mass spectrometry are described. LC/MS is undoubtedly the most frequently used method of quantitation of drugs, their metabolites, and biomarkers in the animal PK samples. A more detailed description of bioanalytical techniques and instrumentation can be found in the literature [121–135].

Basic Concepts of LC–MS/MS Quantitation LC–MS/MS refers to a quantitation method combining liquid chromatography with tandem mass spectroscopy (MS/MS). A typical triple–quadrupole instrument allows for the selection of an ion ("parent" ion) on the first quadrupole followed by fragmentation in a collision cell (second quadrupole), after which the most abundant fragments ("daughter" ions) can be selected using the third quadrupole. Such a double selection of the parent and daughter ions is called single reaction monitoring (SRM) or multiple reaction monitoring (MRM). This monitoring provides LC–MS/MS quantitation as very specific and sensitive and allows for measuring nanomolar and picomolar concentrations of the analytes in very complex biological matrices. Several SRM modes can be combined for simultaneous quantitation of multiple analytes in a multiple reaction monitoring method. LC–MS/MS methodology does not provide high-accuracy or high-precision quantitation.

Calibration Curves, Sensitivity, and Dynamic Range Since the ionization of different compounds may depend on their structure, calibration standards are typically prepared and analyzed in the same or similar biological matrix that is used for PK sample collection. Calibration standards typically cover a broad range of concentrations expected in the PK study samples. A separate calibration curve for each analyte is typically developed based on the best fit of the nominal standard concentrations and the actual MRM signal measured for each standard. Acceptance or rejection of individual calibration standards for each calibration curve is based on the comparison of the fitted (expected) signal intensity and the actual (observed) signal. This comparison characterizes the accuracy of the calibration standards. If multiple calibration standards are prepared and analyzed at the same nominal concentration, the dispersion of their values represents the precision of the method.

Although some LC–MS/MS methods may occasionally have relatively high accuracy and precision, the most frequently used acceptance criteria even for a well-established validated method may be within 15% for all the standards and 20% for the lowest concentration sample representing the lowest level of quantitation (LLOQ) [136]. The highest calibration standard that meets the acceptance criteria is called the upper limit of quantitation (ULOQ).

The ratio of the ULOQ to LLOQ represents the range of concentrations that can be quantified using the calibration curve.

The concentration of the analyte in the study sample is calculated based on comparison of the experimentally measured intensity of the signal in those samples with the calibration curve. If the calculated concentration is lower than the LLOQ, it is considered undetermined and labeled as below the quantitation limit (BQL or BLQ).

If the calculated concentration is higher than the ULOQ, it is considered undetermined and labeled as above the quantitation limit (AQL or ALQ).

If the concentration of the analyte in the study sample is BQL, some additional method development may be necessary to increase the sensitivity of the bioanalysis.

If the concentration of the analyte in the study sample is AQL, the samples may need to be diluted and reanalyzed to provide measurable concentrations of the analyte. This is frequently the case in quantitation of TK samples after administration of a high dose of compound in toxicology studies.

Sample Preparation Only charged analytes can be measured by LC–MS/MS methodology. Some component of the biological matrix may reduce the ability of the analytes to become ionized and have to be removed from the biological sample prior to quantitation. This process is called sample preparation.

There are three most commonly used sample preparation techniques used for PK sample analysis: (a) protein precipitation; (b) solid phase extraction (SPE, either off-line or on-line); and liquid–liquid extraction (LLE) [137]. All three methods allow for quantitation of the total (not free) drug and can be automated to use in a high-throughput manner.

PROTEIN PRECIPITATION Protein precipitation is perhaps the most frequently used method of sample preparation in discovery settings. The concept of the PPX is to denature and remove matrix components (primarily such abundant proteins as albumin) by mixing plasma samples with quenching agents, water-miscible chemicals in which plasma proteins are less soluble than analyte.

Acetonitrile is by far the most commonly used quenching agent in discovery bioanalysis. Other frequently used quenching agents are methanol and ethanol, although there is a potential risk of transesterification for ester-containing prodrugs. It is critical to ensure that the analyte of interest is soluble and stable in the final aqueous-organic mixture formed after protein precipitation by organic-quenching agents. Incomplete solubility of analytes in the aqueous-organic mixture may be a source of low recovery of the samples containing high concentrations of the compounds and their metabolites. Special attention is required for protein precipitation for toxicokinetics sample processing due to higher concentrations of analytes.

Acid-driven protein precipitation (e.g., trichloroacetic acid [TCA]) is a potential alternative to precipitation by organic solvents in the case of very polar analytes stable in acidic conditions.

SOLID PHASE EXTRACTION The SPE sample cleanup is based on the retention of the analyte on a very short reversed-phase chromatographic column. Diluted or quenched biological samples are typically loaded on the SPE device followed by a wash step removing the matrix components. The analyte is eluted with stronger chromatographic solvents. The SPE may require more method development but typically provides cleaner samples than protein precipitation.

The SPE can be used either off-line (typically in 96-well plates) or online [123, 131, 135].

LIQUID–LIQUID EXTRACTION LLE of the analytes by nonwater-miscible organic solvents is perhaps most familiar for medicinal chemists. The LLE usually provides cleaner samples than protein precipitation. However, LLE is usually more labor-intensive unless automated.

An accurate and precise bioanalysis of PK samples may have a significant impact on the quality of PK data and their interpretation.

5.7 ENGINEERING MOLECULES WITH DESIRED ADME PROFILE

This chapter does not describe how key ADME parameters can be "engineered" to improve the quality of drug candidates (see Chapter 2 for a more detailed discussion). There is significant literature that discusses SAR around ADME properties of small molecules from the "Lipinski's rule-of-five" [138] to some rules of thumbs [139–145].

5.A APPENDICES

These appendices contain the normal physiological values for commonly used laboratory animal species and man. These data help discovery scientists for a mechanistic explanation of ADME data. Care should be exercised in using the data. The data should serve as a guide rather than be used in an absolute sense. Additionally, these physiological values are being constantly updated and depending on the species and laboratory conditions, under which they are measured, and can and will differ in many literature sources.

5.A.1 General Morphinometric Data for Different Species

TABLE 5.A.1 General Morphinometric Data for Various Laboratory Animal Species

Parameter	Mouse	Rat	Rabbit	Dog	Monkey	Human
Species weight (kg)	0.02	0.25	2.5	10	5	70
Surface area (m^2)	0.008	0.023	0.17	0.51	0.32	1.85
Mean life span potential (years)	2.7	4.7	8.0	20	22	93
Total plasma protein (g/100 mL)	6.2	6.7	5.7	9.0	8.8	7.4
Plasma albumin (g/100 mL)	3.27	3.16	3.87	2.63	4.93	4.18
Plasma α-1 acid glycoprotein (g/100 mL)	1.25	1.81	0.13	0.37	0.24	0.18
Total ventilation (L/min)	0.025	0.12	0.80	1.50	1.67	7.98
Respiratory rate (min^{-1})	163	85	51	23	38	12
Heart rate (beats per minute)	624	362	213	96	192	65
Oxygen consumption (mL/(h g) of body weight)	1.59	0.84	0.48	0.34	0.43	0.20

Source: Adapted from Ref. 16.

5.A.2 Organ Weights in Different Species

TABLE 5.A.2 Relative Organ Weight (Percent of Body Weight) in Different Species

	Mouse	Rat	Rabbit	Dog	Monkey[a]	Human[b]
Organ						
Adipose tissue						21.42
Adrenals	0.048	0.019		0.009	0.03	0.02
Bone	10.73		0.36	8.10		14.29
Brain	1.65	0.57		0.78	1.38	2.00
GI tract					3.34	1.71
Stomach	0.6	0.46		0.79		0.21
Small intestine	2.53	1.40		2.22		0.91
Large intestine	1.09	0.84		0.67		0.53
Heart	0.50	0.33	0.20	0.78	0.45	0.47
Kidneys	1.67	0.73	0.52	0.55	0.40	0.44
Liver	5.49	3.66	2.87	3.29	2.39	2.57
Lungs	0.73	0.50		0.82	0.92	0.76
Muscle	38.40	40.43		45.65		40.00
Pancreas		0.32		0.23		0.14
Skin	16.53	19.03				3.71
Spleen	0.35	0.20	0.04	0.27	0.08	0.26
Testes			0.109			0.02
Thymus			0.15		0.02	0.03
Thyroid		0.005	0.01	0.008		0.03

[a] Rhesus.
[b] From Ref. 147.
Source: Adapted from Ref. 146.

TABLE 5.A.3 Relative Weights of Brain Regions in Rat and Human (Percent of Total Brain Weight)

Region of Brain	Rat	Human
Cerebrum	51.6	85–88
Cerebellum	14.3	10–12
Midbrain	15.2	
Olfactory lobe	2.8	
Brain stem	16.1	1.9–2.3
Medulla	11.5	
Pons	4.6	

Source: Adapted from Ref. 146.

5.A.3 Organ, Tissue, and Fluid Volumes in Different Species

TABLE 5.A.4 Organ Volumes (mL) and Miscellaneous Volumetric Data in Different Species

	Mouse	Rat	Rabbit	Dog	Monkey[a]	Human
Body weight (kg)	0.02	0.25	2.5	10	5	70
Brain		2.2		72		1,450
Liver	1.3	19.6	100	480	135	1,690
Kidneys	0.34	3.7	15	60	30	280
Heart	0.095	1.2	6	120	17	310
Spleen	0.1	1.3	1	36		192
Lungs	0.1	2.1	17	120		1,170
Gut	1.5	11.3	120	480	230	1,650
Muscle	10.0	245	1,350	5,530	2,500	35,000
Adipose		10.0	120			10,000
Skin	2.9	40.0	110		500	7,800
Blood	1.7	13.5	165	900	367	5,200
Blood (mL/kg)[b]	85	54	66	90	73	74
Plasma	1.0	7.8	110	515	224	3,000
Plasma (mL/kg)[b]	50	31	44	51.5	45	43
Hematocrit	0.45	0.46	0.36	0.42	0.41	0.44
Total body water	14.5	167	1,790	6,036	3,465	42,000
Total body water[b] (mL/kg)	725	668	716	604	693	600
Intracellular fluid		92.8	1,165	3,276	2,425	23,800
Intracellular fluid[b] (mL/kg)		371	466	328	485	340
Extracellular fluid		74.2	625	2,760	1,040	18,200
Extracellular fluid[b] (mL/kg)		297	250	276	208	260

[a] Rhesus.
[b] Calculated based on the values in this table.
Source: Adapted from Refs. [16, 146].

5.A.4 Blood Content in Different Rat Organs

TABLE 5.A.5 Blood Content in Rat Organs and Tissues

	μL Blood/g Tissue [148]	μL Blood/g Tissue [149]
Bone	19.1	45
Brain	13.5	11
Fat (dorsal)	4.6	
Fat (perirental)	7.9	
Gut	10.4	
Intestine		28
Heart	61.0	60

(continued)

TABLE 5.A.5 (*Continued*)

	μL Blood/g Tissue [148]	μL Blood/g Tissue [149]
Kidney	45.9	92
Liver	57.2	99
Lungs	175.0	111
Lymph node	8.2	
Muscle (skeletal)	4.0	4
Pancreas	32.1	
Seminal vesicles	11.0	
Skin	2.1	20
Spleen	321.0	86
Stomach	10.8	
Testis	7.3	6
Thymus	8.8	

5.A.5 Biofluid Flow through the Organs in Different Species

TABLE 5.A.6 Blood, Urine, and Bile Flow through the Body Organs in Laboratory Animals and Humans

Body weight (kg)	Mouse 0.02	Rat 0.25	Rabbit 2.5	Monkey[a] 5	Dog 10	Human 70
		Blood Flow (mL/min)				
Heart	0.28	3.9	16	60	54	240
Cardiac output	8.0	74.0	530	1086	1200	5600
Liver (Q_H)	1.8	13.8	177	218	309	1450
Hepatic artery	0.35	2.0	37	51	79	300
Portal vein	1.45	9.8	140	167	230	1150
Kidneys	1.3	9.2	80	138	216	1240
Brain		1.3		72	45	700
Spleen	0.09	0.63	9	21	25	77
Gut	1.5	7.5	111	125	216	1100
Muscle	0.91	7.5	155	90	250	750
Adipose		0.4	32	20	35	260
Skin	0.41	5.8		54	100	300
		Fluid Flow				
Urine flow (mL/day)	1.0	50.0	150	375	300	1400
Bile flow (mL/day)	2.0	22.5	300	125	120	350
GFR	0.28	1.31	7.8	10.4	61.3	125

[a] Rhesus.

Source: Adopted from Ref. 16.

5.A.6 Anatomical Characteristics of GI Tract in Different Species

TABLE 5.A.7 Relative Weights (Percent of Total Body Weight) of Various Sections of the GI Tract

Segment	Mouse	Rat	Dog	Human
GI tract	4.22	2.37–3.32	4.40	1.65
Stomach	0.60	0.40–0.52	0.65–0.94	0.21
Fore stomach	0.16	0.13		
Glandular stomach	0.44	0.27–0.39		
Small intestine	2.53	0.99–1.93	1.61–2.84	0.91
Duodenum		0.15	0.19–0.25	
Jejunum/ileum		1.24	1.36–1.46	
Large intestine	1.09	0.80–0.89	0.65–0.69	0.53
Cecum	0.30	0.32–0.35		
Colon		0.44–0.54	0.23–0.47	

Source: Adapted from Ref. 146.

TABLE 5.A.8 Anatomical Characteristics of the (Small) Intestine for Various Species

	Rat (Wistar)	Rabbit	Dog	Monkey	Human
Small intestine	0.13	1.51	2.48		6.25
(m)	0.82		4.14		
(% of total)	64	60	85		79
	Diameter (cm)				
Small intestine	0.3–0.5		1	1.2–2	5
Duodenum			2–2.5	1.5–2	3–4
	Region Surface Area Relative to Body Area (%)				
Duodenum	1.8				10.3
Jejunum	19.8				74.9
Ileum	0.4				22.9
Absorption surface area (m^2)					
Duodenum					0.09
Jejunum					60
Ileum					60
Cecum	0.04	0.44	0.08	0.05–0.06	0.15
(m)	0.06	0.61			
(% of total)	31	11	2		2
Colon	0.01	1.23	0.34	0.4–0.5	1.50
(m)	0.26	1.65	0.60		
(% of total)	5	28	13		19

Source: Adapted from Ref. 150.

5.A.7 The pH and Motility of GI Tract in Different Species

TABLE 5.A.9 Intestinal pH in Different Species

	Mouse	Rat (Wistar)	Rabbit	Dog	Monkey	Human
Stomach						
Anterior	4.5[a]					
Posterior	3.1[a]					
Duodenum: fasted (fed)		6.5–7.1 (6.9)	6.0–8.0	6.2–7.5, 4.5–7.5	5.6–6.0, 7–9	5–7, 5.6–6.4
Jejunum: fasted						6–7
Jejunum/ileum: fasted (fed)		(7.8)				
Ileum: fasted (fed)		7.1[a]				7.0, 7.4, 7–8
Cecum: fasted (fed)		6.8 (6.7)	6.6	6.4	5.0	5.9
Colon: fasted (fed)		6.6 (7.1)	7.2	6.5	5.1	5.5–7
Rectum: fasted						7
Feces		6.9[a]	7.2[a]	6.2[a]	5.5[a]	

[a] From Refs. [16, 146] with no specification of meal consumption but most consistent with other data for fasted state.
Source: Adapted from Refs. [150, 151].

TABLE 5.A.10 The GI Tract Motility in Laboratory Animal Species

Parameter	Mouse	Rat	Rabbit	Dog	Monkey	Human
Weight (kg)	0.02	0.25	2.5	10	5	70
Transit time (min)						
Stomach				96		78
Small intestine		88		110		238
Whole gut				770		2350

Source: Adapted from Refs. [16, 146].

5.A.8 Phase I and Phase II Metabolism in Different Species

TABLE 5.A.11 Substrate-Specific P450-Mediated Enzymatic Activity (pmol/(min mg) of protein) in Different Species

	Major Human P450	Dog (Beagle)	Monkey (Cynomolgus)	Monkey (Rhesus)	Human
Ethoxyresorfurin *O*-deethylation	1A1/1A2	46 ± 25	240 ± 85	295 ± 71	21 ± 14
Coumarin 7-hydroxylation	2A6	75 ± 17	678 ± 209	289 ± 125	448 ± 330
Tolbutamide 4-hydroxylation	2C9/10		50 ± 12	47 ± 9	88 ± 37

TABLE 5.A.11 (*Continued*)

	Major Human P450	Dog (Beagle)	Monkey (Cynomolgus)	Monkey (Rhesus)	Human
S-mephentoin 4′-hydroxylation	2C19	12.7 ± 0.4	106 ± 50	30 ± 7	44 ± 30
Bufuralol 1′-hydroxylation	2D6	49 ± 11	530 ± 154	558 ± 189	34 ± 20
N-nitroso dimethylamine *N*-demethylation	2E1	694 ± 220	758 ± 286	610 ± 76	761 ± 319
Erythromycin *N*-demethylation	3A	876 ± 316	2949 ± 298	1997 ± 437	153 ± 74
Midazolam 1′-hydroxylation	3A	1053 ± 257	1330 ± 174	1107 ± 326	320 ± 182

Source: Adapted from Ref. 150.

TABLE 5.A.12 Substrate-Specific P450 Content and Drug Oxidation Activities in Liver Microsomes of Various Animal Species

Parameter	Major Human P450	Rat	Dog	Monkey	Human
Total protein in liver (mg)		1,738 ± 123	43,200 ± 4,199	7,875	222,700
P450 content (pmole P450/mg protein)		673 ± 50	385 ± 36	1,030 ± 106	307 ± 160
Phenacetin *O*-deethylation (pmole/(min mg) protein)	1A2	36 ± 20	28 ± 10	110 ± 20	32 ± 30
Coumarin 7-hydroxylation (pmole/(min mg) protein)	2A6	<1	12 ± 5	209 ± 126	21 ± 22
Pentoxyresorufin *O*-dealkylation (pmole/(min mg) protein)	2B6	70 ± 10	60 ± 10	35 ± 5	5 ± 5
Phenytoin *p*-hydroxylation (pmole/(min mg) protein)	2C9	44 ± 8	84 ± 6	45 ± 12	29 ± 15
Mephenytoin 4-hydroxylation (pmole/(min mg) protein)	2C19	74 ± 15	106 ± 13	144 ± 26	39 ± 23

(*continued*)

TABLE 5.A.12 (*Continued*)

Parameter	Major Human P450	Rat	Dog	Monkey	Human
Bufuralol 1-hydroxylation (pmole/(min mg) protein)	2D6	743 ± 74	12 ± 2	471 ± 58	20 ± 14
Aniline *p*-hydroxylation (pmole/(min mg) protein)	2E1	403 ± 57	280 ± 91	227 ± 165	696 ± 986
Benzphetamine *N*-demethylation (pmole/(min mg) protein)	3A/2B	2,387 ± 639	348 ± 78	940 ± 200	544 ± 427
Ethylmorphine *N*-demethylation (pmole/(min mg) protein)	3A/2B	3,370 ± 621	273 ± 149	1,080 ± 249	423 ± 543
Erythromycin *N*-demethylation (pmole/(min mg) protein)	3A4/5	930 ± 164	144 ± 70	586 ± 101	244 ± 212
Nifedipine oxidation (pmole/(min mg) protein)	3A4/5	820 ± 187	456 ± 126	3,826 ± 131	604 ± 691

Source: Adapted from Ref. 150.

TABLE 5.A.13 Phase II Enzyme Activities in the Liver of Various Animal Species

Phase II Enzyme Activity (pmole/(min mg))	Dog	Monkey (Cynomolgus)	Monkey (Rhesus)	Human
Acetaminophen glucuronyl transferase	407 ± 111	489 ± 93	625 ± 267	78 ± 33
17α-Ethynyl estradiol glucuronyltransferase	142 ± 55	62 ± 32	95 ± 19	85 ± 42
Acetaminophen sulfotransferase	176 ± 36	347 ± 22	360 ± 50	88 ± 28
17α-Ethynyl estradiol sulfotransferase	91 ± 19	44 ± 14	43 ± 16	39 ± 12
6-Mercaptopurine methylase	1.9 ± 0.5	4.1 ± 1.2	3.3 ± 0.6	3.5 ± 0.8
3, 4-Dicholoronitrobenzene glutathione *S*-transferase (nmol/(min mg))	7280 ± 565	2820 ± 560	2720 ± 430	1070 ± 130

Source: Adapted from Ref. 150.

ACKNOWLEDGMENTS

The authors would like to acknowledge our colleagues who by many means (valuable recommendations, checking the accuracy of the information, supplying useful references, and proof reading) improved the quality of this chapter.

Pfizer colleagues: Rajesh V. Devraj, Heather Dowty, Tim Heath, Kathy Hotz Kathy Mandrell, Dean Messing, Scott Obach, Denise K. Pretzer, Yuriy Pyatkivskyy, Charles Stankovic, Joseph W. Strohbach, Jay Wendling, Steve Wene; and MPI Research colleagues: Travis Devlin and Edith M. Luckett.

REFERENCES

1. Dost, F. H. *Der Blutspiegel (Blood Levels)—Kinetic der Knozentrationsablaufe in der Kreislauffussigkeit*, 1953, p. 244.
2. Wagner, J. G. History of pharmacokinetics. *Pharmacol. Ther.* 1981, *12(3)*, 537–562.
3. Gad, S. C. (ed.).; *Animal Models in Toxicology*, 2nd Edition, Gad, S. C. (ed.), CRC Press/ Taylor & Francis Group, LLC, Boca Raton, FL, 2007, p. 933.
4. Peris-Ribera, J. E., et al. General treatment of the enterohepatic recirculation of drugs and its influence on the area under the plasma level curves, bioavailability, and clearance. *Pharm. Res.* 1992, *9(10)*, 1306–1313.
5. Berezhkovskiy, L. M. On the calculation of the concentration dependence of drug binding to plasma proteins with multiple binding sites of different affinities: determination of the possible variation of the unbound drug fraction and calculation of the number of binding sites of the protein. *J. Pharm. Sci.* 2007, *96(2)*, 249–257.
6. Hirayama, M., et al. Pharmacokinetics of RU44403, an active form of newly developed angiotensin-converting enzyme inhibitor (RU44570) in the rat. *Drug Metab. Dispos.* 1994, *22(4)*, 601–606.
7. Meisel, S., Shamiss, A., and Rosenthal, T. Clinical pharmacokinetics of ramipril. *Clin. Pharmacokinet.* 1994, *26(1)*, 7–15.
8. Fuchs, H., et al. Concentration-dependent plasma protein binding of the novel dipeptidyl peptidase 4 inhibitor BI 1356 due to saturable binding to its target in plasma of mice, rats and humans *J. Pharm. Pharmacol.* 2009, *61(1)*, 55–62.
9. Benet, L. Z. and Hoener, B. A. Changes in plasma protein binding have little clinical relevance. *Clin. Pharmacol. Ther.* 2002, *71(3)*, 115–121.
10. Trainor, G. L. Plasma Protein Binding and the Free Drug Principle: Recent Developments and Applications. In *Annual Reports in Medicinal Chemistry*, Macor, J. E. (ed.), Elsevier/ Academic Press, London, 2007, pp. 489–502.
11. Trainor, G. The importance of plasma protein binding in drug discovery. *Expert Opin. Drug Discov.* 2007, *2(1)*, 51–64.
12. Kalvass, J. C. and Maurer, T. S. Influence of nonspecific brain and plasma binding on CNS exposure: implications for rational drug discovery. *Biopharm. Drug. Dispos.* 2002, *23(8)*, 327–338.
13. Kalvass, J. C., Maurer, T. S., and Pollack, G. M. Use of plasma and brain unbound fractions to assess the extent of brain distribution of 34 drugs: comparison of unbound concentration ratios to *in vivo* P-glycoprotein efflux ratios. *Drug. Metab. Dispos.* 2007, *35(4)*, 660–666.

14. Hinderling, P. H. Red blood cells: a neglected compartment in pharmacokinetics and pharmacodynamics. *Pharmacol. Rev.* 1997, *49(3)*, 279–295.
15. Rowland, M. and Tozer, T. N. *Clinical Pharmacokinetics: Concepts and Applications*, 3rd Edition, Williams & Wilkins, Baltimore, MD, 1995, xiv, p. 601.
16. Davies, B. and Morris, T. Physiological parameters in laboratory animals and humans. *Pharm. Res.* 1993, *10(7)*, 1093–1095.
17. Kubitz, R., Helmer, A., and Haussinger, D. Biliary transport systems: short-term regulation. *Methods Enzymol.* 2005, *400*, 542–557.
18. Brockmeier, D. and von Hattingberg, H. M. Mean residence time. *Methods Find Exp. Clin. Pharmacol.* 1986, *8(5)*, 309–312.
19. Gibaldi, M. and Perrier, D. Pharmacokinetics. In *Drugs and the Pharmaceutical Sciences*, 2nd Edition, Vol. 15, Dekker, New York, 1982, viii, p. 494.
20. Shargel, L., Wu-Pong, S. and Yu, A. B. C. *Applied Biopharmaceutics & Pharmacokinetics*, 5th Edition, McGraw-Hill, Medical Publishing Division, New York, 2005, xx, p. 892.
21. Kleiber, M. Body size and metabolic rate. *Physiol. Rev.* 1947, *27*, 511–541.
22. Hu, T. M. and Hayton, W. L. Allometric scaling of xenobiotic clearance: uncertainty versus universality. *AAPS PharmSci.* 2001, *3(4)*, E29.
23. Lave, T., et al. Integration of *in vitro* data into allometric scaling to predict hepatic metabolic clearance in man: application to 10 extensively metabolized drugs. *J. Pharm. Sci.* 1997, *86(5)*, 584–590.
24. Mahmood, I. Application of allometric principles for the prediction of pharmacokinetics in human and veterinary drug development. *Adv. Drug Deliv. Rev.* 2007, *59(11)*, 1177–1192.
25. Hosea, N. A., et al. Prediction of human pharmacokinetics from preclinical information: comparative accuracy of quantitative prediction approaches. *J. Clin. Pharmacol.* 2009, *49(5)*, 513–533.
26. Rowland, M., Balant, L., and Peck, C. Physiologically based pharmacokinetics in drug development and regulatory science: a workshop report (Georgetown University, Washington, DC, May 29–30, 2002). *AAPS Pharm. Sci.* 2004, *6(1)*, E6.
27. Bonate, P. L., Swann, A., and Silverman, P. B. Preliminary physiologically based pharmacokinetic model for cocaine in the rat: model development and scale-up to humans. *J. Pharm. Sci.* 1996, *85(8)*, 878–883.
28. De Buck, S. S., et al. Prediction of human pharmacokinetics using physiologically based modeling: a retrospective analysis of 26 clinically tested drugs. *Drug Metab. Dispos.* 2007, *35(10)*, 1766–1780.
29. Naritomi, Y., et al. Prediction of human hepatic clearance from *in vivo* animal experiments and *in vitro* metabolic studies with liver microsomes from animals and humans. *Drug Metab. Dispos.* 2001, *29(10)*, 1316–1324.
30. Ghibellini, G., et al. *In vitro–in vivo* correlation of hepatobiliary drug clearance in humans. *Clin. Pharmacol. Ther.* 2007, *81(3)*, 406–413.
31. Miners, J. O., et al. *In vitro–in vivo* correlation for drugs and other compounds eliminated by glucuronidation in humans: pitfalls and promises. *Biochem. Pharmacol.* 2006, *71(11)*, 1531–1539.
32. Tabrizi, M. A., et al. Translational strategies for development of monoclonal antibodies from discovery to the clinic. *Drug Discov. Today.* 2009, *14(5–6)*, 298–305.

33. Gan, L.-S., et al. Case Study—Use of ADME Studies for Optimization of Drug Candidates. In *Optimizing the 'Drug-Like' Properties of Leads in Drug Discovery*, Borchardt R. T., et al. (ed.), American Association of Pharmaceutical Scientists, New York, NY, 2006, pp. 81–101.

34. Jewell, C., et al. Specificity of procaine and ester hydrolysis by human, minipig, and rat skin and liver. *Drug. Metab. Dispos.* 2007, *35(11)*, 2015–2022.

35. Hartman, D. A. Determination of the stability of drugs in plasma. *Curr. Protoc. Pharmacol.* 2003, Suppl. 19, 7.6.1–7.6.8.

36. Morissette, S. L., et al. Elucidation of crystal form diversity of the HIV protease inhibitor ritonavir by high-throughput crystallization. *Proc. Natl. Acad. Sci. USA* 2003, *100(5)*, 2180–2184.

37. Huang, L. F. and Tong, W. Q. Impact of solid state properties on developability assessment of drug candidates. *Adv. Drug. Deliv. Rev.* 2004, *56(3)*, 321–334.

38. Gibson, M. (ed.). *Pharmaceutical Preformulation and Formulation: A Practical Guide from Candidate Drug Selection to Commercial Dosage Form*, 2nd Edition, *Drugs and the Pharmaceutical Sciences*, Informa Healthcare, London, 2009, p. 560.

39. Gad, S. C. (ed.). *Preclinical Development Handbook: ADME and Biopharmaceutical Properties. Pharmaceutical Development Series*, Wiley-Interscience, New York, 2008, p. 1352.

40. Hardee, G. E. and Baggot, J. D. (eds.). *Development & Formulation of Veterinary Dosage Forms*. 2nd ed. *Drugs and the Pharmaceutical Sciences*, Vol. 88, Informa HealthCare, London, 1998.

41. Weiner, M. L. and Kotkoskie, L. A. (eds.). *Excipient Toxicity and Safety. Drugs and the Pharmaceutical Sciences*, Vol. 103, Marsel Dekker, New York, Basel, 2000, p.370.

42. Liu, R. (ed.). *Water-Insoluble Drug Formulation*, 2nd Edition, CRC Press, Boca Raton, FL, 2008, p. 669.

43. Lee, Y. C., Zocharski, P. D., and Samas, B. An intravenous formulation decision tree for discovery compound formulation development. *Int. J. Pharm.* 2003, *253(1–2)*, 111–119.

44. Strickley, R. G. Solubilizing excipients in oral and injectable formulations. *Pharm. Res.* 2004, *21(2)*, 201–230.

45. Rowe, R., Sheskey, P., and Weller, P. (eds.). *Handbook of Pharmaceutical Excipients*, 4th Edition, Pharmaceutical Press, London, 2003.

46. Rowe, R., Sheskey, P., and Quinn, M. E. (eds.). *Handbook of Pharmaceutical Excipients*, 6th Edition, Pharmaceutical Press, London, 2009, p. 888.

47. Napaporn, J., et al. Assessment of the myotoxicity of pharmaceutical buffers using an *in vitro* muscle model: effect of pH, capacity, tonicity, and buffer type. *Pharm. Dev. Technol.* 2000, *5(1)*, 123–130.

48. Krzyzaniak, J. F., et al. Lysis of human red blood cells. 4. Comparison of *in vitro* and *in vivo* hemolysis data. *J. Pharm. Sci.* 1997, *86(11)*, 1215–1217.

49. Krzyzaniak, J. F., Raymond, D. M., and Yalkowsky, S. H. Lysis of human red blood cells 1: effect of contact time on water induced hemolysis. *PDA J. Pharm. Sci. Technol.* 1996, *50(4)*, 223–226.

50. Krzyzaniak, J. F. and Yalkowsky, S. H. Lysis of human red blood cells. 3: Effect of contact time on surfactant-induced hemolysis. *PDA J Pharm. Sci. Technol.* 1998, *52(2)*, 66–69.

51. Reed, K. W. and Yalkowsky, S. H. Lysis of human red blood cells in the presence of various cosolvents. *J. Parenter. Sci. Technol.* 1985, *39(2)*, 64–69.
52. Reed, K. W. and Yalkowsky, S. H. Lysis of human red blood cells in the presence of various cosolvents. II. The effect of differing NaCl concentrations. *J. Parenter. Sci. Technol.* 1986, *40(3)*, 88–94.
53. Reed, K. W. and Yalkowsky, S. H. Lysis of human red blood cells in the presence of various cosolvents. III. The relationship between hemolytic potential and structure. *J. Parenter. Sci. Technol.* 1987, *41(1)*, 37–39.
54. Regev, R., et al. Modulation of P-glycoprotein-mediated multidrug resistance by acceleration of passive drug permeation across the plasma membrane. *FEBS J.* 2007, *274(23)*, 6204–6214.
55. Martin-Facklam, M., et al. Dose-dependent increase of saquinavir bioavailability by the pharmaceutic aid cremophor EL. *Br. J. Clin. Pharmacol.* 2002, *53(6)*, 576–581.
56. Suckow, M. A., Weisbroth, S. H., and Franklin, C. L. (eds.). *The Laboratory Rat. American College of Laboratory Animal Medicine Series*, Academic Press, New York, 2006, p. 912.
57. Hau, J. and Hoosier, G. L. V. (eds.). Handbook of Laboratory Animal Science: Essential Principles and Practices. In *Handbook of Laboratory Animal Science*, 2nd Edition, Vol. 2, CRC Press, Boca Raton, FL, 2002, p. 568.
58. Rollin, E. B. and Kesel, M. L. (eds.). The Experimental Animal in Biomedical Research: Care, Husbandry, and Well-Being: An Overview by Species. In *The Experimental Animal in Biomedical Research*, Vol. 1, CRC Press, Boca Raton, FL, 1995, p. 560.
59. Hughes, R. N. Sex does matter: comments on the prevalence of male-only investigations of drug effects on rodent behaviour. *Behav. Pharmacol.* 2007, *18(7)*, 583–589.
60. Imamura, Y. and Shimada, H. Differential pharmacokinetics of acetohexamide in male Wistar-Imamichi and Sprague-Dawley rats: role of microsomal carbonyl reductase. *Biol. Pharm. Bull.* 2005, *28(1)*, 185–187.
61. Louvet, C., et al. Tyrosine kinase inhibitors reverse type 1 diabetes in nonobese diabetic mice. *Proc. Natl. Acad. Sci. USA* 2008, *105(48)*, 18895–18900.
62. Satterwhite, J. H. and Boudinot, F. D. Effects of age and dose on the pharmacokinetics of ibuprofen in the rat. *Drug Metab. Dispos.* 1991, *19(1)*, 61–67.
63. Lin, J. H. Applications and limitations of genetically modified mouse models in drug discovery and development. *Curr. Drug. Metab.* 2008, *9(5)*, 419–438.
64. Cartwright, E. J. Large-scale mouse mutagenesis. *Methods Mol. Biol.* 2009, *561*, 275–283.
65. Gondo, Y. Trends in large-scale mouse mutagenesis: from genetics to functional genomics. *Nat. Rev. Genet.* 2008, *9(10)*, 803–810.
66. Stanley, L. A., et al. Drug transporters: gatekeepers controlling access of xenobiotics to the cellular interior. *Drug Metab. Rev.* 2009, *41(1)*, 27–65.
67. Katoh, M., et al. Chimeric mice with humanized liver. *Toxicology* 2008, *246(1)*, 9–17.
68. Katoh, M. and Yokoi, T. Application of chimeric mice with humanized liver for predictive ADME. *Drug Metab. Rev.* 2007, *39(1)*, 145–57.
69. Katoh, M., et al. *In vivo* drug metabolism model for human cytochrome P450 enzyme using chimeric mice with humanized liver. *J. Pharm. Sci.* 2007, *96(2)*, 428–437.
70. Okumura, H., et al. Humanization of excretory pathway in chimeric mice with humanized liver. *Toxicol. Sci.* 2007, *97(2)*, 533–538.

71. Kacew, S. and Festing, M. F. Role of rat strain in the differential sensitivity to pharmaceutical agents and naturally occurring substances. *J. Toxicol. Environ. Health* 1996, *47(1)*, 1–30.

72. Kacew, S. Confounding factors in toxicity testing. *Toxicology* 2001, *160(1–3)*, 87–96.

73. Lawson, P. T. (ed.). *Assistant Laboratory Animal Technician. ALAT Training Manual*, AALAS, Cordova, TN, 1998, p. 202.

74. Moriyasu, A., et al. *In vivo–in vitro* relationship of methotrexate 7-hydroxylation by aldehyde oxidase in four different strain rats. *Drug Metab. Pharmacokinet.* 2006, *21(6)*, 485–491.

75. Itoh, K., et al. Lack of dimer formation ability in rat strains with low aldehyde oxidase activity. *Xenobiotica* 2007, *37(7)*, 709–716.

76. Yilmazer-Hanke, D. M. Morphological correlates of emotional and cognitive behaviour: insights from studies on inbred and outbred rodent strains and their crosses. *Behav. Pharmacol.* 2008, *19(5–6)*, 403–434.

77. Musick, T. J., et al. Pharmacokinetics, disposition, and metabolism of bicifadine in the mouse, rat, and monkey. *Drug Metab. Dispos.* 2008, *36(2)*, 241–251.

78. Matta, S. G., et al. Guidelines on nicotine dose selection for *in vivo* research. *Psychopharmacology (Berl.)* 2007, *190(3)*, 269–319.

79. Mordenti, J. Man versus beast: pharmacokinetic scaling in mammals. *J. Pharm. Sci.* 1986, *75(11)*, 1028–1040.

80. Guo, Z., et al. Ciclesonide disposition and metabolism: pharmacokinetics, metabolism, and excretion in the mouse, rat, rabbit, and dog. *Am. J. Ther.* 2006, *13(6)*, 490–501.

81. Mordenti, J. Forecasting cephalosporin and monobactam antibiotic half-lives in humans from data collected in laboratory animals. *Antimicrob. Agents Chemother.* 1985, *27(6)*, 887–891.

82. Prescott, M. J. and s.a.o.a.i.P. file, Refining dog husbandry and care. Eighth Report of BVAAWF/FRAME/RSPCA/UFAW Joint Working Groxxxup on Refinement. *Lab. Anim.* 2004, *38(1)*, 1–94.

83. Gipson, C.Animal Care Annual Report of Activities. Fiscal Year 2007, U.S.D.O. Agriculture, A.A.P.H.I. Service, and A. 41-35-075, Editors, 2007, United States Department of Agriculture.

84. Ward, K. W., Nagilla, R., and Jolivette, L. J. Comparative evaluation of oral systemic exposure of 56 xenobiotics in rat, dog, monkey and human. *Xenobiotica.* 2005, *35(2)*, 191–210.

85. Ward, K. W. and Smith, B. R. A comprehensive quantitative and qualitative evaluation of extrapolation of intravenous pharmacokinetic parameters from rat, dog, and monkey to humans. I. Clearance. *Drug. Metab. Dispos.* 2004, *32(6)*, 603–611.

86. Ward, K. W. and Smith, B. R. A comprehensive quantitative and qualitative evaluation of extrapolation of intravenous pharmacokinetic parameters from rat, dog, and monkey to humans. II. Volume of distribution and mean residence time. *Drug Metab. Dispos.* 2004, *32(6)*, 612–619.

87. Hearn, J. P. Primate Priorities—An International Perspective. In *International Perspectives: The Future of Nonhuman Primate Resources, Proceedings of the Workshop*, The National Academies Press, Washington, DC, 2003.

88. Hearn, J. P. Science, ethics and regulation in primate research. *Gynecol. Obstet. Invest.* 2004, *57(1)*, 8–10.

89. Cohen, J. Biomedical research. The endangered lab chimp. *Science* 2007, *315(5811)*, 450–452.

90. VandeBerg, J. L. and Zola, S. M. A unique biomedical resource at risk. *Nature* 2005, *437 (7055)*, 30–32.

91. Varki, A. The uncertain future of research chimpanzees. *Science* 2007, *315(5818)*, 1493–1494.

92. Moore, J. The uncertain future of research chimpanzees. *Science* 2007, *315(5818)*, 1493–1494.

93. Prince, A. M. The uncertain future of research chimpanzees. *Science* 2007, *315(5818)*, 1493–1494.

94. Rowan, A. N. The uncertain future of research chimpanzees. *Science* 2007, *315(5818)*, 1493–1494.

95. Cai, H., et al. A Humanized UGT1 Mouse Model Expressing the UGT1A1*28 Allele for Assessing Drug Clearance by UGT1A1—Dependent Glucuronidation. *Drug. Metab. Dispos.* 2010, doi:10.1124/dmd.109.030130.

96. Sakaeda, T., et al. Blood flow rate in normal and tumor-bearing rats in conscious state, under urethane anesthesia, and during systemic hypothermia. *J. Drug. Target* 1998, *6(4)*, 261–272.

97. Diehl, K. H., et al. A good practice guide to the administration of substances and removal of blood, including routes and volumes. *J. Appl. Toxicol.* 2001, *21(1)*, 15–23.

98. Kurosawa, N., Owada, E., and Ito, K. Avoidance of hepatic first-pass effect in the rabbit via rectal route of administration. *Biopharm. Drug. Dispos.* 1998, *19(9)*, 589–594.

99. Wilhelm, A. J., et al. Analysis of cyclosporin A in dried blood spots using liquid chromatography tandem mass spectrometry. *J. Chromatogr. B Analyt. Technol. Biomed. Life Sci.* 2009, *877(14–15)*, 1595–1598.

100. Spooner, N., Lad, R., and Barfield, M. Dried blood spots as a sample collection technique for the determination of pharmacokinetics in clinical studies: considerations for the validation of a quantitative bioanalytical method. *Anal. Chem.* 2009, *81(4)*, 1557–1563.

101. Balls, M., et al. The three Rs: the way forward: the report and recommendations of ECVAM Workshop 11. *Altern. Lab. Anim.* 1995, *23(6)*, 838–866.

102. Wu, C. Y. and Benet, L. Z. Predicting drug disposition via application of BCS: transport/absorption/elimination interplay and development of a biopharmaceutics drug disposition classification system. *Pharm. Res.* 2005, *22(1)*, 11–23.

103. Martinez, M. N. and Amidon, G. L. A mechanistic approach to understanding the factors affecting drug absorption: a review of fundamentals. *J. Clin. Pharmacol.* 2002, *42(6)*, 620–643.

104. Patel, J. P. and Brocks, D. R. The effect of oral lipids and circulating lipoproteins on the metabolism of drugs. *Expert Opin. Drug. Metab. Toxicol.* 2009, *5(11)*, 1385–1398.

105. Parrott, N., et al. Predicting pharmacokinetics of drugs using physiologically based modeling—application to food effects. *AAPS J.* 2009, *11(1)*, 45–53.

106. Arayne, M. S., Sultana, N., and Bibi, Z. Grape fruit juice–drug interactions. *Pak. J. Pharm. Sci.* 2005, *18(4)*, 45–57.

107. Fleisher, D., et al. Drug, meal and formulation interactions influencing drug absorption after oral administration. Clinical implications. *Clin. Pharmacokinet.* 1999, *36(3)*, 233–254.

108. Paulson, S. K., et al. Pharmacokinetics of celecoxib after oral administration in dogs and humans: effect of food and site of absorption. *J. Pharmacol. Exp. Ther.* 2001, *297(2)*, 638–645.

109. Kojima, S. Factors influencing absorption and excretion of drugs. I. Effect of food on gastrointestinal absorption of amobarbital in rats. *Chem. Pharm. Bull. (Tokyo)* 1973, *21(11)*, 2432–2437.

110. Kohn, D. F. and Lipman, N. S. Anesthesia and Analgesia in Laboratory Animals. In *American College of Laboratory Animal Medicine series*, Academic Press, San Diego, 1997, xvii, p. 426.

111. Carroll, G. L. *Small Animal Anesthesia and Analgesia*, Wiley-Blackwell, New York, 2008, p. 283.

112. Xie, F., et al. Good preclinical bioanalytical chemistry requires proper sampling from laboratory animals: automation of blood and microdialysis sampling improves the productivity of LC/MSMS. *Anal. Sci.* 2003, *19(4)*, 479–485.

113. He, H., et al. A preliminary study on the feasibility of an automated blood-sampling system in conjunction with liquid chromatography/mass spectrometry. *Rapid Commun. Mass Spectrom.* 2001, *15(18)*, 1768–1772.

114. Liu, J. Y., et al. Pharmacokinetic optimization of four soluble epoxide hydrolase inhibitors for use in a murine model of inflammation. *Br. J. Pharmacol.* 2009, *156(2)*, 284–296.

115. Hassan, M., et al. The effect of busulphan on the pharmacokinetics of cyclophosphamide and its 4-hydroxy metabolite: time interval influence on therapeutic efficacy and therapy-related toxicity. *Bone Marrow Transplant*. 2000, *25(9)*, 915–924.

116. Watanabe, T., et al. High-throughput pharmacokinetic method: cassette dosing in mice associated with minuscule serial bleedings and LC/MS/MS analysis. *Anal. Chim. Acta.* 2006, *559(1)*, 37–44.

117. Chen, J., et al. Supercritical fluid chromatography-tandem mass spectrometry for the enantioselective determination of propranolol and pindolol in mouse blood by serial sampling. *Anal. Chem.* 2006, *78(4)*, 1212–1217.

118. Balani, S. K., et al. Effective dosing regimen of 1-aminobenzotriazole for inhibition of antipyrine clearance in guinea pigs and mice using serial sampling. *Drug Metab. Dispos.* 2004, *32(10)*, 1092–1095.

119. Bateman, K. P., et al. Reduction of animal usage by serial bleeding of mice for pharmacokinetic studies: application of robotic sample preparation and fast liquid chromatography-mass spectrometry. *J. Chromatogr. B Biomed. Sci. Appl.* 2001, *754(1)*, 245–251.

120. Fraser, I. J., et al. The use of capillary high performance liquid chromatography with electrospray mass spectrometry for the analysis of small volume blood samples from serially bled mice to determine the pharmacokinetics of early discovery compounds. *Rapid Commun. Mass Spectrom.* 1999, *13(23)*, 2366–2375.

121. Korfmacher, W. A. (ed.). *Using Mass Spectrometry for Drug Metabolism Studies*, 2nd Edition, CRC Press, Boca Raton, FL, 2009, p. 464.

122. Venn, R. F. (ed.). *Principles and Practice of Bioanalysis*, 2nd Edition, CRC Press, Boca Raton, FL, 2008, p. 344.

123. Boyd, R. K., Basic, C., and Bethem, R. A. (eds.). *Trace Quantitative Analysis by Mass Spectrometry*, Wiley, New York, 2008, p. 748.

124. McMaster, M. C. (ed.). *LC/MS: A Practical User's Guide*, Wiley-Interscience, Hoboken, NJ, 2005, p. 184.

125. Dass, C. (ed.). Fundamentals of Contemporary Mass Spectrometry. In *Interscience Series on Mass Spectrometry*, Desederio, D. M. and Nibbering, N. M. M. (eds.), Wiley-Interscience, Hoboken, NJ, 2007, p. 608.

126. Watson, J. T. and Sparkman, O. D. (eds.). *Introduction to Mass Spectrometry: Instrumentation, Applications, and Strategies for Data Interpretation*, 4th Edition, Wiley, Hoboken, NJ, 2007, p. 862.

127. Ramanathan, R. (ed.). *Mass Spectrometry in Drug Metabolism and Pharmacokinetics*, Wiley, Hoboken, NJ, 2009, p. 390.

128. Lavagnini, I., et al. (eds.). *Quantitative Applications of Mass Spectrometry*, Wiley, Hoboken, NJ, 2006, p. 152.

129. Mallet, A. and Down, S. (eds.). *Dictionary of Mass Spectrometry*, Wiley, Hoboken, NJ, 2009, p. 184.

130. Sparkman, D. O. (ed.). *Mass Spectrometry Desk Reference*, 2nd Edition, Global View Publishing, Pittsburgh, PA, 2006, p. 198.

131. Vekey, K., Telekes, A., and Vertes, A. (eds.). *Medical Applications of Mass Spectrometry*, Elsevier Science, The Netherlands, 2008, p. 606.

132. Rossi, D. T. and Sinz, M. (eds.). *Mass Spectrometry in Drug Discovery (Hardcover)*, Marcel Dekker, New York, NY, 2002, p. 432.

133. Lee, M. S. (ed.). *Integrated Strategies for Drug Discovery Using Mass Spectrometry*, Wiley-Interscience, New York, 2005, p. 568.

134. Lee, M. S. *LC/MS Applications in Drug Development*, Wiley-Interscience Series on Mass Spectrometry, New York, 2002, p. 256.

135. Evans, G. (ed.). *A Handbook of Bioanalysis and Drug Metabolism*, CRC Press, Boca Raton, FL, 2004, p. 408.

136. Viswanathan, C. T., et al. Quantitative bioanalytical methods validation and implementation: best practices for chromatographic and ligand binding assays. *Pharm. Res.* 2007, *24(10)*, 1962–1973.

137. Wells, D. A. (ed.). *High Throughput Bioanalytical Sample Preparation*, Elsevier, The Netherlands, 2003, p. 628.

138. Lipinski, C. A., et al. Experimental and computational approaches to estimate solubility and permeability in drug discovery and development settings. *Adv. Drug. Deliv. Rev.* 1997, *23*, 3–25.

139. Gleeson, M. P. Generation of a set of simple, interpretable ADMET rules of thumb. *J. Med. Chem.* 2008, *51(4)*, 817–834.

140. Smith, D. A., Jones, B. C., and Walker, D. K. Design of drugs involving the concepts and theories of drug metabolism and pharmacokinetics. *Med. Res. Rev.* 1996, *16(3)*, 243–266.

141. Kerns, E. and Di, L. (eds.). *Drug-like Properties: Concepts, Structure Design and Methods: From ADME to Toxicity Optimization*, Academic Press, New York, 2008, p. 552.

142. van de Waterbeemd, H. and Gifford, E. ADMET *in silico* modelling: towards prediction paradise? *Nat. Rev. Drug. Discov.* 2003, *2(3)*, 192–204.

143. Dearden, J. C. *In silico* prediction of ADMET properties: how far have we come? *Expert Opin. Drug Metab. Toxicol.* 2007, *3(5)*, 635–639.

144. Lipinski, C. A. Drug-like properties and the causes of poor solubility and poor permeability. *J. Pharmacol. Toxicol. Methods* 2000, *44(1)*, 235–249.

145. Lipinski, C. A., et al. Experimental and computational approaches to estimate solubility and permeability in drug discovery and development settings. *Adv. Drug Deliv. Rev.* 2001, *46(1–3)*, 3–26.

146. Birnbaum, L., et al. *Physiological Parameter Values for PBPK Models*, International Life Science Institute–Risk Science Institute (ILSI–RSI, ILSI@ILSI.org), Washington, DC, 1994, p. III, 87.

147. Kendall, M. D., Johnson, H. R., and Singh, J. The weight of the human thymus gland at necropsy. *J. Anat.* 1980, *131(3)*, p. 483–497.

148. Bernareggi, A. and Rowland, M. Physiologic modeling of cyclosporin kinetics in rat and man. *J. Pharmacokinet. Biopharm.* 1991, *19(1)*, 21–50.

149. Kwon, Y. *Handbook of Essential Pharmacokinetics, Pharmacodynamics and Drug Metabolism for Industrial Scientists*, Kluwer Academic/Plenum Publishers, New York, NY, 2001, p. 291.

150. Zwart, L. d., et al. *Anatomical and Physiological Differences Between Various Species Used in Studies on the Pharmacokinetics and Toxicology of Xenobiotics. A Review of Literature*, National Institute for Public Health and the Environment, Bilthoven, The Netherlands, 1999, p. 100.

151. Horter, D. and Dressman, J. B. Influence of physicochemical properties on dissolution of drugs in the gastrointestinal tract. *Adv. Drug Deliv. Rev.* 2001, *46(1–3)*, 75–87.

6

CARDIAC TOXICITY

RALF KETTENHOFEN AND SILKE SCHWENGBERG

6.1 INTRODUCTION

In the past 30 years, 28% of all approved drugs had to be withdrawn from the market due to cardiac toxicity. These compounds are categorized into two major groups depending on the mechanisms of their toxic action: ion channel-related and nonion channel-related cardiac toxicity. The former group of compounds interferes with the cardiac electrophysiology and are proarrhythmic or induce arrhythmias and sudden cardiac death (SCD). The latter group consists of compounds exhibiting cardiac cytotoxic properties such as induction apoptosis, necrosis, or metabolic disruption.

6.2 ION CHANNEL-RELATED CARDIAC TOXICITY

Functional and regular rhythmic beating of the heart is a prerequisite for the preservation of vital functions of the body and requires a well-defined and subtle interplay between a subset of cardiac ion channels, ion exchangers, and ion pumps. Interference with and perturbation of these intricate processes may cause cardiac toxicity by rising the proarrhythmic risk, inducing atrial and ventricular arrhythmias and fibrillation, and SCD.

The occurrence of life-threatening Torsades de Pointes (TdP) ventricular tachyarrhythmia and SCD in patients treated with approved drugs (e.g., cisapride, terolidine, and terfenadine) lead to the withdrawal of the drugs from the market. Additionally, the incidence rendered the necessity to evolve a generally accepted and harmonized guidance to assess torsadogenic potentials of drug candidates in clinical

ADMET for Medicinal Chemists: A Practical Guide, Edited by Katya Tsaioun and Steven A. Kates trials as well as in preclinical studies. The International Conference on Harmonization (ICH) of technical requirements for registration of pharmaceuticals for human use elaborated and filed the guidelines E14 (clinical) and S7B (preclinical) to address the issues of cardiac safety [1, 2].

The scientific basis for the guidelines benefited from the discovery that patients with congenital long QT syndrome (LQTS) have a higher probability to suffer from TdP tachyarrhythmia. To date, mutations in 12 different genes have been identified, including 8 ion channel α- and β-subunits that are able to cause LQTS. The potential to delay ventricular repolarization has become an accepted surrogate biomarker linked to an enhanced proarrhythmic risk of drug candidates although it is not a necessary condition to provoke life-threatening arrhythmias because other mechanisms are also reported to be proarrhythmic (see 6.2.3 and 6.2.4).

It is discussed that an increase in transmural dispersion of the repolarization (TDR, differential repolarization in the endo-, epi-, and myocard) rather than a delayed ventricular repolarization is predictive and responsible for torsadogenic risk [3]. To date, effects on TDR can be approximated only by *in vivo* or *ex vivo* preparation of perfused ventricular wedges or Langendorff-perfused hearts. These studies are costly and time-consuming that cause early cardiac safety studies to rely on simplified models that are discussed in Section 6.2.5.

In addition to delayed ventricular repolarization, evidence was recently provided and discussed that shortening of ventricular repolarization is a risk factor for ventricular arrhythmias [4–6]. Only a few patients with congenital short QT syndrome (SQTS) have been described to date, but all suffer from an increased vulnerability to atrial and ventricular fibrillation and sudden cardiac death [7]. Mutations in four cardiac ion channels have been identified to have implications in SQTS.

6.2.1 Cardiac Electrophysiology

A short introduction to cardiac electrophysiology is provided to understand the mechanism of ion channel-related cardiac toxicity.

The electrical activity of the heart can be recorded with electrodes from the surface of the body as an electrocardiogram (ECG) (Figure 6.1). The occurring pattern in the ECG is mainly characterized by the P wave, the Q, R, and S spikes (QRS complex), and the T wave.

The QT interval of the ECG describes the time frame starting with the excitation of the ventricle (Q spike) to its relaxation (end of the T wave). The duration of the QT interval has an inverse relationship to the heart rate and has to be normalized to judge drug-induced effects on the heart rate corrected QTc interval. Commonly used correction formulas are described by Fridericia and Bazett although they appear to have some limitations in the correct assessment of drug-induced QTc prolongation [8]. On a single cell level, the QT interval has its counterpart in the action potential duration of a ventricular cardiomyocyte (Figure 6.1).

At rest, the myocyte exhibits an electrochemical gradient across the plasma membrane of the main cardiac ions sodium (Na^+), calcium (Ca^{2+}), and potassium (K^+) with low intracellular Na^+ and Ca^{2+} concentrations ($[Na^+]_i$, $[Ca^{2+}]_i$) and

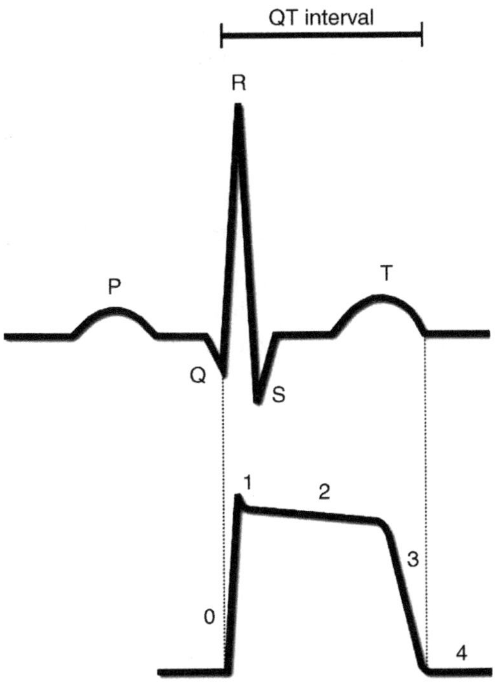

Figure 6.1 Schematic diagram to illustrate the correlation between an ECG and the action potential of a human ventricular myocyte. P: The P wave displays the excitation of the pacemaker and atrium. Q, R, S: The Q, R, and S spikes built a complex, which mirrors the excitation and the propagation of the excitation in the ventricles. T: The T wave reflects the recovery of the ventricles from excitation. The QT interval is the duration from the beginning of the excitation in the ventricles (Q spike) to the end of their recovery (end of T wave). The action potential of a ventricular myocyte starts with depolarization in phase 0 and ends after the membrane potential returned to rest potential in phase 4.

high intracellular K^+ concentrations. These differences in intracellular and extracellular ion concentrations and charges across the plasma membrane are called the electrochemical gradients and generate the driving force of the diffusion-controlled flow of ions through their selective ion channels.

At rest, inwardly rectifying potassium channels are open and keep the membrane potential approximately at –80 mV.

During the excitation of the cardiomyocyte, the membrane potential depolarizes from the rest potential to ~ +40 mV. The membrane is kept at positive potentials throughout phases 0–2 of the action potential due to the subsequent opening of the voltage-gated sodium channel ($Na_v1.5$, gene symbol *SCN5A*) and L-type calcium channels (protein symbol for the pore forming α-subunit is $Ca_v1.2$, gene symbol *CACNA1C*). The opening of these channels leads to a rise in $[Na^+]_i$ and the release of Ca^{2+} from intracellular stores, which subsequently increases $[Ca^{2+}]_i$. The cardiac sodium–calcium exchanger and the ATP-driven pumps sodium–potassium ATPase and calcium ATPase account for the $[Na^+]_i$ and $[Ca^{2+}]_i$ restoration found at rest potentials.

Finally, voltage-gated potassium channels accomplish the repolarization to rest potentials. The primary potassium channel involved in human ventricular repolarization is the human ether a-go-go related gene product (hERG, protein symbol $K_v11.1$, gene symbol *KCNH2*). The current related to this channel is the rapidly activating delayed rectifier current I_{Kr}.

6.2.2 Delayed Repolarization: Mechanisms and Models

6.2.2.1 hERG/I_{Kr} Block Since repolarization is essentially achieved by the hERG/I_{Kr} current, it becomes plausible that a block of this current presumably causes a delay of ventricular repolarization and consequently will increase a torsadogenic risk. A block of hERG/I_{Kr} current is not a sufficient condition to predict neither the potentials of a compound to delay ventricular repolarization nor a torsadogenic risk (see Sections 6.2.2.2–6.2.2.4 and 6.2.3) [4]. Virtually all drugs associated with TdP, however, are hERG/I_{Kr} blockers and prolong QT/QTc intervals of the heart and action potential durations of isolated cardiomyocytes [9]. Consequently, *in vitro* models were developed to address hERG liabilities to assess cardiac risk in an early stage of the drug development process.

hERG blockers comprise compounds with diverse structures and from different therapeutic classes, including antiarrhythmics, antipsychotics, antimicrobials, and antihistamines. In early drug development, ~70% of all compounds have hERG blocker potentials. It is suggested that the presence of multiple aromatic side-chains in the large central cavity of the channel may contribute to the promiscuity of hERG blockers [10–12]. As a safety margin for potential drugs, a 30-fold difference between the maximum therapeutic-free plasma concentration and the IC_{50} for hERG activity is proposed [13].

Impairment of clinically relevant metabolic pathways is able to increase cardiac risk. A key enzyme in the clearance of pharmaceutical drugs is the cytochrome P450 (CYP) 3A4. This enzyme can be affected by a number of compounds including the antifungal drug ketoconazole and grape fruit juice. It was shown that coadministration of these blockers with drugs such as terfenadine, astemizole, cisapride, or pimozide with known hERG blocker properties reveal a higher risk for TdP arrhythmias in patients (Figure 6.2) [14].

A cost-effective high-throughput assay system is the hERG-binding assay. Membrane fractions of cells stably expressing the hERG channel are extracted and incubated with a high affinity hERG channel ligand labeled with radioactive isotope, for example, [^{3}H]astemizole. The nonradioactive test compound is added to the [^{3}H] astemizole-labeled membrane fraction. The decrease of radioactivity with rising concentrations of the test compound is analyzed to determine the IC_{50} values for the inhibition of [^{3}H]astemizole approximation of the dissociation constant K_d and the binding site density B_{max} of the test compound to the hERG channel (Figure 6.3a) [15].

The disadvantage of this assay system is that it only assesses the physical interaction of a compound with the channel and does not provide information regarding the effect on its physiological properties.

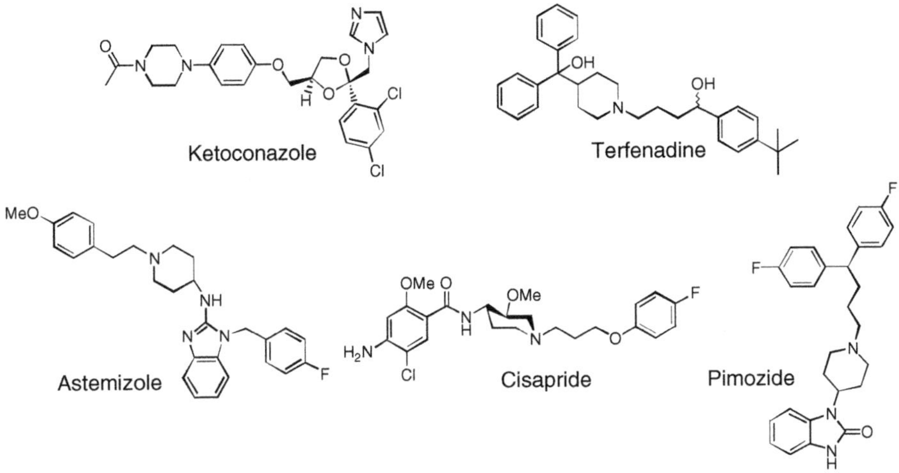

Figure 6.2 Compounds that impair clinically relevant metabolic pathways and increase cardiac risk. Ketoconazole, terfenadine, astemizole, cisapride, and pimozide.

The "gold standard" assay system to display interactions of compounds with the electrical properties of the hERG channel are conventional voltage clamp recordings from recombinant cell lines such as CHO (Chinese hamster ovary) or HEK (human embryonic kidney) cells stably expressing the hERG channel. The typical hERG tail current can be recorded by applying a two-step repolarizing voltage protocol after the initial depolarization. The block of the tail current can be observed by subsequently repeated application of the voltage protocol in the presence of the test compound (Figure 6.3b) [15].

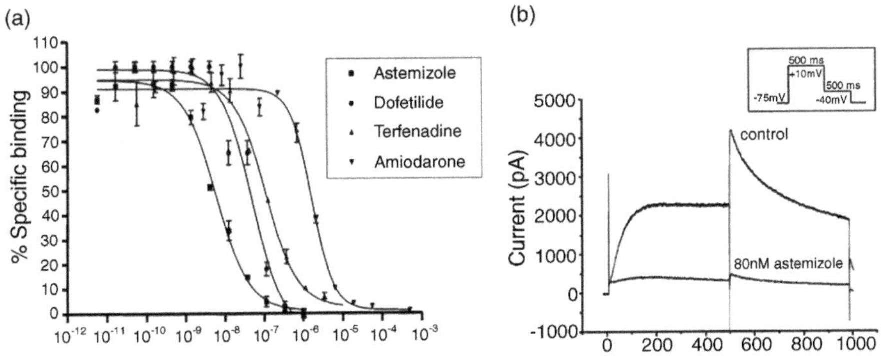

Figure 6.3 (a) Inhibition of [^{3}H]astemizole binding in HERG transfected membranes by typical hERG blocking compounds. (b) A representative hERG/I_{Kr} current tracing before and after astemizole in HERG transfected HEK293 cell (with permission from Dr. Peter Chiu [14]).

Today, the low throughput of conventional patch clamp can be overcome by automated planar patch clamp systems that are able to analyze up to 384 cells in parallel. The throughput of the assay is dependent on the success rate to obtain high quality resistance called "seals" (in the range of giga ohms) of the cell membrane to the patch substrate and whole cells recordings with appropriate current amplitudes. These issues can be overcome by the population patch approach where a single amplifier is able to average the whole-cell currents from multiple cells at once leading to very high success rates (>95%). However, comparisons between conventional and high-throughput patch clamp reveal some significant differences [16, 17].

The hERG assay can be modified to reach high-throughput screening (HTS) capacities by using membrane potential-sensitive fluorescent dyes or the assessment of rubidium (Rb^+) efflux by either spectrophotometric analysis in an atomic absorption spectrometer or using the radioactive nuclide $^{86}Rb^+$. Nonetheless, all these assays provide a decreased sensitivity for compound-induced hERG block and lack an ideal correlation with conventional voltage clamp experiments [16, 18].

The hERG channel blocker effects described above are due to acute (seconds to minutes) compound interactions on the channel itself. Another mechanism, which leads to a block of the I_{Kr} current, is a chronic action (hours to days) on the trafficking of the hERG channel during its synthesis. This provides retention of the protein in the endoplasmatic reticulum, which subsequently decreases the channel density on the cell surface and I_{Kr} currents [19–21]. Drugs with solely chronic blocking capabilities with no acute effect on the electrical properties of the hERG channel were identified [20]. Although these drugs would not be registered by conventional (acute) hERG assays and would be not identified in preclinical cardiac safety assays, no experimental protocols to address this phenomenon are currently issued in the regulatory guidelines.

6.2.2.2 KvLQT1/MinK or IKs Block The slowly activating delayed rectifier potassium current I_{Ks} is involved in ventricular repolarization. This current requires the coupling of the pore forming α-subunit K_vLQT1 (protein symbol K_v7.1, gene symbol *KCNQ1*) with its β-subunit MinK (gene symbol *KCNE1*) to generate functional I_{Ks}. Mutations in the encoding genes *KCNQ1* and *KCNE1* have been linked to the LQT1 or the LQT5 syndromes, respectively. I_{Ks} is a reserve repolarizing current that is activated with increased heart rate and by beta-adrenergic agonists as well as serum- and glucocorticoid-inducible kinase (SGK) 1 [22]. The modulations are dependent on the presence of the functional β-subunit MinK.

It was reported that only a small number of compounds described to be specific I_{Ks} blockers which show benign effects *in vivo* (e.g., chromanol 293B or HMR 1556) can potentiate torsadogenic risk after preceding I_{Kr} block in rabbits [23]. Moreover, more potent I_{Ks} blockers were shown to prolong QT/QTc interval and induce severe TdP arrhythmias in conscious dogs [24].

A higher throughput analysis to record I_{Ks} and address safety pharmacological aspects is established and validated by the application of a recombinant cell line stably expressing both genes, *KCNQ1* and *KCNE1*, in a planar automated patch clamp system [25]. In addition, functional modulation of the current in such recombinant cell lines by adrenergic agonists has been reported [26].

6.2.2.3 Na_v1.5 Activator The excitation of ventricular cardiomyocytes is initiated by the fast activation of voltage-gated sodium channel resulting in inward sodium current (I_{Na}) and the fast upstroke in phase 0 of the cardiac action potential (Figure 6.1). The voltage-gated sodium channel in the heart primarily consists of the pore forming α-subunit Na_v1.5, which largely accounts for the properties of the cardiac sodium current and complex of gene products from all four known β-subunits (gene symbols *SCN1B*, *SCN2B*, *SCN3B*, and *SCN4B*) [27]. The influence of the β-subunits on the properties of the cardiac sodium current is still not defined but the report that a mutation in *SCN4B* causes a Brugada-like LQTS indicates their significance [28].

The fast activation of I_{Na} is responsible for the propagation of the excitation in the heart. Approximately 20% of all patients with Brugada syndrome carry mutations in the gene *SCN5A* encoding the Na_v1.5 channel (LQT3 syndrome), which account for a defective inactivation of the channel and a sustained inward I_{Na} in the late phase of the action potential. The persisting I_{Na} induces delayed ventricular repolarization accompanied by an increased torsadogenic risk [3].

A few compounds including the neurotoxic peptides ATX-II [29], BmK 1 [30], Anthopleurin-C [31], the alkaloid veratridine, and the S-enantiomers of the compounds DPI 201-106 and Carsatrin [32–34] are described to disturb accurate inactivation of cardiac Na_v1.5 and activate persistent late I_{Na} (Figure 6.4). In addition, the α_1-adrenergic agonist Alfuzosin (Figure 6.4), which is approved by the FDA/for the treatment of benign prostatic hyperplasia, revealed QT/QTc interval prolongation properties by activating late I_{Na}[35]. Heterologous expression of cardiac sodium channels Na_v1.5 have been reported to study drug-induced modulations of the gating of channel [31].

6.2.2.4 L-Type Calcium Channel Activator The most important calcium channel in the adult human heart is the voltage-gated L-type (long-lasting activation) calcium channel. The pore forming α-subunit Ca_v1.2 requires coupling to the δ- and β-subunits (α2δ and β2a) to generate functional L-type calcium currents ($I_{Ca,L}$) [36]. Mutations in the exons 8 and 8a in the encoding gene for the α-subunit *CACNA1C* can lead to Timothy's (LQT8) syndrome. These mutations are attributed to cause improper voltage-dependent inactivation of the channel encompassing a prolonged calcium-inward current, a delay in ventricular repolarization with a high risk for sudden cardiac death, and severe complications in other tissues [37]. To date, two compounds have been identified that activate $I_{Ca,L}$ directly, namely FPL 64176 and the (*S*)-(−)-BayK 8644 (Figure 6.5) [38–41]. Both compounds are able to induce TdP-like arrhythmias in perfused cardiac wedges or Langendorff-perfused hearts [42, 43]. Furthermore, β-adrenergic receptor agonists are able to increase $I_{Ca,L}$ currents [44].

Recombinant expression systems have been established and allow the recording of functional L-type calcium channels in planar automated patch clamp systems. Protocols are proposed to overcome typical current run-down effects and (*S*)-(−)-BayK 8644 induced elevation of $I_{Ca,L}$ was revealed [36, 45]. It is still not

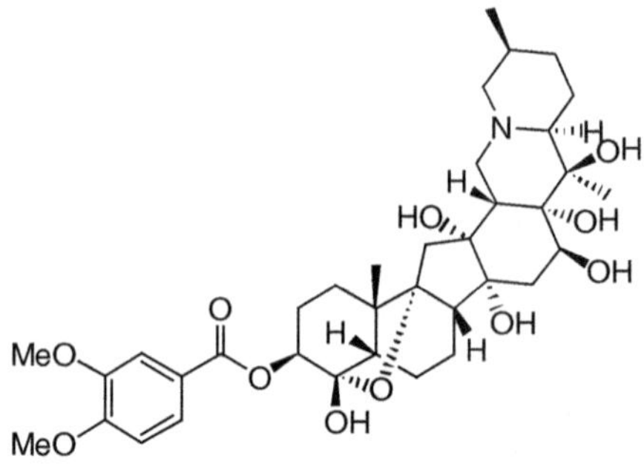

Veratridine

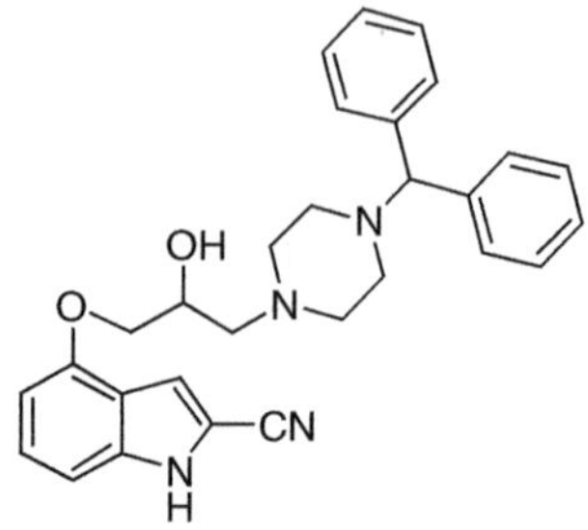

DPI 201-106

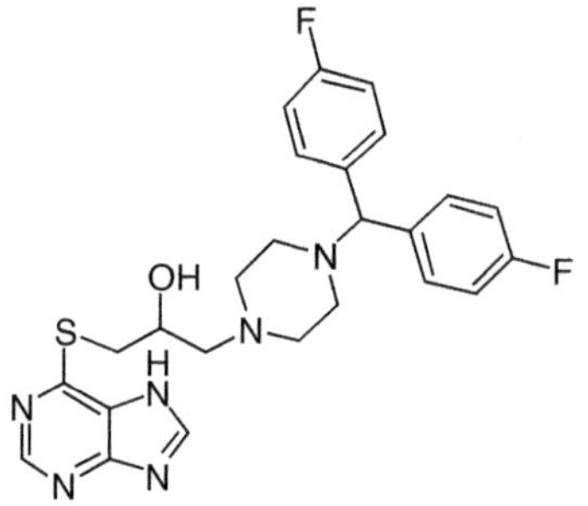

Carsatrin

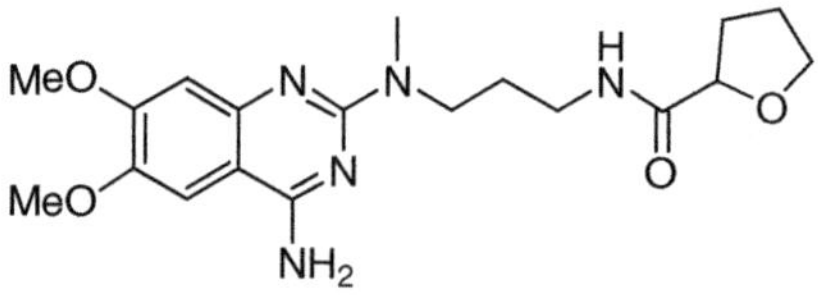

Alfuzosin

Figure 6.4 Compounds that disturb accurate inactivation of cardiac $Na_v1.5$ and/or activate persistent late I_{Na}. Veratridine, DPI 201-106, Carsatrin, and Alfuzosin.

reported if these recombinant cell models are capable of indicating correct GPCR modulation of $I_{Ca,L}$.

6.2.3 Shortened Ventricular Repolarization

The causes for acquired QT shortening have been reported to be hypercalcaemia, hyperkalemia, elevated plasma acetylcholine or catecholamine concentrations, hyperthermia, myocardial ischemia, and VT [46, 47]. Rare incidents for inherited short

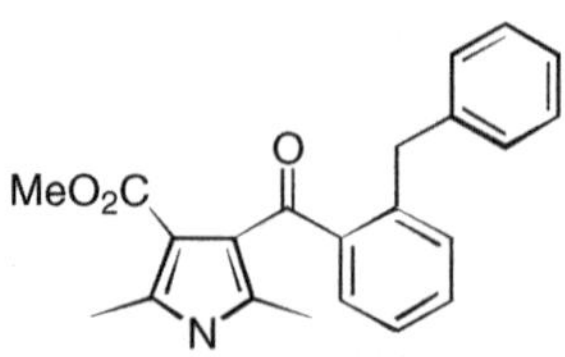

FPL 64176

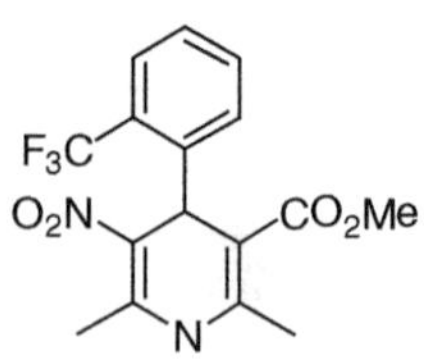

(*S*)-(–)-BayK8644

Figure 6.5 Compounds that activate L-type calcium channels ($I_{Ca,L}$). FPL 64176 and (*S*)-(–)-BayK 8644.

QT syndromes suggest potential targets for drug-induced QT shortening with increased proarrhythmic risk including gain of function mutations in *KCNH2*, *KCNQ1*, or *KCNJ2* and loss of function mutation in the genes *SCN5A*, *CACNA1C*, and *CACNB2B* [5, 48].

It was recently shown that drugs can induce shortening of repolarization, and this effect is also associated with an increased proarrhythmic risk. In the same study, evidence was provided that the *in vitro* hERG assay alone delivers insufficient information to predict potentials to delayed repolarization. From a group of 92 compounds identified as hERG blockers, 28.3% and 16.3% revealed no effect and induced shortening in repolarization assays (either intracellular recordings from isolated rabbit Purkinje fibers or Langendorff-perfused rabbit hearts), respectively. Due to these observations, the shortening of repolarization has to be accounted for cardiac safety studies [4, 5]. There are at least two mechanisms for drug-induced shortening of ventricular repolarization linked to a proarrhythmic risk described in the literature and are discussed in Sections 6.2.3.1 and 6.2.3.2 [5].

***6.2.3.1 hERG/I_{Kr}* Activation** In contrast to the numbers of well-known hERG/I_{Kr} blockers, only a few activators are reported including RPR260243, the two urea derivatives N1643 and N3623, PD-118057, and mallotoxin (Figure 6.6) [49–53]. The compounds increase I_{Kr} current by different mechanism. RPR260243 slows the deactivation and attenuates inactivation of the hERG channel (type-1 agonist). The type-2 agonists, such as PD-118057, attenuate inactivation but do not slow deactivation [49, 54].

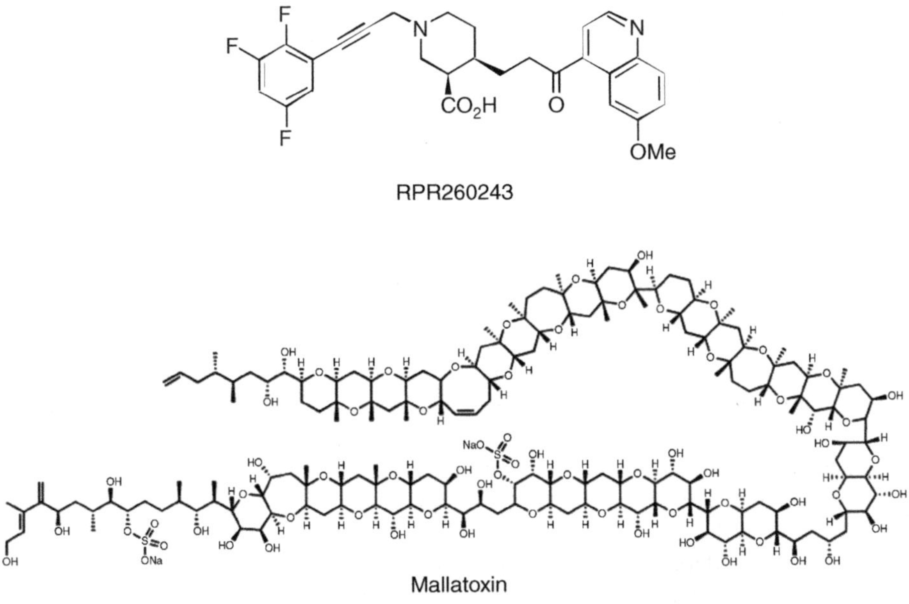

Figure 6.6 Compounds that activate hERG/I_{Kr}. RPR260243 and mallotoxin.

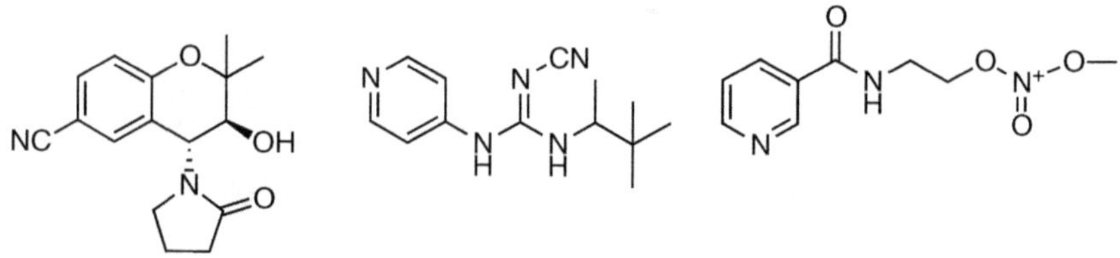

Figure 6.7 Potent activators of the inward rectifier potassium channel Kir6.2. Levcromakalim, pinacidil, and Nicorandil.

Although the hERG activation compounds have been proposed to be potentially antiarrhythmic drugs [52], evidence for the proarrhyhmic potentials have been clearly provided [4].

6.2.3.2 Activation of ATP-Sensitive Inward Rectifier Potassium Currents The α-subunits of inward rectifier potassium channels expressed in the heart belong to the Kir2, Kir3, and Kir6 family. The term "inward rectifier" is related to the electrophysiological properties of the channels. These channels have a high conductance at negative membrane potentials and the conductance does not increase during depolarization when the membrane potential turns to more positive values [55].

I_{KATP} is the only inward rectifier current described to be implicated in drug-induced short QT syndromes. Levcromakalim, pinacidil, and the approved antianginal drug Nicorandil are potent activators of the inward rectifier potassium channel Kir6.2 (Figure 6.7). This channel is the pore-forming α-subunit underlying the cardiac ATP-sensitive potassium current (I_{KATP}) [55]. These compounds induce shortening of repolarization, increased in dispersion of repolarization, and arrhythmia in Langendorff-perfused hearts [4, 56, 57].

In vitro analysis of the current was established in heterologous expression of *KCNJ11* in *Xenopus* oocytes and radioactive $^{86}Rb^{+}$ flux assay with liposomes enriched with purified human Kir6.2 protein, which was expressed in *Saccharomyces cerevisiae* [58, 59].

6.2.4 Alterations in Intracellular Ca^{2+} Handling

L-type calcium channels are activated during the cardiac action potential (Section 6.2.2.4). The influx of calcium ions triggers the calcium release from intracellular stores [calcium-induced calcium release (CICR)] and the contraction of the cardiac myocytes. Mutations in the ryanodine receptor 2 (RyR2) are responsible for catecholaminergic polymorphic ventricular tachyarrhythmias. These are associated with calcium overload, delayed afterdepolarizations, and a higher risk for sudden cardiac death [60].

Delayed after depolarizations (DADs) are caused by $[Ca^{2+}]_i$ overload and/or abnormal spontaneous openings of ryanodine receptors in the diastole. Known drugs, which interfere with the calcium homeostasis are the cardiac glycosides such as

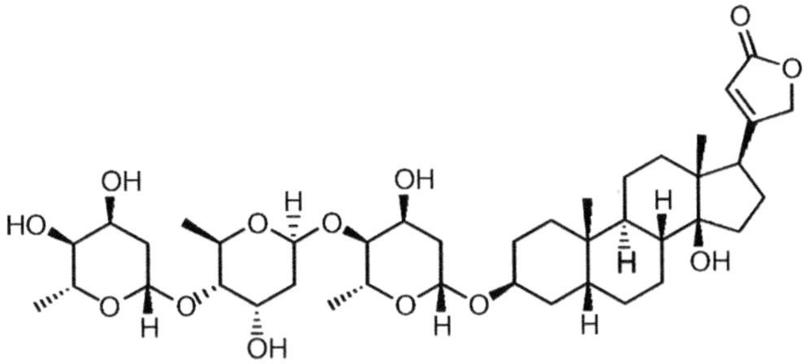

Figure 6.8 Cardiac glycoside, digitoxin, which interferes with calcium homeostasis.

digitoxin (Figure 6.8). A block of the Na^+/K^+-ATPases and subsequently increasing $[Na]_i$ and decreasing the Na^+/Ca^{2+} exchanger in the SR are the supposed proposed mechanisms for the mode of action for this class of compounds. Interestingly, theses drugs cause ventricular arrhythmia without prolongation of the QT/QTc interval and might not be detected in repolarizing assays. For this reason, it is proposed to include assays that monitor the modulation of the calcium handling into cardiac safety studies [61].

6.2.5 Preclinical Models for Assessment of Ion Channel-Related Cardiotoxicity

As outlined above, there are several cardiac ion channels with implication in cardiotoxicity. Recombinant or heterologous expression systems are established for almost all cardiac voltage-gated ion channels to study compound-induced modulation of the currents in different assay systems such as manual or paralleled automated patch clamp, voltage-sensitive fluorescent, or radioactive or nonradioactive rubidium flux assays. These models are necessary to study drug effects on the separated currents in relatively inexpensive assay systems with preferably high throughput and assess potential cardiotoxicity at an early stage in the drug development process.

The results of these *in vitro* assays are now incorporated into *in silico* prediction of drug interaction with ion channels such as the quantitative structure–activity relationship (QSAR) for hERG channel [62–64].

The comprehensive study published in 2008 by Lu and colleagues obviated that assessment of hERG/I_{Kr} current modulation alone was not predictive for drug-induced delay of ventricular repolarization [4]. Moreover, evidence was provided that detection of delayed repolarization was not sufficient to determine proarrhythmic potentials. Lastly, preclinical safety pharmacology studies were suggested to include assessment of the potentials to shorten ventricular repolarization [4–6].

Until recently, there was a gap between the demands to assess the potentials for the modulation of cardiac repolarization in high-content models such as primary cardiac myocytes and tissues or explanted heart and the ability to apply them in high-throughput assay systems. Primary cardiomyocytes derived from either animal or human hearts are difficult to generate in a standardized fashion and their preparation is

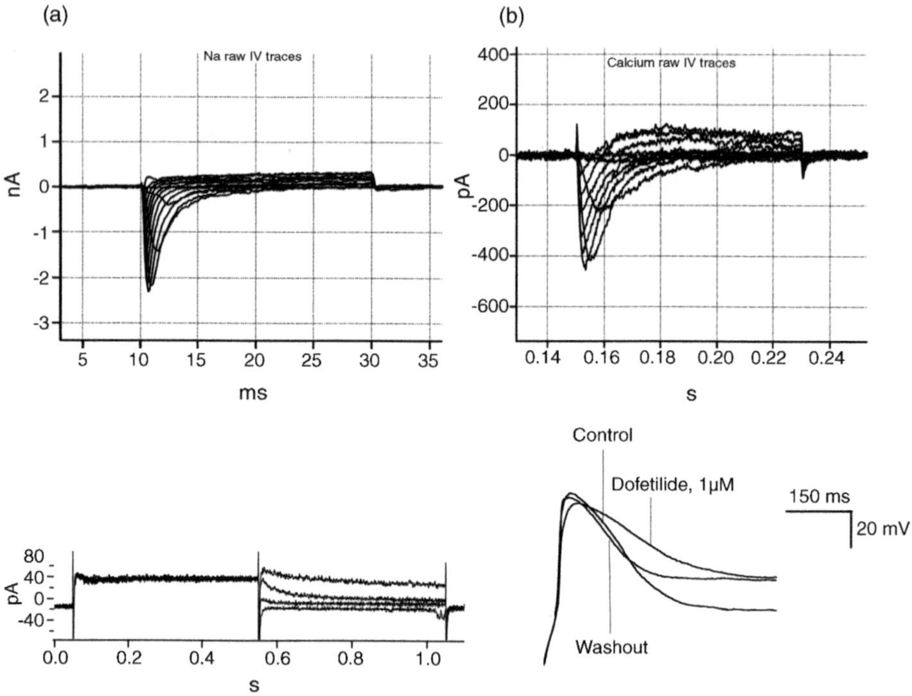

Figure 6.9 Automated patch clamp recordings from selected mouse embryonic stem cell-derived cardiomyocytes (smESCM) in the Patchliner from Nanion (Munich, Germany). a–c: (a) Voltage clamp recordings of I_{Na}, (b) $I_{Ca,L}$, and (c) I_{Kr}. Series of current clamp recording from smESCM in the Port-a-Patch (Nanion) reveals reversible action potential prolongation of the hERG blocker dofetilide.

time consuming and costly. Furthermore, the use of primary adult cardiomyocytes in high-throughput assay systems is hampered by their tendency to dedifferentiate in culture within a few days and the nonhomogeneous nature of the culture.

A promising solution to bridge this gap is provided by the pluripotent stem cell science. Genetically selected mouse embryonic stem cell-derived cardiomyocytes (smESCM) have been shown to be physiologically relevant due to their ability to integrate the cryo-infracted hearts and to recover the contractile function of the injured heart [65]. Moreover, these cells are electrophysiologically characterized and can be applied to automated planar patch clamp systems [66, 67]. Figure 6.9a–c shows typical voltage clamp recording of I_{Na}, $I_{Ca,L}$, and I_{Kr} from smESCM. Moreover, in Figure 6.9D a series of current clamp recording of action potentials in the absence and presence of the hERG blocker dofetilide (Figure 6.10) are provided, which reveal the potential of these cells to monitor I_{Kr} blocker. All patch clamp experiments including the current recordings were conducted with the automated planar patch clamp systems Port-a-Patch and Patchliner from Nanion (Munich, Germany) allowing the assessment of the modulation of cardiac repolarization in a higher throughput.

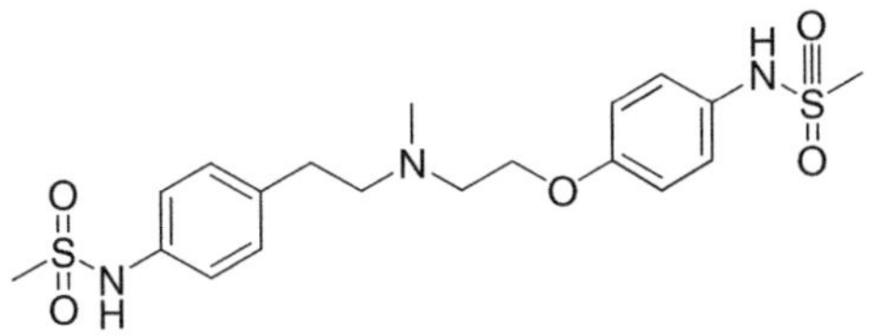

Figure 6.10 hERG blocker dofetilide.

The identification of methods aimed at reprogramming of the human somatic cells to so-called induced pluripotent stem (iPS) offers the possibility to generate tailor-made human cardiomyocytes that will most probably allow the development of ethnical or disease-specific drug actions on cardiomyocytes [68, 69].

These *in vitro* assays based on pluripotent stem cells generated cardiomyocytes in combination with high-throughput assay systems bride the gap to the complex models of primary tissues such as perfused ventricular wedge preparations or Langendorff-perfused hearts [9, 70].

6.3 NONARRHYTHMIC CARDIAC TOXICITY

In addition to cardiac side effects based on interactions of compounds with ion channels causing arrhythmia, nonarrhythmic toxic effects may occur, referred to as cardiac cytotoxicity. The importance of this form of cardiac toxicity is illustrated with the following example.

Some of the most potent cardiotoxic compounds in terms of nonarrhythmic toxicity belong to anthracyclins. Anthracyclins are among the most effective anti-neoplastic agents with broad-spectrum antitumor activity. The first two anthracyclins, doxorubicin and daunorubicin, were discovered over 50 years ago and clinical trials initiated in the 1960s (Figure 6.11). Although there was initial success in the treatment of patients with acute leukemia and lymphoma, it was realized that these anthracyclins induced irreversible cardiac damage in patients on chronic therapy.

In a retrospective analysis of three trials [71], the cumulative percentages of patients developing congestive heart failure after admission of doxorubicin was 5%, 26%, and 48% at a dose of 400, 550, and 700 mg/m^2, respectively. The exact mechanisms of cardiac damage currently remains unclear [72], but mitochondrial damage and the formation of reactive oxygen species have been proposed [73].

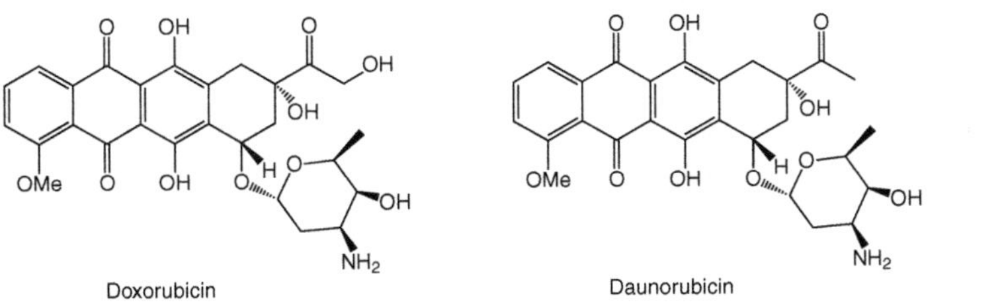

Figure 6.11 Nonarrhythmic cardiotoxic anthracyclins doxorubicin and daunorubicin.

In an attempt to overcome cardiac damage without reducing efficacy, a pegylated form of doxorubicin was developed, which reported a reduction in toxicity [72, 74]. However, chemical modifications of compounds are only successful if predictive test systems are available for screening both efficacy as well as unwanted side effects.

In addition to anthracyclins, anticancer drugs of other classes also exhibit cardiac-specific side effects [75]. The emergence of small molecules acting as inhibitors to kinases will require more demanding relevant toxicological modeling of cardiac side effects to minimizes adverse effects within this organ [76].

6.3.1 Definition of Drug-Induced Cardiac Toxicity

According to Wallace et al. [77], three different types of drug-induced cardiac toxicity can be identified:

(1) structural damage,
(2) functional deficits that may or may not be associated with histopathological changes, and
(3) altered cell or tissue homeostasis in the absence of obvious structural or functional deficits.

Functional deficits of the heart may be assessed *in vivo* using standard techniques (e.g., by MRI). Conversely, structural damage, histopathological changes, and altered cell or tissue homeostasis have to be assessed post mortem, using *ex vivo* or *in vitro* test systems, or *in vivo* by appropriate biomarkers for cardiac damage. Models and techniques to analyze nonarrhythmic cardiac side effects that allow in-depth analysis of different mechanisms of cardiac toxicity are outlined in Sections 6.3.2 and 6.3.3.

6.3.2 Assays for Detection of Nonarrhythmic Cardiac Toxicity

Methods and techniques for measuring functional deficits are described in Section 6.2. To detect nonarrhythmic cardiac toxicity, various models are available, ranging from standard *in vivo* techniques such as ventriculography to sophisticated *in vitro* systems that analyze the molecular basis for a given effect.

For this discussion, the term "*in vivo*" is used for examinations on living animals, either conscious or anesthetized; "*ex vivo*" for experiments on isolated organs and tissue preparations; and "*in vitro*" for investigations using either primary cells isolated from tissue or other suitable cellular models.

6.3.2.1 In Vivo Techniques *In vivo* systems can be used to monitor the mechanic action of the heart, that is, its function as a pump. The key parameter to measure is the ejection fraction, that is, the volume of blood pumped out of the ventricles with every heartbeat. In addition to electrophysiological disturbances, several other events such as loss of functional active cardiomyocytes, myocardial infarction, inflammation, and cardiomyocyte hypertrophy/cardiomyopathy can cause altered cardiac function.

Generally, the left ventricular ejection fraction (LVEF) is used as the marker for correct pumping of the heart. Ejection fraction is defined in Equation 6.1.

$$E_f = \frac{V_{stroke}}{V_{enddia}} = \frac{V_{enddia} - V_{endsys}}{V_{enddia}} \quad (6.1)$$

with V_{stroke} = stroke volume (volume of blood ejected with each heartbeat); V_{enddia} = end diastolic volume (volume of blood within a ventricle immediately before a contraction); and V_{endsys} = endsystolic volume (volume of blood left within the ventricle at the end of contraction).

Measurement of the LVEF can be performed by various methods, most of which are standard clinical diagnostic procedures adapted to the requirements of *in vivo* testing:

Echocardiography is one of the most common diagnostic techniques for detection of cardiac disease. It is possible to monitor the morphology of the heart, detect dysfunction in blood flow as well as hypertrophy-induced cardiomyopathy, and to determine the volume of the ventricles using ultrasound 2D or 3D image analysis and Doppler measurements. The method is noninvasive and usually does not interfere with normal physiological behavior of the heart [78].

Ventriculography is the method in which a dye is injected into the ventricle to stain and visualize the blood volume that is pumped during cardiac action. This can be used either in conjunction with cardiac catheterization, or with magnetic resonance imaging (MRI) (see below).

Cardiac magnetic resonance imaging (*MRI*) is another noninvasive clinical diagnostic tool that can be used to monitor heart function [79] and viability [78] as well as screening for morphological changes such as infarction sites, scars, and fat deposits. The method can be combined with application of contrast dyes for increased visibility of morphological abnormalities and blood flow or imaging agents such as gadolinium for targeted visualization of structures and proteins [80].

Magnetic resonance spectroscopy (*MRS*) can be used to monitor biochemical processes within a given tissue or organ as opposed to MRI to image morphological structures and function. Radioisotopes of standard ions are injected to provide information about cardiac physiology on the molecular level [81]. In contrast to MRI, this method is mainly used for research purposes, and not as a standard diagnostic tool.

The methods described above are adapted from clinical use in patients to preclinical and basic research using animals. Since the physiology (e.g., beating frequency) of laboratory animals can greatly vary from those of humans, modifications have to be applied to allow for reliable and predictive models [82]. Standard animal models for *in vivo* studies include mouse, guinea pig, rabbit, dog, and swine, with the latter usually used sequentially during safety evaluation.

In vivo test systems have drawbacks even though they are a critical component of drug development. The test systems are very costly in terms of time and resources and not suitable for screening of medium or large compound libraries. Many *in vivo* tests lack details concerning the mechanism on the cellular and/or molecular basis. Due to the different species used *in vivo*, interspecies extrapolation of the results is required to conduct risk assessment. Current *in vivo* tests conducted according to protocols that could be revised typically remain unmodified since regulatory acceptance has been obtained.

6.3.2.2 Biomarkers of Cardiac Damage: Cardiac Troponin T as the Gold Standard The detection of a tissue-specific marker in the peripheral blood or any other accessible compartment of the body is another possibility for screening of drug-induced, tissue-specific toxicities. The term "biomarker" was standardized by an NIH working group in 2001 as "a characteristic that is objectively measured and evaluated as an indicator of normal biological processes, pathogenic processes, or pharmacological response to a therapeutic intervention" [83]. Quantification of biomarkers is primarily conducted by an *in vivo* experiment, and may be an ideal supplemental to the methods described above.

As stated by Wallace et al. [77], an "ideal" biomarker for a given toxicity should be

- specific (e.g., not expressed by nontarget tissues, high tissue/serum ratio),
- sensitive (e.g., low baseline level, immediate release after injury, indication of early and reversible toxicity),
- predictive (e.g., release proportional to extent of injury),
- robust,
- noninvasive/accessible, and
- bridge preclinical and clinical findings.

Highly specific and sensitive biomarkers may be difficult to identify if the type of damage is a common cellular event that affects cardiomyocytes as well as other cell types. For example, if cardiomyocytes undergo apoptosis, the same signaling cascades are engaged in other cell types resulting in caspase activation, DNA laddering, and blebbing of the cells. General markers for cell death that can be determined in the circulation of an individual will usually not disclose the type of damage. Moreover, it is more difficult to define an accessible, noninvasive, and robust biomarker as the intricacy and subtleness of a drug-induced change in the physiology increases. Due to these limitations, the key biomarkers for cardiac damage that can be measured in biological samples include cardiac troponin T and cardiac troponin I for myocardial necrosis, ischemia modified albumin (IMA) for ischemia of cardiomyocytes, and type-B natriuretic peptides for acute and chronic cardiac failure (for review, see Ref. 84).

Cardiac troponin is a complex of three proteins (troponin C, troponin I, and troponin T) that are attached to tropomyosin, which prevents binding of myosin to the actin filaments in a relaxed muscle cell. Once the muscle cell becomes excited, calcium ions release from the sarcoplasmatic reticulum leads to conformational changes in the troponin–tropomyosin complex, which enables cross-binding of the actin filament with the myosin proteins [85].

Troponin T is the calcium-binding subunit of the troponin complex. Similar to the other two troponins, it is highly specific, stably released in the circulation upon cardiac muscle damage, and a background level is not detected by common assay systems [77, 86]. The determination of cardiac troponin was therefore established as the "gold standard" for the detection of necrosis of cardiomyocytes [87]. In a patient, cardiac troponins can be released due to different mechanisms of cardiac damage. Myocardial infarction is the most common cause of injury. Nonischemic damage of cardiac tissue such as inflammation, cardiac trauma, and drug-induced necrosis will also result in elevated troponin levels.

In addition to diagnosing heart infarction clinically, several studies have shown that determination of cardiac troponin is also a useful tool for preclinical studies [88, 89]. Due to its high specificity and sensitivity, the release of troponin T highly correlates with histopathological extent of injury, the degree of impairment of cardiac function, and prognosis. This data allows for a direct translation of preclinical development to clinical outcome. Various assays are commercially available for detection of troponin T release in laboratory animals [89] and can be easily implemented in any preclinical strategy for detecting cardiotoxicity. Therefore, the combination of *in vivo* experiments with measurement of troponin levels in the circulation will allow for constant monitoring of nonarrhythmic cardiac side effects. However, for highly predictive results, the biological model (species) and the assay system must be chosen carefully [89].

6.3.2.3 Ex Vivo Test Systems *Ex vivo* test systems either consist of the whole isolated organ (e.g., the Langendorff-perfused heart) or a part of the organ, such as papillary muscle strips [90, 91]. All of these models require highly skilled operators to avoid inter-experimental variations. Moreover, these tests are not capable of medium or high-throughput screening, can be used only for acute experiments, and experimental results may be affected by the procedure that is used to prepare and isolate the material. These test systems are mainly used for screening of ion channel-related cardiac toxicity (Section 6.2). However, monitoring the biochemical and molecular processes of drug-induced cardiac toxicity is also suitable. Explanted rat hearts have been applied to investigate aspects of injuries induced by ischemic reperfusion, for example, apoptosis [92], and anthracycline-induced cardiac toxicity [93]. In contrast to primary cardiomyocytes isolated from the heart, isolated organs or tissue strips retain their natural 3D structure as well as the cell-to-cell contacts, which are necessary for proper physiological behavior [94].

6.3.2.4 In Vitro Test Systems Determination of cardiac-specific toxicity on the cellular, biochemical, or molecular level demands the use of either primary cardiomyocytes isolated from cardiac tissue or cell lines, which mostly resembles cardiomyocyte physiology [95, 96]. In contrast to test systems for detection of ion channel-related cardiac toxicity, the use of artificial cell lines only transfected with cardiac ion channels for determination of cardiac cytotoxicity is not an option.

Primary cardiomyocytes isolated from different species at different stages of development (neonatal, adult) represent established models in toxicological and physiological test systems. Freshly isolated primary cardiomyocytes possessing *in vivo* physiological properties are costly, time-consuming to produce, and difficult to standardize [97, 98]. Moreover, cells are easily damaged during the isolation procedure since strong cell-to-cell connections within the cardiac tissue are formed [94]. Primary cardiomyocyte preparations are usually contaminated with other cells types (e.g., fibroblasts, endothelial cells), which may overgrow the culture of cardiomyocytes within a short time [98]. These contaminations also increase the variability of data and reduce the reliability of test results that are derived from a population of cells as opposed to a single cell. For example, a preparation of primary cardiomyocytes with 70% purity is used in a standard cytotoxicity assay in which 30% of the cells are killed by a given drug at a certain concentration. It is not obvious if the 30% dead cells consist of cardiomyocytes, contaminating cells, or a mixture of both. This limitation can be overcome by more sophisticated read-out systems such as image analysis and high-content screening (HCS) that will break down a given effect to the single cell level.

Cardiomyocytes isolated from either juvenile or adult hearts will not proliferate in culture and tend to dedifferentiate and lose their phenotype within a short time [99]. This limits their use to short-term experiments.

Cardiac cell lines that have been developed to overcome the limitations of primary isolated cardiomyocytes are mainly constructed from immortalized or tumorigenic cardiomyocytes [95, 96]. Although such cell lines have been widely used in recent years, the relevance and predictive ability of drug-induced nonarrhythmic cardiac toxicity is currently not proven.

A promising cellular model that combines the advantages of cell lines (e.g., purity, high standardization, ease of use) with those of primary cells (fully functional, normal physiological behavior) are pluripotent stem cell-derived cardiomyocytes, either from mouse or human origin. Generation of the mouse ES cell line D3 and their differentiation into cardiac myocytes was published in 1985 by Doetschman et al. [100]. Almost 20 years later the generation of human ES cells and differentiation into cardiomyocytes were described [101, 102], followed by the recent development of human-induced pluripotent stem cells [68, 69]. The usefulness, relevance, and predictivity of stem cell-derived cardiomyocytes as well as other cell types for determination of drug-induced toxicity have been well recognized during the past years (for review, [103–105]). Besides their unique primary-like functional behavior, mouse ES cell-derived cardiomyocytes can be produced at 100% purity in large and uniform lot sizes and stockpiled in liquid nitrogen. Their availability allows for full library screening approaches and are suitable for all types of experimental setups and read-outs, that is, standard cytotoxicity assays, apoptosis, and calcium signaling [104, 106–110]. Embryonic stem cell-derived cells and tissues are therefore a perfect tool for cell-based *in vitro* assays and overcome the limitations of the current models such as unspecific cell lines and primary tissue.

6.3.3 Biochemical and Molecular Basis of Drug-Induced Cardiac Toxicity—Impairment of Mitochondrial Function

Recently, it has been acknowledged that toxic effects on mitochondria can be a major cause for the side effects of a drug and subsequently its withdrawal from the market. In

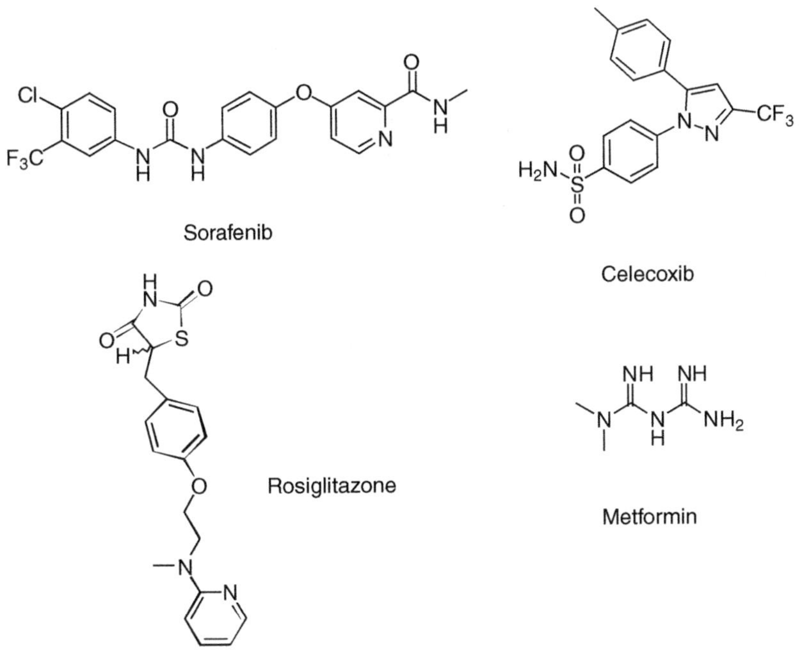

Figure 6.12 Compounds with FDA Black Box Warnings for cardiovascular toxicity with mitochondrial liabilities. Sorafenib, Celecoxib, Rosiglitazone, and Metformin.

a recent review, Dykens and Will reported that ~50% of drugs with FDA Black Box Warnings for cardiovascular toxicity have documented mitochondrial liabilities [111]. Among those drugs are anticancer agents such as anthracyclines and the modern tyrosine kinase inhibitor Sorafenib [112], NSAIDs such as Celecoxib [113], and the antidiabetic drugs Rosiglitazone and Metformin (Figure 6.12) [114].

Mitochondrial dysfunction can be caused either by interaction of a drug with the self-replication of this cell organelle (e.g., by nucleotide reverse transcriptase inhibitors, [115]) or by interference of the drug with the process of oxidative phosphorylation, for example, via inhibition of the electron transport chain or uncoupling of electron transport from ATP synthesis [116–118]. Since cardiomyocytes highly demand oxygen, disturbances in oxidative phosphorylation will immediately cause damage to this cell type, whereas inhibition of mitochondrial DNA synthesis will gradually decrease mitochondrial function.

Historically, it was almost impossible to detect mitochondrial liabilities of drug candidates within the drug development process using common *in vivo* and *ex vivo* test systems. Most often, mitochondrial toxicity was only retrospectively analyzed after clinical reports of unwanted side effects. Although *ex vivo* systems using isolated perfused hearts are suitable to detect mitochondrial toxicity [93, 119], this setup is not capable of medium or high throughput and is therefore not compatible with early stages of drug development and toxicity testing.

Most recently, *in vitro* test systems for mitochondrial function and dysfunction have been developed that can be used either with transformed cell lines, isolated mitochondria from animal tissues, or with primary or ES-cell-derived cardiomyocytes [116, 120, 121]. The current strategy of toxicity testing within drug development will now need to adapt and incorporate these assays that allow high-throughput screening for mitochondrial liabilities.

REFERENCES

1. International Conference on Harmonisation. Guidance on E14 Clinical Evaluation of QT/QTc Interval Prolongation and Proarrhythmic Potential for Non-Antiarrhythmic Drugs; Availability. *Notice. Fed Regist*, 2005, *70(202)*, 61134–61135.
2. International Conference on Harmonisation. Guidance on S7B Nonclinical Evaluation of the Potential for Delayed Ventricular Repolarization (QT Interval Prolongation) by Human Pharmaceuticals; availability. *Notice. Fed Regist*, 2005, *70(202)*, 61133–61134.
3. Antzelevitch, C. Drug-induced spatial dispersion of repolarization. *Cardiol. J.* 2008, *15* (2), 100–121.
4. Lu, H. R., Vlaminckx, E., Hermans, A. N., Rohrbacher, J., Van Ammel, K., Towart, R., Pugsley, M., and Gallacher, D. J. Predicting drug-induced changes in QT interval and arrhythmias: QT-shortening drugs point to gaps in the ICHS7B Guidelines. *Br. J. Pharmacol.* 2008, *154(7)*, 1427–1438.
5. Shah, R. R. Drug-induced QT interval shortening: potential harbinger of proarrhythmia and regulatory perspectives. *Br. J. Pharmacol.* 2009.
6. Holbrook, M., Malik, M., Shah, R. R., and Valentin, J. P. Drug induced shortening of the QT/QTc interval: an emerging safety issue warranting further modelling and evaluation in drug research and development? *J. Pharmacol. Toxicol. Methods* 2009, *59(1)*, 21–28.
7. Gussak, I., Brugada, P., Brugada, J., Wright, R. S., Kopecky, S. L., Chaitman, B. R., and Bjerregaard, P. Idiopathic short QT interval: a new clinical syndrome? *Cardiology* 2000, *94(2)*, 99–102.
8. Indik, J. H., Pearson, E. C., Fried, K., and Woosley, R. L. Bazett and Fridericia QT correction formulas interfere with measurement of drug-induced changes in QT interval. *Heart Rhythm* 2006, *3(9)*, 1003–1007.
9. Gintant, G. A. Preclinical Torsades-de-Pointes screens: advantages and limitations of surrogate and direct approaches in evaluating proarrhythmic risk. *Pharmacol. Ther.* 2008, *119(2)*, 199–209.
10. Sanguinetti, M. C. and Mitcheson, J. S. Predicting drug-hERG channel interactions that cause acquired long QT syndrome. *Trends Pharmacol. Sci.* 2005, *26(3)*, 119–124.
11. Sanguinetti, M. C. and Tristani-Firouzi, M. hERG potassium channels and cardiac arrhythmia. *Nature* 2006, *440(7083)*, 463–469.
12. Lagrutta, A. A., Trepakova, E. S., and Salata, J. J. The hERG channel and risk of drug-acquired cardiac arrhythmia: an overview. *Curr. Top. Med. Chem.* 2008, *8(13)*, 1102–1112.
13. Redfern, W. S., Carlsson, L., Davis, A. S., Lynch, W. G., MacKenzie, I., Palethorpe, S., Siegl, P. K., Strang, I., Sullivan, A. T., Wallis, R., Camm, A. J., and Hammond, T. G.

Relationships between preclinical cardiac electrophysiology, clinical QT interval prolongation and torsade de pointes for a broad range of drugs: evidence for a provisional safety margin in drug development. *Cardiovasc. Res.* 2003, *58(1)*, 32–45.

14. Dresser, G. K., Spence, J. D., and Bailey, D. G. Pharmacokinetic-pharmacodynamic consequences and clinical relevance of cytochrome P450 3A4 inhibition. *Clin. Pharmacokinet.* 2000, *38(1)*, 41–57.
15. Chiu, P. J., Marcoe, K. F., Bounds, S. E., Lin, C. H., Feng, J. J., Lin, A., Cheng, F. C., Crumb, W. J., and Mitchell, R. Validation of a [^{3}H]astemizole binding assay in HEK293 cells expressing HERG K^+ channels. *J. Pharmacol. Sci.* 2004, *95(3)*, 311–3119.
16. Sorota, S., Zhang, X. S., Margulis, M., Tucker, K., and Priestley, T. Characterization of a hERG screen using the IonWorks HT: comparison to a hERG rubidium efflux screen. *Assay Drug Dev. Technol.* 2005, *3(1)*, 47–57.
17. Finkel, A., Wittel, A., Yang, N., Handran, S., Hughes, J., and Costantin, J. Population patch clamp improves data consistency and success rates in the measurement of ionic currents. *J. Biomol. Screen* 2006, *11(5)*, 488–496.
18. Netzer, R., Bischoff, U., and Ebneth, A. HTS techniques to investigate the potential effects of compounds on cardiac ion channels at early-stages of drug discovery. *Curr. Opin. Drug Discov. Dev.* 2003, *6(4)*, 462–469.
19. Zhou, Z., Gong, Q., and January, C. T. Correction of defective protein trafficking of a mutant HERG potassium channel in human long QT syndrome. Pharmacological and temperature effects. *J. Biol. Chem.* 1999, *274(44)*, 31123–31126.
20. Wible, B. A., Hawryluk, P., Ficker, E., Kuryshev, Y. A., Kirsch, G., and Brown, A. M. HERG-Lite: a novel comprehensive high-throughput screen for drug-induced hERG risk. *J. Pharmacol. Toxicol. Methods* 2005, *52(1)*, 136–145.
21. van der Heyden, M. A., Smits, M. E., and Vos, M. A. Drugs and trafficking of ion channels: a new pro-arrhythmic threat on the horizon? *Br. J. Pharmacol.* 2008, *153(3)*, 406–409.
22. Seebohm, G., Strutz-Seebohm, N., Ureche, O. N., Henrion, U., Baltaev, R., Mack, A. F., Korniychuk, G., Steinke, K., Tapken, D., Pfeufer, A., Kaab, S., Bucci, C., Attali, B., Merot, J., Tavare, J. M., Hoppe, U. C., Sanguinetti, M. C., and Lang, F. Long QT syndrome-associated mutations in KCNQ1 and KCNE1 subunits disrupt normal endosomal recycling of IKs channels. *Circ. Res.* 2008, *103(12)*, 1451–1457.
23. Michael, G., Dempster, J., Kane, K. A., and Coker, S. J. Potentiation of E-4031-induced torsade de pointes by HMR1556 or ATX-II is not predicted by action potential short-term variability or triangulation. *Br. J. Pharmacol.* 2007, *152(8)*, 1215–1227.
24. Towart, R., Linders, J. T., Hermans, A. N., Rohrbacher, J., van der Linde, H. J., Ercken, M., Cik, M., Roevens, P., Teisman, A., and Gallacher, D. J. Blockade of the I(Ks) potassium channel: an overlooked cardiovascular liability in drug safety screening? *J. Pharmacol. Toxicol. Methods* 2009, *60(1)*, 1–10.
25. Trepakova, E. S., Malik, M. G., Imredy, J. P., Penniman, J. R., Dech, S. J., and Salata, J. J. Application of PatchXpress planar patch clamp technology to the screening of new drug candidates for cardiac KCNQ1/KCNE1 (I Ks) activity. *Assay Drug Dev. Technol.* 2007, *5(5)*, 617–627.
26. Imredy, J. P., Penniman, J. R., Dech, S. J., Irving, W. D., and Salata, J. J. Modeling of the adrenergic response of the human IKs current (hKCNQ1/hKCNE1) stably expressed in HEK-293 cells. *Am. J. Physiol. Heart Circ. Physiol.* 2008, *295(5)*, H1867–H1881.

27. Meadows, L. S. and Isom, L. L. Sodium channels as macromolecular complexes: implications for inherited arrhythmia syndromes. *Cardiovasc. Res.* 2005, *67(3)*, 448–458.

28. Medeiros-Domingo, A., Kaku, T., Tester, D. J., Iturralde-Torres, P., Itty, A., Ye, B., Valdivia, C., Ueda, K., Canizales-Quinteros, S., Tusie-Luna, M. T., Makielski, J. C., and Ackerman, M. J. SCN4B-encoded sodium channel beta4 subunit in congenital long-QT syndrome. *Circulation* 2007, *116(2)*, 134–142.

29. Shimizu, W. and Antzelevitch, C. Sodium channel block with mexiletine is effective in reducing dispersion of repolarization and preventing torsade des pointes in LQT2 and LQT3 models of the long-QT syndrome. *Circulation* 1997, *96(6)*, 2038–2047.

30. Feng, X. H., Chen, J. X., Liu, Y., and Ji, Y. H. Electrophysiological characterization of BmK I, an alpha-like scorpion toxin, on rNav1.5 expressed in HEK293t cells. *Toxicol. In Vitro* 2008, *22(6)*, 1582–1587.

31. Richard Benzinger, G., Tonkovich, G. S., and Hanck, D. A. Augmentation of recovery from inactivation by site-3 Na channel toxins. A single-channel and whole-cell study of persistent currents. *J. Gen. Physiol.* 1999, *113(2)*, 333–346.

32. Tsushima, R. G., Kelly, J. E., Salata, J. J., Liberty, K. N., and Wasserstrom, J. A. Modification of cardiac Na(+) current by RWJ 24517 and its enantiomers in guinea pig ventricular myocytes. *J. Pharmacol. Exp. Ther.* 1999, *291(2)*, 845–855.

33. Romey, G., Quast, U., Pauron, D., Frelin, C., Renaud, J. F., and Lazdunski, M. Na + channels as sites of action of the cardioactive agent DPI 201-106 with agonist and antagonist enantiomers. *Proc. Natl. Acad. Sci. USA* 1987, *84(3)*, 896–900.

34. Nilius, B., Benndorf, K., Markwardt, F., and Franke, T. Modulation of single cardiac sodium channels by DPI 201-106, *Gen. Physiol. Biophys.* 1987, *6(5)*, 409–424.

35. Lacerda, A. E., Kuryshev, Y. A., Chen, Y., Renganathan, M., Eng, H., Danthi, S. J., Kramer, J. W., Yang, T., and Brown, A. M. Alfuzosin delays cardiac repolarization by a novel mechanism. *J. Pharmacol. Exp. Ther.* 2008, *324(2)*, 427–433.

36. Xia, M., Imredy, J. P., Koblan, K. S., Bennett, P., and Connolly, T. M. State-dependent inhibition of L-type calcium channels: cell-based assay in high-throughput format. *Anal. Biochem.* 2004, *327(1)*, 74–81.

37. Splawski, I., Timothy, K. W., Sharpe, L. M., Decher, N., Kumar, P., Bloise, R., Napolitano, C., Schwartz, P. J., Joseph, R. M., Condouris, K., Tager-Flusberg, H., Priori, S. G., Sanguinetti, M. C., and Keating, M. T. Ca(V)1.2 calcium channel dysfunction causes a multisystem disorder including arrhythmia and autism. *Cell* 2004, *119(1)*, 19–31.

38. Liu, L., Gonzalez, P. K., Barrett, C. F., and Rittenhouse, A. R. The calcium channel ligand FPL 64176 enhances L-type but inhibits N-type neuronal calcium currents. *Neuropharmacology* 2003, *45(2)*, 281–292.

39. Bechem, M. and Hoffmann, H. The molecular mode of action of the Ca agonist (−) BAY K 8644 on the cardiac Ca channel. *Pflugers Arch.* 1993, *424(3–4)*, 343–53.

40. Bechem, M. and Schramm, M. Calcium-agonists. *J. Mol. Cell Cardiol.* 1987, *19(2)*, 63–75.

41. Lacerda, A. E. and Brown, A. M. Nonmodal gating of cardiac calcium channels as revealed by dihydropyridines. *J. Gen. Physiol.* 1989, *93(6)*, 1243–1273.

42. Sicouri, S., Glass, A., Ferreiro, M., and Antzelevitch, C. Transseptal dispersion of repolarization and its role in the development of torsade de pointes arrhythmias. *J. Cardiovasc. Electrophysiol.* 2009.

43. Cheng, H. C. and Incardona, J. Models of torsades de pointes: effects of FPL64176, DPI201106, dofetilide, and chromanol 293B in isolated rabbit and guinea pig hearts. *J. Pharmacol. Toxicol. Methods* 2009, *60(2)*, 174–184.

44. Hulme, J. T., Westenbroek, R. E., Scheuer, T., and Catterall, W. A. Phosphorylation of serine 1928 in the distal C-terminal domain of cardiac CaV1.2 channels during beta1-adrenergic regulation. *Proc. Natl. Acad. Sci. USA* 2006, *103(44)*, 16574–16579.

45. Balasubramanian, B., Imredy, J. P., Kim, D., Penniman, J., Lagrutta, A., and Salata, J. J. Optimization of Ca(v)1.2 screening with an automated planar patch clamp platform. *J. Pharmacol. Toxicol. Methods* 2009, *59(2)*, 62–72.

46. Nierenberg, D. W. and Ransil, B. J. Q-aTc interval as a clinical indicator of hypercalcemia. *Am. J. Cardiol.* 1979, *44(2)*, 243–248.

47. Karjalainen, J. and Viitasalo, M. Fever and cardiac rhythm. *Arch. Intern. Med.* 1986, *146* (6), 1169–11671.

48. Patel, C. and Antzelevitch, C. Pharmacological approach to the treatment of long and short QT syndromes. *Pharmacol. Ther.* 2008, *118(1)*, 138–151.

49. Kang, J., Chen, X. L., Wang, H., Ji, J., Cheng, H., Incardona, J., Reynolds, W., Viviani, F., Tabart, M., and Rampe, D. Discovery of a small molecule activator of the human ether-a-go-go-related gene (HERG) cardiac K^+ channel. *Mol. Pharmacol.* 2005, *67(3)*, 827–836.

50. Hansen, R. S., Diness, T. G., Christ, T., Demnitz, J., Ravens, U., Olesen, S. P., and Grunnet, M. Activation of human ether-a-go-go-related gene potassium channels by the diphenylurea 1, 3-bis-(2-hydroxy-5-trifluoromethyl-phenyl)-urea (NS1643). *Mol. Pharmacol.* 2006, *69(1)*, 266–277.

51. Hansen, R. S., Diness, T. G., Christ, T., Wettwer, E., Ravens, U., Olesen, S. P., and Grunnet, M. Biophysical characterization of the new human ether-a-go-go-related gene channel opener NS3623 [*N*-(4-bromo-2-(1H-tetrazol-5-yl)-phenyl)-N'-(3'-trifluoromethylphenyl)urea]. *Mol. Pharmacol.* 2006, *70(4)*, 1319–1329.

52. Zhou, J., Augelli-Szafran, C. E., Bradley, J. A., Chen, X., Koci, B. J., Volberg, W. A., Sun, Z., and Cordes, J. S. Novel potent human ether-a-go-go-related gene (hERG) potassium channel enhancers and their in vitro antiarrhythmic activity. *Mol. Pharmacol.* 2005, *68(3)*, 876–884.

53. Zeng, H., Lozinskaya, I. M., Lin, Z., Willette, R. N., Brooks, D. P., and Xu, X. Mallotoxin is a novel human ether-a-go-go-related gene (hERG) potassium channel activator. *J. Pharmacol. Exp. Ther.* 2006, *319(2)*, 957–962.

54. Perry, M., Sachse, F. B., Abbruzzese, J., and Sanguinetti, M. C. PD-118057 contacts the pore helix of hERG1 channels to attenuate inactivation and enhance K^+ conductance. *Proc. Natl. Acad. Sci. USA* 2009, *106(47)*, 20075–20080.

55. Ehrlich, J. R. Inward rectifier potassium currents as a target for atrial fibrillation therapy. *J. Cardiovasc. Pharmacol.* 2008, *52(2)*, 129–135.

56. Robert, E., Delye, B., Aya, G., Peray, P., Juan, J. M., Sassine, A., de La Coussaye, J. E., and Eledjam, J. J. Comparison of proarrhythmogenic effects of two potassium channel openers, levcromakalim (BRL 38227) and nicorandil (RP 46417): a high-resolution mapping study on rabbit heart. *J. Cardiovasc. Pharmacol.* 1997, *29(1)*, 109–118.

57. Milberg, P., Tegelkamp, R., Osada, N., Schimpf, R., Wolpert, C., Breithardt, G., Borggrefe, M., and Eckardt, L. Reduction of dispersion of repolarization and prolongation

of postrepolarization refractoriness explain the antiarrhythmic effects of quinidine in a model of short QT syndrome. *J. Cardiovasc. Electrophysiol.* 2007, *18(6)*, 658–664.

58. Shimomura, K., Girard, C. A., Proks, P., Nazim, J., Lippiat, J. D., Cerutti, F., Lorini, R., Ellard, S., Hattersley, A. T., Barbetti, F., and Ashcroft, F. M. Mutations at the same residue (R50) of Kir6.2 (KCNJ11) that cause neonatal diabetes produce different functional effects. *Diabetes* 2006, *55(6)*, 1705–1712.

59. D'Avanzo, N., Cheng, W. W., Xia, X., Dong, L., Savitsky, P., Nichols, C. G., and Doyle, D. A. Expression and purification of recombinant human inward rectifier K(+) (KCNJ) channels in *Saccharomyces cerevisiae*. *Protein Expr. Purif.* 2010.

60. Priori, S. G., Napolitano, C., Tiso, N., Memmi, M., Vignati, G., Bloise, R., Sorrentino, V., and Danieli, G. A. Mutations in the cardiac ryanodine receptor gene (hRyR2) underlie catecholaminergic polymorphic ventricular tachycardia. *Circulation* 2001, *103(2)*, 196–200.

61. Pasquie, J. L. and Richard, S. Prolongation in QT interval is not predictive of Ca^{2+}-dependent arrhythmias: implications for drug safety. *Expert Opin. Drug Saf.* 2009, *8(1)*, 57–72.

62. Ekins, S., Crumb, W. J., Sarazan, R. D., Wikel, J. H., and Wrighton, S. A. Three-dimensional quantitative structure–activity relationship for inhibition of human ether-a-go-go-related gene potassium channel. *J. Pharmacol. Exp. Ther.* 2002, *301(2)*, 427–434.

63. Cavalli, A., Poluzzi, E., De Ponti, F., and Recanatini, M. Toward a pharmacophore for drugs inducing the long QT syndrome: insights from a CoMFA study of HERG K(+) channel blockers. *J. Med. Chem.* 2002, *45(18)*, 3844–3853.

64. Gavaghan, C. L., Arnby, C. H., Blomberg, N., Strandlund, G., and Boyer, S. Development, interpretation and temporal evaluation of a global QSAR of hERG electrophysiology screening data. *J. Comput. Aided Mol. Des.* 2007, *21(4)*, 189–206.

65. Kolossov, E., Bostani, T., Roell, W., Breitbach, M., Pillekamp, F., Nygren, J. M., Sasse, P., Rubenchik, O., Fries, J. W., Wenzel, D., Geisen, C., Xia, Y., Lu, Z., Duan, Y., Kettenhofen, R., Jovinge, S., Bloch, W., Bohlen, H., Welz, A., Hescheler, J., Jacobsen, S. E., and Fleischmann, B. K. Engraftment of engineered ES cell-derived cardiomyocytes but not BM cells restores contractile function to the infarcted myocardium. *J. Exp. Med.* 2006, *203(10)*, 2315–2127.

66. Choy, N., Davis, A., Brugger, S., and Liang, S. The Sixth Annual Ion Channel Retreat Vancouver, Canada, June 23-25 2008. *Assay Drug Dev. Technol.* 2008 *6(6)*, 759–764.

67. Kettenhofen, R. Pluripotent Stem Cell-derived Cardiomyocytes as Suitable Substrates For Automated Ion Channel and Electrophysiological Analysis Systems, in *The Seventh Annual Ion Channel Retreat*. 2009, Vancouver.

68. Takahashi, K. and Yamanaka, S. Induction of pluripotent stem cells from mouse embryonic and adult fibroblast cultures by defined factors. *Cell* 2006, *126(4)*, 663–676.

69. Yu, J., Vodyanik, M. A., Smuga-Otto, K., Antosiewicz-Bourget, J., Frane, J. L., Tian, S., Nie, J., Jonsdottir, G. A., Ruotti, V., Stewart, R., Slukvin, I. I., and Thomson, J. A. Induced pluripotent stem cell lines derived from human somatic cells. *Science* 2007, *318(5858)*, 1917–1920.

70. Hondeghem, L. M. and Hoffmann, P. Blinded test in isolated female rabbit heart reliably identifies action potential duration prolongation and proarrhythmic drugs: importance of

triangulation, reverse use dependence, and instability. *J. Cardiovasc. Pharmacol.* 2003, *41(1)*, 14–24.

71. Swain, S. M., Whaley, F. S., and Ewer, M. S. Congestive heart failure in patients treated with doxorubicin: a retrospective analysis of three trials. *Cancer* 2003, *97(11)*, 2869–2879.
72. Minotti, G., Menna, P., Salvatorelli, E., Cairo, G., and Gianni, L. Anthracyclines: molecular advances and pharmacologic developments in antitumor activity and cardiotoxicity. *Pharmacol. Rev.* 2004, *56(2)*, 185–229.
73. Bruynzeel, A. M., Abou El Hassan, M. A., Torun, E., Bast, A., van der Vijgh, W. J., and Kruyt, F. A. Caspase-dependent and -independent suppression of apoptosis by monoHER in Doxorubicin treated cells. *Br. J. Cancer* 2007, *96(3)*, 450–456.
74. Safra, T. Cardiac safety of liposomal anthracyclines. *Oncologist* 2003, *8(2)*, 17–24.
75. Jones, R. L. and Ewer, M. S. Cardiac and cardiovascular toxicity of nonanthracycline anticancer drugs. *Expert Rev. Anticancer Ther.* 2006, *6(9)*, 1249–1269.
76. Force, T. and Kerkela, R. Cardiotoxicity of the new cancer therapeutics--mechanisms of, and approaches to, the problem. *Drug Discov. Today* 2008, *13(17–18)*, 778–784.
77. Wallace, K. B., Hausner, E., Herman, E., Holt, G. D., MacGregor, J. T., Metz, A. L., Murphy, E., Rosenblum, I. Y., Sistare, F. D., and York, M. J. Serum troponins as biomarkers of drug-induced cardiac toxicity. *Toxicol. Pathol.* 2004, *32(1)*, 106–121.
78. Wu, K. C. and Lima, J. A. Noninvasive imaging of myocardial viability: current techniques and future developments. *Circ. Res.* 2003, *93(12)*, 1146–1158.
79. Dulce, M. C., Mostbeck, G. H., Friese, K. K., Caputo, G. R., and Higgins, C. B. Quantification of the left ventricular volumes and function with cine MR imaging: comparison of geometric models with three-dimensional data. *Radiology* 1993, *188(2)*, 371–376.
80. Jaffer, F. A. and Weissleder, R. Seeing within: molecular imaging of the cardiovascular system. *Circ. Res.* 2004, *94(4)*, 433–445.
81. Horn, M. Cardiac magnetic resonance spectroscopy: a window for studying physiology. *Methods Mol. Med.* 2006, *124*, 225–248.
82. Chacko, V. P., Aresta, F., Chacko, S. M., and Weiss, R. G. MRI/MRS assessment of in vivo murine cardiac metabolism, morphology, and function at physiological heart rates. *Am. J. Physiol. Heart Circ. Physiol.* 2000, *279(5)*, H2218–H2224.
83. Biomarkers and surrogate endpoints: preferred definitions and conceptual framework. *Clin. Pharmacol. Ther.* 2001, *69(3)*, 89–95.
84. Collinson, P. O. and Gaze, D. C. Biomarkers of cardiovascular damage and dysfunction—an overview. *Heart Lung Circ.* 2007, *16(3)*, S71–S82.
85. Farah, C. S. and Reinach, F. C. The troponin complex and regulation of muscle contraction. *FASEB J.* 1995, *9(9)*, 755–767.
86. Collinson, P. O., Boa, F. G., and Gaze, D. C. Measurement of cardiac troponins. *Ann. Clin. Biochem.* 2001, *38(5)*, 423–449.
87. Myocardial infarction redefined—a consensus document of The Joint European Society of Cardiology/American College of Cardiology Committee for the redefinition of myocardial infarction. *Eur. Heart J.* 2000, *21(18)*, 1502–1513.
88. O'Brien, P. J. Cardiac troponin is the most effective translational safety biomarker for myocardial injury in cardiotoxicity. *Toxicology* 2008, *245(3)*, 206–218.

89. O'Brien, P. J., Smith, D. E., Knechtel, T. J., Marchak, M. A., Pruimboom-Brees, I., Brees, D. J., Spratt, D. P., Archer, F. J., Butler, P., Potter, A. N., Provost, J. P., Richard, J., Snyder, P. A., and Reagan, W. J. Cardiac troponin I is a sensitive, specific biomarker of cardiac injury in laboratory animals. *Lab. Anim.* 2006, *40(2)*, 153–171.

90. Heavner, J. E. Cardiac toxicity of local anesthetics in the intact isolated heart model: a review. *Reg. Anesth. Pain Med.* 2002, *27(6)*, 545–555.

91. Skrzypiec-Spring, M., Grotthus, B., Szelag, A., and Schulz, R. Isolated heart perfusion according to Langendorff—still viable in the new millennium. *J. Pharmacol. Toxicol. Methods* 2007, *55(2)*, 113–126.

92. Mocanu, M. M., Baxter, G. F., and Yellon, D. M. Caspase inhibition and limitation of myocardial infarct size: protection against lethal reperfusion injury. *Br. J. Pharmacol.* 2000, *130(2)*, 197–200.

93. Platel, D., Pouna, P., Bonoron-Adele, S., and Robert, J. Comparative cardiotoxicity of idarubicin and doxorubicin using the isolated perfused rat heart model. *Anticancer Drugs* 1999, *10(7)*, 671–676.

94. Woodcock, E. A. and Matkovich, S. J. Cardiomyocytes structure, function and associated pathologies. *Int. J. Biochem. Cell Biol.* 2005, *37(9)*, 1746–1751.

95. Hescheler, J., Meyer, R., Plant, S., Krautwurst, D., Rosenthal, W., and Schultz, G. Morphological, biochemical, and electrophysiological characterization of a clonal cell (H9c2) line from rat heart. *Circ. Res.* 1991, *69(6)*, 1476–1486.

96. Wang, Y. C., Neckelmann, N., Mayne, A., Herskowitz, A., Srinivasan, A., Sell, K. W., and Ahmed-Ansari, A. Establishment of a human fetal cardiac myocyte cell line. *In Vitro Cell Dev. Biol.* 1991, *27(1)*, 63–74.

97. Tytgat, J. How to isolate cardiac myocytes. *Cardiovasc. Res.* 1994, *28(2)*, 280–283.

98. White, S. M., Constantin, P. E., and Claycomb, W. C. Cardiac physiology at the cellular level: use of cultured HL-1 cardiomyocytes for studies of cardiac muscle cell structure and function. *Am. J. Physiol. Heart Circ. Physiol.* 2004, *286(3)*, H823–H829.

99. Nag, A. C. and Cheng, M. Biochemical evidence for cellular dedifferentiation in adult rat cardiac muscle cells in culture: expression of myosin isozymes. *Biochem. Biophys. Res. Commun.* 1986, *137(2)*, 855–862.

100. Doetschman, T. C., Eistetter, H., Katz, M., Schmidt, W., and Kemler, R. The in vitro development of blastocyst-derived embryonic stem cell lines: formation of visceral yolk sac, blood islands and myocardium. *J. Embryol. Exp. Morphol.* 1985, *87*, 27–45.

101. Itskovitz-Eldor, J., Schuldiner, M., Karsenti, D., Eden, A., Yanuka, O., Amit, M., Soreq, H., and Benvenisty, N. Differentiation of human embryonic stem cells into embryoid bodies compromising the three embryonic germ layers. *Mol. Med.* 2000, *6 (2)*, 88–95.

102. Thomson, J. A., Itskovitz-Eldor, J., Shapiro, S. S., Waknitz, M. A., Swiergiel, J. J., Marshall, V. S., and Jones, J. M. Embryonic stem cell lines derived from human blastocysts. *Science* 1998, *282(5391)*, 1145–1147.

103. Davila, J. C., Cezar, G. G., Thiede, M., Strom, S., Miki, T., and Trosko, J. Use and application of stem cells in toxicology. *Toxicol. Sci.* 2004, *79(2)*, 214–223.

104. Kettenhofen, R. and Bohlen, H. Preclinical assessment of cardiac toxicity. *Drug Discov. Today* 2008, *13(15–16)*, 702–707.

105. McNeish, J. Embryonic stem cells in drug discovery. *Nat. Rev. Drug Discov.* 2004, *3(1)*, 70–80.

106. An, D., Kewalramani, G., Chan, J. K., Qi, D., Ghosh, S., Pulinilkunnil, T., Abrahani, A., Innis, S. M., and Rodrigues, B. Metformin influences cardiomyocyte cell death by pathways that are dependent and independent of caspase-3. *Diabetologia* 2006, *49(9)*, 2174–2184.

107. Braam, S. R., Tertoolen, L., van de Stolpe, A., Meyer, T., Passier, R., and Mummery, C. L. Prediction of drug-induced cardiotoxicity using human embryonic stem cell-derived cardiomyocytes. *Stem Cell Res.* 2010, *4(2)*, 107–1016.

108. Cainarca, S., Fenu, S., Ferri, C., Nucci, C., Arioli, P., Menegon, A., Piemonti, L., Lohmer, S., Wrabetz, L., and Corazza, S. A photoprotein in mouse embryonic stem cells measures Ca^{2+} mobilization in cells and in animals. *PLoS One* 2010, *5(1)*, e8882.

109. Farokhpour, M., Karbalaie, K., Tanhaei, S., Nematollahi, M., Etebari, M., Sadeghi, H. M., Nasr-Esfahani, M. H., and Baharvand, H. Embryonic stem cell-derived cardiomyocytes as a model system to study cardioprotective effects of dexamethasone in doxorubicin cardiotoxicity. *Toxicol. In Vitro* 2009, *23(7)*, 1422–1428.

110. Pouton, C. W. and Haynes, J. M. Embryonic stem cells as a source of models for drug discovery. *Nat. Rev. Drug Discov.* 2007, *6(8)*, 605–616.

111. Dykens, J. A. and Will, Y. The significance of mitochondrial toxicity testing in drug development. *Drug Discov. Today* 2007, *12(17–18)*, 777–785.

112. Wallace, K. B. Doxorubicin-induced cardiac mitochondrionopathy. *Pharmacol. Toxicol.* 2003, *93(3)*, 105–115.

113. Jendrossek, V., Handrick, R., and Belka, C. Celecoxib activates a novel mitochondrial apoptosis signaling pathway. *FASEB J.* 2003, *17(11)*, 1547–1549.

114. Brunmair, B., Staniek, K., Gras, F., Scharf, N., Althaym, A., Clara, R., Roden, M., Gnaiger, E., Nohl, H., Waldhausl, W., and Furnsinn, C. Thiazolidinediones, like metformin, inhibit respiratory complex I: a common mechanism contributing to their antidiabetic actions? *Diabetes* 2004, *53(4)*, 1052–1059.

115. Arnaudo, E., Dalakas, M., Shanske, S., Moraes, C. T., DiMauro, S., and Schon, E. A. Depletion of muscle mitochondrial DNA in AIDS patients with zidovudine-induced myopathy. *Lancet* 1991, *337(8740)*, 508–510.

116. Hynes, J., Marroquin, L. D., Ogurtsov, V. I., Christiansen, K. N., Stevens, G. J., Papkovsky, D. B., and Will, Y. Investigation of drug-induced mitochondrial toxicity using fluorescence-based oxygen-sensitive probes. *Toxicol. Sci.* 2006, *92(1)*, 186–200.

117. Krause, M. M., Brand, M. D., Krauss, S., Meisel, C., Vergin, H., Burmester, G. R., and Buttgereit, F. Nonsteroidal antiinflammatory drugs and a selective cyclooxygenase 2 inhibitor uncouple mitochondria in intact cells. *Arthritis Rheum.* 2003, *48(5)*, 1438–1444.

118. Nadanaciva, S., Bernal, A., Aggeler, R., Capaldi, R., and Will, Y. Target identification of drug induced mitochondrial toxicity using immunocapture based OXPHOS activity assays. *Toxicol. In Vitro* 2007, *21(5)*, 902–911.

119. Tokarska-Schlattner, M., Lucchinetti, E., Zaugg, M., Kay, L., Gratia, S., Guzun, R., Saks, V. A., and Schlattner, U. Early effects of doxorubicin in perfused heart: transcriptional profiling reveals inhibition of cellular stress response genes. *Am. J. Physiol. Regul. Integr. Comp. Physiol.* 2010, *298*, R1075–R1088.

120. Gerencser, A. A., Neilson, A., Choi, S. W., Edman, U., Yadava, N., Oh, R. J., Ferrick, D. A., Nicholls, D. G., and Brand, M. D. Quantitative microplate-based respirometry with correction for oxygen diffusion. *Anal. Chem.* 2009, *81*, 6868–6878.
121. Will, Y., Hynes, J., Ogurtsov, V. I., and Papkovsky, D. B. Analysis of mitochondrial function using phosphorescent oxygen-sensitive probes. *Nat. Protoc.* 2006, *1(6)*, 2563–2472.

7

GENETIC TOXICITY: *IN VITRO* APPROACHES FOR MEDICINAL CHEMISTS

RICHARD M. WALMSLEY AND DAVID ELDER

7.1 INTRODUCTION

7.1.1 Scope of this Chapter

Positive genetic toxicity data in preclinical development can terminate the development path of a compound. Although this should be a very rare occurrence, at present it occurs for 10–15% of compounds. Currently genotoxicity assessment mostly is conducted by preclinical safety assessment experts, who perform labor-intensive assays on very small numbers of compounds. However, it is now possible to envisage a situation in which the potent genotoxins are identified by high-throughput assays and even computer programs similar to other ADME/Tox liabilities. The increasing appearance of publications that discuss genotoxicity in an earlier screening context reflects a growing willingness to consider genotoxicity hazard assessment early in the discovery process.

This chapter explains why failure due to genotoxic hazard in safety assessment should, and could, be reduced to 2% or lower if genotoxicity assessment were a part of routine hit-to-lead and lead optimization screening. A basic introduction to the fundamentals, mechanisms, and practices of genetic toxicology is provided, along with brief descriptions of the regulatory GLP assays and the newer pre-GLP screening methods. The chemistry of genotoxins and the use of *in silico* methods for the prediction of genotoxicity are reviewed. Some examples of approaches to genotoxicity issues are provided. Finally, the current guidelines for regulatory genotoxicity

ADMET for Medicinal Chemists: A Practical Guide, Edited by Katya Tsaioun and Steven A. Kates

assessment are discussed along with the prospects for change in the future, and how these might affect screening strategies.

7.1.2 Definitions

For the purposes of this chapter, genotoxins are defined as agents that cause genome damage. This damage includes all quantifiable changes in DNA base sequence (mutagenesis), chromosome number (aneugenesis), and chromosome content (translocation) as well as single- and double-strand DNA breaks (clastogenesis). Direct damage to DNA may be caused by a compound, or its metabolic product, reacting or interacting with DNA, either to form adducts or through subsequent processing to alter a DNA base, etc. Indirect damage is a consequence of interference with either the enzymes associated with DNA replication and repair, or with the ordered segregation of chromosomes during mitosis. The term "indirect damage" can also apply to processes which lead to the generation of reactive oxygen species, which can damage DNA. Some authors use the term "indirect acting agents," to describe promutagens/progenotoxins—compounds which become genotoxins following metabolism—but for this chapter the former is used. To detect these many different types of DNA/genome damage, a variety of methods have evolved. In this chapter, these will be considered in terms of their utility as early screening methods.

Early in the development of this field, there was an assumption that if a compound was a carcinogen, then any dose would pose a hazard. However, it has become clear that for some compounds there is a threshold dose, up to which there is no hazard. This is particularly important in the assessment of pharmaceutical safety. If a compound is pharmacologically active at a very low dose, but has been shown to carry a genotoxic liability threshold, it might be argued successfully that the intended dose and exposure for the patient are acceptable.

Sensitivity, specificity, and concordance are the terms most frequently used to define the performance of the genotoxicity assays. Sensitivity is defined as the proportion of *in vivo* genotoxins or genotoxic carcinogens, which give a positive result in an assay. Specificity is defined as the proportion of noncarcinogens, which give a negative result in an assay. Concordance is defined as the overall proportion of correct positive and negative results obtained. In order to compare figures for concordance between different assays, there should either be approximately equal numbers of positive and negative compounds in the studies, or results from the same collection should be compared.

7.1.3 Positive Genotoxicity Data is not Uncommon and Very Costly

A recent study reported that serious safety concerns arise from genotoxicity in about 15% of drug candidates [1]. Such compounds might be abandoned, writing off the huge expenses of discovery and early development. However, the prevalence of misleading positive *in vitro* genotoxicity results, discussed later in this chapter, indicates that compounds with positive data can often be taken safely to market providing that there is an adequate risk-benefit balance for the patient. The costs of additional animal studies that might assure human safety are dwarfed by the costs of delayed clinical trials —and even these costs become insignificant, compared with the loss of revenue from delays to market. The extent of these problems is reflected in the US Physicians Desk Reference [2], where about 25% of compounds have adverse genotoxicity labeling [3]. These have been taken to market for nonlife threatening therapies because the observed genotoxicity was not found to present hazard to humans. These include Acyclovir (over the counter antiviral), Citalopram (antidepressant), Claritin (over the counter antiallergy), Griseofulvin (antifungal), theophylline (bronchodilator), and Zolmitriptan (antimigraine medicine). There are currently efforts from many international agencies to address the "false positive" problem and these issues are also addressed in this chapter.

7.1.4 Why Genome Damage is Undesirable

The genome stores information encoded by DNA. Compounds which cause corruption in either the information itself or the control of its use can lead to serious illnesses including cancer and inherited susceptibility to illness. Genetic toxicologists are concerned with the identification of such genotoxic compounds and the mechanism by which they exert their effects. In general, and in this chapter, the focus is on those compounds that either directly or indirectly causes alteration to the genome sequence and organization. There are also semipermanent changes in gene expression, which can be linked to local changes in the normal patterns of DNA and histone modification, as well as epigenetic changes, or the expression of interfering microRNA molecules. Compounds that affect such changes are often nongenotoxic carcinogens. This latter class is less well understood and is currently not part of the genetic toxicologist's domain. The reader is referred to a recent review [4].

7.1.5 The Inherent Integrity of the Genome and its Inevitable Corruption

During physiological development, information in the genome is used to control cell division and differentiation into different tissue/cell types. This differentiation is a consequence of the selective activation and inactivation of genes. Selective cell killing/suicide or apoptosis is also programmed part of development, and occurs during such diverse processes as neuron development and the separation of fingers and toes. However, apoptosis is also part of the evolved response to overwhelming DNA damage. This is perhaps the most extreme, but most effective limitation to the potentially harmful overaccumulation of mutations during the natural life span.

There are some evolved exceptions to conservation of sequence. These exceptions are found within the cells of the immune system, the germ cells of the ovary and testis, and at the telomeres, the ends of the chromosomes. Cells in the immune system have evolved to deliberately shuffle subsets of information, generating diversity in the antibodies that protect the body from a variety of exogenous agents. During meiosis, the germ cells make different combinations of the diverse maternal and paternal genes that came together in the individual. This process allows the segregation of genuinely new information sets, and hence diversity in subsequent generations. The ends of chromosomal DNA molecules are protected by the repetitive DNA sequences of the telomere and their associated proteins. Telomeres shorten with age, and eventually lose their protective properties. This leads to cell death, which contributes critically to the aging process. At approximately 52 sequential cell divisions, most cells lose the ability to divide further.

During active cell division, individual cells will steadily accumulate random mutations. These will arise from the rare errors in DNA replication prior to cell division, as well from the oxidative DNA damage caused by the reactive oxygen species generated by the dependence on oxidative metabolism. These are unavoidable hazards which contribute to the overall risk of cancer. Toxin-induced cell damage and cell death lead to extra cell divisions to replace lost tissue, so repeated or long-term exposure to a variety of poisons leads to increased accumulation of random mutations caused by increased cell division. The longer a human lives, the more errors accumulate, and the increased likelihood of corrupting the genes which ensure that proper cell division occurs. This is part of the reason for the increased incidence of tumors found in populations as the average age at death increases. There is essentially no selection against age-related diseases that emerge postreproductively.

7.1.6 Many Chemicals can Cause Cancer, but do not Pose a Significant Risk to Humans

There are a few well-known and often avoidable genotoxic hazards. For example, ionizing radiation and ultraviolet radiation both increase the incidence of genome damage and tumorigenesis. However, there are countless less well-known hazards, including the almost countless xenobiotics that humans inhale, eat, and drink. It is not uncommon to read of the genotoxicity of common food from bread and chips (French fries) to barbequed meat. It has been estimated that a human consumes gram quantities of genotoxins every day [5], though as with any potential poison, the actual risk is a function of dose/exposure. The carcinogenicity potency data base [6] shows that nearly 70% of all natural and synthetic compounds that have been tested are rodent carcinogens. However, for most of these compounds, it would be difficult for a human to consume the same dose that caused tumors in the rodents. For many, the additional cell divisions caused by high toxic doses in early LD_{50} studies were presumably the reason for the observed tumors rather than genotoxic effects.

7.1.7 The False Positives: Many Chemicals Produce Positive Genotoxicity Data that are neither Carcinogens nor *In Vivo* Genotoxins

Most of the current *in vitro* mammalian assays were developed for late-stage safety assessment, with full appreciation of the limitations in nonanimal systems. For many years there was an emphasis on developing high sensitivity without corresponding attention to specificity. The result has been the establishment of tests generating a high prevalence of positive data, within collections of noncarcinogens as well as carcinogens. As previously noted, about 25% of pharmaceuticals in Physicians Desk Reference, registered for use with clinical indications, excluding antineoplastic and antiviral drugs, have positive data from *in vitro* mammalian genotoxicity tests. The positive results were concluded not to be relevant to humans. Subsequent studies of data from both drug submissions [7] and other chemicals in the public domain [8]

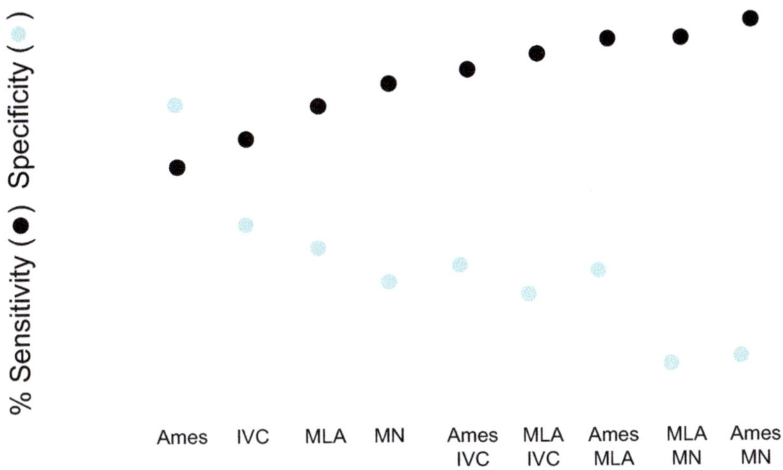

Figure 7.1 The sensitivity and specificity of the *in vitro* regulatory tests in the prediction of rodent carcinogenicity. Upper dark circles, sensitivity; lower light circles, specificity; IVC, *in vitro* chromosome aberration; MLA, mouse lymphoma assay; MN, micronucleus test.

reveal the same pattern. It is clear that while the Ames test and *in vivo* chromosome aberration assessments have high specificity, the *in vitro* mammalian tests for mutation and chromosome aberration have poor specificity. These tests produce misleading positive results for many noncarcinogens (Figure 7.1, derived from data in Ref. 8). Perhaps the most alarming statistic to emerge from that study was that the most frequently used combination of the Ames test and the micronucleus test, produced twin negative results for only 5% of noncarcinogens. At the regulatory level, this problem has been recognized in proposed revisions to the ICH S2 guidance [9], which include a new option for the registration of new pharmaceuticals whereby the Ames test is the only required *in vitro* assay (Table 7.1). The implications for this are discussed in Section 7.5. Fortunately, recognition of the poor specificity problem has also stimulated assay developers to improve the methodologies for existing tests and to develop new high-specificity tests. These are addressed in later sections.

7.1.8 Defense Against Genotoxic Damage

The hazards associated with exposure to genome-damaging agents are met by highly evolved and largely conserved cellular mechanisms for the recognition of damage, and its repair. These involve the repair of double-strand breaks by recombinational repair or nonhomologous endjoining, as well as base excision and nucleotide excision repair for damage that does not cause breakage. The detection of DNA damage also triggers a delay in cell division so that repair can be completed before chromosomes are segregated. If these processes are overwhelmed, apoptosis (programmed cell death, or cell suicide) may be triggered. Damage/change to the genes encoding the proteins of DNA repair active in these processes can also lead to tumorigenesis.

TABLE 7.1 Comparison of Current and Proposed Revised ICH Guidelines

	ICH S2 (R1)	
ICH S2B	Option 1	Option 2
Ames and repeat 5 mg per plate	Ames one complete assay Tested to first precipitating dose	Ames one complete assay Tested to first precipitating dose
In vitro mammalian cell assay	*In vitro* mammalian cell assay	No *in vitro* mammalian assay
Chromosome aberrations, OR *tk* mutations in mouse lymphoma cells	Chromosome aberrations, OR *tk* mutations in mouse lymphoma cells OR *in vitro* micronucleus assay	
10 mM	1 mM or 0.5 mg/mL top concentration	
In vivo cytogenetic assay	*In vivo* cytogenetic assay integrated into 28 day rodent toxicity study, provided it is adequate to support clinical trials and sampling within a day of last day of dosing	*In vivo* cytogenetic assay and a second *in vivo* endpoint, integrated with 28 day rodent assay and first *in vivo* endpoint if possible

There are also the more generic metabolic responses to xenobiotics. These are generally described as mechanistically distinct phases, though there may be quite complex reactions involving both phases. In Phase 1, oxidative reactions catalyzed by the cytochrome P450 monooxygenase enzymes, may activate target molecules. The resulting molecules may be more reactive and/or genotoxic than the original compound. In Phase 2, the Phase 1 oxidation products are conjugated, for example, to glutathione, glucuronic acid, or to acyl, methyl, or sulfate groups. Xenobiotics that are themselves oxidative may be conjugated directly by Phase 2 enzymes. These products may then be targeted for exclusion by the kidneys.

Humans are diverse, and each individual's genome contains unique variations, which might occur in the genes encoding the enzymes of DNA replication, repair, or the genes encoding the metabolic enzymes of xenobiotic defense. These variations can affect our susceptibility to genotoxin-induced illnesses, and the identification of such variations is just one of the challenges for personalized medicine. This is of particular significance when the treatment of a life-threatening disease might involve the use of genotoxic chemicals.

7.1.9 Mechanisms of Genotoxic Damage

The chemistry of genotoxins is diverse, and discussed in a later section. However, the underlying mechanisms of direct DNA damage are limited—DNA is a fairly homogeneous target.

Oxidative damage can modify bases, particularly guanine. Modified bases that are not excised can lead to replication errors due to failures in base pairing. Oxidative damage can also cause DNA double-strand breaks (clastogenesis).

Intrinsic, programmed alkylation of DNA is a normal frequent phenomenon. However, inappropriate alkylation of bases such as methylation can lead to replication errors and mutation. Repair of methylated bases can also lead to single-strand breaks, which can become double-strand breaks during replication.

Hydrolysis of bases can lead to depurination, depyrimidination, and deamination, which in turn can lead to error prone repair and mutation/damage.

The covalent linking of xenobiotic molecules to DNA, adduct formation, is often associated with their conversion to reactive molecules by metabolism. The cytochrome P450 monooxygenase enzymes are particularly active in this respect. Adducts that are not removed can also lead to collapse of replication forks and replication errors.

Proteins provide many indirect targets for genotoxins. Interference or inhibition of the enzymes of DNA metabolism, including those required for replication, repair, and precursor supply as well as the topoisomerase enzymes, can lead to mutation or clastogenesis depending on the target. Interference with proteins of the mitotic machinery, for example, tubulins that are polymerized and repolymerized during the functioning of the mitotic spindle apparatus, can lead to loss of chromosome attachment, missegregation, and aneugenesis.

7.1.10 Genotoxicity Assessment Occurs after Medicinal Chemistry Optimization

Until recently, genotoxicity has been conducted during preclinical safety assessment where GLP test results are generated for regulatory submission. This is often preceded by relatively small scale screening exercises with a subset of compounds (~25) from a discovery program. The compound collection represents a limited number of chemistries. The screen reduces the number of compounds to a main candidate and a backup in the same chemistry as well as an example from a different chemistry. These screens are usually streamlined, pre-GLP versions of the regulatory assays. The results provide some basic mechanistic classification for safety assessment of a drug candidate (mutagen, clastogen, or aneugen). At this stage in a development program, active chemical optimization by medicinal chemists has been completed. In the earlier screening stage of a program, generally a broader chemical space is considered. More importantly, it is still possible then to engineer chemical modifications during hit-to-lead and lead optimization phases.

If there was genetic toxicology hazard information during earlier phases of active chemistry, then routine strategies could be implemented to separate useful pharmacology from a genotoxic hazard. Instead, the discovery of genotoxicity during preclinical safety assessment leads to either abandonment of the candidate (or a whole program) or additional mechanistic studies and *in vivo* testing to better evaluate human risk. The costs of these studies are high, but dwarfed by the costs of delay in bringing a product to market. For these reasons, it appears to be valuable to obtain genotoxicity data early in discovery, to ensure that candidate pharmaceuticals carry a low risk of genotoxicity failure during preclinical safety assessment.

7.2 LIMITATIONS IN THE REGULATORY *IN VITRO* GENOTOXICITY TESTS

Aside from the confounding effects of poor specificity, there are other practical and technical limits to the data that genetic toxicology can supply for the medicinal chemist. They require hundreds of milligrams of compound, are labor-intensive and time-consuming. These alone serve as significant barriers to their use in screening. However, there are also limitations to their biological utility. These and other challenges are explored below.

7.2.1 Biology Limitations of *In Vitro* Tests

Bacterial and mammalian cells can both produce viable models for the identification of direct-acting genotoxins. Bacteria are prokaryotes and provide a less complete model for the detection of indirect agents and aneugens that are expected to affect human or eukaryotic cells. Prokaryotic cells lack the membrane-bound nucleus of the eukaryotes, have less complex packaging of DNA and have a single circular chromosome. Together these properties have led to the evolution of structurally different enzymes that interact with DNA, compared with the multiple linear chromosomes in eukaryotes and their more complex chromatin. Agents that affect replication, recombination, and repair of DNA in bacteria might not have similar effects in mammals. Bacteria also lack mitosis, the conservative segregation of replicated chromosomes during cell division, and meiosis. They are therefore deficient in the detection of important events in the development of cancer, including karyotype instability and aneugenesis. Finally, the mechanisms for chemical defense have followed evolutionarily different pressures between the free-living bacteria and the often more protected metazoan eukaryotic cells. This is partially reflected by differences in xenobiotic metabolism that can impact on the relevance of genotoxicity results from different species.

Even within the eukaryotes, different evolutionary paths indicate that individual targets for particular genotoxic compounds are not present in all cell types, or even in all mammals. The corollary to this is that no single test is effective in the identification of all genotoxins. For pharmaceutical safety assessment, *Homo sapiens* is the species of interest, but genetic toxicologists are ultimately constrained by the use of different animal models. These models do not always reproduce human patterns of tumor development and chemical sensitivity. As a result, broader differences in drug absorption, receptor distribution, distribution, excretion, and metabolism are obtained (Chapter 4). The assessment of metabolites often requires complex preclinical studies, and cell-based assays are not particularly effective in reproducing the *in vivo* metabolism of the human liver or other tissues. The rodent S9 liver extracts used as an exogenous source of metabolism are incomplete metabolic surrogates and their properties are inappropriate for handling on an automated HTS no need of the expanded form platform.

7.2.2 Hazard and Safety Assessment have Different Requirements

The need to use more than one test is not a problem when assessing low numbers of compounds. However, in larger scale screening exercises when there are still perhaps thousands of hits, a reliable positive hazard result from just one assay (i.e., a positive result that is predictive of *in vivo* genotoxicity/carcinogenicity) can be extremely valuable. It can trigger a round of chemistry development, or be used as an attrition tool. Breadth of chemistry and clinical indication dictate the choice of leads in a discovery campaign. Any drug discovery program needs the genotoxicity hazard screening assays with high specificity. Wrongly classifying noncarcinogens as carcinogens could lead to the loss of potentially valuable drugs.

In later candidate selection (safety), when there may be fewer than 20 compounds left in contention, reliable safety results (i.e., a negative result that is accurately predictive of negative *in vivo* genotoxicity/carcinogenicity) are required to carry the drug forward into development and FTIH (first time in human) studies. Thus, safety assessment groups require high sensitivity, wrongly classifying carcinogens as noncarcinogens will allow compounds to continue their ever more expensive progress to the clinic via animal studies before the liability is identified.

The medicinal chemist is concerned with activity, attrition, and hazard, while the safety expert is concerned with saving compounds, and hence the relevance of the underlying hazard mechanisms to humans. The safety expert's concerns are obviously much more costly to address. In reality, there is a trade-off between specificity and sensitivity. High specificity often comes at the expense of sensitivity. This is less concerning in a strategy without the early screen, since in later GLP studies missed genotoxins will be detected, albeit in fewer compounds. This compromise needs to be understood and recognized when developing testing strategies at different stages in discovery and development.

7.2.3 The Data from Genetic Toxicologists

Genetic toxicity testing generates quantitative data. Genotoxic compounds may generate no-effect levels (NOELS) and lowest effective concentrations (LECs). These might be in the submicromolar or millimolar range for potent or weak genotoxins, respectively. The measured effects also vary in magnitude that reflect increases in mutation rate, the incidence of chromosome abnormalities, or increased expression of genes associated with the response to DNA damage. In making a safety assessment, both exposure and dose are considered, that is, a weak genotoxin might be an acceptable drug if the therapeutic dose is low enough. In addition, genotoxicity in pharmaceuticals can be tolerated in the case of life-threatening diseases. In the particular cases of antivirals and antineoplastic agents, genotoxicity can also be a consequence of the mechanism of action.

7.3 PRACTICAL ISSUES FOR GENOTOXICITY PROFILING

7.3.1 Vehicle

The practical aim of screening for genotoxic potential much earlier than safety assessment should be to identify potent genotoxins. Those active at low concentrations would be the most challenging to carry forward in safety assessment. The *in vitro* tests described in this chapter are performed in living cells. Hence, samples stored in 100% DMSO need diluting to around 1% DMSO to be tolerated by living cells. Generally, a pharmaceutical library will be prepared between 10 and 50 mM in >98% DMSO. Dilution sets the upper limit for testing between 100 and 500 μM, which is considerably below the current 10 mM requirements for the regulatory tests. Thus, a screen performed on such library cannot be expected to give an accurate prediction of regulatory testing. Instead compounds will be identified that are potent genotoxins at low concentrations, which is ultimately a goal for medicinal chemists.

7.3.2 Dilution Range

In contrast to the true high-throughput screening paradigm of single point data, genotoxicity data is best derived from a range of compound concentrations. This is because genotoxins usually kill cells at concentrations where genome damage becomes overwhelming. In eukaryotic cells, this is often observed as a reduced growth rate caused by cell cycle delay or death through apoptosis. Given the wide range of potencies amongst known genotoxins, testing at a single concentration is unlikely to coincide with the concentration at which genotoxicity is detected. It might only allow the conclusion that a compound allows growth, or causes growth inhibition or death. A range of concentrations provides the opportunity to generate useful actionable data. In a lead optimization program, a range of exposures allows the selection of modifications that progressively reduce genotoxicity or separates genotoxic effects from pharmacological efficacy.

The NIH set up the National Chemical Genomics Center (NCGC) in 2007 to reproduce the state of the art in the pharmaceutical industry screening facilities. NCGC runs a variety of tests at 15 dilutions from a highest concentration of about 92 μM. Such screen conducted with the purpose of detecting genotoxins would detect the genotoxicity of the most potent compounds, but not the least potent.

7.3.3 Purity

Purity, or potential impurity, can be a confounding factor for any *in vitro* screen and poses a theoretical risk as a result of *in silico* predictions as well as synthetic chemistry. There are particular issues with purity that are relevant to genotoxicity screening. While most useful drugs are nonreactive by design, the synthesis of novel small molecules is almost inevitably achieved through the use of reactive chemicals, which might persist as contaminants in the library samples. Many compounds such as alkylators, aromatic nitro, and aromatic amines are commonly active in mutagenicity assays. A potent genotoxic impurity might falsely identify the test compound as hazardous.

A related challenge is the presence of intermediates in synthesis. Both readily anticipated impurities, such as structural isomers, as well as unanticipated intermediates might pose a genotoxic hazard. The increased scale of production that is required once a compound reaches development often follows a different synthetic route and/or allows for greater investment in purity. In such cases, a positive result for a discovery compound that arose because of an intermediate is not at all relevant.

This topic has been the subject of industry-wide discussion, leading to proposals for the determination, testing, and control of specific impurities in pharmaceuticals [10] as well as some investigation of how structure-based assessment can support safety assessment of impurities [11] (see below). The actual risk posed by an impurity or intermediate will depend on whether or not it is actually present and in what quantities. If the *in silico* prediction is to be followed up, the purification or *de novo* synthesis of the intermediate for *in vitro* or *in vivo* testing requires the development of new analytical methods to detect and measure the compound. A similar scenario arises from the consideration of genotoxic metabolites that might either be predicted, or detected in *in vitro* studies under metabolic activation conditions (e.g., with S9 fractions), or is inferred or detected in animals.

Detailed reiteration of other issues related to impurities is beyond the scope of the present discussion. It is relevant, however, to consider the concept of a threshold of toxicological concern (TTC) as it relates to genotoxicity. A TTC defines a level of acceptable exposure to known carcinogens. It is expressed as a level of daily dose that would increase the number of cancers in the population by only a negligible level. The European Medicines Agency has proposed that "a TTC value of 1.5 μg/day intake of a genotoxic impurity is considered to be associated with an acceptable risk (excess cancer risk of <1 in 100,000 over a lifetime) for most pharmaceuticals. From this threshold value, a permitted level in the active substance can be calculated based on the expected daily dose. Higher limits may be justified under certain conditions such as "short-term exposure periods" [12]. Delaney [13] summarized a variety of reasons to view this as an overcautious limit, including inappropriate linear extrapolation from TD_{50} values, and reliance on carcinogenicity data from rodent studies that substantially overestimates human risk. A more direct focus on the absurdity of this virtually zero-risk approach is that the actual lifetime risk of all cancers in human is 30–40,000 per 100,000, and that humans consume gram quantities of known rodent carcinogens every day [5].

7.4 COMPUTATIONAL APPROACHES TO GENOTOXICITY ASSESSMENT: THE *IN SILICO* METHODS

7.4.1 General Considerations

Accurate *in silico* (computational) methods provide cost-effective and fast virtual screening for drug candidates that allow profiling molecules for genotoxicity before a compound has been synthesized. Thus, chemists can theoretically avoid the time and expense of synthesis of compounds with readily predictable liabilities, and instead focus their efforts on compounds with reduced risks. The current predictive power of computational methods derives from traditional regulatory genotoxicity datasets and generally tends to overpredict *in vivo* hazard. *In silico* methods should be used in concert with accurate *in vitro* genotoxicity assays. The results of such tests can then feed back into the development of ever more sophisticated tools.

The prediction of genotoxicity based on chemical structure began in earnest after Ashby and Tennant [14, 15] established that there are correlations between chemical structure, *Salmonella* mutagenicity and carcinogenicity. Their work produced the theoretical "supermutagen" (Figure 7.2), which remains a valuable reference of how not to design a new drug! The distinction between genotoxic and nongenotoxic carcinogens does not follow the same rules. In the subsequent early development of *in silico* methods there was an inevitable reliance on the Ames and rodent carcinogenicity data because these provided the most readily available datasets. This is a rapidly evolving field, but before considering the state-of-the-art, the challenges that are now being addressed such as the biological relevance of the carcinogenicity and genotoxicity test data used to construct models and the breadth of chemistry in the molecular structures should be explored.

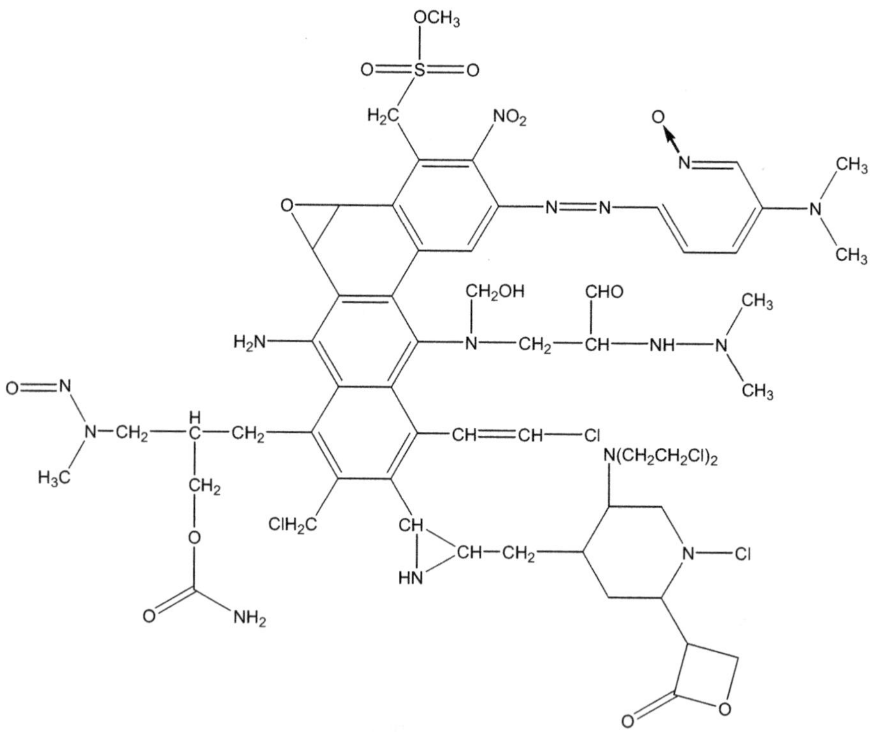

Figure 7.2 Theoretical "Supermutagen."

As mentioned above, historical carcinogenicity data was often derived from animals exposed to chronic sublethal doses of a test chemical. This can lead to cell damage and cell death, which in turn requires cell division to replace lost cells. DNA replication is intrinsically very accurate, but mutations occur in every cell at every division and can increase the risk of cancer independently of the cause of increased cell division. An expectation that a molecule will never reach such concentrations in man is likely to overestimate this hazard. Similar problems arise from the *in vitro* data. The Ames test has high specificity, so Ames positive compounds are quite likely to be genotoxic carcinogens and their structures are of value in modeling. However, its relatively low sensitivity indicates that there are many Ames negative compounds, which are both *in vitro* and *in vivo* genotoxins and carcinogens. Without data from these Ames negative genotoxic compounds, the predictive model will be deficient. This gap is increasingly filled by the inclusion of data from the current regulatory *in vitro* mammalian genotoxicity tests, though their poor specificity contributes to the risk of a model generating false predictions of hazard.

From a chemical perspective, reactive molecules are not generally good drug candidates. The original Ashby and Tennant rules were derived from industrial chemicals including pesticides, herbicides, and others chemicals of environmental concern as opposed to drug-like molecules. These are often highly electrophilic and reactive. While drug-like molecules are usually nonreactive, reactive molecules are important in the synthesis of drugs as reactants or intermediates and may remain as impurities. They may also be generated by the metabolism of drugs. Putative reactive derivatives might not exist and be detectable, and can certainly be challenging and costly to synthesize. However, a study of the potential value of *in silico* methods in risk assessment of impurities found that *in silico* methods are actually quite effective in this application [11].

Snyder and coauthors [16] analyzed the extent to which the above limitations might influence the accuracy of three different *in silico* methods (DEREK for Windows, TOPKAT, and MCASE) by using them to predict the genotoxicity of 394 marketed pharmaceuticals. Their general conclusions were that the *in silico* methods had poor sensitivity in the prediction of genotoxicity of pharmaceuticals. Since this report there have been concerted efforts to improve the models by populating the chemical structure databases with more drug-like molecules, and collecting data from chemical classes that have alerting structures, but are not all genotoxic or carcinogenic.

Two branches of genotoxicity assessment based on molecular structure have emerged. The first branch is based on mathematical algorithms, which generate a statistical assessment of risk by the definition of quantitative structure–activity relationships (QSAR), based on correlations between molecular structure and genotoxicity endpoints. Examples of these are MC4PC (MultiCASE), MDL-QSAR (MDL), BioEpisteme (Prous Science), and Predictive Data Miner (Lead-Scope) [17, 18]. In general, these methods have high specificity and low sensitivity. The second branch adds research information gathered by human experts to the structure. These include molecular context of the alert, as well as mechanisms of genotoxicity, activities, and reactivities to build knowledge-based expert system rules for correlation with genotoxicity endpoints (DEREK for Windows, LHASA). These methods have a lower specificity but higher sensitivity. Similar to the *in vitro* tests, presumably the best strategy is to consider a combination of *in silico* approaches [18].

Yang and coauthors [18] have undertaken a comprehensive effort to integrate genotoxicity data from multiple databases, incorporating private databases from four private industrial sources, including pharmaceuticals. The latter considerably increases coverage of pharmaceutical space despite only using general structure feature statistics rather than actual chemical structures. Principal component analysis (PCA) was applied to reveal multiple domain correlations between chemical structures/features with semimechanistic data from the following genotoxicity tests: Bacterial (Ames) and mammalian (MLA) mutation, *in vitro* chromosome aberration, and *in vivo* (rodent) micronucleus formation. The broader chemical space and multiple genotoxicity endpoints should result in generation of an *in silico* genotoxicity hazard profile containing a recommendation on follow-up testing.

7.4.2 The Chemistry of Genotoxins

To ascertain the cancer risk of specific structural moieties in a molecular substrate, it is essential to understand the relationship (if any) between those structural alerts and mutagenicity and/or carcinogenicity. It is generally recognized that there are approximately 30 alerting groups based on structural motifs [15, 19–21]. The different classes expand or contract, depending on the perspectives of different research groups. These moieties are cataloged in Table 7.2.

Electrophilic compounds (including those derived via metabolic activation) have long been associated with carcinogenic potential [22, 23]. Cheeseman and colleagues [20] found that if they removed those compounds containing highly alerting structures from the 709 compounds (in their database) exhibiting carcinogenicity, that the median adjusted log value (MALV) of remaining compounds within the database fell to 4.85 (the same value as for substances testing negative in the Ames assay); whereas, the MALV for those containing a structural motif of concern increased to 6.18. The authors indicated that there was a 20-fold decrease in potency between those compounds with structural alerting motifs compared with those that did not contain these moieties. The authors contended that this allowed regulatory bodies to build structural alerts database that could trigger a level of concern even in the absence of alerting biological data.

Cheeseman and colleagues [20] examined highly alerting structural motifs and demonstrated that 8 out of 19 subgroups in their database alerted for carcinogenicity. These subgroups were further scrutinized and stricter controls were proposed. These included *N*-nitroso compounds, endocrine disrupters, strained heterocyclics, for example, epoxides and aziridines, heavy metals, α-nitrofuryl compounds, hydrazines (and related triazenes, azides, and azoxy compounds), polycyclic amines, and organophosphorous compounds.

TABLE 7.2 Structural Alerts Leading to High Risks of Carcinogenicity

Number	Structural Motif Alerting for Carcinogenicity	Metabolic Activation (if any)
1	Primary alky halides[a]	
2	Aryl amines and alkylated aryl amines	*In situ* formation of nitrenium ion
3	Aromatic nitro (and some aliphatic nitro)	*In situ* formation of nitrenium ion
4	Azo compounds[b]	Via reduction and *in situ* formation of diazonium ion
5	Unsymmetrical hydrazines[b]	*In situ* formation of carbocation or diazonium species
6	Di-substituted hydrazines[b]	Via reduction and *in situ* formation of diazonium ion
7	Alkyl aldehydes	
8	Epoxides (both alkyl and aryl)[c]	
9	Aziridines (both alkyl and aryl)[c]	
10	*N*-nitroso	Via formation of carbocation or diazonium species
11	Esters of sulfonic and phosphonic acids (both alkyl and aryl)[a]	
12	Aza *N*-oxides, Aryl *N*-oxides	
13	*N*-chloro amines[a]	Accumulation possible
14	Michael reagents (amides, e.g., acrylamide, nitriles, α,β-unsaturated esters)[b]	
15	Carbamate derivatives (urethanes)	
16	*N*-methyol derivatives	
17	*N*- and *S*-mustards (β-haloethyl)	
18	Propiolactones (and their thiolated derivatives, propiosultones)	
19	Monohaloalkenes	
20	Heavy metal compounds[d]	
21	Polycyclic amines	*In situ* formation of nitrenium ion
22	Organophosphorous compounds[d]	
23	Aflatoxin-like compounds[c]	*In situ* formation of epoxide
24	Azoxy compounds[b]	Via reduction and *in situ* formation of diazonium ion
25	Benzidine compounds[e]	*In situ* formation of nitrenium ion
26	Steroid-like compounds[f]	
27	Tetra-halogenated dibenzodioxins and dibenzofurans[f]	Accumulation possible
28	Vinyl-containing compounds[c]	*In situ* formation of epoxide
29	*N*-hydroxy aminoaryls	
30	*N*-acetylated aminoaryls	

[a]Part of miscellaneous Ashby alerts [21].
[b]Part of Cheeseman's original hydrazine grouping [20].
[c]Part of Cheeseman's original strained ring grouping [20].
[d]Often viewed separately under neurotoxic classification [21].
[e]Benzidine is often included in polycyclic amine grouping [21].
[f]Part of Cheeseman's original endocrine disrupters grouping [20].

The *N*-nitroso compounds would be expected to demonstrate toxicity via metabolic activation to either the carbocation or diazonium ions via similar pathways. These compounds are about 100-fold more potent (MALV = 6.79) compared to the nonalerting elements in the database.

The endocrine disruptors include estrogen mimetics that disrupt endocrine-mediated biological pathways and include substituted dibenzodioxins, tetra-substituted dibenzofurans, ergot-derived alkaloids, flavenoids, and polychlorinated pesticides. Other researchers have divided this original subgroup into four further subgroups: steroids, highly chlorinated compounds, organotin compounds, and tetra-halogenated dibenzodioxins and structurally similar compounds [21]. Some members of this original endocrine disruptor class have the common 1,2-cyclopentanophenathrene ring system which is characteristic of the steroids and the structurally related motifs observed in the flavone ring systems and ergot alkaloids. Other related structural moieties include the multiple substituted dibenxodioxins and dibenzofurans and the polychlorinated ring systems in some pesticides. These findings are in broad agreement with the structural motifs required to bind to the endocrine receptor sites [24]. These compounds are about 40-fold more potent (MALV = 6.45) versus the nonalerting elements in the database.

The strained heterocyclic ring compounds include those that do not require metabolic activation, for example, epoxides, aziridines, strained lactones, and alkyl imines; as well as those undergoing bioactivation to produce these structures *in vivo*, for example, polycyclic aromatic hydrocarbons and the extremely potent aflatoxins. These compounds are about 10 times more potent (MALV = 5.95) versus the nonalerting elements in the database. Subsequently, other research groups have subdivided this original class into epoxides and aziridines (strained ring systems) and three additional groups of compounds that are established as expressing their toxicology after metabolic activation via strained ring metabolites, for example, aflatoxin-like compounds, polycyclic aromatic hydrocarbons, and compounds containing a vinyl structural moiety [21].

In a similar fashion to *N*-nitroso analytes, the aromatic nitro (and related aromatic amine) compounds undergo metabolic activation to form the very reactive nitrenium ions. Cheeseman and colleagues [20] narrowed this group to a nitro-substituted furan ring with the substituent alpha to the heterocyclic oxygen and, for example, the related nitrogen-substituted imidazole and sulfur-substituted thienyl compounds. However, as other researchers have indicated, the whole class of aromatic nitro groups are highly alerting for mutagenicity and carcinogenicity. The MALV (5.90) for this more restricted class of nitroaromatics shows 10-fold greater potency than the nonalerting elements in the database.

The heavy metals, exemplified by lead, cadmium, mercury, and some of the precious metals, for example, platinum and palladium have been long recognized as being highly toxic. It is also probable that this class also forms a significant subset of the potent neurotoxins, as well as alerting for mutagenicity and carcinogenicity. The MALV (5.91) is very similar to the previous class of alerting compounds.

Hydrazines, azoarenes, and related triazenes, azides, and azoxy compounds all share a common structural alert and, similar to the *N*-nitroso group, demonstrate toxicity via metabolic activation to either the carbocation or diazonium ions. The MALV (5.88) is again about 10 times more potent than the nonalerting elements in the database. Latterly, other researchers have concluded that this grouping is too broad and have recommended a subdivision into hydrazines, azoxy compounds, and azo compounds [21].

Polycyclic amines, which include polyheterocyclic amines, biphenyl amines, aromatic acetamides, benzidines as well as the ubiquitous polycyclic aromatic amines are often encountered in nature via overcooked meats, fish, and poultry. Their toxicity is via bioactivation to form the highly reactive nitrenium ion in a similar fashion to nitroarenes. Benzidine is one of the more potent subgroups in this group causing carcinogenicity after even limited exposure and is sometimes extracted as a separate group. The MALV (5.82) is again about 10 times more potent than the nonalerting elements in the database.

Finally, organophosphorous compounds are the least potent of this highly alerting subgroup, with a MALVof 5.67. They act via their intrinsic ability to phosphorylate or alkylate biomolecules. Similar to the heavy metals, organophosphorous compounds are neurotoxic in nature and anticholinesterase substrates due to phosphorylation of this neurotransmitter.

Different authors have advocated that heavy metals and organophosphorous compounds should be excluded from any databases predicting solely for mutagenicity and carcinogenicity. These compounds, particularly organophosphates, should be extracted into a separate neurotoxicant database to avoid biases towards high potency based on both numbers of compounds and high toxicity [21].

Kroes and colleagues [21] identified five different high concern groups: aflatoxin-like, *N*-nitroso, azoxy, steroids, and polyhalogenated compounds, for example, halogenated dibenzo-*p*-dioxins and dibenzofurans and defined these as the "cohort of concern". Steroids and polyhalogenated compounds are considered to be non-genotoxic carcinogens with thresholded-toxicity.

In addition to the structurally alerting motif, metabolic, and other toxicokinetic considerations should be evaluated. Besides the functional groups present, for example, nitro, epoxide, and so on; the potential of that group to be metabolically activated is critical [25]. This is exemplified by the decision tree used for the safety evaluation of flavors [26, 27]. This identified structural motifs with a high potential for toxicity. These included (1) safrole-like structural motifs, (2) unionized moieties containing elements in addition to C,H,N, O, divalent S, for example, halide substituted compounds, (3) strained ring systems, for example, aziridines, epoxides, (4) α,β-unsaturated lactone, or fused lactones, (5) aliphatic secondary nitrile, quaternary *N*, amino, *N*-nitroso, diazo, and so on, (6) aryl unsubstituted groups, and (7) multifunctional groupings, excluding methoxy groups and classifying esters and acids as one functional grouping.

Most structurally alerting compounds are rapidly metabolized and do not pose a threat towards accumulation. However, halogenated molecules (where halogen is directly substituted onto carbon atom) are poorly metabolized. These substituents may block normal metabolism at that carbon or at the adjacent carbon atoms, for example, α-C atom. Structural moieties that particularly alert for accumulation are multiple halogenated substituted alkyl groups, for example, CF_3, CHF_2, and so on, and multisubstituted aryl halides, where either all ring substituents are halides or are adjacent to halide-substituted ring carbon atoms, for example, C_6Cl_6, hexachlorophene [27].

Some authors advocated additional structural groupings, for example, aromatic amines and aromatic nitro groups based on structural alerts identified previously by Ashby and Tennant [15]. As with all rule-based Expert systems, some of the generic structural alerts appear to be quite nonspecific such as the generic alert for aromatic amines [28]. It was proposed by other researchers that the various alkylating agents, for example, *N*-chloro amines, alkyl chlorides, sulfonate, and phosphonate esters were combined into a group labeled "miscellaneous Ashby alerts" [21].

Dobo and colleagues [11] evaluated 272 pharmaceutical starting materials and intermediates using structure based analysis (DEREK for Windows [29]; TOX-NET [30]; and SCIFINDER [31]). These compounds had already being tested for mutagenicity using Ames tests. However, on a blinded basis, without the benefit of this biological information, these materials were then classified into five separate categories (see Table 7.3).

Based on the Ames test data there were 18% (48) mutagens contained in the data set. The percentage concordance of the actual mutagenicity (based on Ames testing) versus the predicted mutagenicity (based on structure–activity relationships) was then evaluated for each of the five categories; with the exception of category 3, where no predictions were undertaken. The data showed a very high degree of concordance, with 100% predictivity for category 1 ($n = 2$), 76% for category 2 ($n = 25$), 96% for category 4 ($n = 67$), and 94% for category 5 ($n = 111$). The overall predictivity within the data set was 92%, with a higher predictivity value for negative concordance (94%) versus positive concordance (74%).

Based on the available Ames test data for the category 3 data set ($n = 67$), 25% were actually mutagenic. The authors [11] assessed within each category the occurrence of a particular alerting motif that is either known or suspected of

TABLE 7.3 Compound Classification with Respect to Mutagenicity or Carcinogenicity

Classification	Mutagenicity or Carcinogenicity
1	Literature precedent for mutagenicity or carcinogenicity
2	Known mutagens, but with unknown carcinogenic potential or the chemical structure gave a positive alert for mutagenicity and a closely related structural analogue was identified as a known mutagen
3	Alerting structure for mutagenicity or carcinogenicity, without the necessary supporting evidence to confirm/deny biological relevance of data
4	Alerting structure for mutagenicity or carcinogenicity, with data on related compounds that demonstrate negative Ames tests and are consequently considered to be nonmutagenic
5	No alerting structure for mutagenicity or carcinogenicity

Based on Ref. 11.

bestowing mutagenicity (or carcinogenicity) onto the structure. In those cases where more than one alerting moiety was present, then the motif that gave the highest alert for mutagenicity (or carcinogenicity) was selected. The data are summarized in Table 7.4.

Both of the category 1 structural motifs were aniline derivatives. In contrast, in category 2 just over half of the alerting structures were comprised of aromatic nitro

TABLE 7.4 The Percentage Frequency of an Alerting Structural Motif in each Category

Category	Alerting Structural Motif	Percentage Frequency
1	Aromatic amine	0.74
2	Aromatic nitro	4.78
	Aromatic amine	1.48
	Secondary amine	1.48
	Alkylating agent	0.37
	α-Haloether	0.37
	Acid halide	0.37
	Hydrazine	0.37
3	Aromatic nitro	5.15
	Alkylating agent	4.78
	Aromatic amide	4.41
	Aromatic amine	2.57
	Halogenated quinoline	1.48
	Michel acceptors	1.48
	Aliphatic nitro	0.74
	Halogenated heterocyclic	0.74
	Pyridine dialdehyde	0.74
	Acid halide	0.37
	Alkyl ester	0.37
	α-Haloether	0.37
	Epoxide	0.37
	Hydrazine	0.37
	N-methyol derivative	0.37
	Oxime	0.37
4	Secondary amine	9.93
	Aromatic amide	4.41
	Aromatic amine	2.94
	Aldehyde	1.47
	Alkyl aldehyde	1.47
	Dialdehyde	1.10
	Vinyl ketone	1.10
	Aliphatic carboxylic acid	0.74
	Hydroxamic acid	0.74
	Halogenated alkene	0.37
	Alkyl carbamate	0.37
5	No alerting structural motif	40.80

Based on Ref. 11.

compounds (52%) and just under a third comprised of amines (30%). The rest were a very diverse group of structural moieties (16 in total). In category 3, 21% of the alerting structures were comprised of aromatic nitro compounds, with similar representation from alkylating agents (19%) and aromatic amides (18%) and 10% were aromatic amines. The remainder alerting structures were less common. Similarly, in category 4, 40% of the total comprised of secondary amines, 18% comprised of aromatic amides and 12% were aromatic amines. The remainder of the group comprised of less common structural motifs. Finally, category 5 compounds were represented by aromatic/aliphatic ring systems with a wide ranging of carboxylic and heterocyclic ring structures.

Dobo and colleagues [11] reported that although the concordance analysis gave highly predictive outcomes, 25% of the compounds were allocated into category 3 where mutagenic potential was not easily predictable. This was attributed to the complexity as well as the novelty of the compound with few literature precedent structures. However, the authors indicated that this should not be considered surprising. They cited the work of Shimizu et al. [32], who related the position of substituents on the aromatic ring and Vance and Levin [33], who related the number of ring systems to the overall mutagenicity of aromatic nitro groups. The authors concluded that there was little literature precedence for nitro-substituted heterocycles. In a similar fashion, Ninomiya et al. [34] had previously demonstrated that the structure of both the alkyl and the sulfonic acid moieties were intrinsically linked with mutagenicity of alkyl sulfonates.

The FDA has initiated an Informatics and Computational Safety Analysis Staffing (ICSAS) group within the Office of Pharmaceutical Science (OPS) to provide QSAR assessment of the safety implications of structural motifs (both known and unknown). This group has constructed QSAR models for molecules where both individual and groups of genotoxic and reproductive toxicity (reprotoxic) tests data are available and correlated those results with the findings of rodent carcinogenicity bioassays [35, 36]. The group used *in silico* experiments based on MultiCASE, MC4PC software program [37], which was selected because of proven predictability for correlating mutagenicity with rodent carcinogenicity data [7, 8, 38]. This program identifies QSAR motifs and/or molecular fragments that correlate with either enhanced or reduced biological activity for groups of chemicals sharing a common structural alert. Interestingly, the associated physicochemical attributes of the molecule, for example, log P are considered to be fairly inconsequential in comparison to a significant structural alert.

The authors utilized a database with a total of 7205 compounds, comprising of 4961 with genotoxic end points, 2173 with reprotoxic end points, and 2173 with rodent carcinogenicity bioassay end points. The correlation of genotoxic and reprotox end points with carcinogenicity data was evaluated using a correlation indicator (CI) which is defined as the average of high specificity (SP), positive predictivity value (PPV), and low false positive (FP) rates. Of the 27 genotoxic and reprotoxicity tests evaluated, just over 50% (14/27) showed high CI values and 48% (13/27) were suitable for QSAR modeling using the MC4PC program. The authors found four alerting structures (aziridine, epoxide, *N*-nitroso, and sulfonate esters) that alerted in multiple genotoxic and reprotoxic animal models and termed these trans-genera alerts. The majority of trans-genera alerts were the same types of polar electrophilic molecules that are also identified in human expert systems [15, 19].

Although this exercise demonstrated high correlation (80.9% CI, 83.1% SP, 78.6% PPV, and 16.9% FP), most of the QSAR assessments were of low sensitivity. This was based on two underlying factors: the relatively small size of the training data sets coupled with the comparatively rigid expert rules within the MC4PC program. Relaxing the expert rules of the system inevitably increases FP and lowers the specificity. The latter can be addressed by increasing the size of the training data set, using multiple validated QSAR programs to predict toxicity, and by combination of the results of related toxicological endpoints to predict the overall toxicity of the chemical.

Medicinal chemists are now actively encouraged to avoid structures with embedded genotoxic moieties. A good example of the changing perceptions of chemists can be ascertained by looking at the structural evolution of the dihydropyridine (DHP) calcium channel blockers. The first generation of DHPs, for example, nifedipine (2,6-dimethyl-4-(2-nitrophenyl)-1,4-dihydropyridine-3,5-dicarboxylate) had a 2-subsituted aryl nitro group. Pharmacological activity is linked to noncoplanarity of the two ring systems. Initially bulky nitro groups in the *ortho* position were utilized to facilitate this requirement, but this does have a structural alert for genotoxicity. In contrast, the third generation DHPs, for example, amlodipine (3-ethyl-5-methyl (4*RS*)-2-[(2-aminoethoxy)methyl]-4-(2-chlorophenyl)-6-methyl-1,4-dihydropyridine-3,5-dicarboxylate) replaced the alerting structural motif with a 2-chlorophenyl moiety. This substitution was still bulky to prevent coplanarity but without the genotoxic liability.

7.5 GENOTOXICITY ASSAYS FOR SCREENING

In this section, regulatory genotoxicity assays are briefly introduced in the context of early profiling and are contrasted with the distinctive properties of discovery-stage screening assays. Table 7.5 provides a summary of the properties of tests suitable for early screening. The regulatory assays are summarized and the reader is referred to published guidelines for detailed information. The various regulatory and screening tests are considered in three basic classes according to the endpoint of the assay: (1) gene mutation; (2) chromosome damage, including single and double-strand breaks and aneugenesis; and (3) genotoxin-induced gene expression. Screening assays that have been derived from regulatory assays are described noting protocol differences from the parent assays, as well as the strengths and weaknesses of all the assays, which might be considered for use in the profiling context.

The current ICH tripartite guideline for genotoxicity testing of pharmaceuticals (S2B) defines a battery of standard *in vitro* and *in vivo* tests. The 3-test battery consists of the following:

TABLE 7.5 Properties of Tests Suitable for Profiling

Test Endpoint	Category	Validation: Transfer	Application	Throughput
Bacterial mutation	Ames II	Yes: Yes	Candidates/ leads	50/week; 2,500/year
Bacterial mutation	Biolum	Yes: No	Candidates	20/week; 1,000/year
Bacterial reporter	*Escherichia SOS*	Yes: Yes	Candidates/ leads	180/week; 9,000/year
Yeast deletion	DEL	Yes: No	Candidates	Unknown
Yeast reporter	RAD54-GFP	Yes: Yes	Candidates/ leads	160/week; 8,000/year
Mammalian DNA damage	MNT imaging	Yes: Yes	Candidates	55/week; 2,750/year
Mammalian DNA damage	MNT flow	Yes: Yes	Candidates	40/week; 2,000/year
Mammalian DNA damage	Comet	Yes: Yes	Candidates	30/week; 1,500/year
Mammalian reporter	GADD45a-GFP	Yes: Yes	Candidates/ leads	200/week; 10,000/year

1. bacterial gene mutation test (Ames)
2. *in vitro* mammalian cell test (cytogenetic evaluation of chromosomal damage or mouse lymphoma forward mutation thymidine kinase (TK) assay)
3. *in vivo* test for genetic damage.

The *in vivo* assays suggested to be most useful are based in rodent hematopoietic cells and comprise either assessment of chromosomal damage in bone marrow cells or micronuclei in bone marrow or peripheral blood erythrocytes. If all the tests in the battery give negative results then this is usually considered sufficient to demonstrate the lack of potential human genotoxic activity. However, according to the current guideline, compounds yielding positive results may require more extensive testing, provided in the form of the ICH S2A "Guidance on Specific Aspects of Regulatory Genotoxicity Tests for Pharmaceuticals." This current guidance suggests that for a compound producing biologically relevant positive results in one or more *in vitro* tests, further useful information may be obtained by performing another *in vivo* test in an alternative tissue. The target tissue for the compound and the endpoint measured in the *in vitro* test both impact on the choice of the additional *in vivo* test.

In 2008, the ICH proposed revisions to its S2 battery guideline and issued guidance on specific aspects [9]. In the combined revision, S2(R1), there is a new option for regulatory submissions in which the bacterial mutation assay is the only required *in vitro* test, but two *in vivo* endpoints are required [9]. Table 7.1 provides a summary of existing and proposed testing regimes (see also Section 7.9). Further advice is offered on the choice of *in vivo* test and top concentration for testing. ICH guidelines do not intend to affect the development of an effective early screening strategy. It is not anticipated that early profiling and screening will replace the regulatory battery in the near future. Instead, they are complimentary strategies that allow for safer compounds to be promoted from discovery to regulatory testing stage.

7.5.1 Bacterial Gene Mutation Assays

The bacterial and mammalian cell assays for gene mutation were developed to measure statistically significant increases in mutation rate. Mutations are infrequent ($< 10^{-5}$) so many millions of exposed cells must be plated out to provide robust assessment. This generates hundreds of Petri dishes for counting cells and is not practical for profiling. The *Salmonella typhimurium* reverse mutation assay ("Ames" test) is carried out in a variety of different mutant strains selected to identify the various classes of mutation. For example, TA98 and TA1537 for frameshift mutations, TA100 for base pair mutations, TA102 for oxidative damage, and TA1535 for base pair substitution.

The "mouse lymphoma assay" (MLA) is one of several mammalian cell mutations assays. MLA assesses mutation at the TK locus in murine lymphoma cells (L5178Y), though TK mutation data are produced in the human lymphoblastoid cell line TK6, and from the HGPRT (hypoxanthine–guanine phosphoribosyl-transferase) locus in Chinese Hamster ovary or lung (V79) cells and mouse lymphoma cells. Since Ames mutation data and often mammalian cell mutation data may cause the abandonment of a drug, efforts have been made to increase throughput of the tests and apply them appropriately during the candidate selection stage.

The Ames Test Variants Many laboratories use streamlined versions of the regulatory Ames test in which a reduced set of strains is used, and a smaller number of colonies may be counted to estimate mutation rate [39]. While practical for candidate selection, this is still not suitable for profiling assessments. A more recent development is the Pfizer "BioLum" test [1]. In this assay, bacterial mutation assays are incorporated into the *Salmonella* tester strains of a gene encoding a light-emitting protein under the control of the constitutively expressed kanamycin resistance gene. Cells that can form even small colonies (for the Ames test, revertant mutant colonies selected for histidine prototrophy) will emit light and are readily counted using electronic imaging systems. This allows higher cell densities to be plated in microplate format with the concomitant reduction in use of plastic ware and test article [1]. Initial validation work was performed in 24-well microplates with a throughput of around 20 compounds per week in the authors' laboratories. The authors believe that the simple protocol and amenability to automation should mean that significantly higher throughputs are possible.

Fluctuation Tests Mutation rate can also be estimated using fluctuation tests (cited in OECD 471). Multiple wells containing a specified number of cells are scored for growth in selective media. The mutation rates are derived from the number of cells where growth occurs. A further improvement in the efficiency of these methods is the use of "mixes" of tester strains in addition to single strains. After a series of handling and treatment steps in larger volumes, cells are transferred to 384-well microplates for incubation and scoring. Assay preparation can be efficiently handled robotically. Cell proliferation can be detected with colorimetric indicators of cell growth (e.g., purple to yellow change), permitting the use of spectrophotometric plate readers for data collection. The method can be established independently, but is also available commercially as either "Ames MPF™" or "Ames II™" (Xenometrix by Endotell GmbH). The difference between the two commercially available assays lies in the *Salmonella* strains employed: Ames MPF uses up to 4 of the classical TA strains (98, 100, 1535, and 1537). Ames II uses TA98 and then a TA mix, consisting of the TA700X series of strains.

The Ames II test is reported to use at least threefold less test compound and sixfold less plastic ware than the traditional Ames test. This assay may be developed into a rather high-throughput test: one study reported screening 2698 compounds in a little more than a year [40]. An interlaboratory "ring trial" with 19 coded compounds concluded that the method provides an effective reproducible and reliable higher throughput screening alternative to the standard Ames test [41].

7.5.2 Mammalian Cell Mutation Assays

The mouse lymphoma assay detects gene mutations as well as chromosomal mutations with the difference inferred from colony size and confirmed by secondary assays. Both colony-counting and well-counting methods are used in microplate format for the calculation of mutant frequency. Cells are first exposed to the test chemical, then after a wash step are allowed an expression/recovery phase before an estimate of cell growth. This is followed by another wash step, plating for growth, colony counting, and derivation of mutation rate. Small and large colony types are identified by inspection. The assay requires weeks rather than hours or days. The slower growth of mammalian cells coupled with the complex handling protocols make these the least promising assays to adapt for use in hit and lead profiling. At present there are no reports of these assays being used routinely earlier than preclinical drug candidate selection.

7.5.3 Saccharomyces cerevisiae ("Yeast") Mutation Assays The use of yeast cells, as a eukaryotic complement to the prokaryotic Ames test led to the development of several new protocols for the detection of mutation, gene conversion, and recombination. The formal introduction of methods [42], followed by much development work from Dr. Zimmermann's laboratory, led to large systematic studies [43, 44] and OECD guidelines for the test battery (OECD 480, 481). However, those early assays are now rarely used partially due to concerns over low sensitivity presumably from limited permeability of the cell wall.

An intrachromosomal recombination assay ("DEL") based on a genetically engineered *HIS3* locus in *S. cerevisiae* [45] has been developed both as a colony-counting and a well-counting assay. Nine chemicals were used in a proof of principle for higher throughput screening in 96- or 384-well format that had been modified into a colorimetric assay [46]. The assay is reported to detect carcinogenic compounds including those for which a genotoxicity mechanism has not previously been reported. At present, the assay is not widely available.

7.5.4 Chromosome Damage and Aberration Assays

Chromosome damage and aberration assays may be classified into two classes: (1) chromosome aberration tests in which all the chromosomes in a cell are examined and (2) micronucleus tests in which chromosomes outside the nucleus in smaller micronuclei are examined. In the first class, gross rearrangements of chromosomes are examined including translocations, large insertions/deletions, the loss or gain of whole chromosomes, and double- or single-stranded DNA breakage. Since chromosomes only condense and become visible during mitosis, most test protocols require treatment with a mitotic poison that causes cells to accumulate at metaphase (such cytochalasin B). In this procedure, all cells in the exposed population can be scored rather than the subpopulation in mitosis at the analytical time point (OECD 473). Some tools and systems are on the market for aiding mitotic indexing and chromosome aberration scoring (Pathfinder™ technology from IMSTAR, Paris, France). Metasystems GmbH (Altlussheim, Germany) also provides a metaphase locating software called Metafer MSearch. Such systems have the potential to speed up the identification of metaphase cells, and use chromosome "painting" to help identify the type of aberration. At present, automated high-throughput scoring of translocations, insertions, and deletions has not replaced microscopic examination and it remains unclear how widespread such systems will become. In a recent review of methods focusing on human cells, the authors commented that "Even the best automated system may never replace a skilled observer" [47]. These methods are not yet sufficiently mature for profiling.

The micronucleus test (MNT) is effective in the automated detection of clastogens and aneugens. Nuclear membrane forms around chromosomes and chromosome fragments that fail to segregate into nuclei during anaphase. This might be a consequence of failures in the mitotic machinery or chromosome breakage that generates fragments without centromeres. These smaller "micronuclei" can be identified and counted using two quite different approaches: high-resolution imaging and flow cytometry. In both cases, DNA-specific dyes are crucial in resolving nuclei and micronuclei. Imaging is reliant on careful optimization of the parameters used to distinguish DNA-containing bodies from other membrane-bound compartments.

Diaz and coworkers [48] published an evaluation of an automated MNT assay using fluorescent microscopy coupled with image analysis software from Cellomics (Pittsburg, KS, USA). The results showed high concordance with data collected by manual scoring. The speed of scoring limited throughput to 11 compounds per day (at multiple dilutions, with and without S9 activation). This throughput approaches the minimum levels required for screening. Although the sample preparations remain relatively complex, the ever-increasing processing power and data storage available to developers will increase the assay throughput. Alternative imaging systems and analysis software are also available. IMSTAR and Metasystems reduce analysis times to 4–5 min per slide rather than the 25 min to score manually.

Flow cytometric assessment generates results that reproduce microscopic methods for the *in vivo* assessment of micronucleus frequency in peripheral blood micronucleated reticulocytes [49] and the method is increasingly applied in *in vitro* assessments. Litron Laboratories (Rochester, NY, USA) recently launched their "MicroFlow® *In Vitro*" kit for the *in vitro* micronucleus test following a six compound interlaboratory evaluation [50]. This method permits 50 samples to be analyzed over the course of 3.5 h including incubation times, leading to a possible throughput of 40 compounds per week or 2000 compounds per year.

It is important for the screener to recognize the inherent problems in specificity observed in chromosome aberration assays. Only about 50% of compounds with positive results are likely to be hazardous to rodents (or humans).

7.5.5 The "Comet" Assay

The electrophoresis of the nuclear content of individual cells followed by DNA staining provides microscopic images reminiscent of comets hurtling across the night sky—giving the name to the comet assay. It identifies strand-breaking agents. Although it has several handling steps, it is a relatively simple assay. The comet "head" contains giant (75 μm) supercoiled loops of DNA liberated from higher order chromatin packaging by high salt treatment. The "tail" contains loops in which there has been at least one single-stranded break leading to a more extended relaxed supercoil. More single-strand breaks lead to the formation of more relaxed loops and a greater proportion of staining migrates into the tail. Under alkaline conditions, double-strand breaks, or two single-strand breaks in the same loop, lead to fragmentation of the loops and altered tail structure. Smaller fragments of DNA including mitochondrial DNA (5.6 μm) and apoptotic fragments are beyond the resolution of the gels, and do not contribute to the head or tail staining. Thus, the comet assay, in alkaline or neutral conditions, should detect single- and double-stranded breaks, but not "pure" aneugens. In alkaline conditions, breakage can occur at alkaline labile sites including sites where the base has been lost from the sugar/phosphate backbone. Modified assays in which lesion-specific nuclease treatment is included can be used to reveal oxidative damage. Readers are referred to Collins and coworkers [51] for more detail on data generation and interpretation.

In the routine comet assay, a user can operate at a maximum throughput of 8–12 compounds per week, limited by sample and cell preparation, imaging, and scoring. There are a number of imaging and software analysis solutions currently available from companies such as IMSTAR, Metasystems, and Perceptive Instruments Ltd (Haverhill, UK). The assay has also been developed into a higher throughput format that accommodates four compounds each tested at 10 dilutions in a 96-well microplate. In this method, cells are still transferred to slides for scoring [52], and with robotic handling data from six compounds per day can be analyzed. A new protocol in development utilizes a multichamber plate that can be used for both cell treatment and electrophoresis [53]. The throughput is potentially 1500 compounds per year, which approaches the minimum requirements for late profiling.

7.5.6 DNA Adduct Assessment

A general and sensitive approach for the measurement of DNA lesions formed with nonradioactive carcinogens has been described. Normal and adducted nucleotides, generated by nuclease digests of DNA modified *in vivo* or *in vitro* with a compound of interest, are labeled with ^{32}P and detected and quantified after thin-layer chromatography (TLC). Such analysis of DNA adducts is used in mechanistic studies but presently not suited to profiling because of the complexities in sample preparation and analysis and subsequent low throughput. There are no formal guidelines for testing.

7.5.7 Gene Expression Assays

Microbes and metazoans are exposed to a variety of toxic stresses and have evolved appropriate defenses and repair mechanisms. Some of these systems are regulated at the protein level and others are regulated at the transcriptional level, allowing the development of reporter assays. These transcriptional responses can be used to provide an earlier marker for genotoxin exposure in a whole population of cells. This is opposed to the detection of the endpoints discussed above in which genotoxic stress leads to fixation of mutations or chromosomal aberrations/damage in a small subpopulation.

Prokaryotic The first generation of reporters exploited the DNA damage inducible genes of the SOS operon [54] in bacteria. These genes variously encode proteins involved in excision repair, recombinational repair, and DNA polymerase. Reporters for both the *sfiA* gene (SOS chromotest, [55]) and *umuC* [56] have been used to drive β-galactosidase synthesis which can be assessed using a colorimetric assay. A review of SOS chromotest data from 751 compounds [57] revealed that for the 452 compounds, which also had Ames data, there was agreement between the tests for 82% of compounds. A number of alternative SOS reporters have been developed to drive expression of the *lux* operon, which allows luminometric data collection. These include reporters for *recA*, *uvrA*, *alkA* [58], and *umuC* [59] as well as the commercially available Vitotox assay (Gentaur Molecular Products BVBA, Brussels, Belgium), which exploits the *recN* gene [60]. In a limited comparison of data from seven genotoxins and six environmental samples generated using *recA*-lux, *umuC*, and *sfi* reporter assays, the *umuC* test performed the best [61]. Although these systems are less accurate in prediction of Ames data than the more cumbersome fluctuation tests, their simplicity and low compound requirement are advantages for use.

The SOS-*umuC* assay allows three compounds to be assessed over seven dilutions on a 96-well microplate. A user can prepare up to 15 assay microplates per day translating to ~180 compounds profiled per week, or around 10,000 per year.

Eukaryotic (Yeast Cells) The first eukaryotic gene regulation assay (GreenScreen GC, Gentronix Ltd, UK), used Green Fluorescent Protein (GFP) as a reporter for induction of the yeast *RAD54* gene—a member of the recombinational repair family of genes [62]. A screening validation study [63] demonstrated that the assay detected a different spectrum of compounds to bacterial genotoxicity assays. It was suggested that in conjunction with a high-throughput bacterial screen, the two assays would provide an effective preview of the regulatory battery of genotoxicity tests. This proposal was subsequently justified in a study of 2698 proprietary compounds from the Johnson & Johnson (J&J) compound library [40]. Four compounds per 96-well microplate were tested with robust host cells and rapid assay time. It was possible to assess up to 160 compounds per week even without automation. Beyond this throughput, compound supply and data collection become the rate-limiting factors. An alternative *RAD54* reporter has also been described [64].

7.5.7.1.3 Eukaryotic (Human Cells) Broader reservation about yeast tests led to the development of a human cell assay in which GFP was used as a reporter for induction of the *GADD45a* gene [65]. Significantly, the human TK6 cell line was chosen not only because of its origins, but also due to its wild-type p53 status. Other mammalian cell lines used commonly are insufficient or deficient in p53 and this compromises the effectiveness of the DNA damage response. The resultant GADD45a-GFP assay (GreenScreen HC, Gentronix Ltd) responds to all classes of genotoxin including S9-generated metabolites [66]. In contrast to the regulatory *in vitro* mammalian assays, the results demonstrate high specificity without compromising sensitivity. This 96-well microplate assay is becoming widely employed and its transfer to other laboratories has been systematically evaluated [67]. The format of the GADD45a-GFP assay is very similar to the yeast assay. Four compounds are tested on a 96-well microplate although the assay incubation time is longer (48 h instead of 16 h) due to longer doubling time of the host cells. Manually, a compound throughput of 80–100 per operator per week is possible. This can be significantly improved using robotics and/or a reduced number of compound dilutions. In a recent study using this higher throughput assay format, a library of 1266 pharmacologically active compounds (LOPAC, Sigma-Aldrich Co. Ltd) was screened [68]. The potential throughput from this assay format could be as high as 36,000 compounds per year.

A second p53 responsive reporter has been described. This reporter exploits elements of the *p53R2* gene, which encodes a subunit of ribonucleotide reductase linked to a luciferase gene [69, 70]. It has been validated against diverse mechanistic classes of genotoxin. To perform this assay, the p53 wild-type cell line MCF-7 is transiently transfected with two plasmids: one with the *p53R2* reporter and the second with constitutively expressed control (driven by elements of CMV promoter). Between 4 and 6 h after transfection, cells are exposed to test materials (five dilutions) for 24 h, then washed three times, lysed, and assayed. It is not yet known how well the assay transfers to other laboratories, and the protocol is quite complex for adaptation to high throughput.

7.6 THE "OMICS"

The completion of the human genome project has led to new disciplines within genetic toxicology—the "omics." The study of global gene expression from transcription and translation, to a protein's various posttranslational states and intracellular location(s), as well as tools that are beginning to give clues about the more common toxicological response patterns, increasingly provide techniques for novel drug target identification. These technologies and the interpretation of their data are not yet sufficiently developed for screening at the throughput required for profiling and are not discussed in this chapter. However, in an integrated approach to safety assessment, genetic toxicologists will increasingly have access to data from broader toxicogenomic approaches. This data is already becoming useful in confirming mechanism of drug action and adverse reaction. There have already been proposals for a "new paradigm" in preclinical safety assessment in which *in vitro* and *in silico* approaches are combined [71].

7.7 USING DATA FROM *IN VITRO* PROFILING: CONFIRMATORY TESTS, FOLLOW-UP TESTS, AND THE LINK TO SAFETY ASSESSMENT AND *IN VIVO* MODELS

The principal aim of a genotoxicity screening program is to reduce the proportion of compounds that give positive results in IND-enabling GLP studies. The default action for a compound with a positive genotoxicity result during profiling tests would be removal from the collection. Profiling occurs when the properties of compounds identified in other screening tests are already channeling into the strategy of chemistry lead optimization. A positive result may not end a program, but would immediately reduce the ranking of the compound and provide valuable actionable information to the medicinal chemistry team. Only in very particular cases would a potent genotoxin be carried forward. If the choice of compounds is not broad due to the therapeutic indication, discovery, or patent strategy or the nature of the target, then there will be two avenues for immediate follow-up of a positive result. First, lead optimization chemists can be alerted to the need to focus on the segregation of useful pharmacology from unwanted genotoxicity facilitated by knowledge of the known structural alerting motifs (Section 7.4.2). Second, the compound profile should be annotated or flagged to indicate the possible need for follow-up by safety assessment teams to consider mechanism of action.

7.7.1 Annotations from Screening Data

All annotations/alerts should carry basic information including the assay type, the result, the top dose tested, the solvent, and any additional information generated such as control, lowest effective concentration, magnitude of effect, and associated toxicity data. Annotations and appropriate alerts should be included even where the result is negative and should be specific to the screening strategy. For a strategy based solely on mutation endpoints, a negative result should generate an alert that genotoxicity assessment is incomplete, and aneugenicity and clastogenicity have not been assessed. For a strategy based solely on aneugenicity or clastogenicity, a negative result should generate an alert that assessment is incomplete and an *in vitro* mutation has not been assessed. For a strategy using a reporter assay that is not endpoint-specific, a negative result should generate an alert for a complementary assay such as a bacterial assay after a eukaryotic screen or a eukaryotic assay after a bacterial screen.

Most of the *in vitro* assays are described with an additional protocol for the assessment of metabolites generated by the monooxygenases (CYPs) and various conjugation systems. It is unclear whether genuine high-throughput screening assays would be performed routinely with a source of exogenous metabolism such as the rodent liver extract S9. This seems unlikely because of S9 handling difficulties in a high-throughput situation: S9 is heat labile and frozen samples create problems associated with rethawing, etc. If there are no data from assays incorporating S9, then an alert should be generated to reflect that metabolites have not been investigated. This alert might be strengthened by linkage to data from metabolic liability assays or *in silico* approaches. In due course it is expected that there will be validated, metabolically competent cell lines for metabolite assessment.

7.7.2 Can a Genetic Toxicity Profile Assist with *In Vivo* Testing Strategies?

Current regulatory practice already requires that a positive *in vitro* result is followed up with two *in vivo* tests. The first regulatory *in vivo* assay is routinely the micronucleus test using either bone marrow or peripheral blood cells from only one sex in a rodent. With appropriate planning it is generally possible to use different tissues from the same animals for the second test. This is generally selected to assess the *in vivo* significance of the result of the *in vitro* test giving a positive result. Thus a positive result from a mutation assay suggests the use of an *in vivo* test for DNA damage/mutagenesis such as unscheduled DNA synthesis (UDS OECD 486), or ^{32}P-postlabelling to detect DNA adduct formation (no OECD guideline). If the positive result is only in the presence of metabolic activation, further metabolism studies are often instigated to determine if the metabolite formed *in vitro* (by a rat liver extract) is actually formed or is inactivated *in vivo*.

A recent review identified 120 rodent carcinogens where the *in vivo* MNT gave negative or equivocal results, and there were other *in vivo* data to consider. It was apparent that UDS has very poor sensitivity [72] and adduct assessment is generally reserved for compounds where reactive metabolites are suggested. The alkaline comet assay is now considered an appropriate alternative. The other alterative is to use one of the genetically engineered rodent mutation assays (Muta™Mouse, Big Blue), though these are expensive and time-consuming, so unlikely to be used routinely for both tissues/endpoints. Advice regarding choice of tissue will be dependent on other factors such as the target tissue of the drug. This information may not be available when screening alerts are recorded and is beyond the scope of this chapter.

Most recently attention has been drawn to the assessment of PigA mutations [73,74]. This X-linked gene provides a readily scored mutant phenotype as a consequence of its essential role in the anchoring of GPI proteins in the membrane. Mutant cells are distinguished by their inability to bind GPI-linked proteins such as CD59, CD55, and CD24. Furthermore, wild-type cells are killed by Aerolysin, a bacterial toxin that uses the GPI anchor to mediate lysis. Thus, aerolysin resistance is a direct selection for PigA mutants that can be cloned and sequenced to determine the nature of the mutation.

A positive result from a chromosome aberration assay (MNT, cytogenetic analysis, or small colonies in MLA), suggests a second *in vivo* assay for clastogenesis or aneugenesis. Centromere and DNA staining of mitotic cells allows the distinction of aneugens and clastogens.

If positive results in reporter assays specifically developed for profiling screening are obtained, *in vivo* MNT is conducted as a follow-up. Additional information may also be generated during the regulatory *in vitro* testing. Kirkland and Speit [72] recommend the comet assay as a second *in vivo* test, because the limited data available suggests that this assay identifies more of the carcinogens missed by MNT.

7.8 WHAT TO TEST, WHEN, AND HOW

Genotoxicity data should become an important part of a compound's profile. It can provide value in decision making at all stages in discovery from libraries containing millions of compounds to leads progressing to candidate selection. For entire libraries, screening could allow segregation of genotoxins into a sublibrary. If a new therapeutic campaign is initiated where genotoxicity is allowable or expected, such as antineoplastics or antivirals, then those compounds are included; if genotoxicity is unacceptable, then these compounds are excluded. As previously discussed, no screen detects all genotoxins. Conducting a library screen does not eliminate genotoxicity concerns and appropriate alerts remain for unassessed hazards. Furthermore, the chemical differences that evolve from hit to lead to drug-like candidate introduce new structural motifs.

None of the genotoxicity assays described above has yet been used for large libraries. Although most assay developers have access to the instrumentation required for developing HTS or ultra-HTS methods, a progressive longer term strategy to collect the data over a period of at least a year is a feasible approach for screening large sets.

Hit profiling is more feasible as it is generally anticipated that the initial target screen will generate $\sim <1\%$ hits (10,000–100,000 compounds per year). All compounds would benefit from the early inclusion of genotoxicity data in the profile. Only four of the assays discussed have the capacity for this screening scale: the bacterial Ames II, SOS reporters, the yeast RAD54-GFP reporter and the human GADD45a-GFP reporter. The bacterial

Ames II and SOS reporters provide an early warning for Ames positives. The yeast RAD54-GFP reporter and the human GADD45a-GFP reporter preview human aneugens and clastogens, missed by Ames. The most effective approach to screening would combine the bacterial, yeast, and now the human tests. As early as 2004, Kitching et al. [75] compiled validation data for 71 compounds from the GreenScreen GC (yeast) test with published SOS/*umu* data. The results were as follows:

- 54 compounds (76%) had positive data in cancer studies.
- 32 compounds (45%) were positive in GreenScreen GC.
- 32 compounds (45%) compounds were positive with SOS/*umu*.
- 22 compounds (31%) were positive for both tests.
- Each test had 10 unique positives.

Subsequently J&J assessed 2698 potential drug candidates through the Green-Screen yeast assay during preregulatory screening [40]. Two thousand three hundred fifty one compounds were also tested with Ames II. One hundred sixty four (7%) of the 2351 compounds were positive in Ames II, with and/or without S9 metabolic activation and 176 (7.5%) were positive in the GreenScreen. Twelve (7%) of the 176 GreenScreen-positive compounds were positive in Ames II. These results emphasize that the Ames II and GreenScreen assays each detect a different but overlapping spectrum of genotoxins, reflecting both the differences between pro-karyotic and eukaryotic test organisms and their different endpoints (mutation and DNA damage-induced transcription, respectively). Recently, the same group tested 1684 compounds using the GreenScreen HC (human cells) and Ames II assays (data not published). There was a 31 compound overlap between the two assays. This again confirms the different endpoints covered by bacterial and mammalian cell tests and reveals how genotoxicity results can vary for different compound collections.

A combination of two genotoxicity tests is a better screening strategy than conducting one assay. At earlier stages of discovery when chemical development is still in progress, one test is presumably sufficient. Given that *in silico* methods are quite effective in the identification of Ames-positive compounds based on structural alerts, a single eukaryotic screening test is preferred.

Profiling during lead optimization might generate 2,000–10,000 compounds per year. Genetic toxicity screening using eukaryotic models such as GreenScreen HC is already occurring at this level in some of the larger pharmaceutical companies.

7.9 CHANGES TO REGULATORY GUIDELINES CAN INFLUENCE SCREENING STRATEGY

The current ICH S2B guidelines require both Ames and *in vitro* mammalian test data. Since Ames data causes the greatest concern, most screening methods use one of the bacterial screens as well as one of the MNT screening tests using flow cytometry or imaging readouts. Early mammalian genotoxicity screens provide a useful preview of the regulatory MNT. However, MNT is known to have high prevalence of positive results (35% or more) in which many are false positives, not confirmed in *in vivo* testing. Consequently, many potentially valuable nonhazardous leads might be discarded based on MNT results before the selection of candidates is complete or require a large follow-up effort. To reduce this risk, a secondary screen of MNT positives with the higher specificity GADD45a-GFP (GreenScreen HC) test would identify the subset of compounds liable to give positive results in later *in vivo* tests. Many of the remaining GADD45a-GFP negatives could become useful drugs once mechanistic studies establish the nonrelevance of the positive MNT data.

The problems generated by the poor specificity of the current regulatory *in vitro* mammalian tests has led to the proposal of new testing strategies published in the US Federal Register as/or ICH S2(R1). These proposals contain two significant changes (Table 7.1). First, the maximum testing dose in the *in vitro* mammalian tests should be reduced from 10 to 1 mM to reduce the generation of misleading positive results due to high toxicity. The second change is that two different options for data submission are proposed. Option one is essentially the same as the current requirement except for the lower dosing. Option two is more radical: The submission requires Ames test for *in vitro* data and two different *in vivo* endpoints. It is proposed that these endpoints can be obtained from the same animal exposure study. For compound discovery and development, option 2 may be preferred since there is value in generating profiling data in *in vitro* mammalian assays during screening. The bacterial screens are valuable in as a preview of the regulatory Ames test results. Hence, there is now a broad selection of assays available that help avoid *in vivo* failures by compounds inevitably undetected by Ames. In the absence of informative *in silico* data, a high-specificity eukaryotic test would be preferred.

7.10 SUMMARY

There are now highly specific genotoxicity screening assays that can provide reliable hazard warnings, data early enough for medicinal chemists. Individual prokaryotic and eukaryotic tests detect different but overlapping classes of genotoxins. It has been demonstrated that the overall level of genotoxicity in a library that can be detected by these approaches is similar to the level of candidate attrition due to genotoxicity. This strategy can be facilitated using *in silico* approaches to identify embedded genotoxic structural moieties that can be potentially avoided. This suggests that early profiling will lead to development of more predictive *in silico* tools, which in turn will cause a significant reduction in late stage failure due to genotoxicity. It also offers an overall increase in efficiency in later regulatory genotoxicity safety assessment by providing an early alert for projects likely to require mechanistic investigation.

ACKNOWLEDGMENT

Andy Scott (Unilever) is thanked for the preparation of Figure 7.1. Nick Billinton is thanked for his contributions to the screening sections.

REFERENCES

1. Aubrecht, J., Osowski, J. J., Persaud, P., Cheung, J. R., Ackerman, J., Lopes, S. H., and Ku, W. W. Bioluminescent *Salmonella* reverse mutation assay: a screen for detecting mutagenicity with high throughput attributes. *Mutagenesis* 2007, *22*, 335–342.
2. *Physicians' Desk Reference*, 55th Edition, Medical Economics Co. Inc., Montvale, NJ, 2001.
3. Snyder, R. D. and Green, J. W. A review of the genotoxicity of marketed pharmaceuticals. *Mutat. Res.* 2001, *488*, 151–169.
4. Esteller, M. Epigenetics in cancer. *N. Engl. J. Med.* 2008, *358(11)*, 1148–1159.
5. Ames, B. N. and Gold, L. S. Paracelsus to parascience: the environmental cancer distraction. *Mutat. Res.* 2000, *447*, 3–13.
6. Available at http://potency.berkeley.edu/
7. Matthews, E. J., Kruhlak, N. L., Cimino, M. C., Benz, R. D., and Contrera, J. F. An analysis of genetic toxicity, reproductive and developmental toxicity, and carcinogenicity data: I. Identification of carcinogens using surrogate endpoints. *Regul. Toxicol. Pharm.* 2006, *44*, 83–96.
8. Kirkland, D., Aardema, M., Henderson, L., and Muller, L. Evaluation of the ability of a battery of three *in vitro* genotoxicity tests to discriminate rodent carcinogens and non-carcinogens I. Sensitivity, specificity and relative predictivity. *Mutat. Res.* 2005, *584*, 1–256.
9. US Federal Register. International Conference on Harmonisation: Draft Guidance on S2 (R1) Genotoxicity Testing and Data Interpretation for Pharmaceuticals Intended for Human Use; availability, 2008, 73, p. 59.
10. Müller, L., Mauthe, R. J., Riley, C. M., Andino, M., De Antonis, D., Beels, C., DeGeorge, J., De Knaep, F., et al. A rationale for determination, testing and control of genotoxic impurities. *Regul. Toxicol. Pharm.* 2006, *44*, 198–211.
11. Dobo, K. L., Greene, N., Cyr, M. O., Caron, S., and Ku, W. W. The application of structure-based assessment to support safety and chemistry diligence to manage genotoxic impurities in active pharmaceutical ingredients during drug development. *Regul. Toxicol. Pharm.* 2006, *44*, 282–293.
12. EMEA Guideline on the limits of genotoxic impurities. Available at http://www.emea.europa.eu/pdfs/human/swp/519902en.pdf.
13. Delaney, E. J. An impact analysis of the application of the threshold of toxicological concern concept to pharmaceuticals. *Regul. Toxicol. Pharmacol.* 2007, *49*, 107–124.
14. Ashby, J. Fundamental structural alerts to potential carcinogenicity or non-carcinogenicity. *Environ. Mutagen.* 1985, *7*, 919–921.
15. Ashby, J. and Tennant, R. W. Definitive relationships among chemical structure, carcinogenicity and mutagenicity for 301 chemicals tested by the U. S. NTP. *Mutat. Res.* 1991, *257*, 229–306.
16. Snyder, R. D., Pearl, G. S., Mandakas, G., Choy, W. N., Goodsaid, F., and Rosenblum, I. Y. Assessment of the sensitivity of the computational programs DEREK, TOPKAT, and MCASE in the prediction of the genotoxicity of pharmaceutical molecules. *Environ. Mol. Mutagen.* 2004, *43*, 143–158.
17. Matthews, E. J., Kruhlak, N. L., Benz, R. D., Contrera, J. F., Marchant, C. A., and Yang, C. Combined Use of MC4PC, MDL-QSAR, BioEpisteme, Leadscope PDM, and Derek for

windows software to achieve high-performance, high-confidence, mode of action-based predictions of chemical carcinogenesis in rodents. *Toxicol. Mech. Methods* 2008, *18*, 189–206.

18. Yang, C., Hasselgren, C. H., Boyer, S., Arvidson, K., Aveston, S., Dierkes, P., Benigni, R., and Benz, R. D., et al. Understanding genetic toxicity through data mining: the process of building knowledge by integrating multiple genetic toxicity databases. *Toxicol. Mech. Methods* 2008, *18*, 277–295.
19. Ashby, J. and Tennant, R. W. Chemical structure, Salmonella mutagenicity and extent of carcinogenicity as indicators of genotoxic carcinogenesis among 222 chemicals tested in rodents by U. S. NCI/NTP. *Mutat. Res.* 1988, *204*, 17–118.
20. Cheeseman, M. A., Machuga, E. J., and Bailey, A. B. A tiered approach to threshold of regulation. *Food Chem. Toxicol.* 1999, *37*, 387–412.
21. Kroes, R., Renwick, A. G., Cheeseman, M., Kleiner, J. Mangelsdorf, I. Piersma, A., Schilter, B., Schletter, J., van Schothorst, F., Vos, J. G., and Wűrtzen, G. Structure-based thresholds of toxicological concern (TTC). Guidance for application to substances present at low levels in the diet. *Food Chem. Toxicol.* 2004, *42*, 65–83.
22. Prestera, T. and Talay, P. Electrophile and antioxidant regulation of enzymes that detoxify carcinogens. *Proc. Natl. Acad. Sci. USA.* 1995, *92*, 8965–8969.
23. Williams, G. M. and Weisburger, J. H. Chemical Toxicology. In *Casarett and Douell's Toxicology. The Basic Science of Poisons*, Amdur, M. O., Doull, J.,and Claasen, C.D. (eds.), 4th Edition, McGraw-Hill, London, 1991, pp. 127–200.
24. Tong, W., Perkins, R., Strelitz, R., Collantes, E. R., Keenan, S., Welsh, W. J., Branham, W. S., and Sheehan, D. M. Quantitative structure–activity relationship (QSAR) for estrogen binding to the estrogen receptor. Predictions across species. *Environ. Health Perspect.* 1997, *105*, 1116–11124.
25. Cramer, G. F. M., Ford, R. A., and Hall, R. L. Estimation of toxic hazard—a decision tree approach. *Food Cosmetic Toxicol.* 1978, *16*, 255–276.
26. Cramer, G. F. M., and Ford, R. A. Evaluation of Certain Food Additives and Contaminants. Procedure for the Safety Evaluation of Flavouring Agents. 49th Report of the Joint FAO/WHO Expert Committee on Food Additives (JECFA). WHO Technical Report Series 884. World Health Organization, Geneva, 1999.
27. Munro, I. C., Ford, R. A., Kennepohl, E., and Kroes, R. Correlation of structural class with no-observed-effect levels: a proposal for establishing a threshold of concern. *Food Chem. Toxicol.* 1996, *34*, 829–867.
28. Cash, G. G., Anderson, B., Mayo, K., Bogaczyk, S., and Tunkel, J. Predicting genotoxicity of aromatic and heteroaromatic amines using electropological state indices. *Mutat. Res.* 2005, *585*, 170–183.
29. DEREK. Available at http://www.chem.leeds.ac.uk/luk/derek/.
30. TOXNET. Available at http://www.toxnet.nim.nih.gov/.
31. SCIFINDER. Available at http://www.cas.org/SCIFINDER/scicover2.html.
32. Shimizu, M., Yasui, Y., and Matsumoto, N. Structural specificity of aromatic compounds with special reference to mutagenic activity in *Salmonella typhimurium*—a series of chloro- or fluoronitrobenzene derivatives. *Mutat. Res.* 1983, *116*, 217–238.
33. Vance, W. A. and Levin, D. E. Structural features of nitroaromatics that determine mutagenic activity in *Salmonella typhimurium*. *Environ. Mutagen.* 1984, *6*, 797–811.

34. Ninomiya, S.-I., Kohda, K., and Kawazoe, Y. Studies on chemical carcinogens and mutagens. XXV. Chemoselectivity of the alkyl sulfonates toward 4-(p-nitrobenzyl)pyridine (NBP) in phosphate buffer. *Chem. Pharm. Bull.* 1984, *32*, 1326–1132.

35. Matthews, E. J., Kruhlak, N. L., Cimino, M. C., Benz, R. D., and Contrera, J. F. An analysis of genetic toxicology, reproductive and developmental toxicity, and carcinogenicity data: I. Identification of carcinogens using surrogate endpoints. *Reg. Tox. Pharm.* 2006, *44*, 83–96.

36. Matthews, E. J., Kruhlak, N. L., Cimino, M. C., Benz, R. D., and Contrera, J. F. An analysis of genetic toxicology, reproductive and developmental toxicity, and carcinogenicity data: II. Identification of genotoxicants, reprotoxicants and carcinogens using *in silico* methods. *Reg. Tox. Pharm.* 2006, *44*, 97–110.

37. MultiCASE, MC4PC. Available at http://www.multicase.com/products/prod01.hym.

38. Matthews, E. J. and Contrera, J. F. A new highly specific method for predicting the carcinogenic potential of pharmaceuticals in rodents using MCASEQSAR software. *Reg. Tox. Pharm.* 1998, *28*, 242–264.

39. Burke, D. A., Wedd, D. J., and Burlinson, B. Use of the Miniscreen assay to screen novel compounds for bacterial mutagenicity in the pharmaceutical industry. *Mutagenesis*, 1996, *11*, 201–205.

40. van Gompel, J., Woestenborghs, F., Beerens, D., Mackie, C., Cahill, P. A., Knight, A. W., Billinton, N., and Tweats, D. J., et al. An assessment of the utility of the yeast GreenScreen assay in pharmaceutical screening. *Mutagenesis* 2005, *20*, 449–454.

41. Flückiger-Isler, S., Baumeister, M., Braun, K., Gervais, V., Hasler-Nguyen, N., Reimann, R., Van Gompel, J., and Wunderlich, H., et al. Assessment of the performance of the Ames II™ assay: a collaborative study with 19 coded compounds. *Mutat. Res.* 2004, *558*, 181–197.

42. Mortimer, R. K. and Manney, T. R. Mutation induction in yeast. In *Chemical Mutagens: Principles and Methods for their Detection*, Vol. *1*, Hollaender, A. (ed.), Plenum Press, New York, 1971.

43. Zimmermann, F. K., von Borstel, R. C., von Halle, E. S., Parry, J. M., Siebert, D., Zetterberg, G., Barale, R., and Loprieno, N. Testing of chemicals for genetic activity with *Saccharomyces cerevisiae,* in Report to the US Environmental Protection Agency Gene-Tox Program. *Mutat. Res.* 1984, *133*, 199–244.

44. Parry, E. M. and Parry, J. M. The Assay of Genotoxicity of Chemicals Using the Budding Yeast *Saccharomyces cerevisiae*. In Mutagenicity Testing: A Practical Approach, Venitt, S. and Parry, J. M. (eds.), IRL Press, Oxford, 1985.

45. Schiestl, R. H., Gietz, R. D., Mehta, R. D., and Hasting, P. J. Carcinogens induce intrachromosomal recombination in yeast. *Carcinogenesis* 1989, *10*, 1445–1455.

46. Hontzeas, N., Hafer, K., and Schiestl, R. H. Development of a microtiter plate version of the yeast DEL assay amenable to high-throughput toxicity screening of chemical libraries. *Mutat. Res.* 2007, *634*, 228–234.

47. Mateuca, R., Lombaert, N., Aka, P. V., Decordier, I., and Kirsch-Volders, M. Chromosomal changes: induction, detection methods and applicability in human biomonitoring. *Biochimie* 2006, *88*, 1515–1531.

48. Diaz, D., Scott, A., Carmichael, P., Shi, W., and Costales, C. An assessment of the performance of an automated scoring system (Cellomics) for the *in vitro* micronucleus assay in CHO-K1 cells. *Mutat. Res.* 2007, *630*, 1–13.

49. Witt, K. L., Livanos, E., Kissling, G. E., Torous, D. K., Caspary, W., Tice, R. R., and Recio, L. Comparison of flow cytometry- and microscopy-based methods for measuring micronucleated reticulocyte frequencies in rodents treated with nongenotoxic and genotoxic chemicals. *Mutat. Res.* 2008, *649*, 101–113.

50. Bryce, S. M., Avlasevich, S. L., Bemis, J. C., Lukamowicz, M., Elhajouji, A., Van Goethem, F., De Boeck, M., Beerens, D., et al. Interlaboratory evaluation of a flow cytometric, high content *in vitro* micronucleus assay. *Mutat. Res.* 2008, *650*, 181–195.

51. Collins, A. R., Oscoz, A. A., Brunborg, G., Gaivão, I., Giovannelli, L., Kruszewski, M., Smith, C. C., and Stetina, R. The comet assay: topical issues. *Mutagenesis* 2008, *23*, 143–151.

52. Kiskinis, E., Suter, W., and Hartmann, A. High throughput Comet assay using 96-well plates. *Mutagenesis* 2002, *17*, 37–43.

53. Witte, I., Plappert, U., de Wall, H., and Hartmann, A. Genetic toxicity assessment: Employing the best science for human safety evaluation part III: The comet assay as an alternative to *in vitro* clastogenicity tests for early drug candidate selection. *Toxicol. Sci.* 2007, *97*, 21–26.

54. Radman, M. SOS repair hypothesis: Phenomenology of an inducible DNA repair which is accompanied by mutagenesis. *Basic Life Sci.* 1975, *5A*, 355–367.

55. Quillardet, P., Huisman, O., D'Ari, R., and Hofnung, M. SOS Chromotest, a direct assay for induction of an SOS function in *Escherichia coli* K-12 to measure genotoxicity. *Proc. Natl. Acad. Sci. USA* 1982, *79*, 5971–5975.

56. Reifferscheid, G. and Heil, J. Validation of the SOS/*umu* test using test results of 486 chemicals and comparison with the Ames test and carcinogenicity data. *Mutat. Res.* 1996, *369*, 129–145.

57. Quillardet, P. and Hofnung, M. The SOS chromotest: a review. *Mutat. Res.* 1993, *297*, 235–279.

58. Vollmer, A. C., Belkin, S., Smulski, D. R., Van Dyk, T. K., and LaRossa, R. A. Detection of DNA damage by use of *Escherichia coli* carrying *recA'::lux, uvrA'::lux,* or *alkA'::lux* reporter plasmids. *Appl. Environ. Microbiol.* 1997, *63*, 2566–2571.

59. Schmid, C., Reifferscheid, G., Zahn, R. K., and Backmann, M. Increase in sensitivity and validity of the SOS/umu-test after replacement of the beta-galactosidase reporter gene with luciferase. *Mutat. Res.* 1997, *394*, 9–16.

60. Verschaeve, L., Van Gompel, J., Thilemans, L., Regniers, L., Vanparys, P., and van der Lelie, D. VITOTOẌ bacterial genotoxicity and toxicity test for the rapid screening of chemicals. *Environ. Mol. Mutagen.* 1999, *33*, 240–248.

61. Flegrova, Z., Skarek, M., Bartos, T., Cupr, P., and Holoubek, I. Usefulness of three SOS-response tests for genotoxicity detection. *Fresenius Environ. Bull.* 2007, *16*, 1369–1376.

62. Walmsley, R. M., Billinton, N., and Heyer, W.-D. Green fluorescent protein as a reporter for the DNA damage-induced gene RAD54 from *Saccharomyces cerevisiae. Yeast* 1997, *13*, 1535–1545.

63. Cahill, P. A., Knight, A. W., Billinton, N., Barker, M. G., Walsh, L., Keenan, P. O., Williams, C. V., Tweats, D. J., et al. The GreenScreen genotoxicity assay: a screening validation programme. *Mutagenesis* 2004, *19*, 105–119.

64. Westerink, W. M., Stevenson, J. C., Lauwers, A., Griffioen, G., Horbach, G. J., and Schoonen, W. G. Evaluation of the Vitotox and RadarScreen assays for the rapid

assessment of genotoxicity in the early research phase of drug development. *Mutat. Res.* 2009, *401*, 6391–6318.

65. Hastwell, P. W., Chai, L.-L., Roberts, K. J., Webster, T. W., Harvey, J. S., Rees, R. W., and Walmsley, R. M. High-specificity and high-sensitivity genotoxicity assessment in a human cell line: Validation of the GreenScreen HC *GADD45a-GFP* genotoxicity assay. *Mutat. Res.* 2006, *607*, 160–175.
66. Jagger, C., Tate, M., Cahill, P. A., Hughes, C., Knight A. W., Billinton, N., and Walmsley, R. M. Assessment of the genotoxicity of S9-generated metabolites using the GreenScreen HC GADD45a–GFP assay. *Mutagenesis* 2009, *1*, 35–50.
67. Billinton, N., Hastwell, P. W., Beerens, D., Birrell, L., Ellis, P., Maskell, S., Webster, T. W., Windebank, R. M., et al. Interlaboratory assessment of the GreenScreen HC GADD45a-GFP genotoxicity screening assay: an enabling study for independent validation as an alternative method. *Mutat. Res.* 2008, *653*, 23–33.
68. Knight, A. W., Birrell, L., and Walmsley, R. M. Development and validation of a higher throughput screening approach to genotoxicity testing using the *GADD45a-GFP* Green-Screen HC assay. *J. Biomol. Screen.* 2009, *14*, 16–30.
69. Ohno, K., Taaka-Azuma, Y., Yoneda, Y., and Yamada, T. Genotoxicity test system based on p53R2 gene expression in human cells: examination with 80 chemicals. *Mutat. Res.* 2005, *588*, 45–57.
70. Ohno, K., Ishihata, K., Tanaka-Azuma, Y., and Yamada, T. A genotoxicity test system based on p53R2 gene expression in human cells: assessment of its reactivity to various classes of genotoxic chemicals. *Mutat. Res.* 2008, *656*, 27–35.
71. Ku, W. K., Aubrecht, J., Mauthe, R. J., Schiestl, R. H., and Fornace, A. J. Jr. Genetic toxicity assessment: employing the best science for human safety evaluation part VII: why not start with a single test: a transformational alternative to genotoxicity hazard and risk assessment. *Toxicol. Sci.* 2007, *99*, 20–25.
72. Kirkland, D. and Speit, G. Evaluation of the ability of a battery of three *in vitro* genotoxicity tests to discriminate rodent carcinogens and non-carcinogens III. Appropriate follow-up testing *in vivo*. *Mutat. Res.* 2008, *654*, 114–132.
73. Kawagoe, K., Takeda, J., Endo, Y., and Kinoshita, T. Molecular cloning of murine Pig-a, a gene for GPI-anchor biosynthesis, and demonstration of interspecies conservation of its structure, function, and genetic locus. *Genomics* 1994, *23*, 566–574.
74. Bryce, S.M., Bemis, J.C., and Dertinger, S.D. In vivo mutation assay based on the endogenous Pig-a locus. *Env. Mol. Mutagen* 2008, *49*, 256–264.
75. Kitching, J., Burlinson, B., Wing, M.G., and Walmsley, R.M. Finding the optimum approach for genetic toxicology screening. *Toxicologist* 2004, *78*, 132.

8

HEPATIC TOXICITY

JINGHAI JAMES XU AND KEITH HOFFMASTER

8.1 INTRODUCTION

Drug-induced liver injury (DILI) has been a significant challenge limiting the utility of many otherwise quite efficacious medications since the beginning of the modern pharmaceutical industry. The usage of a variety of medications including the nonsteroidal anti-inflammatory drugs (NSAIDs) nimesulide, antidepressant nefazodone, antifungal trovafloxacin, antidiabetic troglitazone, and antiviral drug nevirapine, have been associated with fatal cases of DILI even after successful completion of preclinical and clinical safety testing of these compounds in animals, healthy humans and human patients [1]. DILI is the number one reason for drug withdrawals after regulatory approval for marketing [2]. Hepatotoxicity is also a major cause of drug failures or attritions in the preclinical and clinical phases of drug development [3]. The problem of DILI is exacerbated by the fact that preclinical animal species such as rats, dogs, and monkeys combined only predict 55% of drugs that show hepatotoxicity in humans, according to a pharmaceutical industry-wide study [4]. As a result, the regulatory agencies in both the United States and Europe have developed guidelines for preclinical and clinical evaluations of DILI. These guidance documents can be found from the web sites of the Food and Drug Administration (http://www.fda.gov/) and the European Medicines Agency (http://www.emea.europa.eu/).

Since it takes on average 10–15 years and costs almost $1 billion to successfully develop an efficacious and safe drug *de novo* [5], earlier and better predictions of DILI before costly late-stage attritions becomes necessary to sustain continuous growth of the pharmaceutical industry and discovery of novel medicines. Better predictions of

ADMET for Medicinal Chemists: A Practical Guide, Edited by Katya Tsaioun and Steven A. Kates

DILI require focused effort by academics, industry, and government. Within the industry, close collaborations among medicinal chemists, pharmacologists, toxicologists, drug metabolism, and pharmacokinetic scientists, are key to de-risk the potential toxicity of a new chemical entity (NCE) or new molecular entity (NME) in order to be safely administered to human patients. This chapter will focus on our current understanding of DILI mechanisms and strategies to identify safer drug candidates.

8.2 MECHANISMS OF DILI

Clinical phenotypes of DILI include: necrosis, cholestasis, steatohepatitis, and other mixed types of injury. Liver injury manifests clinically by increased serum biomarkers, that is, alanine aminotransferase (ALT) levels more than three times the upper limit of normal (>3× ULN), and a total bilirubin level of more than twice the upper limit of normal (>2× ULN) [6]. Clinical patterns of liver necrosis are typically associated with a predominant initial elevation of ALT, as a result of the death of liver parenchymal cells (i.e., the hepatocytes). The clinical patterns of steatohepatitis can include an initial silent steatosis (i.e., fatty liver), followed by elevated ALT in patients blood. According to the late Dr. Hyman Zimmerman, elevations in serum enzyme levels (ALT, aspartate aminotransferase (AST), and alkaline phosphatase (ALP) are indicators of liver injury, whereas increases in both total and conjugated bilirubin levels are measures of overall liver dysfunction. If a drug causes sufficient hepatocyte injury to affect global liver function and, in particular, to cause jaundice (i.e., elevated total bilirubin in the blood because of impaired bilirubin excretion by the liver), the offending drug could lead to a 10–50% patient mortality rate depending on when the drug is stopped and other patient host factors. Dr. Zimmerman's observation, which was subsequently validated by multiple independent studies, is known as the Hy's law [7].

Different from hepatocellular necrosis (or death of the liver parenchymal cell type, the hepatocyte), cholestasis is defined as a condition where bile and/or bile constituents are disrupted from normal flow through the liver. Extrahepatic cholestasis usually manifests as a result of mechanical blockage of bile flow to the intestine or due to the presence of a gallstone or tumor, and is not considered to be caused by drug therapy. Intrahepatic cholestasis, however, can result from either blockage of the small canalicular ducts within the liver from underlying liver disease (e.g., hepatitis), or from therapeutic agents that interact with active mechanisms of bile secretion, for example, inhibition of bile salt transport mechanisms. Clinical symptoms of cholestasis include jaundice, light-colored stools, and dark urine (due to lack of bilirubin excretion into the bile/feces and compensatory excretion to the urine by the kidney), and severe cases can result in pruritus when bile constituents accumulate in the skin. Whereas elevated levels of serum ALT enzymes often suggest hepatocellular damage, ALP levels >3× the upper limit of normal (>3× ULN) often are diagnostic of cholestasis.

DILI does not occur in every single patient administered an offending hepatotoxic drug. Often, the incidence of DILI is so rare that only about 1 in 100 to 1 in

1000 patients experiences transient elevations of liver enzymes in serum (including ALT, ALP, etc.), and only 1 in 1000 to 1 in 10,000 patients goes on to develop irreversible liver injury. The term "idiosyncratic liver injury" is often used to describe this rare incidence of hepatotoxicity. Such patient idiosyncrasy, on top of the lack of good predictivity of animal models mentioned earlier [4], has made it even more challenging to identify the exact mechanism(s) of DILI in a particular patient and drug situation. It is well-known that the normal human liver has an incredible ability to adapt to injury. However, in susceptible patients with particular circumstances (such as underlying disease and conditions), continuous toxicant insult could eventually lead to "full-blown" liver injury. There is now general recognition that several potential mechanisms of DILI are frequently associated with hepatotoxic drugs, sometimes with multiple mechanisms within the same patient and drug situation. These mechanisms include repeated and excessive generation of reactive metabolites that cannot be cleared, mitochondrial inhibition and/or dysfunction that cannot be regenerated, generation of excessive oxidative stress leading to oxidative damage that cannot be sufficiently repaired, and disruption of bile acid homeostasis that cannot be counterbalanced [8]. Notice the deliberate mention of both concepts of "damage" and "repair" in each mechanism. While "damage" may be initiated by a drug, lack of sufficient "repair" may be largely determined by a patient's host factors. The job of medicinal chemists is to find drugs that are less likely to cause damage (i.e., first do no harm). Better understanding of these drug "damage" mechanisms have led to the development of experimental models and assay systems suitable for both characterizing such toxic mechanisms, and selecting better drug candidates in the earlier phases of drug discovery and development.

8.2.1 Reactive Metabolite Formation

A large amount of circumstantial evidence suggests that reactive metabolites of a drug, rather than the parent drug itself, are often responsible for many idiosyncratic hepatotoxicity [9]. One of the liver's main physiological roles is the metabolism of lipophilic xenobiotics into hydrophilic metabolites to facilitate their excretion. As a consequence of such drug transformation and excretion, the liver is typically exposed to a much higher local concentrations of drugs and metabolites than the systemic blood after oral drug administration. This phenomenon is termed the "first-pass" effect. In this physiological process, orally administered drugs are absorbed through the intestinal enterocyte (i.e., epithelial cells lining the intestinal wall) into the portal circulation (i.e., blood that normally transports nutrients from intestine to the liver), delivered as a concentrated amount to the liver for the "first-pass" metabolism and excreted into bile and/or blood; only then the remaining drug and/or metabolites are mixed with systemic blood circulation (hence another dilution effect), and delivered to the rest of the body.

The parenchymal cells of the liver, the hepatocytes, express an abundance of drug-metabolizing enzymes, consisting of both phase-I (typically oxidative) and phase-II (typically conjugative) enzymes. Cytochrome P450 (CYP450) enzymes are the major players in the phase-I metabolism of an incredibly diverse range of xenobiotics, including therapeutic agents as well as endogenous substances. In general, the stable metabolites after phase-I metabolism are more hydrophilic than the parent molecules and exhibit less toxicity. However, for some drugs, CYP450-mediated enzymatic reactions generate unstable or more toxic species. These so-called reactive metabolites can subsequently covalently bind to cellular proteins, a process known as bioactivation of proteins. These "bioactivated proteins" have the potential to trigger an immune-mediated response including the generation of antibodies to these drug-modified and sometimes even the native cellular proteins. The best example of the *in vivo* detection of antidrug antibodies that are associated with DILI is the case of tienilic acid. Tienilic acid (TA) or ticrynafen is a diuretic drug originally marketed for the treatment of hypertension. It was withdrawn in 1982, shortly after its introduction to the market, after several case reports of hepatotoxicity. Subsequently, it was found that the reactive metabolites of tienilic acid can covalently modify CYP2C9 and CYP2C11, both protein family members of CYP450. In addition, antibodies were detected in sera from patients with TA hepatotoxicity. These antibodies can recognize both drug-modified CYP2C11 as well as the native/unchanged CYP2C9 [10]. The proof that these antibodies that recognize drug–protein adducts are ultimately the major cause of drug-induced hepatotoxicity (as opposed to a bystander of drug exposure to the patient host) remains somewhat circumstantial [11].

According to the more "chemistry-centric" view of toxicology, the phenotype of toxicity can be traced back to a "toxicon," or a single toxic chemical structure. Less toxicity will result if a chemical structure that is more prone to converting to a reactive metabolite and thus the formation of covalent protein adducts be abolished or masked. A number of potential "toxicon scaffolds" or "toxicophores" have been identified, which medicinal chemists nowadays try to avoid during the design of a new chemical entity. These toxicophores include furans, thiophenes, and certain aromatic amines [12]. The presence or absence of such toxicophores can be inspected "visually" by computer algorithms or medicinal chemistry experts familiar with the drug metabolism field (i.e., automated or manual structural alerts). The formation of reactive metabolites also can be measured experimentally using a variety of *in vitro* CYP450-containing test systems coupled with sensitive analytical chemistry detection methods [12–16]. These test systems have been utilized by some research organizations to proactively screen molecules to minimize the formation of reactive metabolites [17].

Reactive metabolites can be formed by most, if not all, of the enzymes that are involved in drug metabolism. A variety of phase-I enzymes including CYP450, monoamine oxidase (MAO), and peroxidases can bioactivate nitrogen-containing chemicals. These biochemical reactions involve either direct oxidation on the nitrogen atom leading to reactive intermediates, or by oxidation at an alternate site in the molecule but with participation by the nitrogen atom in a subsequent reaction [18]. However the mere presence of such nitrogen-containing molecules or other "structural alerts," for that matter, is often not a reliable predictor of the ultimate toxicity outcome. Whether bioactivation will occur for a given molecule *in vivo* depends on several key factors: (i) does the molecule possess a toxicophore that is susceptible to bioactivation; (ii) is there an alternative (higher affinity but innocuous) route of metabolism within the molecule that minimizes the potential bioactivation of the toxicophore; and (iii) are there parallel competing detoxification pathways that can scavenge the reactive metabolite or its precursor [19]. Furthermore, whether tissue injury will occur as a result of bioactivation depends on additional host factors such as toleration to injury and adaptability to tissue repair. Hence, it is exceptionally challenging (if not impossible) to establish a direct correlation between bioactivation findings *in vitro* and toxicity outcomes *in vivo*.

Several major limitations of placing too much emphasis on the "avoidance of bioactivation" approach include:

(1) There are five major families of drug-metabolizing CYP450 enzymes (1A, 2C, 2D, 2E, and 3A), and each with several subfamily members. The types of structures that these enzymes can recognize are quite diverse. The number of *potential* "toxicophores" that these enzymes could recognize can be quite substantial and will inevitably overlap with "pharmacophores" required for a given drug's efficacy.

(2) The relationship between the generation of reactive metabolite or "bioactivation" and the occurrence of hepatotoxicity is not simple, as explained above. It is possible for drugs to undergo bioactivation in the liver without causing hepatotoxicity. The widely used analgesic acetaminophen is well-known to generate reactive metabolites via the reactions of CYP1A2, 2E1, and 3A4, but it only becomes hepatotoxic in a subset of patients at high therapeutic or supratherapeutic doses.

(3) There are still other and different mechanisms of DILI that are dependent on the parent drug molecules (as opposed to reactive metabolites). Examples include inhibition of the bile salt export protein (BSEP) in cholestatic injury with flutamide [20] and troglitazone [21], mitochondrial dysfunction with nefazodone [22], generation of reactive oxygen species with nimesulide [23], and lipid peroxidation by perhexiline, amiodarone, and 4,4′-diethylaminoethoxyhexestrol [24].

Indeed, if one examines sufficient numbers of both hepatotoxic and nonhepatotoxic drugs, reactive metabolite and/or covalent protein modification in an *in vitro* setting does not discriminate these two drug cohorts sufficiently to support a general application of such a proactive screening approach [25, 26]. Increasing evidence now exists for the multifactorial nature of DILI, in particular the role played by mitochondria, oxidative stress, bile acid transport (include BSEP), and tissue repair and immune adaptability [8, 27].

8.2.2 Mitochondrial Dysfunction and Oxidative Stress

Mitochondrial dysfunction has increasingly been recognized as an important mechanism of DILI [28–31]. The mammalian mitochondrion serves a variety of important cellular physiological roles including energy production, oxidative–reductive signaling, and apoptosis.

Mitochondria generate 95% of the cell's energy. This occurs in the electron transport chain, which contains four oxidative phosphorylation (OXPHOS) complexes (or complex I–IV) and an ATPase (or complex V). Oxidizable substrates from glycolysis, fatty acid, or protein catabolism enter the mitochondrion in the form of acetyl-CoA, or as other intermediaries of the Krebs cycle. Reducing equivalents in the form of NADH and FADH pass electrons to complex I (NADH-ubiquinone oxidoreductase), or complex II (succinate dehydrogenase) of the electron transport chain, respectively. Electrons pass from complex I and II to complex III (ubiquinol-cytochrome c oxidoreductase) and then to complex IV (cytochrome c oxidase), accumulating four electrons in the process. The four electrons then tetravalently reduce O_2 to water. Protons are pumped into the inner membrane space at complexes I, II, and IV, and then diffuse down their concentration gradient through the ATPase or complex V where their potential energy is captured in the form of ATP. ATP formation is coupled to electron transport and the formation of water, a process termed OXPHOS) (recently reviewed by Ref. 32).

Under ideal circumstances, all the electrons entering the electron transport system will reduce oxygen to water at complex IV. However, electrons can "leak" from several sites along the way, predominantly complexes I and III, and ubiquinone, resulting in univalent reduction of O_2 to form the superoxide radical ($O_2^{-\bullet}$). The superoxide radical can dismutate to form hydrogen peroxide H_2O_2, either spontaneously or more by the enzyme superoxide dismutase (SOD). These oxidative by-products of normal cellular metabolism form the basis of normal oxidative stress of cells, and cells have evolved several enzymatic systems (e.g., SOD) and antioxidant reserves (e.g., glutathione) to cope with these reactive species. The mitochondrion is the major hub of redox activities in mammalian cells, and the major source of endogenous oxidative stress in these cells [33]. If drug insults increase the electron "leak" by blocking the normal functions of the mitochondrial complex, this could lead to increased oxidative stress of the cell, and mitochondrial and cellular damages can ensue if there is no sufficient compensatory increase in SOD activity [34–36].

Drugs of many important classes can undermine mitochondrial function via direct and indirect effects. The former arise acutely via direct interference with mitochondrial function, and the latter over longer periods via interference with mitochondrial transcription/translation, and/or acceleration of free radical production. Drugs can inhibit the functions of multiprotein mitochondrial complexes. Impairment of mitochondrial beta-oxidation leads to accumulation of fat resulting in steatosis, and ensuing lipid peroxidation can lead to steatohepatitis [24]. With regard to indirect effect, mitochondria contain the only extranuclear genomic DNA (mtDNA), and it encodes 13 proteins using a genetic code different from that in the nucleus. These proteins are key components of OXPHOS complexes I, III, IV, and V. Inhibition of mtDNA transcription as well as expression of mitochondrial proteins will therefore lead to loss of OXPHOS function. The best-known drugs that inhibit mtDNA synthesis are the nucleotide reverse transcriptase inhibitors (NRTIs), such as zalcitabine, didanosine, and stavudine, all of which cause hepatic DNA depletion, and liver toxicity in susceptible patients (recently reviewed by Ref. 29).

8.2.3 Bile Flow, Drug-Induced Cholestasis, and Inhibition of Biliary Efflux Transporters

The flow of bile from the liver into the small intestine serves several important physiologic roles. Bile contains high levels of bile acids which serve to aid in the digestion of fat and nutrients from dietary intake. In the liver, these bile acids help in the solubilization and subsequent elimination of cholesterol across the canalicular membrane and prevent the formation of gallstones in the biliary ducts and gall bladder. Bile flow also represents the predominant pathway for elimination of bilirubin and bilirubin glucuronide, the breakdown product of hemoglobin. The proper maintenance of biliary flow relies upon mechanisms of uptake of biliary constituents from the blood across the sinusoidal membrane, fluid flow through the hepatocyte, and subsequent active and passive processes of excretion across the canalicular membrane into the bile duct. Conjugated and unconjugated bile acids are actively transported into the bile predominantly via the bile salt export pump or BSEP, localized at the canalicular membrane of the hepatocyte. In addition to BSEP, other transport mechanisms are important for the proper excretion of components into the bile. These include ABCG5/ABCG8, the heterodimer protein responsible for the excretion of cholesterol directly from the liver, MDR3, the flippase responsible for the movement of phosphatidyl choline from the inner to the outer leaflet of the canalicular membrane, and ATP8B1, the flippase responsible for the translocation of phosphatidyl serine from the outer to the inner leaflet of the bilayer [37–39]. Genetic disorders that result in the lack of function of BSEP, ATP8B1, or MDR3 all result in the clinical manifestation of cholestasis in some form (reviewed in Refs. 40 and 41).

In addition to its intrinsic physiologic functions, bile flow and biliary excretion can play a key role in the elimination of xenobiotics. Many drugs and metabolites of drugs have been shown to be eliminated into the bile via active transport mechanisms. For example, the muscle relaxant vecuronium [42] and the cardiac glycoside digoxin are extensively excreted into the bile by P-glycoprotein (MDR1) [43]. The canalicular transporter MRP2 plays a role in the excretion of several HMG-CoA reductase inhibitors including pravastatin [44] and the breast cancer resistance protein (BCRP) has been shown to be important for the biliary excretion of several fluoroquinolones [45]. Although MDR1, MRP2, and BCRP are thought to be responsible for the biliary excretion of most drugs and their metabolites, some recent results have implicated BSEP in the direct excretion of pravastatin into the bile [46]. Several studies also highlight the overlapping role of these transporters to facilitate the excretion of xenobiotics and their metabolites [47–49].

Potential interactions of therapeutic agents with the endogenous mechanisms of bile flow and biliary excretion include decreased drug clearance as a result of reduced biliary function due to underlying cholestatic disease as well as direct interaction of a drug with hepatobiliary function, resulting in bland cholestasis. Several reports have described the impact of hepatic disease on the disposition of drugs and mechanisms of hepatobiliary excretion [50, 51], and should be considered in the drug development process to understand the potential that these patient populations will be targeted in routine clinical treatment. The ability of drugs to inhibit the normal excretion of bile from the liver can lead to the accumulation of bile acids within the cell [52, 53]. Although compensatory mechanisms (e.g., multidrug resistance-associated protein 3, MRP3) at the sinusoidal membrane of the liver may help transport bile acids from the hepatocyte back into the blood, some drugs and their metabolites have been shown to inhibit multiple mechanisms of transport within the liver, at sinusoidal and canalicular membranes [54, 55]. Due to their detergent like properties, cellular accumulation of bile acids and their conjugates can lead to hepatic necrosis [56]. As mentioned above, genetic mutations in BSEP result in intrahepatic cholestasis. Analogous to genetic disruption, inhibition of BSEP by drugs and their metabolites has been shown to result in cholestasis *in vivo*. BSEP inhibition by compounds such as cyclosporine, nefazodone, bosentan, glibenclamide, and troglitazone (described in Section 8.4) has been suggested to contribute to the underlying mechanism of hepatotoxicity observed clinically [56–60].

8.3 ASSAYS AND TEST SYSTEMS TO MEASURE VARIOUS TYPES OF DILI

Assays and test systems to measure various types of DILI are discussed with attention to *in vitro* assay systems with sufficient predictivity and throughput for lead optimization programs of the drug discovery process.

Since the normal human liver has an enormous capacity to adapt, repair and regenerate itself, any *in vitro* system that lacks the ability to adapt to injury can only be viewed as restricted to investigating the initial chemical insult(s) to the liver. Whole cell-based models typically have more capability to cellular defense and repair than cell-free systems, and are increasing utilized to study DILI mechanisms and processes. Human liver cell-based systems, due to the presence of human-specific liver transporters and drug-metabolizing enzymes, are becoming more mainstream as well as cells isolated from animal species (e.g., rat, dogs, monkeys) [61, 62].

Human liver cell lines (exemplified by the HepG2 hepatocarcinoma cell line), despite their limitations in drug-metabolizing capacity (low) and cell cycle status (proliferating cells), are still frequently used to study the general cytotoxic potential of the parent drug molecule. Cellular necrosis can be measured by the amount of intracellular ATP levels left after a period of drug treatment, as only healthy cells can produce ATP. Since the mitochondrion is the major source of cellular ATP, this simple assay can be an initial surrogate assay (although not a definitive test) for drug-induced mitochondrial injury. Since the parental HepG2 cell line has low levels of CYP450 enzymatic activity, engineered HepG2 cell lines have been used to express various CYP450 enzymes (although not engineered in the same cell line). In addition to the HepG2 line, other cell lines include the HepaRG (a clonal selection of the HepG2 cell line) [63, 64], the THLE (an SV40 tumor antigen immortalized human liver cells) [65], and their CYP450-expressing daughter cell lines [65]. These CYP450-expressing cell lines may be used to investigate CYP450 metabolite-specific toxicities to these cells. Most of these cell lines can only be used to study drug- or metabolite-induced necrosis or apoptosis, but not cholestasis.

Primary cells, in particular, primary hepatocytes cultured in defined media, can sustain differentiated liver morphology and function for extended culture time (typically at 1 week or more). These differentiated liver-specific traits include: nondividing and polynuclear phenotypes, expression of phase-I and -II drug-metabolizing enzymes that are inducible, and expression of drug uptake and efflux transporters that are responsive to perturbations. Primary human hepatocytes cultured in the sandwiched configuration (either Collagen/Collagen, or Collagen/Matrigel sandwich, with hepatocytes between two layers of matrix), reestablish cellular polarity over time in culture where functional sinusoidal and canalicular transporters are localized to the proper membrane surfaces of the hepatocytes. These transporters are capable of facilitating vectorial transport of compounds across the hepatocyte and compound accumulation within the cellular compartment and the bile canaliculi compartment can be quantified. Therefore, the primary hepatocyte sandwiched model is an optimal *in vitro* model to study both hepatobiliary drug transport [49, 66] and drug-induced cholestasis [67, 68].

Other *in vitro* methodologies have been developed to complement the whole cell sandwich-cultured hepatocyte model. BSEP-transfected Sf9 membrane vesicles are a useful tool to understand the intrinsic potential for a compound to directly inhibit BSEP-mediated bile acid transport across the canalicular membrane [69, 70]. This system does however have the potential to incorrectly predict the true impact of BSEP inhibition *in vivo* since in the intact liver, compounds must first cross the sinusoidal membrane of the hepatocyte to gain access to the proposed site of inhibition. Compounds such as estradiol-17β-D-glucuronide do not appear to directly inhibit BSEP, rather, may cause endocytic retrieval of the transporter in intact cells, suggesting that the entire complement of cellular machinery is required to elicit the true impact of bile acid transport inhibition [71]. Some data support that compound excretion into the canalicular space is required to inhibit BSEP, so-called trans-inhibition that has been observed by metabolites of progesterone as well as estradiol-17 β-D-glucuronide [72, 73]. Membrane vesicles derived from the canalicular membranes of intact hepatocytes have also been utilized to demonstrate the potential for xenobiotics to inhibit mechanisms of bile acid transport [58]. Although these systems integrate the function of other transport proteins present at the apical membrane of the hepatocyte, technical challenges regarding purity and the absence of a sinusoidal membrane may limit the ultimate translation of these data to the *in vivo* setting.

While the simple cellular ATP measurement provides a rapid screen without much mechanistic insight, other more informative assays can measure more subtle insult to cellular health, and provide more insights toward mechanistic understandings of DILI. Cellular imaging aimed at measuring prelethal events (as opposed to simple cell loss due to cell detachment from the cell culture surface), can provide both a direct correlation to histopathology and information on intracellular organelles affected by such drug insults. In cellular imaging, cells are typically treated with drug or metabolite with or without imaging dyes. When drug is treated without dyes, the imaging reagents can be added post drug treatment to highlight organelle morphology. These imaging reagents can highlight specific cellular phenotypes relevant to toxicology such as apoptosis (programmed cell death), steatosis (neutral lipid accumulation), phospholipidosis (phospholipid accumulation), oxidative stress (production of reactive oxygen species), mitochondria stress (mitochondria membrane potential), and cholestasis (decreased bile acid flux) [74]. These cellular morphologies are either inspected manually under an appropriate microscope, or more commonly, rapidly captured and digitized by an automated microscope equipped with a semiautomated image analysis algorithm. The image analysis algorithms can continuously capture and measure any objects of interest, and can be programmed to alert the researcher on any "abnormal" or "findings of interest" at the cellular-, field-, well-, treatment-, or compound-level. This whole field of efficient cellular imaging analysis, termed high-content screening (HCS, as opposed to HTS for high-throughput screening), have practically exploded in the past decade to a highly sophisticated and organized scale to discover both novel pharmacology, toxicology, systems biology, and systems medicine [74–79]. In the spirit of "seeing is believing," high-content screens provide or enable:

(a) visual proof for a given biological conclusion,
(b) multiple cellular phenotypes that can be measured at the same time from within the same cell, thus lending the technology endless possibilities to investigate cellular dynamics and processes in pharmacology and toxicology,
(c) drug precipitate, fluorescent or colored compound, that can be easily deciphered, minimizing both false positives and false negatives in traditional HTS,
(d) accurate cell count from a treated sample, thus any "findings of interest" can be normalized by cell count, minimizing false conclusions derived due to the loss of cell attachment, and
(e) probably the most significant, *in vitro* correlation to *in vivo* histopathology.

Detailed primary hepatocyte cell culture, staining, imaging, and image analysis protocols have recently been published [80–82]. The hepatocyte imaging assay technology (HIAT), identified over half of the hepatotoxic drugs tested including many idiosyncratic hepatotoxicants, while maintaining a low false-positive rate of 0–5%, in a validation study using over 300 drugs [80]. The HIAT utilized a combination of epifluorescent molecules to simultaneously probe the intensity and location of several intracellular organelles and species. Nuclei count, shape, and intensity were stained by the DNA-specific anthraquinone dyes Draq5 [83] (Figure 8.1a). Intrahepatocyte levels and distributions of reduced glutathione were imaged by monochlorobimane [84] (Figure 8.1b); monochlorobimane is a nonfluorescent hydrophobic probe that readily permeates into cells and is conjugated with glutathione to form the fluorescent glutathione bimane, an organic anion [85]. This fluorescent glutathione conjugate displayed a strong cytosolic fluorescence in healthy hepatocytes. It is also a substrate for the canalicular multispecific organic anion transporter MRP2, which mediates the ATP-dependent secretion of a wide range of organic anions over the canalicular membrane into bile. The primary human hepatocytes were cultured in a confluent sandwiched culture that facilitates the

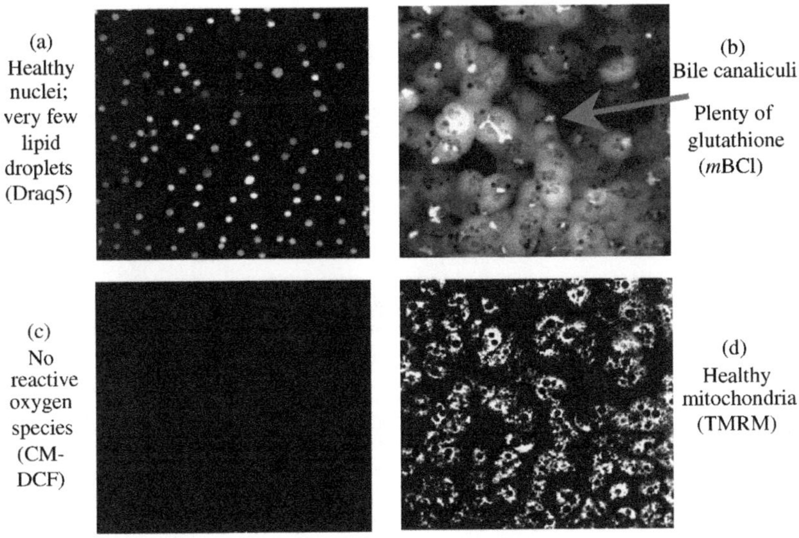

Figure 8.1 Representative epifluorescence images of healthy hepatocytes from the HIAT.

formation of bile canaliculi (BC) and the function of a family of multispecific transporters including MRP2, MDR1, and BSEP in between two adjacent hepatocytes (Figure 8.1b) [86]. The maintenance of normal hepatobiliary efflux function of such transporter can also be measured by the signal intensity of the bimane fluorescence in the BC region (Figure 8.1b). In addition, HIAT utilizes a fluoresceine-based probe for reactive oxygen species, and a potential-sensitive dye to measure mitochondrial membrane potential [87]. Healthy hepatocytes exhibit normal nuclear morphology (Figure 8.1a), strong intracellular glutathione fluorescence with even stronger signals in the BC regions (Figure 8.1b), very little reactive oxygen species (Figure 8.1c), and strong mitochondrial membrane potential (Figure 8.1d). Deviations from such normal morphology upon drug treatment can signal one or more potential mechanisms of drug-induced liver injury [80]. Some examples of such morphological deviations are shown in Figure 8.2a–d. Drug-induced inhibition of BSEP can be quantitatively measured by the efflux of a BSEP-selective fluorescent probe, cholyl–lysyl fluoresceine (CLF), into the bile canaliculi space of similarly sandwiched cultured human hepatocytes [81].

For any test system to be useful for lead optimization, it is important that the system is robust enough for assay optimization. The field of HTS has benefited from both laboratory automation and development of sensitive imaging instruments [88]. Image analysis algorithms have been sufficiently automated to allow meaningful extraction of data from a large number of cellular features over many cellular samples [79, 88, 89]. The intelligent combination of these technologies enabled automated statistical mining of cellular images for novel cellular phenotype combinations relevant for both drug efficacy [79, 90] and drug toxicity [80, 89]. A new era of phenotype-based drug screening has been born, but now it is fully dependent on novel combinations of

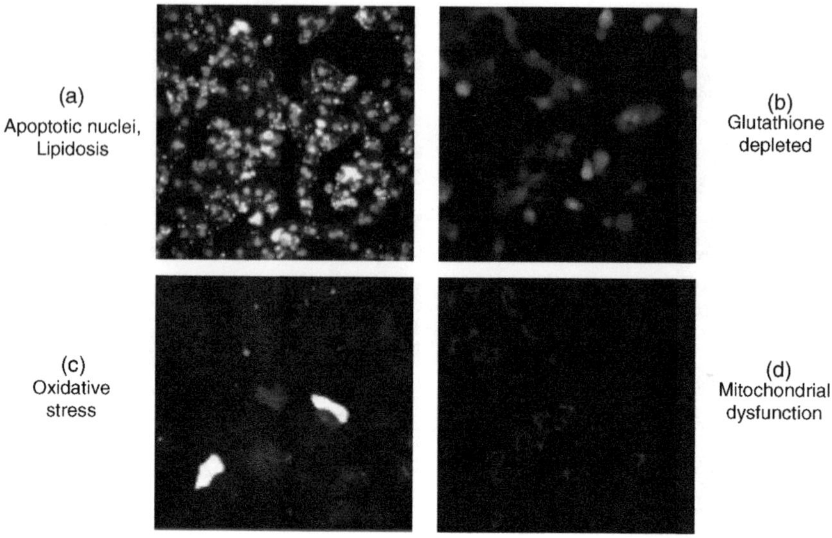

Figure 8.2 Representative epifluorescence images of abnormal hepatocytes from the HIAT.

molecular probes and systems biology, as opposed to the heritage of phenotypic descriptions.

It is important to maintain a low false-positive rate for any toxicological assay system to be useful for lead optimization. Since a false-positive finding or false alarm on an otherwise quite safe drug in the lead optimization stage, could potentially lead to disinterest or even abandonment of viable drug candidate, it is imperative that any assay systems be subject to thorough evaluation and validation using a sufficient number of "safe" drugs. It is quite common that there exists an imbalance in the number of toxic versus safe drugs in many scholarly publications on potential assay and test systems for DILI [91–94]. Since the number of toxic drugs outnumbers the safe ones by a very wide margin in these studies, a potential side effect of optimizing the assay sensitivity as much as possible is decreased specificity (i.e., increasing false-positive rate without truly knowingly). In a few recent studies with more balanced number of safe (i.e., negative) drugs, the findings are quite illuminating [25, 26, 80, 95, 96].

There is no shortage of clinically beneficial drugs that can cause a transient increase in serum ALT activity, no increase in total serum bilirubin (TBL) concentration, and do not cause serious hepatotoxicity in the clinic. Well-known examples of such drugs include the Alzheimer's medication tacrine, HMG-CoA reductase inhibitors or statins such as simvastatin, widely used pain killers such as aspirin, effective antidepressants such as fluoxetine, paroxetine, and buspirone, the antihypertensive drug propranolol, and the selective estrogen receptor modulator (SERM) raloxifene [97–99]. These drugs should be classified as DILI negatives, and should be included in the drug validation list of any test systems to better assess their false-positive rate, before such test systems can be used for routine testing or prospective prediction of DILI. All of these drugs were classified as DILI negatives by the

HIAT testing paradigm [80]. Hence the final conclusions from HIAT are distinct from what have been published about these compounds in the past [100–108].

The reason for the high specificity of the HIAT may be a combination of: (1) the drug concentrations used have reasonable relevance to the *in vivo* situation (e.g., using a common scaling factor of 100× to account for higher liver drug exposure to the liver for an orally dosed drug and other patient-related idiosyncratic variables), (2) primary hepatocytes in culture are nondividing cells and compared to hepatoma cell lines are less sensitive to agents that may perturb the cell cycle [109]; and (3) primary hepatocyte culture in the sandwiched configuration maintains more normal and balanced drug metabolizing and transporter functions [86, 110–112]. HIAT was evaluated against a large number of drugs (>300 in total) with over a hundred DILI negative drugs, including those that cause a transient increase in ALT but not TBL (as discussed above). As a result the low false-positive rate of the HIAT system is more likely than other testing systems to be translated to a "real world" scenario. The high positive predictive value toward the ultimate *in vivo* outcome (in this case serious DILI) is a striking contrast to the current *in vitro* tests for drug-induced genotoxicity [96] or developmental toxicity [95], and should be a continued emphasis in developing, evaluating, and implementing *in vitro* test systems for the prediction of other drug-induced toxicity.

8.4 MEDICINAL CHEMISTRY STRATEGIES TO MINIMIZE DILI

Hepatotoxic drugs can sometimes cause DILI by a multitude of mechanisms. Because of their role in insulin resistance, the family of PPARs—specifically PPARγ, have been leveraged as therapeutic targets for type-II diabetes mellitus. Several thiazolidinediones have been developed that are effective in controlling insulin levels in diabetic patients. First reported in 1982, ciglitazone was the first molecule in this class to show promise in preclinical models of diabetes [113] and subsequent optimization of this series of molecules resulted in compounds such as troglitazone (Rezulin®), pioglitazone (Actos®), and rosiglitazone (Avandia®) (Figure 8.3).

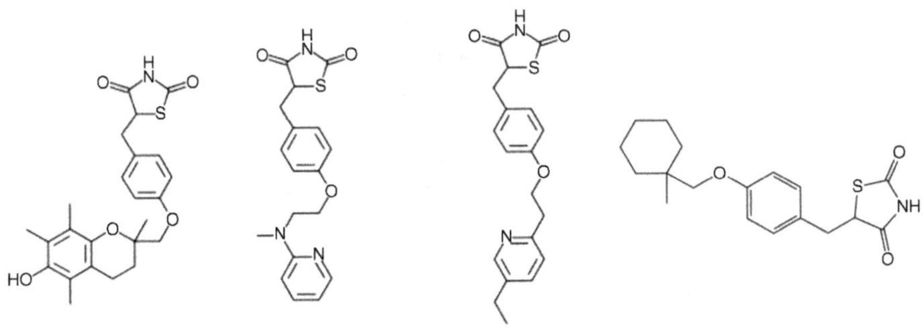

Troglitazone Rosiglitazone Pioglitazone Ciglitazone

Figure 8.3 Chemical structures of thiazolidinediones developed for the treatment of type-II diabetes mellitus. Troglitazone and ciglitazone exhibited more hepatotoxicity than rosiglitazone or pioglitazone in the clinic.

Troglitazone was removed from the United States market in 2000 due to several reports of hepatotoxicity, whereas the latter two are still prescribed to patients in the United States. Following these reports of adverse events with troglitazone, several mechanistic studies probed the underlying reasons behind the toxicity observed. Several hypotheses have since been proposed to explain the incidence of clinical hepatotoxicity. Troglitazone, but not the other three glitazones, was shown to produce a reactive metabolite in the presence of human liver microsomes [114]. In addition, troglitazone and ciglitazone, but not rosiglitazone or pioglitazone, can induce mitochondrial permeability transition (MPT) and cause mitochondrial dysfunction [115]. Recently, in a murine model of silent mitochondrial stress, troglitazone treatment induces first an initial adaptive response, followed by a toxic response involving oxidant injury to mitochondrial proteins [116]. Troglitazone and its metabolite troglitazone sulfate were shown to be potent inhibitors of the bile salt export pump *in vitro* in canalicular liver plasma membrane vesicles and *in vivo* in rats [58]. Snow et al. demonstrated the potential for pioglitazone and rosiglitazone to also inhibit BSEP-mediated transport of bile salts in a dose-dependent manner, suggesting that the core thiazolidinedione moiety may represent a class effect on bile acid homeostasis *in vivo* [117]. However, the earlier studies clearly indicated that the sulfate metabolite of troglitazone was ~10-fold more potent inhibitor of transport than troglitazone itself, with an apparent IC_{50} value of 0.4 μM for inhibition of BSEP-mediated taurocholate transport in membrane vesicles. *In vivo*, troglitazone is predominantly metabolized to this sulfate conjugate, whereas 62% of the dose of rosiglitazone is excreted unchanged into the urine [118].

Target-based SAR of the thiazolidinediones has been well described (see Ref. 119 for extensive reviews). Structurally, all three of the PPARγ activators contain the core thiazolidinedione moiety with a single carbon linking a phenyl group. All three structures also contain an ether functionality linking a lipophilic tail. This lipophilic tail differentiates troglitazone and ciglitazone from the others, and by deduction could therefore be at least in part, responsible for the observed toxicity. Troglitazone has differentiated itself in a variety of *in vitro* experimental systems from pioglitazone and rosiglitazone, as summarized above. Recent data from Huh-7 cells showed that troglitazone, not pioglitazone or rosiglitazone, was capable of modulating the farnesoid X receptor, a key transcription factor responsible for the regulation of target genes responsible for bile acid homeostasis (e.g., BSEP) [21]. Although not directly related to mechanisms of bile acid transport, troglitazone has been shown to be a more potent inducer of CYP3A4 and CYP2B6, and is a more potent inhibitor of CYP3A4-, CYP2C8-, and CYP2C9-mediated metabolism than pioglitazone or rosiglitazone [120]. Given that clinical doses of troglitazone result in plasma C_{max} values two- to fourfold higher than pioglitazone or rosiglitazone, the increased potency to modulate several P450 mechanisms coupled with these higher systemic concentrations could further contribute to the hepatotoxicity observed. Overall, the absolute mechanisms responsible for the toxicity of the thiazolidinediones still remain somewhat debated [121]. It is clear that emerging data do support the differentiation of troglitazone from other analogs that have shown limited signals of hepatic dysfunction clinically.

The case of four glitazones highlights the need for medicinal chemists to improve the potency of the molecule toward its intended target (i.e., from ci- and tro- to rosi-, and pioglitazone), while at the same time maintain the simplicity of the molecule's structure (e.g., the more lipophilic tail in troglitazone may be a reason why it is associated with the more promiscuity toward a variety of "off-targets" by the troglitazone molecule). In general, medicinal chemists will be well-advised to consider these strategies to minimize a molecule's propensity to induce hepatotoxicity:

(a) Increasing drug potency without introducing excessive molecular size, lipophilicity, and ionization state:

Despite the now well-known publication of the concept of drug-likeness, such as the "rule of five" [122], it has been recognized that both the calculated 1-octanol–water partition coefficient (i.e., clog *P*, which is a measure of a drug's lipophilicity) and the median molecular weight (i.e., MW, which is a general measure of a drug's molecular size) have been increasing since around 1985 [123]. Lipophilicity of a drug molecule reflects its likelihood to transfer from aqueous phase to cell membranes and to protein binding sites, which are mostly hydrophobic in nature. Some degree of lipophilicity is obviously needed for a drug molecule to engage its intended target. If lipophilicity is too high, there is an increased likelihood of binding to multiple targets and resultant pharmacological promiscuity, or toxicity, as well as poor solubility and metabolic clearance. Pharmacological promiscuity is predominantly controlled by lipophilicity and ionization state, with bases being more promiscuous than acids, neutral compounds, or zwitterions [123].

It is proposed that the essence of lead optimization is to increase potency without increasing lipophilicity or excessive molecular mass at the same time [123]. In this regard, two useful metrics to guide the progress of lead optimization are "ligand efficiency" (LE, Equation 8.1) and "ligand-lipophilicity efficiency" (LLE, Equation 8.2):

$$\mathrm{LE} = \mathrm{pIC}_{50}(\text{or } \mathrm{p}K_{\mathrm{i}}) \div \text{number of heavy atoms} \tag{8.1}$$

$$\mathrm{LLE} = \mathrm{pIC}_{50}(\text{or } \mathrm{p}K_{\mathrm{i}}) - \mathrm{c}\log P(\text{or} \log D) \tag{8.2}$$

The average oral drug with a clog $P \sim 2.5$ and potency in the range ~1–10 nM suggests an LLE target of ~5–7 or greater [123]. Increased LE and LLE during the lead optimization stage are expected to increase the overall therapeutic index of the lead series.

(b) Leverage noncompetitive binding, especially, for targets with a high concentration of endogenous ligands, to lower drug exposure required for *in vivo* efficacy.

Although the importance of good drug-like physicochemical properties cannot be underestimated, these properties alone may not always be responsible for the lack of success in a target class. It is recognized that biochemical mechanisms of drug action is as important as, if not more so, for the translation into a better therapeutic index [124]. If IC_{50} is the concentration required to inhibit the functional response by one half, and K_i is the binding affinity of the drug for the target, the biochemical efficiency or BE can be defined by Equation 8.3. Equation 8.4 is the equivalent of Equation 8.3, for the case of agonism mechanism as opposed to antagonism. The *in vivo* therapeutic effective dose, ED_{50}, or the dose required to inhibit the functional response by one half, is related to IC_{50} or EC_{50}, and specific pharmacokinetic (PK) factors, as in Equations 8.5 and 8.6 [124].

$$IC_{50} = K_i/BE \qquad \text{((8.3) for antagonists)}$$

$$EC_{50} = K_d/BE \qquad \text{((8.4) for agonists)}$$

$$ED_{50} = PK(IC_{50}) \qquad \text{((8.5) for antagonists)}$$

$$ED_{50} = PK(EC_{50}) \qquad \text{((8.6) for agonists)}$$

In essence, BE is dependent upon the biochemical mechanism of action (e.g., competitive, noncompetitive, irreversible, quasiirreversible, etc.). BE is inversely related to the potency, consistent with concept that the less efficient a drug's mechanism of action, the greater the concentrations of drug (thus IC_{50} or EC_{50}) required to achieve the required potency. High drug concentrations may compromise the safety of the drug and decrease the therapeutic window. Therefore, another metric of successful lead optimization is to increase a drug candidate's BE. One way to achieve this goal is to leverage noncompetitive or nonequilibrium mode of biochemical modulation [124]. This is especially important when the concentration of the endogenous ligand of the intended target is high or highly fluctuating in an open biological system (e.g., concentration of ATP for kinase inhibitors, concentration of other endogenous substrates, and cofactors for other enzymes).

(c) Take therapeutic C_{max} into consideration when predicting DILI.

Since the liver is potentially exposed to a higher effective C_{max} for an orally administered drug, pharmaceutical scientists should not be misled by the apparent low IC_{50}, K_i, or K_d in a cell-free and plasma protein-free test system *in vitro*. As demonstrated by recently published studies of over 300 drugs, the toxicological response of the liver is largely driven by *in vivo* liver C_{max} exposure, which is higher than measured systemic C_{max} values for an orally administered drug [80]. In the preclinical and drug discovery phase, the "systemic C_{max} needed" to ensure continuous efficacy of a drug candidate in the simplest case can be estimated from the minimal efficacious *in vivo* concentration (C_{min}), projected half-life ($T_{1/2}$), and intended dosing interval (I), by Equations 8.7 and 8.8, assuming one-compartment kinetics:

$$A = I/T_{1/2} \tag{8.7}$$

$$\text{Systemic } C_{max} \text{ needed} = C_{min}(2^A) \tag{8.8}$$

Therefore, a successful lead optimization and drug candidate selection program can be further guided by ultimately lowering the C_{max} needed to elicit a desired *in vivo* response in experimental animal models first, followed by later human proof of concept trials. The strategies and metrics proposed in (a), (b), and (c) herein are highly correlated and consistent in guiding principles, that is, toward the widening of a drug's therapeutic index, lowering of drug doses and its required clinical C_{max}, and increasing *in vivo* potency. High *in vivo* potency has advantages in addition to cost-of-goods benefits: when the total dose in humans is low, adventitious compound-related toxicity is less of an issue. It has been stated that very few idiosyncratic drug reactions have been observed with drugs given at a dose of 10 mg or less [125].

(d) Use predictive assays to minimize hepatotoxicity.

Since DILI remains a major challenge in late-stage drug attritions, it is important to apply some form of well-characterized predictive hepatotoxicity test systems. Specifically, application of assays and scoring algorithms with sufficient sensitivity and high specificity (i.e., low false-positive rate) is a must in the lead optimization and drug candidate selection stage. While the broad application of hepatotoxicity assays prospectively on all drug candidates may not be as mature as applying the Ames test for genotoxicity [126, 127] or hERG inhibition test for cardiotoxicity [128, 129], it is well advised to apply some of the more established and better-characterized hepatotoxicity tests [80] in programs with previously documented hepatotoxicity findings. For example, the mitogen-activated protein kinase (MAPK) p38α is a Ser/Thr kinase, originally isolated from lipopolysaccharide (LPS)-stimulated monocytes. p38α kinase is involved in the biosynthesis of the cytokines tumor necrosis factor-alpha (TNF-α) and interleukin-1beta (IL-1β) at the translational and transcriptional level. MAPK p38α represents a point of convergence for multiple signaling processes that are activated during inflammation, making it a key potential target for the modulation of cytokine production. Many pharmaceutical companies have tried to develop p38α inhibitors as potential treatments for inflammatory diseases. However few p38α inhibitors were chosen, largely because of side effects in the liver (e.g., elevated liver enzymes in serum) and skin (e.g., skin rash) [130]. In our past experience, by integrating data and knowledge from the human HIAT assay, human lymphocytes TNFα assay, and kinase selectivity data, a whole new series of MAPK p38α kinase inhibitors were identified with much wider therapeutic index for liver injury signals.

8.5 FUTURE OUTLOOKS

The success of a new pharmaceutical entity depends on potency and a sufficient therapeutic window between drug efficacy and safety (i.e., wide enough margin between toxic dose/concentration and efficacious dose/concentration). The validity of a sufficient therapeutic window can only be ascertained by the completion of large-scale clinical trials and possibly even by years of postmarketing experience in the case of rare forms of idiosyncratic injury. The early prediction of a therapeutic window will be critical to sustain an industry with such a long product development cycle, costly research and development (R&D) investments, and unusually low success rate. To correct the course of increased R&D spending and low NCE approvals will likely require both conceptual and organizational adjustments. In the target identification and validation stage, the efficiency of the target in modulating the disease as well as the normal function of the target in the context of human physiology need to be better understood. The biochemical and cellular mechanism or mode of target modulation need to be efficient in the presence of competing endogenous ligands [124]. In the hit-to-lead stage, it is troubling that despite the widespread acceptance of guidelines related to desirable physicochemical properties of small-molecule oral drugs, key properties such as clog *P* and molecular mass of drug leads generated by HTS continue to exceed such properties of approved drugs [131]. In today's highly competitive world, the ingenuity of medicinal chemists and close collaborations with pharmacologists, ADME/PK scientists, and toxicologists will continue to be imperative to engineer a compound with desirable pharmacokinetics and a sufficient and optimal therapeutic window.

ACKNOWLEDGMENT

The authors gratefully extend their acknowledgement to many past collaborators at Pfizer Global Research and Development (PGRD), especially Margaret Dunn, Arthur Smith, David de Graaf, Jeffrey Chabot, Peter Henstock, Jonathan Cyr, Yvonne Will, James Dykens, David Duignan, Amit Kalgutkar, and Scott Obach.

REFERENCES

1. Kaplowitz, N. Idiosyncratic drug hepatotoxicity. *Rev. Drug Discov.* 2005, *4(6)*, 489–499.
2. FDA. Available at http://www.fda.gov/cder/livertox/. Accessed May 28th, 2007.
3. Schuster, D., Laggner, C., and Langer, T. Why drugs fail—a study on side effects in new chemical entities. *Curr. Pharm. Des.* 2005, *11(27)*, 3545–3559.
4. Olson, H., et al. Concordance of the toxicity of pharmaceuticals in humans and in animals. *Regul. Toxicol. Pharmacol.* 2000, *32(1)*, 56–67.
5. DiMasi, J. A., Hansen, R. W., and Grabowski, H. G. The price of innovation: new estimates of drug development costs. *J. Health Econ.* 2003, *22(2)*, 151–185.
6. Navarro, V. J. and Senior, J. R. Drug-related hepatotoxicity. *N. Engl. J. Med.* 2006, *354(7)*, 731–739.

7. Temple, R. Hy's law: predicting serious hepatotoxicity. *Pharmacoepidemiol. Drug Saf.* 2006, *15(4)*, 241–243.
8. Lee, W. M. Drug-induced hepatotoxicity. *N. Engl. J. Med.* 2003, *349(5)*, 474–485.
9. Antoine, D. J., Williams, D. P., and Park, B. K. Understanding the role of reactive metabolites in drug-induced hepatotoxicity: state of the science. *Expert Opin. Drug Metab. Toxicol.* 2008, *4(11)*, 1415–1427.
10. Robin, M. A., et al. Antigenic targets in tienilic acid hepatitis. Both cytochrome P450 2C11 and 2C11-tienilic acid adducts are transported to the plasma membrane of rat hepatocytes and recognized by human sera. *J. Clin. Invest.* 1996, *98(6)*, 1471–1480.
11. Neuberger, J. and Williams, R. Immune mechanisms in tienilic acid associated hepatotoxicity. *Gut* 1989, *30(4)*, 515–519.
12. Kalgutkar, A. S., et al. A comprehensive listing of bioactivation pathways of organic functional groups. *Curr. Drug Metab.* 2005, *6(3)*, 161–225.
13. Williams, D. P. and Naisbitt, D. J. Toxicophores: groups and metabolic routes associated with increased safety risk. *Curr. Opin. Drug Discov. Devel.* 2002, *5(1)*, 104–115.
14. Zhou, S., et al. Drug bioactivation, covalent binding to target proteins and toxicity relevance. *Drug Metab. Rev.* 2005, *37(1)*, 41–213.
15. Prakash, C., et al. *In vitro* screening techniques for reactive metabolites for minimizing bioactivation potential in drug discovery. *Curr. Drug Metab.* 2008, *9(9)*, 952–964.
16. Nassar, A. E. and Lopez-Anaya, A. Strategies for dealing with reactive intermediates in drug discovery and development. *Curr. Opin. Drug Discov. Devel.* 2004, *7(1)*, 126–136.
17. Doss, G. A. and Baillie, T. A. Addressing metabolic activation as an integral component of drug design. *Drug Metab. Rev.* 2006, *38(4)*, 641–649.
18. Kalgutkar, A. S., et al. On the diversity of oxidative bioactivation reactions on nitrogen-containing xenobiotics. *Curr. Drug Metab.* 2002, *3(4)*, 379–424.
19. Xu, J. J., et al. Predicting Drug-Induced Hepatotoxicity: *In vitro*, *In Silico* and *In Vivo* Approaches. In *Hit and Lead Profiling*, Urban, B. F. a. L. (ed.), Wiley-VCH, Weinheim, 2009, pp. 345–385.
20. Iwanaga, T., et al. Involvement of bile salt export pump in flutamide-induced cholestatic hepatitis. *Biol. Pharm. Bull.* 2007, *30(4)*, 739–744.
21. Kaimal, R., et al. Differential modulation of farnesoid X receptor signaling pathway by the thiazolidinediones. *J. Pharmacol. Exp. Ther.* 2009, *330(1)*, 125–134.
22. Dykens, J. A., et al. *In vitro* assessment of mitochondrial dysfunction and cytotoxicity of nefazodone, trazodone and buspirone. *Toxicol. Sci.* 2008, *103(2)*, 335–345, doi: 10.1093/toxsci/kfn056.
23. Ong, M., et al. Nimesulide-induced hepatic mitochondrial injury in heterozygous Sod2 (+/−) mice. *Free Radic. Biol. Med.* 2006, *40(3)*, 420–429.
24. Robin, M. A., et al. Steatohepatitis-inducing drugs trigger cytokeratin cross-links in hepatocytes. Possible contribution to Mallory-Denk body formation. *Toxicol. In Vitro* 2008, *22(6)*, 1511–1519.
25. Bauman, J. N., et al. Can *in vitro* metabolism-dependent covalent binding data distinguish hepatotoxic from nonhepatotoxic drugs? An analysis using human hepatocytes and liver S-9 fraction. *Chem. Res. Toxicol.* 2009, *22(2)*, 332–340.
26. Obach, R. S., et al. Can *in vitro* metabolism-dependent covalent binding data in liver microsomes distinguish hepatotoxic from nonhepatotoxic drugs? An analysis of 18 drugs

with consideration of intrinsic clearance and daily dose. *Chem. Res. Toxicol.* 2008, *21(9)*, 1814–1822.

27. Zimmerman, H. *Hepatotoxicity: The Adverse Effects of Drugs and Other Chemicals on the Liver*, 2nd Edition, Lippincott Williams & Wilkins, Baltimore, MD, 1999, p. 789.
28. Kashimshetty, R., et al. Underlying mitochondrial dysfunction triggers flutamide-induced oxidative liver injury in a mouse model of idiosyncratic drug toxicity. *Toxicol. Appl. Pharmacol.* 2009, *238(2)*, 150–159.
29. Labbe, G., Pessayre, D. and Fromenty, B. Drug-induced liver injury through mitochondrial dysfunction: mechanisms and detection during preclinical safety studies. *Fundam. Clin. Pharmacol.* 2008, *22(4)*, 335–353.
30. Kass, G. E. Mitochondrial involvement in drug-induced hepatic injury. *Chem. Biol. Interact.* 2006, *163(1–2)*, 145–159.
31. Jaeschke, H., et al. Mechanisms of hepatotoxicity. *Toxicol. Sci.*, 2002, *65(2)*, 166–176.
32. Dykens, J. and Will, Y. *Drug-Induced Mitochondrial Dysfunction*, Wiley, Hoboken, NJ, 2008.
33. Kakkar, P. and Singh, B. K. Mitochondria: a hub of redox activities and cellular distress control. *Mol. Cell Biochem.* 2007, *305(1–2)*, 235–253.
34. Yuan, L. and Kaplowitz, N. Glutathione in liver diseases and hepatotoxicity. *Mol. Aspects Med.* 2009, *30(1–2)*, 29–41.
35. Sato, N. Central role of mitochondria in metabolic regulation of liver pathophysiology. *J. Gastroenterol. Hepatol.* 2007, *22(1)*, S1–S6.
36. Pessayre, D., Fromenty, B. and Mansouri, A. Mitochondrial injury in steatohepatitis. *Eur. J. Gastroenterol. Hepatol.* 2004, *16(11)*, 1095–1105.
37. Kidambi, S. and Patel, S. B. Cholesterol and non-cholesterol sterol transporters: ABCG5, ABCG8 and NPC1L1: a review. *Xenobiotica* 2008, *38(7–8)*, 1119–1139.
38. Trauner, M., Fickert, P., and Wagner, M. MDR3 (ABCB4) defects: a paradigm for the genetics of adult cholestatic syndromes. *Semin. Liver Dis.* 2007, *27(1)*, 77–98.
39. Paulusma, C. C., et al. ATP8B1 requires an accessory protein for endoplasmic reticulum exit and plasma membrane lipid flippase activity. *Hepatology* 2008, *47(1)*, 268–278.
40. Jansen, P. L. and Sturm, E. Genetic cholestasis, causes and consequences for hepatobiliary transport. *Liver Int.* 2003, *23(5)*, 315–322.
41. Kullak-Ublick, G. A. and Meier, P. J. Mechanisms of cholestasis. *Clin. Liver Dis.* 2000, *4 (2)*, 357–385.
42. Smit, J. W., et al. Hepatobiliary and intestinal clearance of amphiphilic cationic drugs in mice in which both mdr1a and mdr1b genes have been disrupted. *Br. J. Pharmacol.* 1998, *124(2)*, 416–424.
43. Hedman, A., et al. Interactions in the renal and biliary elimination of digoxin: stereoselective difference between quinine and quinidine. *Clin. Pharmacol. Ther.* 1990, *47(1)*, 20–26.
44. Nakai, D., et al. Human liver-specific organic anion transporter, LST-1, mediates uptake of pravastatin by human hepatocytes. *J. Pharmacol. Exp. Ther.* 2001, *297(3)*, 861–867.
45. Ando, T., et al. Involvement of breast cancer resistance protein (ABCG2) in the biliary excretion mechanism of fluoroquinolones. *Drug Metab. Dispos.* 2007, *35(10)*, 1873–1879.

46. Hirano, M., et al. Bile salt export pump (BSEP/ABCB11) can transport a nonbile acid substrate, pravastatin. *J. Pharmacol. Exp. Ther.* 2005, *314(2)*, 876–882.

47. Kitamura, S., et al. Involvement of multiple transporters in the hepatobiliary transport of rosuvastatin. *Drug Metab. Dispos.* 2008, *36(10)*, 2014–2023.

48. Vlaming, M. L., et al. Functionally overlapping roles of Abcg2 (Bcrp1) and Abcc2 (Mrp2) in the elimination of methotrexate and its main toxic metabolite 7-hydroxymethotrexate *in vivo*. *Clin. Cancer Res.* 2009, *15(9)*, 3084–3093.

49. Hoffmaster, K. A., et al. Multiple transport systems mediate the hepatic uptake and biliary excretion of the metabolically stable opioid peptide [D-penicillamine 2,5]enkephalin. *Drug Metab. Dispos.* 2005, *33(2)*, 287–293.

50. Geier, A., et al. Principles of hepatic organic anion transporter regulation during cholestasis, inflammation and liver regeneration. *Biochim. Biophys. Acta* 2007, *1773 (3)*, 283–308.

51. Trauner, M., et al. Molecular regulation of hepatobiliary transport systems: clinical implications for understanding and treating cholestasis. *J. Clin. Gastroenterol.* 2005, *39 (4)*, S111–S124.

52. Trauner, M., Meier, P. J., and Boyer, J. L. Molecular pathogenesis of cholestasis. *N. Engl. J. Med.* 1998, *339(17)*, 1217–1227.

53. Funk, C., et al. Troglitazone-induced intrahepatic cholestasis by an interference with the hepatobiliary export of bile acids in male and female rats. Correlation with the gender difference in troglitazone sulfate formation and the inhibition of the canalicular bile salt export pump (Bsep) by troglitazone and troglitazone sulfate. *Toxicology* 2001, *167(1)*, 83–98.

54. Slitt, A. L., et al. Regulation of transporter expression in mouse liver, kidney, and intestine during extrahepatic cholestasis. *Biochim. Biophys. Acta* 2007, *1768(3)*, 637–647.

55. Mennone, A., et al. Mrp4$^{-/-}$ mice have an impaired cytoprotective response in obstructive cholestasis. *Hepatology* 2006, *43(5)*, 1013–1021.

56. Gores, G. J., et al. Induction of the mitochondrial permeability transition as a mechanism of liver injury during cholestasis: a potential role for mitochondrial proteases. *Biochim. Biophys. Acta* 1998, *1366(1–2)*, 167–175.

57. Kadmon, M., et al. Inhibition by cyclosporin A of adenosine triphosphate-dependent transport from the hepatocyte into bile. *Gastroenterology* 1993, *104(5)*, 1507–1514.

58. Funk, C., et al. Cholestatic potential of troglitazone as a possible factor contributing to troglitazone-induced hepatotoxicity: *in vivo* and *in vitro* interaction at the canalicular bile salt export pump (Bsep) in the rat. *Mol. Pharmacol.* 2001, *59(3)*, 627–635.

59. Fattinger, K., et al. The endothelin antagonist bosentan inhibits the canalicular bile salt export pump: a potential mechanism for hepatic adverse reactions. *Clin. Pharmacol. Ther.* 2001, *69(4)*, 223–231.

60. Stieger, B., et al. Drug- and estrogen-induced cholestasis through inhibition of the hepatocellular bile salt export pump (Bsep) of rat liver. *Gastroenterology* 2000, *118 (2)*, 422–430.

61. Tuschl, G., Lauer, B., and Mueller, S. O. Primary hepatocytes as a model to analyze species-specific toxicity and drug metabolism. *Expert Opin. Drug Metab. Toxicol.* 2008, *4(7)*. 855–870.

62. Li, A. P. Human hepatocytes: isolation, cryopreservation and applications in drug development. *Chem. Biol. Interact.* 2007, *168(1)*, 16–29.

63. Guillouzo, A., et al. The human hepatoma HepaRG cells: a highly differentiated model for studies of liver metabolism and toxicity of xenobiotics. *Chem. Biol. Interact.* 2007, *168(1)*, 66–73.
64. Josse, R., et al. Long-term functional stability of human HepaRG hepatocytes and use for chronic toxicity and genotoxicity studies. *Drug Metab. Dispos.* 2008, *36(6)*, 1111–1118.
65. Pfeifer, A. M., et al. Simian virus 40 large tumor antigen-immortalized normal human liver epithelial cells express hepatocyte characteristics and metabolize chemical carcinogens. *Proc. Natl. Acad. Sci. USA* 1993, *90(11)*, 5123–5127.
66. Liu, X., et al. Biliary excretion in primary rat hepatocytes cultured in a collagen-sandwich configuration. *Am. J. Physiol.* 1999, *277(1 Pt 1)*, G12–G21.
67. Kemp, D. C., Zamek-Gliszczynski, M. J., and Brouwer, K. L. Xenobiotics inhibit hepatic uptake and biliary excretion of taurocholate in rat hepatocytes. *Toxicol. Sci.* 2005, *83(2)*, 207–214.
68. Kostrubsky, V. E., et al. Evaluation of hepatotoxic potential of drugs by inhibition of bile-acid transport in cultured primary human hepatocytes and intact rats. *Toxicol. Sci.* 2003, *76(1)*, 220–228.
69. Byrne, J. A., et al. The human bile salt export pump: characterization of substrate specificity and identification of inhibitors. *Gastroenterology* 2002, *123(5)*, 1649–1658.
70. Noe, J., Stieger, B., and Meier, P. J. Functional expression of the canalicular bile salt export pump of human liver. *Gastroenterology* 2002, *123(5)*, 1659–1666.
71. Crocenzi, F. A., et al. Estradiol-17 beta-D-glucuronide induces endocytic internalization of Bsep in rats. *Am. J. Physiol. Gastrointest. Liver Physiol.* 2003, *285(2)*, G449–G459.
72. Vallejo, M., et al. Potential role of trans-inhibition of the bile salt export pump by progesterone metabolites in the etiopathogenesis of intrahepatic cholestasis of pregnancy. *J. Hepatol.* 2006, *44(6)*, 1150–1157.
73. Huang, L., et al. Mrp2 is essential for estradiol-17beta(beta-D-glucuronide)-induced cholestasis in rats. *Hepatology* 2000, *32(1)*, 66–72.
74. Xu, J. J., Dunn, M. C., and Smith, A. R. "Seeing is believing": perspectives of applying imaging technology in discovery toxicology. *Comb. Chem. High Throughput Screen* 2009, *12(9)*, 827–837.
75. Eggert, U. S. and Mitchison, T. J. Small molecule screening by imaging. *Curr. Opin. Chem. Biol.* 2006, *10(3)*, 232–237.
76. Megason, S. G. and Fraser, S. E. Imaging in systems biology. *Cell* 2007, *130(5)*, 784–795.
77. Megason, S. G. In toto imaging of embryogenesis with confocal time-lapse microscopy. *Methods Mol. Biol.* 2009, *546, 317–332.*
78. Jaffer, F. A., et al. Molecular imaging of myocardial infarction. *J. Mol. Cell Cardiol.* 2006, *41(6)*, 921–933.
79. Perlman, Z. E., et al. Multidimensional drug profiling by automated microscopy. *Science* 2004, *306(5699)*, 1194–1198.
80. Xu, J. J., et al. Cellular imaging predictions of clinical drug-induced liver injury. *Toxicol. Sci.* 2008, *105(1)*, 97–105.
81. Feng, B., et al. Role of hepatic transporters in the disposition and hepatotoxicity of a HER2 tyrosine kinase inhibitor CP-724,714. *Toxicol. Sci.* 2009, *108(2)*, 492–500.

82. Cosgrove, B. D., et al. Synergistic drug-cytokine induction of hepatocellular death as an *in vitro* approach for the study of inflammation-associated idiosyncratic drug hepatotoxicity. *Toxicol. Appl. Pharmacol.* 2009, *237(3)*, 317–330.

83. Edward, R. Use of DNA-specific anthraquinone dyes to directly reveal cytoplasmic and nuclear boundaries in live and fixed cells. *Mol. Cells* 2009, *27(4)*, 391–396.

84. Stevenson, D., et al. Measurement of the intracellular distribution of reduced glutathione in cultured rat hepatocytes using monochlorobimane and confocal laser scanning microscopy. *Toxicol. In Vitro* 2002, *16(5)*, 609–619.

85. Oude Elferink, R. P., et al. Accumulation of organic anion in intracellular vesicles of cultured rat hepatocytes is mediated by the canalicular multispecific organic anion transporter. *Hepatology* 1993, *17(3)*, 434–444.

86. Bi, Y. A., Kazolias, D., and Duignan, D. B. Use of cryopreserved human hepatocytes in sandwich culture to measure hepatobiliary transport. *Drug Metab. Dispos.* 2006, *34(9)*, 1658–1665.

87. Qu, B., et al. Mechanism of clofibrate hepatotoxicity: mitochondrial damage and oxidative stress in hepatocytes. *Free Radic. Biol. Med.* 2001, *31(5)*, 659–669.

88. Taylor, D. L. Past, present, and future of high content screening and the field of cellomics. *Methods Mol. Biol.* 2007, *356, 3–18.*

89. Xu, J. J., Dunn, M. C., and Ryley, L. C.Automated *in vitro* cellular imaging assays for micronuclei and other target objects. Available at http://www.patentlens.net/patentlens/structured.cgi?patnum=WO_2004/099773_A1#show. Pfizer, 2004.

90. Fenistein, D., et al. A fast, fully automated cell segmentation algorithm for high-throughput and high-content screening. *Cytometry A* 2008, *73(10)*, 958–964.

91. Noor, F., et al. An integrated approach to improved toxicity prediction for the safety assessment during preclinical drug development using Hep G2 cells. *Toxicol. Appl. Pharmacol.* 2009, *237(2)*, 221–231.

92. Elferink, M. G., et al. Microarray analysis in rat liver slices correctly predicts *in vivo* hepatotoxicity. *Toxicol. Appl. Pharmacol.* 2008, *229(3)*, 300–309.

93. Suter, W., Predictive value of *in vitro* safety studies. *Curr. Opin. Chem. Biol.* 2006, *10(4)*, 362–366.

94. Takakusa, H., et al. Covalent binding and tissue distribution/retention assessment of drugs associated with idiosyncratic drug toxicity. *Drug Metab. Dispos.* 2008, *36(9)*, 1770–1779.

95. Paquette, J. A., et al. Assessment of the embryonic stem cell test and application and use in the pharmaceutical industry. *Birth Defects Res. B. Dev. Reprod. Toxicol.* 2008, *83(2)*, 104–111.

96. Kirkland, D., et al. How to reduce false positive results when undertaking *in vitro* genotoxicity testing and thus avoid unnecessary follow-up animal tests: report of an ECVAM Workshop. *Mutat. Res.* 2007, *628(1)*, 31–55.

97. FDA. Drug-Induced Liver Injury: Premarketing Clinical Evaluation. Available at http://www.fda.gov/Cder/guidance/7507dft.htm, 2007.

98. Lee, W. M. and Senior, J. R. Recognizing drug-induced liver injury: current problems, possible solutions. *Toxicol. Pathol.* 2005, *33(1)*, 155–164.

99. Senior, J. R. Drug hepatotoxicity from a regulatory perspective. *Clin. Liver Dis.* 2007, *11(3)*, 507–524.

100. Galisteo, M., et al. Hepatotoxicity of tacrine: occurrence of membrane fluidity alterations without involvement of lipid peroxidation. *J. Pharmacol. Exp. Ther.* 2000, *294(1)*, 160–167.

101. O'Brien, P. J., et al. High concordance of drug-induced human hepatotoxicity with *in vitro* cytotoxicity measured in a novel cell-based model using high content screening. *Arch. Toxicol.* 2006, *80(9)*, 580–604.

102. Tavintharan, S., et al. Reduced mitochondrial coenzyme Q10 levels in HepG2 cells treated with high-dose simvastatin: a possible role in statin-induced hepatotoxicity? *Toxicol. Appl. Pharmacol.* 2007, *223(2)*, 173–179.

103. Pessayre, D., et al. Hepatotoxicity due to mitochondrial dysfunction. *Cell. Biol. Toxicol.* 1999, *15(6)*, 367–373.

104. Laville, N., et al. Effects of human pharmaceuticals on cytotoxicity, EROD activity and ROS production in fish hepatocytes. *Toxicology* 2004, *196(1–2)*, 41–55.

105. Xu, J., Ma, M., and Purcell, W. M. Characterisation of some cytotoxic endpoints using rat liver and HepG2 spheroids as *in vitro* models and their application in hepatotoxicity studies. II. Spheroid cell spreading inhibition as a new cytotoxic marker. *Toxicol. Appl. Pharmacol.* 2003, *189(2)*, 112–119.

106. Chen, Q., et al. Cytochrome P450 3A4-mediated bioactivation of raloxifene: irreversible enzyme inhibition and thiol adduct formation. *Chem. Res. Toxicol.* 2002, *15(7)*, 907–914.

107. Zhao, S. X., et al. NADPH-dependent covalent binding of [3H]paroxetine to human liver microsomes and S-9 fractions: identification of an electrophilic quinone metabolite of paroxetine. *Chem. Res. Toxicol.* 2007, *20(11)*, 1649–1657.

108. Kalgutkar, A. S., et al. Bioactivation of the nontricyclic antidepressant nefazodone to a reactive quinone-imine species in human liver microsomes and recombinant cytochrome P450 3A4. *Drug Metab. Dispos.* 2005, *33(2)*, 243–253.

109. Holownia, A. and Braszko, J. J. Tamoxifen cytotoxicity in hepatoblastoma cells stably transfected with human CYP3A4. *Biochem. Pharmacol.* 2004, *67(6)*, 1057–1064.

110. Page, J. L., et al. Gene expression profiling of extracellular matrix as an effector of human hepatocyte phenotype in primary cell culture. *Toxicol. Sci.* 2007, *97(2)*, 384–397.

111. Gross-Steinmeyer, K., et al. Influence of Matrigel-overlay on constitutive and inducible expression of nine genes encoding drug-metabolizing enzymes in primary human hepatocytes. *Xenobiotica* 2005, *35(5)*, 419–438.

112. Hoffmaster, K. A., et al. P-glycoprotein expression, localization, and function in sandwich-cultured primary rat and human hepatocytes: relevance to the hepatobiliary disposition of a model opioid peptide. *Pharm. Res.* 2004, *21(7)*, 1294–1302.

113. Fujita, T., et al. Reduction of insulin resistance in obese and/or diabetic animals by 5-[4-(1-methylcyclohexylmethoxy)benzyl]-thiazolidine-2,4-dione (ADD-3878, U-63,287, ciglitazone), a new antidiabetic agent. *Diabetes* 1983, *32(9)*, 804–810.

114. Madsen, K. G., et al. Electrochemical oxidation of troglitazone: identification and characterization of the major reactive metabolite in liver microsomes. *Chem. Res. Toxicol.* 2008, *21(10)*, 2035–2041.

115. Masubuchi, Y., Kano, S., and Horie, T. Mitochondrial permeability transition as a potential determinant of hepatotoxicity of antidiabetic thiazolidinediones. *Toxicology* 2006, *222(3)*, 233–239.

116. Lee, Y. H., et al. Troglitazone-induced hepatic mitochondrial proteome expression dynamics in heterozygous Sod2(+ / −) mice: two-stage oxidative injury. *Toxicol. Appl. Pharmacol.* 2008, *231(1)*, 43–51.

117. Snow, K. L. and Moseley, R. H. Effect of thiazolidinediones on bile acid transport in rat liver. *Life Sci.*, 2007, *80(8)*, 732–740.

118. Avandia product insert, G.

119. Hulin, B. McCarthy, P. A., and Gibbs, E. M. *Curr. Pharm. Design* 1996, *2, 85–102.*

120. Sahi, J., et al. Comparative effects of thiazolidinediones on *in vitro* P450 enzyme induction and inhibition. *Drug Metab. Dispos.* 2003, *31(4)*, 439–446.

121. Chojkier, M. Troglitazone and liver injury: in search of answers. *Hepatology* 2005, *41(2)*, 237–246.

122. Lipinski, C. A., et al. Experimental and computational approaches to estimate solubility and permeability in drug discovery and development settings. *Adv. Drug. Deliv. Rev.* 2001, *46(1–3)*, 3–26.

123. Leeson, P. D. and Springthorpe, B. The influence of drug-like concepts on decision-making in medicinal chemistry. *Nat. Rev. Drug Discov.* 2007, *6(11)*, 881–890.

124. Swinney, D. C. Biochemical mechanisms of drug action: what does it take for success? *Nat. Rev. Drug. Discov.* 2004, *3(9)*, 801–808.

125. Uetrecht, J. Idiosyncratic drug reactions: current understanding. *Annu. Rev. Pharmacol. Toxicol.* 2007, *47, 513–539.*

126. Kirkland, D. J., et al. *In vitro* approaches to develop weight of evidence (WoE) and mode of action (MoA) discussions with positive *in vitro* genotoxicity results. *Mutagenesis* 2007, *22(3)*, 161–175.

127. Thybaud, V., et al. Strategy for genotoxicity testing: hazard identification and risk assessment in relation to *in vitro* testing. *Mutat. Res.* 2007, *627(1)*, 41–58.

128. Dumotier, B. M., et al. Relevance of *in vitro* SCREENIT results for drug-induced QT interval prolongation *in vivo*: a database review and analysis. *Pharmacol. Ther.* 2008, *119(2)*, 152–159.

129. Pollard, C. E., Valentin, J. P., and Hammond, T. G. Strategies to reduce the risk of drug-induced QT interval prolongation: a pharmaceutical company perspective. *Br. J. Pharmacol.* 2008, *154(7)*, 1538–1543.

130. Xu, J. J., et al. Multiple effects of acetaminophen and p38 inhibitors: towards pathway toxicology. *FEBS Lett.* 2008, *582(8)*, 1276–1282.

131. Keseru, G. M. and Makara, G. M. The influence of lead discovery strategies on the properties of drug candidates. *Nat. Rev. Drug Discov.* 2009, *8(3)*, 203–212.

9

IN VIVO TOXICOLOGICAL CONSIDERATIONS

John P. Devine, Jr.

9.1 INTRODUCTION

The role of a medicinal chemist is to design molecules with a therapeutic benefit. Thus, in time the molecule will need to be evaluated for safety before being introduced to humans. While chemists that design such therapeutic molecules are presumably knowledgeable in their field, many have not necessarily been exposed to the toxicology aspect of drug development. This chapter provides a basic framework for submitting a NME (novel molecular entity) for an IND (investigational new drug) by discussing the process for selecting the route of administration for the intended therapeutic and determining the compound requirements for toxicological studies as it relates to different species. Issues related to formulation such as overage, spillage, stability, reactivity/compatibility with glassware, infusion equipment and method validation, and sample analysis will be presented and the design and interpretation of IND supporting toxicology studies and species selection for different therapeutic indications will also be reviewed.

9.2 ROUTE OF ADMINISTRATION

In toxicology, the route of administration (ROA) is the path by which a drug is introduced into a biological test system. A review of the FDA website reveals more than 100 recognized routes of administration. Therefore, the method of delivering a molecule to the intended target must be given careful consideration. In addition to

ADMET for Medicinal Chemists: A Practical Guide, Edited by Katya Tsaioun and Steven A. Kates

TABLE 9.1 Examples of Various Routes of Administration

Topical	Enteral	Parenteral
Epicutaneous (local anesthesia)	Orally (tablets or suspensions)	Intravenous
Inhalation (asthma medications and inhaled insulin)	Gastric feeding tube	Intra-arterial (vasodilators)
Intranasal route (nasal spray)	Rectally (suppository or enema)	Intramuscular (vaccines and antibiotics)
Eye drops (antibiotics)		Subcutaneous (insulin)
Ear drops (corticosteroids)		Intraperitoneal (peritoneal dialysis)

the molecule being transported from the point of entry to the intended site of action, the pharmacokinetic properties of the molecule (i.e., those related to the processes of absorption, distribution, metabolism, and elimination) must be evaluated as these factors are influenced by the route of administration. Additionally, economic factors may also influence decisions regarding the ROA since if provided a choice between similar drugs delivered either orally or subcutaneously, most patients would select an oral formulation.

The various routes of administration may be categorized into three groups:

- topical—applied directly to site of action
- enteral—administered via the digestive tract
- parenteral—administered via routes other than the digestive tract

Examples of various routes of administration are provided in Table 9.1.

When designing preclinical toxicology studies, for most cases the ROA will be the same as the intended clinical route. Since the data generated from these preclinical toxicology assays will be extrapolated to humans, using the same ROA eliminates an unnecessary variable. Often, the ROA will be determined by the therapeutic indication of the compound. Treatments for localized skin disorders are usually applied dermally, while a compound intended for use as an emergency treatment for acute poisoning will likely be given intravenously. If similar drugs are already on the market, then the ROA should be the same or less invasive than the current drug to be a viable contender, as illustrated by the various oral and inhaled therapeutics that are intended to replace injectable formulations.

9.2.1 Oral Route

The intended therapeutic route of administration for most compounds is oral, and this route is mimicked in many preclinical toxicology studies. The drug to be tested may either be weighed into inert, gelatin capsules or suspended or dissolved in a vehicle/carrier for delivery to the animal model. The rate of dissolution of the compound is the rate-limiting step for drug absorption and is determined by drug solubility (water), pH of the environment, the chemical structure or form of the drug, and the drug formulation (excipients, binders, enteric coating).

Following dissolution, the drug must pass through the semipermeable membrane between the lumen of the gastrointestinal tract and the systemic circulation by passive diffusion, active transport, or facilitated transport [1]. Passive diffusion follows a concentration gradient and requires no energy, while active transport uses energy to move compounds against the concentration gradient. Facilitated transport moves molecules along the concentration gradient, across the cell membrane *via* special transport proteins that are embedded within the cellular membrane, but at a much faster rate than passive diffusion. Small molecules may be absorbed by either mechanism. Molecules such as glucose, amino acids, and carbohydrates are transported by active or facilitated transport.

The pH of the gastrointestinal environment also affects the relative bioavailability by altering the diffusion rates of compounds in the stomach and intestines. The rate of diffusion is directly related to the ionization of the compound. The proportion of a substance that is ionized at a given pH is determined using the Henderson–Hasselbalch equation. In the stomach, drugs that are weak acids (such as aspirin) will be present mainly in their nonionic form, and weak bases will be in their ionic form. As nonionic compounds diffuse more readily through cell membranes, weak acids will have a higher absorption in the highly acidic stomach. However, in the basic environment of the intestines weak bases such as caffeine will diffuse more readily since weak bases will be nonionic.

In addition to pH, the anatomical differences between the stomach and the small and large intestines may influence the absorptive rates of compounds. The smooth epithelium of the stomach and relatively fast gastric emptying rate ($t_{1/2} = 20$–180 min in the dog) [2] offers less opportunity for absorption when compared with the highly invaginated small intestine, with a relatively long residence time of 4–6 h. For these reasons, the small intestine is considered the most important absorptive site for drugs administered orally.

Occasionally, animal studies are conducted to determine food effects (fasted versus fed) on the absorption of the compound. Food may cause delayed or reduced absorption, accelerated or increased absorption, or may have no effect on absorption. The food effects on drug absorption must be determined before the compound is introduced to humans. Basic animal model study designs provide for oral administration of a compound to one group of fasted animals and one group of animals that had ingested a known amount of food. Samples are collected to determine absorption and the groups are rotated the following week from fed to fasted and the process is repeated. Relative bioavailability is determined and the food effect is evaluated. Fenofibrate is an example of a compound due to its poor affinity for water and to its hydrophobic nature that is much better absorbed after ingestion of food than in fasting conditions [3].

9.2.2 Intravenous Route

Some compounds that cannot be readily absorbed via the gastrointestinal tract or must bypass the acidic conditions of the stomach (e.g., proteins) or delivered to the site of action immediately (i.e., emergency care drugs) are administered directly to the circulatory system, usually intravenously. Whether delivered directly to a vein as a bolus injection or infused over a period of time such as many of the chemotherapies, study designs for compounds intended to be administered intravenously must be given special considerations. For example, compounds may be administered to mice intravenously, but their small size presents challenges that may confound the results of the assay. Alternatively, the lack of easily accessible peripheral veins in guinea pigs may limit their use on intravenous studies. For other species, either a temporary peripheral catheter or a surgically implanted, indwelling venous access port may be utilized to facilitate intravenous administration.

While bolus intravenous administration may be accomplished by skilled technicians, the use of catheters is recommended as it minimizes the chance of extravasation, accidental administration into the surrounding tissue. If the ROA is expected to be intravenous infusion, surgically implanted venous access ports may be used in preclinical studies to mimic the clinical route. The port is a central venous line attached to a small reservoir that is covered with silicone rubber and is implanted under the skin. Compounds are administered, usually with the aid of an infusion pump, by connecting the pump to the port with an external catheter. Certain risks are inherent with intravenous administration and include local or systemic infection and phlebitis as well as irritation of a vein caused by the mechanical effects of the IV catheter. Rodent studies require animals to be tethered, while ambulatory pumps are used for delivery in larger mammals.

9.2.3 Dermal Route

The intended therapeutic indication for some compounds may require application directly to the skin or dermally. In several cases, the intended site of action is the skin such as Retin A compounds used to treat acne. Other examples include pain medication, birth control, and other treatments delivered in a dermal patch in which systemic absorption is the intended route. In either case, dermal application in the preclinical toxicology studies can present challenges.

As with other routes of administration, the formulation of creams, gels, or ointments may greatly influence the exposure levels to the animal model. Since low viscosity preparations may be difficult to keep isolated at the dose site for the duration of the dose period, a viscous preparation is preferred. Dermal application of these types of preparations usually involves application with a syringe or tongue depressor to the dorsal surface of the animal. Prior to the first application, the dose site should be clipped free of hair to maximize skin contact and the site should represent approximately 10% of the total body surface of the animal. Although a variety of jackets and collars are available to minimize the animal's access to dose sites, formulations with low viscosity may lead to inadvertent oral ingestion by the animal. Obviously, this inadvertent ingestion would confound the toxicology and pharmacokinetic results and could invalidate the entire study.

Another option for dermal delivery is the use of a transdermal patch with the patch affixed to the dose site by means of an adhesive or hypoallergenic tape. This route of administration offers a more consistent and uniform delivery than applying a cream or gel and the opportunities for inadvertent oral ingestion are reduced. If an adhesive is used to secure the patch, care must be taken to determine if any observed dermal irritation can be attributed to the test article or the adhesive. This irritation may be minimized by rotating application sites on the animal.

9.3 FORMULATION ISSUES

The route of delivery will play a key role in determining the formulation. Compounds intended to be delivered orally generally pose fewer problems than those administered via a parenteral route since the latter need to be solutions. Additionally, this formulation will ultimately be used in human clinical trials, thus any vehicle or excipient in the formulation must be selected as to not interfere with the toxicological interpretation.

To comply with GLP guidelines, the API (active pharmaceutical ingredient) should have an accompanying certificate of analysis (C of A). It is critical for the compound to have a purity of close to 100%. However, any unknown impurities in the API may confound the results of the assay and may require additional testing to determine if toxicity is caused by the test article or the impurity. Additionally, the storage conditions for the API and the control and test article formulations must be controlled and documented.

A variety of vehicles are available for use, but it is advisable to use vehicles with a known toxicity profile. For compounds to be administered orally, the test compound may be dissolved (e.g., water, 0.9% saline) or suspended (e.g., 0.5% methylcellulose) at the desired concentration levels with the target concentration levels based on the actual purity of the compound or free base/free base acid content. If a suspension is used, the mixture should be stirred continuously throughout the dosing process to maintain homogeneity and prevent precipitation. Intravenous formulations are commonly prepared with physiological compatible vehicles such as 0.9% saline or lactated ringer's solution. If the solution requires sterile filtration, solution samples should be collected and analyzed before and after filtration to determine if the compound adheres to the filter membrane.

Once the above issues have been addressed, the process for verifying the formulation must be established. A requirement of all GLP toxicology studies is verification of the concentration, stability, and homogeneity of the dose formulations under their conditions of use. This task may be accomplished by pulling samples of the dosing formulations, including the control material, immediately following preparation and again at the end of the period of use for that particular batch. If the formulation is a suspension, multiple samples would be required to demonstrate homogeneity within the formulation container. These samples are then analyzed using a validated analytical method according to GLP standards with the results included in the study report. The results should demonstrate the following:

- initial concentrations were within acceptable range of theoretical,
- suspensions were relatively homogenous,

- all formulations were stable over the period of use,
- the absence of test compound in the control material.

9.4 COMPOUND REQUIREMENTS

The amount of test article required to complete the IND supporting studies is often either overlooked or underestimated. One must consider the size of the animal model, the route of administration, and the proposed dose levels when calculating the amount of required material cognizant that dose levels are based on toxicity and not efficacy.

Selection of animal models will be discussed in more detail in Section 9.5, but for most IND filings, two models will be used, one rodent (mouse or rat) and one nonrodent. Assuming an average body weight of 250 g for a rat, 10 animals/sex/group, and dose levels of 10, 50, and 100 mg/kg of body weight, estimated requirements for the rodent study given orally for 28 days would be near 23 g of the test article (Table 9.2).

For the nonrodent species, common options include rabbits, dogs, monkeys, pigs, and more frequently mini-pigs, with dogs and monkeys being the most commonly selected nonrodent species. The daily compound requirement is calculated for a standard oral dog study assuming 5 animals/sex/group, average weight of 8 kg/dog, and dose levels of 10, 50, and 100 mg/kg of body weight. Using these assumptions, the daily compound requirements would be 12.8 g/day or 358.4 g for a 28 day study (Table 9.3).

These estimates reflect only the theoretical amount delivered to the animals and do not account for additional factors that will influence the actual amount. GLP studies require a retention sample for all studies of longer than 4 weeks duration although an amount is not specified (BASi generally retains 0.5 g). For studies that are delivered via a solution or suspension, periodic samples of the formulated material will need to be collected and analyzed using a GLP validated analytical method. The volume of formulated material prepared must exceed the expected volume requirement to avoid an interruption in the dosing regimen. The occurrence of unexpected spills can further increase drug requirements. Many labs multiply the theoretical drug amount by a factor of 1.5 to compensate for these unknowns. For the example cited above, the total drug requirement to complete a 28 day oral toxicology studies in rats and dogs at

TABLE 9.2 Compound Requirement for a Standard Rat Study

Group ID	Dose Level (mg/kg)	Animals/Group	Total Group Weight (kg)	Total (mg/day)
Control	0	20	5	0
Low dose	10	20	5	50
Mid dose	50	20	5	250
High dose	100	20	5	500
				800

TABLE 9.3 Compound Requirement for a Standard Dog Study

Group ID	Dose Level (mg/kg)	Animals/Group	Total Group Weight (kg)	Total (mg/day)
Control	0	10	80	0
Low dose	10	10	80	800
Mid dose	50	10	80	4000
High dose	100	10	80	8000
				12,800

dose levels of 10, 50, and 100 mg/kg of body weight would be (23 + 358.4)1.5 or approximately 572 g of active compound which does not include a correction for purity, water, salt weight, and so on.

9.5 ANIMAL MODELS

As with ROA, drug formulation and material requirements discussed in Sections 9.2, 9.3, and 9.4, respectively, selection of the animal models for the preclinical studies requires some forethought. With some exceptions, such as large molecules, IND requirements for the US Food and Drug Administration (FDA) require testing in two species, one rodent and one nonrodent. Prior to selection of the animal models, the ROA, physiological species variations and/or similarities, therapeutic indication, and historical sensitivity to the class of compounds must be considered.

9.5.1 Mouse

The mouse is the most ubiquitous of the lab animals with a variety of inbred, outbred, and genetically modified strains available along with volumes of historical data. First utilized in the early 1900s as a laboratory model for genetic research, mice continue to be used extensively for the study of genetics as well as research for cancer, toxicology, metabolic disease, obesity, aging, and cardiovascular disease [4]. The recent mapping of the mouse genome along with the ability to manipulate gene expression in mice make the mouse unique to biomedical researchers and toxicologists. Their small size reduces compound requirements and their short reproductive cycle adds to their value as a research model. Mice are also relatively economical to acquire and maintain in the laboratory compared with larger species and space requirements for housing are minimal. One disadvantage of the mouse model is the minimal blood volume, which can present difficulties in collecting multiple samples for toxicokinetics, hematology, and clinical chemistry. Even with recent improvements in micromethodology, approximately 0.5 mL that can be collected with a survival procedure is usually insufficient to conduct more than a few of the endpoints. Dose administration can also present challenges. Intravenous administration, often using a lateral tail vein which is quite small, requires considerable practice. Oral gavage or compound admixed into the feed is the ROA for many 2 year oncogenecity studies, and with a lifespan of 2–3 years, the mouse, along with the rat, is the species of choice for these types of studies.

9.5.2 Rat

Rats, in addition to being used for oncogenecity studies, are also used for a variety of studies to support biomedical research. As with the mouse, many inbred and outbred strains have been developed since rats were first domesticated in the 1800s and an extensive historical database is available [5]. As rats are generally larger than mice, the test article requirements are slightly increased. The size of a rat does allow for multiple blood sampling and easier access to the venous system. As a result, this animal is the more prevalent rodent model used in support of an IND application. Among the species variations of the rat to consider during the study design process are their inability to regurgitate and their lack of a gall bladder. In addition, the rat's coprophagic behavior may have an impact on the test article exposure, particularly if the compound is excreted in the feces. Lastly, in my experience, rats are also easier to handle and manipulate. Compared with mice, incidents of rat bites are fairly uncommon.

9.5.3 Dog

Centuries of selective breeding have created hundreds of breeds of dog that differ in size, shape, and behavior, but the beagle dog remains the most commonly used breed for toxicology studies. The beagle dog offers several advantages for use in research:

1. their size and disposition allow for collection of multiple blood samples and reduce the difficulty of dose administration;
2. an extensive historical database is available;
3. less expensive than nonhuman primates.

Similar to the rat and humans, dogs are obligate nasal breathers, which leads to their use for inhalation studies, and aerosol deposition in the alveolar region of the dog lung also closely correlates with humans (6). Among the disadvantages for the dog model is their propensity for emesis following oral and often intravenous administration. Any emesis following an oral dose may confound study results.

9.5.4 Swine

The use of swine as the nonrodent model has increased significantly since the development of the miniature swine in the 1950s [7]. The availability of several breeds of mini-pigs (Gottingen, Hanford, Yucatan, Sinclair, and others) and public pressure to avoid using dogs and monkeys has contributed to this trend. While most often considered for use on dermal studies, the pig is a suitable surrogate for many other types of toxicology studies, particularly drugs intended to treat cardiac disease. In addition, since pigs and humans are both omnivores, the digestive system of the pig is physiologically similar to that of humans and may be helpful in evaluating compounds with an intended clinical route of oral administration. Economically, mini-pigs are similar to dogs relative to the cost of acquiring and maintaining, but depending on the breed, they will necessitate increased compound requirements.

9.5.5 Nonhuman Primates

Nonhuman primates (NHP) are physiologically more similar to humans than any other laboratory species and are used for a variety of general toxicology studies to support registration of small molecules. In the last several years, breeding programs have been established for the cynomolgus monkey, which has led to a readily available supply of healthy animals. Rhesus monkeys and marmosets are also used occasionally. The relatively small size of marmosets present challenges in multiple blood collections and these animals tend to be less hardy than either the rhesus or cynomolgus. The average weight of cynomolgus monkeys used for toxicology studies often ranges from 2 to 4 kg. Compared with other nonrodent models such as dog (8–10 kg) or mini-pig (Gottingen—8–12 kg) compound requirements may be reduced but animal cost may be two to three times higher for NHPs. Difficulties in restraint and handling, concerns over zoonotic diseases including Herpes B, and sensitivity to the pressures of animal rights activist all must be considered when opting to use an NHP model.

9.6 IND-SUPPORTING TOXICOLOGY STUDIES

A typical toxicology package to support filing an IND contains data from the following studies:

- Acute toxicity profile in rodent and one or more nonrodent species.
- A dose ranging finding study in rodent and one or more nonrodent species.
- A repeat dose toxicity study with recovery in one rodent and one nonrodent species.
- Genotoxicity battery consisting of Ames test, chromosomal aberration, and micronucleus assay.

9.6.1 Single-Dose Studies

Often the first mammalian toxicology studies will involve single-dose administrations to mice or rats. While the specific names of the tests can vary based on the specific design (i.e., dose range finding, dose escalation, etc.), these studies can generally be categorized as acute studies as a single dose is typically involved. The objective of the acute studies is to characterize the potential toxic effects of the compound as well as establish dose levels for multiple dose studies. The study should be designed to provide data on a range of dose levels delivered *via* the intended therapeutic ROA.

One example of an acute toxicology study is a dose escalation design. A dose escalation study is designed to deliver a single dose to a group of animals (e.g., 4–10 rats/group, 1–3 dogs/group) and closely observe the animals for several days for changes in body weight and/or behavior. Following the dose administration, the animals are returned to their cages and any unusual clinical signs of toxicity are documented. It is imperative that all changes are noted accurately as this information is useful in determining the possible site and mechanisms of action of the compound.

Based on the results of this initial dose administration, subsequent dose levels will be either decreased or increased with the goal of predicting dose levels in repeat dose studies that will produce moderate toxicity in the high dose and no toxicity in the low dose.

In some designs, blood sampling is added to the acute study to provide information related to the kinetics of the compound. This information may be useful, especially if correlated to clinical signs of toxicity. Unfortunately, the stress of blood collection to the animal may confound results so the risk versus benefit should be considered.

Upon completion of single-dose studies, the results are evaluated to determine dose levels for repeat-dose studies. Obviously dosages in the acute studies that caused mortality or more than minimal toxicity following a single dose would not be suitable for repeat-dose studies. The goal for selecting dose levels in repeat-dose studies is to demonstrate a no-effect level at the lowest dose whereas establishing the potential toxic effects of the compound at the highest dose level.

9.6.2 Repeat-Dose Studies

9.6.2.1 Objectives With the exception of drugs with an intended therapeutic use as a single administration, most drugs require a series of repeated dose administrations before the first dose to humans. The fundamental concept of repeat-dose studies is administration of the drug by the anticipated ROA to multiple groups of experimental animals, one dose level per group for a period of days to weeks. The actual duration of the studies may be 7 days up to 90 days, but the clinical dosing regimen may not exceed the duration of the preclinical studies. A variety of endpoints may be evaluated and the design of each repeat-dose study should be adapted on the basis of information specific to each compound. Fundamental points that should be addressed in a study protocol and specific parameters are tabulated in Table 9.4 and are described below.

9.6.2.2 Test System The animal models, acquired from approved commercial vendors, should be laboratory strains of young healthy adult animals and the females should be nonpregnant. The initial dose administration should ideally begin before the animals are 9 weeks old (rats) or 8 months old (dogs), and physical examinations must prove animals to be healthy for study inclusion. Animals found suitable for inclusion to the study should be randomly assigned to the control or treated groups. The animal weights should be stratified among groups with a target of $\pm 20\%$ of the mean weight of each sex.

9.6.2.3 Identification Appropriate animal identification methods such as permanent tattoos, ear tags, or subcutaneous transponders must be used to uniquely label each animal individually, thereby minimizing mis-dosing of the animals and ensuring the validity of the data. To reduce the effects of stress, animals should be acclimated to their room and cage assignments several days before the first dose administration.

9.6.2.4 Study Groups At least 20 rodents (10 female and 10 male) and 6 nonrodents (3 female and 3 male) should be used at each dose level and consideration

TABLE 9.4 Fundamental Repeat Dose Study Protocol and Specific Parameters

	Rodent	Nonrodent
Number of groups	Control and low, mid, and high	Control and low, mid, and high
Number of main study animals	10/sex/group	3/sex/group
Number of recovery animals	5/sex/group	2/sex/group
Number of satellite animals	10/sex/group	None
Body weight and feed consumption	Yes	Yes
Daily clinical observations	Yes	Yes
Hematology	• White blood cell count • Absolute differential leukocyte count • Red blood cell count • Hemoglobin • Hematocrit • Mean cell volume • Mean cell hemoglobin • Mean cell hemoglobin concentration • Platelet count • Reticulocyte count	
Clinical chemistry	• Sodium • Potassium • Chloride • Alkaline phosphatase • Alanine aminotransferase • Aspartate aminotransferase • Glucose • Blood urea nitrogen • Creatinine • Total cholesterol • Triglycerides • Total protein • Albumin • Globulin (calculated) • Albumin/globulin ratio (calculated) • Calcium • Inorganic phosphorus • Total bilirubin	
Coagulation	• Prothrombin time • Activated partial thromboplastin time	
ECGs	None	Pretest and study termination
Macroscopic examination of tissues	Yes	Yes
Standard organ weights	Yes	Yes
Histology	48–65 tissues/animal	48–65 tissues/animal
Pathology	All animals	All animals

should be given to an additional satellite group of animals for at least 14 days check Webster for all such entries posttreatment to observe for reversibility or delayed toxicity [8, 9]. Generally, at least three test groups and a control group should be used with dosages calculated from the range-finding studies. Except for treatment with the test article, animals in the control group should be handled the same as the animals given the test article. Preferably, all animals should receive the same volume with dosages adjusted by varying the concentration of the dose formulation. If a study design incorporates a vehicle to administer the test substance and different dose volumes are used, the control group should receive the vehicle in the highest dose volume.

9.6.2.5 Justification of Doses All existing toxicity and kinetic data available for the test compound or related compounds should be considered when selecting dose levels. The highest dose level should be selected with the intent of eliciting toxic effects but not mortality or severe toxicity. Once the high dose is selected, a descending sequence of dose levels should be chosen. Two- to fourfold intervals are frequently used for setting the descending dose levels, but the lowest dose level should demonstrate a no-observed-adverse effect (NOAEL).

9.6.2.6 Dosing The control or test article is administered to each animal daily for a period of up to 28 days. In some cases, the dosing regimen may be altered to mimic the intended clinical use such as chemotherapy drugs, which may be given as an infusion once or twice a week for 4 weeks. Regardless of the ROA, changes in dosages should be achieved by adjusting the concentration as opposed to altering dose volumes between groups.

9.6.2.7 Body Weight and Food Consumption Body weight and food consumption data are collected periodically to assess the health of the animal and to calculate dosages (body weight). Baseline body weight values are collected during the pretest period and then daily or weekly during the dose administration phase. Food consumption is quantitated by weighing the feeder either daily or weekly and subtracting the ending weight of the feeder with the initial weight and dividing by the number of days the feed was offered. Occasionally, for species such as rabbits, monkeys, and swine, only a limited amount of food is offered to control weight gain and prevent food wastage.

9.6.2.8 Clinical Observations Careful observation of animals following dose administration should always be included in a study design. The observer must be trained to recognize normal animal behavior, and it is also helpful to note individual behaviors a few days before dose administration has commenced. A standardized menu of common clinical observations is useful in maintaining consistency and accuracy in the recorded clinical signs of toxicity. These observations should "include, but not be limited to, changes in skin, fur, eyes, mucous membranes, occurrence of secretions and excretions and autonomic activity (e.g. lacrimation, piloerection, pupil size, unusual respiratory pattern). Changes in gait, posture and response to handling as well as the presence of clonic or tonic movements, stereotypes (e.g. excessive grooming, repetitive circling) or bizarre behavior (e.g. self mutilation, walking backwards) should also be recorded." [10] no changes in quoted text

9.6.2.9 Clinical Pathology Many options are available for evaluating clinical pathology. Common tests include hematology, coagulation, clinical chemistry, and urinalysis testing. For larger species, baseline samples are collected at pretest and periodically during the dosing and recovery period. In consideration of blood volume restrictions, sampling for rodent studies is often restricted to a terminal sample collected at necropsy. The results from the clinical pathology coupled with clinical observations recorded during the dosing period and gross and microscopic observation of the tissues at the end of the study can be useful in determining organs or organ systems affected by administration of the test compound.

9.6.2.10 Electrocardiograph Electrocardiograph (ECG) data is usually restricted to larger mammals although recent advances in technology have enabled researchers to collect data from rodents. ECG data may be collected from either conscious animals or animals that have been anesthetized. One or two ECGs are collected before the first dose administration to screen for preexisting conditions and establish baseline information, once following the first dose to capture acute changes, and at periodic intervals during the study. If pharmacokinetic information is available, design the study to collect ECGs on Day 1 at approximate $C_{\max}$ to maximize the opportunity to observe potential cardiotoxicity.

9.6.2.11 Postmortem Procedures and Evaluations At the end of the dosing or recovery period, animals must be humanely euthanized and subjected to a gross necropsy. The AVMA has published guidelines on acceptable methods of euthanasia and review of this document is recommended [11]. The actual method of euthanasia may cause gross and microscopic changes in tissues (i.e., sodium pentobarbital—enlarged spleens in dogs), so euthanasia of the control and treated animals should be identical. Immediately following euthanasia, appropriate blood and urine samples should be collected and then all organs examined grossly. During this process, organs or tissues as specified in the study protocol will be harvested and either fixed in formalin or weighed and then fixed. A complete description of any abnormal tissue or lesion is recorded and the finding is collected to ensure that the tissue will be examined microscopically. Target organs may often be identified during the gross necropsy process.

9.6.2.12 Organ Weight Immediately following tissue collection, organ weight data is collected and recorded. The weight of the organ or tissue is recorded following complete exsanguination and trimming of extraneous fat and tissue. Care must be taken to be consistent in the trimming of tissues to increase the validity of the results. The data are often reported as actual weights, relative to brain weight, or relative to body weight with the latter requiring a fasted body weight. In the absence of control data for comparison, organ weight data for animals found dead or sacrificed moribund are not normally collected.

9.6.2.13 Microscopic Pathology Once tissues have been preserved in 10% neutral buffered formalin or another fixative, representative samples (3–5 mm) are taken from each tissue and processed. Tissue processing involves taking tissue from a water-based state, dehydrating it and infiltrating it with paraffin. Following processing, the tissues are embedded in paraffin blocks or other embedding media and thin slices of tissue are transferred to microscope slides. A variety of specialized stains are available today, but the most common stain is hematoxylin and eosin (H&E) stain. This staining method involves application of the basic dye hematoxylin, which colors basophilic structures with blue–purple hue, and alcohol-based acidic eosin Y, which colors eosinophilic structures bright pink. The slides are then evaluated, preferably by a board certified veterinary pathologist, to determine what changes, if any, can be attributed to the administration of the test compound.

9.7 STUDY RESULT INTERPRETATION

The challenge of evaluating and interpreting data generated by a toxicology study is an important process to recognize. Data collected from treated animals are compared, either individually or by group, to correlating data collected from control animals to determine physiological or pathological alterations that can be attributed to administration of test compound. Group mean values may be analyzed statistically, but it is equally important to evaluate any "outliers" that may artificially skew the group mean. Each study design will be adapted to the specific compound to be tested based on discovery data, therapeutic area, method or mode of action, and results of studies conducted on similar class compounds and the endpoints from these designs may be extensive. A few of the fundamental endpoints are discussed below.

9.7.1 Clinical Observations

Careful observation of animals periodically during the study may reveal valuable information as to the toxicity of the compound and the site of action. Technicians are carefully trained to observe and record behavioral data following administration of the test compound, preferably at or near $C_{\max}$ and periodically throughout the study. Evaluation of these observations may indicate whether the compound affects systems such as digestive (diarrhea, emesis, dark stool), nervous (ataxia, convulsions, paralysis), renal (urine output and coloration), anogenital (estrus, rectal prolapse), oral/nasal (nasal discharge, discolored mucous membranes), and respiratory (dyspnea, cyanosis). In addition to recording the presence of the observation, it is equally important to document the time (relative to dose administration) the observation was noted, the severity of the observation, and when and if the observation resolved.

9.7.2 Body Weight/Feed Consumption

Examination of body weight and feed consumption data may often provide the first indication of toxicity in repeat dose studies. Young healthy animals should exhibit daily weight gain until they reach the adult stage. Thus, body weight loss may indicate subtle toxicity that is otherwise not apparent. While decreased feed consumption usually accompanies a decrease in body weight, some compounds may cause weight reduction while normal feed consumption is maintained, either by increasing the metabolism or increasing the rate of peristalsis. Reduced body weight coupled with reduced food consumption could indicate inappetance due to either a neurological effect or gastrointestinal irritation or blockage. Review of the clinical observations, in particular incidences of loose stool/diarrhea, emesis, or no stool should be utilized to differentiate this occurrence. Alternatively, a reduced/increased body weight coupled with unchanged food consumption may indicate a metabolic change.

9.7.3 Clinical Pathology

Hematology test usually references a complete blood count (CBC) (with reticulocyte count, platelet count, mean cellular volume (VCM), and differential leukocyte count). This test includes the quantification of red blood cells (RBCs) and hemoglobin and calculation of the percentage of blood volume that is occupied by RBCs (hematocrit). Potential toxic effects include decreases in red blood cells, hemoglobin, and/or hematocrit, which may be indicative of anemia, caused by hemorrhage, red cell destruction, or decreased red cell production (bone marrow suppression). Anemia is the most common hematologic change noted in toxicology studies [12]. Results from the clinical observations and gross necropsy can usually identify the source of blood loss, while evaluation of the reticulocytes or red cell distribution width (RDW) may be used to distinguish cell destruction from cell production. Reticulocyte production should increase as a normal adaptive response in anemic condition. Sometimes the intended therapeutic use of a compound may cause anemia, such as the immunosuppressant drug Azathioprine [13] and other chemotherapy drugs. In rare cases, increases in red blood cells, hemoglobin, and/or hematocrit are noted, but these increases are usually related to hemoconcentration caused by dehydration.

The CBC also includes quantification and differentiation of leucocytes (neutrophils, lymphocytes, monocytes, eosinophils, and basophils). Changes in the number of leukocytes or white blood cells may indicate an immune response to infection or disease, effects of physiological stress, or may be a sign of immunotoxicity. Examination of the changes in the numbers of each type of cell provides additional information as to the cause or source of the effect. When interpreting the differential results, the absolute counts as opposed to relative or percent counts are evaluated since the latter have no inherent value in assessing the condition of an animal [14].

9.7.4 Clinical Chemistry

The analysis of serum may detect toxicity of the hepatic-biliary function, renal function, carbohydrate, protein, and lipid metabolism, and balance of electrolytes.

Elevations of alanine aminotransferase and aspartate aminotransferase may indicate hepatic injury while increased alkaline phosphatase may be a sign of cholestasis or biliary hyperplasia. Although uncommon, bilirubin increases suggest hepatic injury, cholestasis, or both. Serum urea nitrogen and creatinine levels are used to evaluate renal function but are not sensitive to subtle changes. Serum proteins (albumin and globulin), glucose, and serum lipids (total cholesterol and triglycerides) are monitored to detect toxic effects on metabolism. Changes in serum levels of the electrolytes (sodium, potassium, and chloride) may be attributed to dehydration from emesis or diarrhea, decreased food intake, or renal failure. The clinical chemistry data are often compared statistically (control versus treated groups) to determine if any changes reach significance. For individual or groups of animals that do exhibit a significant change, it is equally important to compare with pretest or historical data to verify the biological significance of the finding.

9.7.5 Electrocardiograms

The ECG data collected from animals in a toxicology study are ideally analyzed by a board certified veterinary cardiologist with the results appended as a contributing scientific report. Cardiovascular (hemodynamic) function is part of the safety pharmacology tests and limited to detecting cardiotoxicity following single administrations. These tests are not designed to capture cardiac changes caused by repeated administrations. Baseline readings collected once or twice pretest indicate the absence of preexisting abnormalities and are compared to a reading collected following one dose and readings collected following multiple doses such as on Day 13 for a 2 week study. Parameters for evaluation may include blood pressure (diastolic, mean, and systolic), heart rate, P duration, PR interval, QRS interval, R amplitude, and QT interval. If it is determined that cardiac changes are present and appear to be related to administration of the test article, ECG data should be collected from recovery animals to determine the reversibility of the noted changes.

9.7.6 Organ Weights

Careful examination of organ weight data may often illustrate the site of action of a drug as well as identify target organs for microscopic evaluation. After careful trimming and removal of residual blood, organ weight data are collected. As a means to normalize the data, the organ weights are also expressed relative to fasted body weight and brain weight. One common finding noted in many studies is the incidence of increased liver weights due to the relatively high doses that are used for toxicology studies. This increase is not necessarily indicative of hepatic injury, but can typically be attributed to increased activity of the drug-metabolizing enzymes present in the liver [15]. The method of euthanasia may also affect organ weights. For example, splenic weights from dogs euthanized with pentobarbital are increased. It is best practice to evaluate all of the three options (actual organ weights, organ weight relative to body weight, and organ weights relative to body) at the same time to differentiate if any noted changes are due to actual changes in the weight of the organ or possibly related to changes in weight gain. The data from microscopic examination of the tissues may be used to help assess the biological relevance of any differences between organ weights that appear to be affected by drug administration.

9.7.7 Pathology

Similar to the evaluation of electrocardiograms, pathology slides are ideally examined by an expert in the field such as a board-certified veterinary pathologist. Experience is invaluable in the evaluation of pathology slides. The decision between reporting a lesion as drug induced as opposed to a tissue collection or processing artifact is not trivial and may be the determining factor for advancing into clinical trials versus shelving the compound. The pathology report should be clear in stating what lesions were present and whether these lesions were drug related, dose dependent, and reversible. If results are questionable, it is advisable to consider using a peer review pathologist to resolve any issues. The peer review process utilizes an independent pathologist to review the slides and original report to verify or question the findings. Upon review, the peer review pathologist consults with the original pathologist to discuss any findings that may be questionable. In my experience, the peer review process adds value to a study when pathology findings are spurious and not supported by clinical pathology or organ weights.

9.8 GENETIC TOXICOLOGY STUDIES

In addition to the general toxicology studies, most small molecule IND applications will also require inclusion of the results from a series of genetic toxicology tests. A brief description of the guidelines promulgated by the ICH "Standard Battery of Genotoxicity Testing of Pharmaceuticals" and its role in an IND submission are presented. For a more detailed discussion, see Chapter 7. Three standard tests are required

1. gene mutation test in bacteria;
2. *in vitro* test with evaluation of chromosomal damage in mammalian cells or *in vitro* mouse lymphoma assay;
3. *in vivo* test to screen for chromosomal damage using rodent hematopoietic cells.

9.8.1 Gene Mutation

The objective of the gene mutation or Ames assay is to evaluate the genotoxicity potential of a drug by measuring its ability to induce reverse mutations at selected loci in several bacterial strains in the presence and absence of a rat-liver-derived metabolizing system (S9 mix). Several strains of *Salmonella typhimurium* and/or *Escherichia coli* are genetically modified to require amino acids for growth. These strains are then exposed to the drug along with appropriate positive and negative controls and evaluated for colonies that restore the functional capability to synthesize the required amino acid [16]. Drugs that promote reverse mutations may be classified as mutagens.

9.8.2 Chromosomal Aberration

Screening for chromosomal aberrations may be conducted either *in vivo* or *in vitro*. The mouse lymphoma-TK assay is the standard *in vivo* test to examine mutations at the thymidine kinase locus caused by base-pair changes, frameshift, and small deletions [17]. Mutant cells, deficient in thymidine kinase due to the forward mutation in the TK locus, are resistant to the cytotoxic effect of pyrimidine analogues such as 5-trifluorothymidine (TFT). The mutagenicity of the test article is indicated by the increase in the number of mutants after treatment with test article.

The *in vitro* chromosome aberration test uses cultured mammalian cells to identify test articles that cause structural chromosome aberrations. Two types of structural aberrations may be observed: chromosome or chromatid [18]. The majority of chemical mutagens are chromatid-induced aberrations. Some chromosome-type aberrations also occur. While there is evidence that chromosome mutations causing alterations in oncogenes and tumor-suppressor genes are involved in cancer induction in humans and experimental animals, the incidence of false positives continues to fuel debate on the validity of this assay.

9.8.3 *In Vivo* Mouse Micronucleus

The micronucleus test is used to screen for potential genotoxic compounds. There are two versions of this test: *in vivo* and *in vitro*. The *in vivo* test is commonly used in support of an IND. Groups of mice are exposed to control material or test article with bone marrow smears collected from the mice at 24 or 48 h following administration. One smear from each animal is examined for the presence of micronuclei in polychromatic erythrocytes. The ratio of polychromatic to normochromatic erythrocytes is assessed by examination. The values from the treated animals are compared with control values. Detection of damage induced by the test substance to the chromosomes or the mitotic apparatus of erythroblasts is reported [19]. This assay is useful in predicting genotoxic carcinogens, that is, carcinogens that act by causing genetic damage.

9.9 CONCLUSION

The toxicology studies to support filing of an IND are an integral part of the drug development process for a new chemical entity. It is critical that all key aspects of the plan be considered beforehand to prevent loss of time and resources and to avoid mistakes that may prevent a drug from moving forward into clinical trials. This chapter reviewed key aspects to consider based on my years of experience in the field of drug development. While timing is always an important factor in filing an IND, the time and effort to prepare a well-thought and comprehensive IND plan will, in most cases, save time and resources. Failure to consider these aspects may result in costly (money and time) mistakes, which sometimes requires studies to be repeated.

REFERENCES

1. Nogrady, T. and Weaver, D. F., *Medicinal Chemistry, A Biochemical Approach*, Oxford University Press, New York, 1988, pp. 431–432.
2. Dunlop, R. H. and Malbert, C. H., *Veterinary Pathophysiology*, Wiley, New York, 2004, pp. 113–114.
3. Brunton, L., Blumenthal, D., Buxton, I., and Parker, K., *Goodman and Gilman's Manual of Pharmacology and Therapeutics*, McGraw-Hill, New York, 2008, p. 619.
4. Suckow, M. A., Danneman, P., and Brayton, C., *The Laboratory Mouse*, CRC Press, Boca Raton, FL, 2001.
5. Sharp, P. E., LaRegina, M., and LaRegina, M. C., *The Laboratory Rat*, CRC Press, Boca Raton, FL, 1998.
6. Hall, R. L., *Principles and Methods of Toxicology*, Hays, A. W. (ed.), CRC Press, Boca Raton, FL, 2007, p. 1321.
7. Bollen, P., Hansen, A., and Rasmussen, H., *The Laboratory Swine*, CRC Press, Boca Raton, FL, 2000.
8. OECD Guideline for the Testing of Chemicals 407—Repeated Dose 28-day Oral Toxicity Study in Rodents, Adopted by the Council on 27th July 1995.
9. OECD Guideline for the Testing of Chemicals 409—Repeated Dose 90-day Oral Toxicity Study in Non-Rodents, Adopted by the Council on 21st September 1998.
10. Code of Federal Regulations. Title 9: Animals and animal products. US Government Printing Office. Revised 1 January 1998.
11. AVMA Guidelines on Euthanasia June 2007.
12. Jacobson-Kram, D., and Keller, K. A., *Toxicology Testing Handbook: Principles, Applications, and Data Interpretation*, Marcel Dekker, New York, 2001, pp. 62–68.
13. Maddison, J. E., Page, S., and Church, D., *Small Animal Clinical Pharmacology*, Elsevier Health Sciences, Amsterdam, The Netherlands, 2002, p. 234.
14. Hall, R. L.(Author) and Hayes, A. W. (Editor), *Principles and Methods of Toxicology*, CRC Press, Boca Raton, FL, 2001, pp. 1019, 1023.
15. Amacher, D. E., Schomaker S. J., and Burkhardt, J. E. The relationship among microsomal enzyme induction, liver weight and histological change in rat toxicology studies. *Food Chem. Toxicol.*, 1998, *36(9–10)*, pp. 831–839.
16. OECD Guideline for the Testing of Chemicals 471—Bacterial Reverse Mutation Test, Adopted by the Council on 21st July 1997.
17. OECD Guideline for the Testing of Chemicals 476—*In Vitro* Mammalian Cell Gene Mutation Test, Adopted by the Council on 21st July 1997.
18. OECD Guideline for the Testing of Chemicals 473—*In Vitro* Mammalian Chromosome Aberration Test, Adopted by the Council on 21st July 1997.
19. OECD Guideline for the Testing of Chemicals 474—Mammalian Erythrocyte Micronucleus Test, Adopted by the Council on 21st July 1997.

10

PRECLINICAL CANDIDATE NOMINATION AND DEVELOPMENT

NILS BERGENHEM

10.1 INTRODUCTION

The generic discovery phase starts with identifying a target, screening for compounds that affect the target, identifying hits, understanding the structure–activity relationship to be able to modify the hits into potent lead molecules, and finally optimizing those lead molecules to be as drug like and efficacious as possible (Figure 10.1). The activities in this phase are performed under non-GLP (Good Laboratory Practice) conditions, and involve a lot of problem solving and novel thinking. This is the phase when the drug is invented.

With the selection of the preclinical candidate, the more constrained development phase is initiated. In development, all the boxes are checked to insure that the drug is likely to be safe when dosed in humans. The activities in this phase are performed under GLP conditions to ensure the quality of the results meets the requirements of the investigational new drug (IND) application. Moving a candidate into development will initiate a cascade of activities that are quite costly. Also, for preclinical development to proceed as rapidly as possible, activities occur in parallel, leading the process to be difficult to discontinue if a problem is identified. Therefore, the selection of a preclinical development candidate is a critical step in drug discovery and development.

ADMET for Medicinal Chemists: A Practical Guide, Edited by Katya Tsaioun and Steven A. Kates

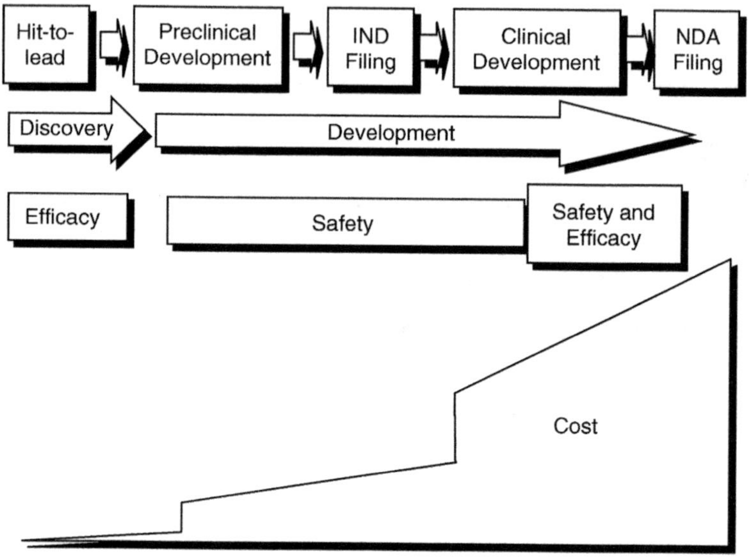

Figure 10.1 The efficacy of a drug candidate is assessed during discovery and Phase 2 and 3 clinical trials. The safety of a drug candidate is assessed in preclinical development and Phase 1 clinical trial. The cost increases dramatically during initiation of preclinical clinical development.

10.2 INVESTIGATIONAL NEW DRUG APPLICATION AND CLINICAL DEVELOPMENT

While this chapter describes preclinical candidate selection and preclinical development, the outcome is the nomination of a clinical candidate, and a basic understanding of the clinical development phases is required to establish the goals for preclinical development.

The goal of preclinical development is to generate the data and documentation of the drug candidate required to complete an IND application. To administer a drug candidate to a human, an (IND) application has to be approved by the FDA that provides guidance for the content and format of the application [1]. Interestingly, the IND application is a request for an exemption from the Federal statute that prohibits an unapproved drug from being transported across state lines, which is typically required to ship and subsequently provide clinical investigators drug product. An IND is the documentation the Sponsor of the clinical trial submits to the FDA for this exemption.

The IND application includes data and information in three broad areas:

- Chemistry, Manufacturing, and Control (CMC) Information;
- Animal Pharmacology and Toxicology Studies; and
- Clinical Protocols and Investigator Information

10.2.1 Chemistry, Manufacturing, and Control Information

Information related to the composition, manufacturing, stability, packaging, and controls used to produce the drug substance and the drug product is detailed in the CMC section of the application. Documentation in the CMC section ensures consistent batches of the drug candidate for production and packaging.

10.2.2 Animal Pharmacology and Toxicology Studies

Preclinical data assessing whether the product is likely to be efficacious and most importantly safe for testing in humans is the primary focus of this section.

10.2.3 Clinical Protocols and Investigator Information

Protocols for the proposed clinical studies to insure subjects are not exposed to unnecessary risks, and information regarding the qualification of the clinical investigators who will oversee the administration of the experimental drug are described in these sections.

10.2.3.1 Clinical Trials Phase 1–3 [2] In addition to Phase 1–3, there are also Phase 0 (exploratory) and Phase 4 (post marketing) clinical trials; both not discussed further in this chapter.

10.2.3.2 Phase 1 In a Phase 1 trial, a small (20–80) number of healthy volunteers are dosed to assess the safety, tolerability, pharmacokinetics, and pharmacodynamics of a drug. It is rare that any indication of the efficacy of the drug candidate can be assessed in a Phase 1 trial. A typical Phase 1 study design is a single ascending dose (SAD) in which a single dose is administered, and if no adverse effects are observed, a higher single dose is given. Dosing continues until either the plasma drug levels reach those estimated to be safe from the preclinical studies or side effects are noticed (maximum tolerated dose (MTD)). In a multiple ascending dose (MAD) study, a group of healthy volunteers are administered multiple doses of the drug. If no side effects are noticed, a second group is given a higher dose, and the process is continued until the dose calculated to be safe from the preclinical studies are reached, or side effects are noticed. Administering the drug under fasting and fed conditions and determining the effects of food on drug concentration in blood levels is also investigated.

The two main endpoints of a Phase 1 trial are determining the blood levels of the drug versus time after dosing (pharmacokinetics) and establishing the MTD

10.2.3.3 Phase 2 Phase 2 trials are designed with a larger group of volunteers (20–300 patients) to continue to establish safety and to begin to assess the efficacy of a drug candidate. Doses selected are believed to be safe, either based upon the MTD found in Phase 1 or the Phase 1 pharmacokinetics in conjunction with the preclinical pharmacokinetic and toxicological studies. In addition to being safe, the selected doses administered to patients are also predicted to be efficacious based upon the efficacy established in animal and human cell or tissue studies during the discovery phase of the project.

10.2.3.4 Phase 3 Phase 3 trials involve several clinical centers with a large number of patients (300–3000 or more depending upon the disease/medical condition studied). The aim is to assess the safety and efficacy of the drug candidate compared to the standard of care treatment for the disease indication. The length of the studies will vary depending on the disease indication. For example, according to the FDA guidelines [4], in an obesity trial, patients are dosed for 12 months which provides a complex and costly study to conduct.

A new drug application (NDA) can be submitted to the FDA based upon the data obtained from one or several Phase 3 studies. Upon FDA approval, the drug can be marketed.

10.3 STRATEGIC GOALS FOR THE PRECLINICAL DEVELOPMENT

The attrition rate of drug discovery and development candidates (Figure 10.2) is key to the strategic goals for selecting a preclinical candidate. There are two major decreases in the number of compounds advancing from one stage to the next. The first and largest decline is the number of drug candidates in discovery advancing to the clinic. Based on the data set, only 1 out of every 150 drug candidates in discovery enters clinical development (Figure 10.2). Once a drug candidate has been shown to be sufficiently efficacious in animal models of the disease, and safe in preclinical development for the FDA to approve the IND application, the average likelihood for the drug candidate to reach market is about 1 in 10. For a pharmaceutical company,

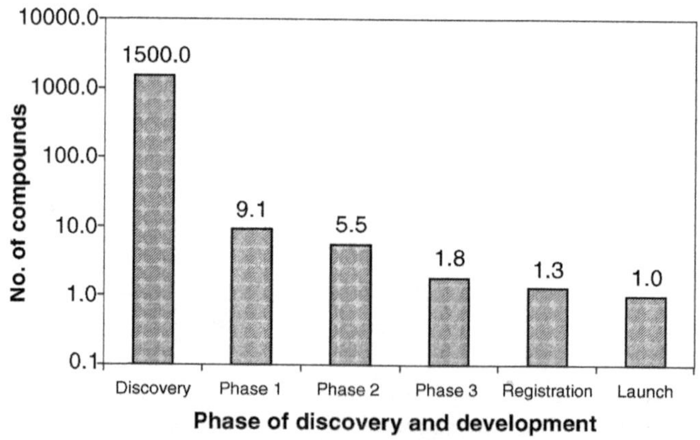

Figure 10.2 *Attrition rate of drug candidates.* The number of compounds prepared versus the phase of development is plotted. For 1500 compounds in discovery, only 9 enter a Phase 1 clinical trial. Data from Ref. 3.

there is increased motivation to support the project and drive the drug candidate forward toward the market. For a smaller company, compounds in the clinic will significantly increase the chance of attracting investors willing to provide the capital required to continue development, close an attractive licensing deal, or sell the asset or company.

In the latter case, a business plan may incorporate preclinical studies early in the development plan to initiate a Phase 1 clinical study even if these preclinical studies need to be supplemented to initiate Phase 2 and 3 studies. For most indications, the efficacy endpoints of a clinical study (Phase 2 and 3) will involve dosing for months to years. The preclinical toxicological studies have to support this length of human dosing, which requires long and costly preclinical toxicological studies. If the business strategy is to place a compound into the clinic and conduct a Phase 1 study early in the development plan, 1 month toxicological studies are all that is required. These preclinical studies are substantially less time and money consuming than a preclinical package that may be required to support Phase 2 and 3 clinical trials. Thus the clinical development plan must account for the risk for conducting a Phase 1 trial before the entire preclinical data package has been completed.

10.4 SELECTION OF PRECLINICAL DEVELOPMENT CANDIDATE

The cost and the precise IND enabling preclinical toxicology and pharmacology studies will vary depending on the disease indication. Typically, one should budget ~$1.5 million with a timeline of 9–12 months to complete the studies required for an IND submission. It is therefore unrealistic to conduct IND enabling studies for several candidates and strategies to select one candidate are necessary.

The reasons for drug candidates to fail in development have evolved over time. In 1991, the major reasons for failure where attributed to issues with PK and bioavailability. Since then, assays to assess these parameters prior to selecting a preclinical candidate have been developed. In 2000, the number of clinical failures due to poor PK or bioavailability was less than 10%; poor efficacy, problems with toxicology or safety, and commercial reasons attributed to the majority of failures [5]. It is clear that assessment of PK, efficacy, and safety and toxicology should be evaluated prior to selecting a candidate for preclinical development (commercial reasons are beyond the scope of this chapter).

10.4.1 Efficacy

The efficacy of the drug candidate is measured in the discovery phase (Figure 10.1). As the compound advances to preclinical and Phase 1 clinical development, the drug candidate is evaluated for safety as opposed to efficacy.

Based upon *in vitro* efficacy, the most potent molecules are the preferred candidates for development. However, molecules that are potent *in vitro* may not be the most potent and efficacious *in vivo*. A number of parameters such as cell permeability, stability in plasma, plasma protein binding, and clearance from plasma will determine the concentration of the drug candidate at the molecular target *in vivo*. These parameters are also considered when selecting leads to be tested for efficacy *in vivo*. The most potent and efficacious lead *in vivo* are selected as the preclinical candidates. The more potent the drug candidate, the lower the dose will be, which presumably reduces the risk for off-target side effects.

A clear relationship between the pharmacokinetics (plasma/tissue levels of the drug or active metabolites versus time after dosing) and pharmacodynamics (efficacy) of the drug candidate should be known. If a drug candidate interacts with a molecular target with an EC_{50} of 1 nM, in principle, the free fraction (not bound to plasma proteins) of the drug candidate needs to be in the low nanomolar range for as long after dosing as the drug candidate shows efficacy. Alternatively, the efficacy of a drug candidate may depend on a more or less complete inhibition of a target and thus the drug concentrations for that target need to be greater. Lastly, the efficacy may involve activating a target that leads to a cascade of events that is sustained even after the drug levels are below target activation. Regardless of the mechanism for efficacy, the PK/PD relationship needs to be described for the preclinical candidate.

The FDA will not approve a drug that is inferior to a drug already marketed thus establishing the goal for efficacy. For an indication that does not have any marketed drugs, efficacy may be based upon estimates for what can be successfully marketed. At project initiation, a target profile should be established to favorably compare a preclinical candidate to marketed benchmarks for the desired indication. All lead compounds for preclinical development should be at least as efficacious as the target profile dictates.

If a drug candidate has the same target as an already marketed drug, the drug candidate must be at least as efficacious in pharmacological models of the disease, more potent to the target and possess a greater safety margin. Statins are an excellent example of a class of drugs in which different compounds have been successfully developed and commercialized. Bayer's Baycol was initially marketed until severe side effects removed the drug from patients [6]. Merck's Zocor is on the market and is metabolized by a single Cyp(3A4) [7], which increases the risk of drug–drug interactions. Astra Zeneca's Crestor is more potent than Zocor, and is not metabolized [8]. These improvements over previously marketed drugs have allowed Crestor to gain a substantial market share.

Another example of efficacy guiding the selection of a preclinical candidate is OSI Prosidion's PSN602, a monoamine reuptake inhibitor with 5-HT1A agonism [9]. In this case Abbott's Meridia (Sibutramine) [10] is the benchmark. Sibutramine is a dual serotonin (5-HT)/norepinephrine (NE) reuptake inhibitor approved for the treatment of obesity. The drug is associated with elevations in blood pressure and heart rate in some patients limiting the dose that can be used. By designing a 5-HT1A agonist in conjunction with monoamine reuptake inhibition, OSI Prosidion PSN602 was as efficacious as sibutramine at reducing body weight in a rodent model of obesity, but exhibits a more favorable cardiovascular safety profile after single doses.

It is more difficult to set the efficacy criteria if the molecule under development is first-in-class. Metabolex MBX-2982 [11] targets the G-protein coupled receptor 119 (GPR119) as a therapy for Type-2 diabetes [12] and is currently in Phase 1 clinical studies. Most likely, Metabolex aims to advance MBX-2982 to Phase 2 as soon as possible to generate proof-of-concept efficacy data in terms in patients. Concurrently, Metabolex is developing second-generation compounds as an improvement to the properties of MBX-2982. If the human efficacy data indicates that MBX-2982 is a validated target for Type-2 diabetes, Metabolex may terminate the development of MBX-2982 and initiate the clinical development with an improved second-generation molecule.

10.4.2 Safety/Tolerance

In addition to efficacy (discussed in Section 10.4.1), safety is another parameter to be thoroughly assessed in guiding the selection of a preclinical candidate. There are a number of assays that are both inexpensive and may be used under non-GLP conditions to generate data on several representatives from a chemical lead series to help selection of a preclinical candidate with a strong probability of passing the preclinical filter in terms of safety parameters (Table 10.1)

10.4.2.1 HGPRT Forward Mutation, Ames Test, and Herg Channel Inhibition For most disease indications a positive HGPRT forward mutation, Ames, or Herg channel inhibition test is a "show stopper" for a drug candidate and the compound should not be considered for future development. However, there are exceptions such as the cancer drug Sutent. Sutent inhibits the Herg channel [13], and yet is approved and marketed. Nevertheless, it is advisable to generate data on these assays mentioned above at an early stage to be able to screen compounds that do not warrant any further testing.

10.4.2.2 Receptor Binding and Kinase Panels To assess the possibility for off-target side effects, the drug candidate is screened against a panel of receptors and kinases. If the drug candidate does interact with some of the receptors in the panel, the risk for off-target effects is greater than if there were no interactions with the

TABLE 10.1 Non-GLP Assays to Assess Safety of a Chemical Lead

In Vitro	*In Vivo*
HGPRT forward mutation	Pharmacokinetics
Ames test	Non-GLP toxicological study
Herg channel	
Receptor binding and kinase panels	
Cyp inhibition, induction, and metabolism	
Protein binding	

receptors. A drug candidate's interaction with receptors does not necessarily "kill" the compound since there still may be a range for on-target efficacy. However, positive results in any nontarget assay raises concerns about the compound and the data may assist the selection of a candidate among a series of molecules. For example, assessing the effects on as many kinases as possible is valuable to develop a selective kinase inhibitor per-clinical candidate.

10.4.2.3 Cyp Inhibition, Induction, and Metabolism A drug candidate that affects CYP inhibition, CYP induction, or is metabolized by a single CYP should be "flagged" as a potential issue. As an example, the drug candidate inhibits an isoform of CYP metabolizing other drug substances. Thus, upon administration of the drug candidate, the metabolism of any compound which is a substrate for this CYP will be reduced, presumably leading to higher drug levels, and prolonged exposure of these compounds. This drug–drug interaction can then effectively lead to an overdose of the compounds metabolized by the particular CYP. Inhibition of the major human drug metabolizing CYPs [14] 3A4, 2D6, 2C19, 1A2, 2A6, 2B6, 2C8, 2C9, and 2E1 should be examined. A positive result may not "kill" the compound but should be carefully reviewed before advancing the candidate further.

A compound that induces a CYP has the potential to have an opposite effect. If a drug candidate induces a CYP, any drugs the patient is taking that is metabolized by this CYP will presumably be eliminated faster, and effectively be under dosed.

If a compound is metabolized solely by one CYP, there will be a greater risk for drug–drug interactions. Examples on the market displaying this phenomenon include Zocor which is metabolized solely by CYP 3A4. In this case, in addition to the risk for drug–drug interactions, the drug should not be taken with grape fruit juice. Drinking grape fruit juice will inhibit CYP3A4 and cause a substantial increase in the plasma concentrations of Zocor [7] as well as other marketed drugs metabolized by CYP3A4. Drugs metabolized by one CYP can also be strongly affected by CYP polymorphisms in the population. These variations include different expression levels or activities of CYPs and can lead to variations in drug concentration levels.

10.4.2.4 Protein Binding Binding of a drug candidate to plasma proteins will lower the free fraction of the compound available to a target. A compound possessing strong protein binding typically requires an increase in dose to affect the target. Also, strong binding to plasma proteins poses a risk for drug–drug interactions. If a large fraction of a molecule is bound to plasma proteins and a second molecule is introduced binding to the same site on the plasma proteins, the competition for binding can result in a significant increase in the free-drug concentration. For example, if 99% of a molecule is protein bound and competition by a second molecule reduces protein binding to 90%, there will be a 10-fold increase in the free-drug concentration of the first molecule.

Conversely, binding to plasma proteins is not necessarily an undesired property. Novo Nordisk GLP-1 analog Liraglutide is designed to bind to albumin. Bound to albumin, Liraglutide is protected from proteolysis by dipeptidyl peptidase-4 that results in prolonging the plasma half-life of the drug candidate [15]

10.4.3 PK

Determination of the bioavailability, half-life, and clearance of a drug candidate and the ability to correlate the plasma concentration of the drug candidate with potency on the target are important to select a lead compound. With several potential lead candidates, these parameters are used to prioritize compounds with the bioavailability and clearance rates that support the desired dosing regimen. To obtain these PK parameters, typical studies include a single dose administered by intravenous and the expected route of administration (i.e., oral).

In addition to single-dose PK studies, a multiple dose PK study will determine the dose proportionality of the drug candidate. Plasma levels of the drug candidate should increase linearly with dose. If the plasma concentrations of the drug do not increase above a certain dose, presumably the absorption of the drug limits the exposure. The highest dose producing an increase in plasma concentration of the drug will be the highest dose that can be used in toxicological studies in this species. Since doses proposed to be tested in humans need to be supported by toxicological studies in animals, this will limit the doses than can be tested in the clinic. Ideally, repeat dosing of a drug candidate should not change the PK parameters. If there is an increase in drug concentration in plasma due to repeat dosing, this in conjunction with protein binding is correlated with the efficacy of the compound (PK/PD relationship).

The cost of non-GLP repeat dose PK studies with a few select drug candidates is rather nominal compared to the IND enabling studies.

10.4.4 Non-GLP Toxicological Study

The *in vivo* efficacy studies in discovery should generate data at varied doses to identify a minimum efficacious dose (MED) and an MTD. The difference between an MED and an MTD should be as large as possible to decrease the likelihood of side effects at efficacious doses. The assessment of an MTD varies with the disease indication and target. In some cases, an MTD is defined by off-target effects and an assessment is made based upon measures of gross toxicology; change in organ weights, animals behavior, morbidity, or mortality. Alternatively, an MTD may be driven by the efficacy on the target. For example, a molecule increasing the secretion of insulin may lower blood glucose levels below physiological levels causing hypoglycemia.

In addition to these fundamental assessments of toxicology, prior to selecting a final preclinical candidate, conducting a 14-day non-GLP formal toxicological study in rats at several doses will identify any potential issues associated with the drug candidate before costly GLP studies are initiated.

From the analysis of the toxicological screening data, drug candidates may be ranked. There are no generic rules to rank compounds based on this data since the disease indication will dictate the safety or allowable side effect. Oncology drugs often are associated with rather severe side effects. Alternatively, a recent FDA guidance document requires data demonstrating that antidiabetic drugs will not result in an unacceptable increase in cardiovascular risk [16].

10.5 CMC

There are several factors in a CMC section that may be assessed under non-GLP conditions at a modest cost in time and money to help select a successful preclinical candidate.

10.5.1 Solubility

Typically compounds with low solubility are more difficult to develop since this impacts testing the activity of the compound *in vitro* and *in vivo* for activity and safety. Thus for compounds with equal other properties, it is advisable to select a candidate with high solubility.

There are examples of drugs with very low solubility that were commercialized. The COX-2 inhibitor Vioxx (rofecoxib) (removed from the market due to cardiovascular issues) had high bioavailability (>90%) for a dose of <50 mg [17].

10.5.2 Solutions Stability

A drug candidate needs to be stable in solution. Typically, a high-performance liquid chromatography (HPLC) method analyzes the concentration of a compound at varying pH values to assess its stability. An acid-labile compound planned to be dosed orally might need to be formulated in a capsule to prevent degradation in the stomach, while a compound which is not very stable at any pH is potentially problematic.

10.5.3 Synthetic Feasibility, Solid-State Stability, and Hygroscopicity

The large-scale synthesis required for GMP production is typically different from the laboratory-scale synthetic route. In some instances, it is difficult to evaluate the final synthetic route at an early stage; however, understanding the cost of goods is essential for selecting a drug candidate.

Large-scale synthesis can produce material that is different in the solid state compared to laboratory-scale material. These polymorphs of a compound can behave differently chemically and biologically. Solid-state stability may be assessed with micro calorimetry and an accelerated stability program will provide data that may assist in selecting a preclinical candidate. A hygroscopic compound is more difficult to manufacture and formulate and should not be selected as a lead compound.

10.5.4 Patent Position

Although patents are not part of the IND application *per se*, the intellectual property of the invention is a commercially important factor and should be addressed in the hit-to-lead stage. Typically, claiming the composition of matter for a drug candidate is the most critical claim. Ironically, there are examples in which a development candidate without a strong patent position was advanced to the clinic. Biostratum had completed Phase 2 clinical trials with Pyridorin with promising efficacy when it became evident the active ingredient was commercially available via the internet, eventually leading to the failure of the company [18]. The rights to Pyridorin have since been acquired by Nephrogenex (http://www.nephrogenex.com), and the drug candidate is still in clinical development.

10.6 PRECLINICAL STUDIES

Although IND application has three general areas as discussed above, different disease indications differ in terms of the details that are required for each section. While guidance can be found on the Center for Drug Evaluation and Research (CDER) website [19], the requirements are under constant evaluation, and changes are often implemented. It is important to arrange to meet with the FDA to review the plans for generating an IND package in a pre-IND meeting to ensure that the planned studies will provide the data needed. If a company does not have a designated development organization, there are contract research organizations (CROs) that can design and conduct the required studies. Preclinical studies require chemical, animal pharmacology, and medical knowledge for the CMC, nonclinical pharmacology and toxicology, and clinical sections, respectively. It is advisable to designate an in-house project manager with some experience, or to work closely with a consultant with experience in preclinical development.

It is important to realize that preclinical drug development is a process in which data are collected aimed at terminating a compounds development. The drug candidate needs to pass the battery of safety and toxicology analysis. As mentioned above, some of the parameters analyzed are precautionary and should not end a compounds development. The whole process is designed to filter out compounds that are not suitable to be tested in humans since no improvements are made to the drug candidate once in this process.

It is not possible to design one generic preclinical study package. There are indications such as antiinfectives in which case the drug needs to be safe, and most likely will be administered for one or a few weeks. In this case, 1 month toxicological studies will suffice. Conversely, the safety and toxicological hurdles for an oncology drug candidate, while typically administered for a longer period of time than an antiinfective, will be lower than for most indications. Tarceva, marketed by OSI Pharmaceuticals and Roche for advanced nonsmall cell lung cancer and pancreatic cancer causes a rather significant rash which would not be acceptable for most other indications [20].

Alternatively, drugs for diabetes presumably will be dosed daily for most or the remainder of the patient's life and the toxicological studies need to include dosing for 1 year. For some classes of diabetes drug candidates, such as peroxisome proliferator-activated receptor (PPAR) agonists, the FDA requires a 2 year carcinogenicity study in two species to be completed before dosing in man for longer than 6 months [21].

10.6.1 Example 1: IND Enabling Data Package to Support 1 Month Dosing in Man

A generic IND enabling data package for the animal pharmacology and toxicology studies to dose humans for 1 month is displayed in Figure 10.3. This preclinical data package can be generated within 1 year with the toxicity studies requiring the longest duration (~9 months).

10.6.2 Example 2: Peroxisome Proliferator-Activated Receptor Agonist for Type-2 Diabetes

A generic IND enabling data package for the animal pharmacology and toxicology studies to dose a PPAR agonist for Type-2 diabetes in humans for more than 6 months is displayed in Figure 10.4. Due to chronic toxicity studies that require >2 years to generate data, this preclinical data package is assembled in ~3.5 years.

There have been several failures for PPAR agonists in late stage clinical trials due to an increase in the incidence of cancers. This has led FDA to request the 2 year carcinogenicity study to be completed in two species before the drug is given to humans for more than 6 months. Since Phase 3 trials will include dosing for more than 6 months, the carcinogenicity studies have to be completed before the Phase 3 trials can be initiated. A 2 year carcinogenicity study actually requires 3 years to complete. Hence, assuming Phase 1 and 2 studies require 2.5–3 years to complete, the carcinogenicity studies should be initiated approximately at the time of IND filing to avoid a delay in development. Sine carcinogenicity studies may cost as much as fivefold the cost of an initial Phase 1 study, candidate selection for development is critical at a very early stage.

A complete set of experiments for an IND enabling package is displayed in Table 10.2. Rat and dog are assumed as the two species for toxicological assessments. Although many of the items outlined in Table 10.1 are conducted to select a preclinical candidate, the tests need to be repeated under GLP conditions to be included in an IND application.

Below are brief discussions of the parameters that were not discussed previously.

10.6.3 Mass Balance

A radiolabeled sample of the compound is synthesized for a mass balance study. Typically, rats are dosed with the radiolabeled compound and urine and feces are collected over a period of time for analysis of radioactivity. Recovery of the radiolabel as the intact compound or metabolite in urine, feces as well as tissue and organs should be ~100% to account for absorption, distribution, metabolism, and excretion of the compound.

10.6.4 Animal Pharmacology and Toxicology Studies

For a detailed discussion on animal pharmacology and toxicology studies, see Chapter 7.

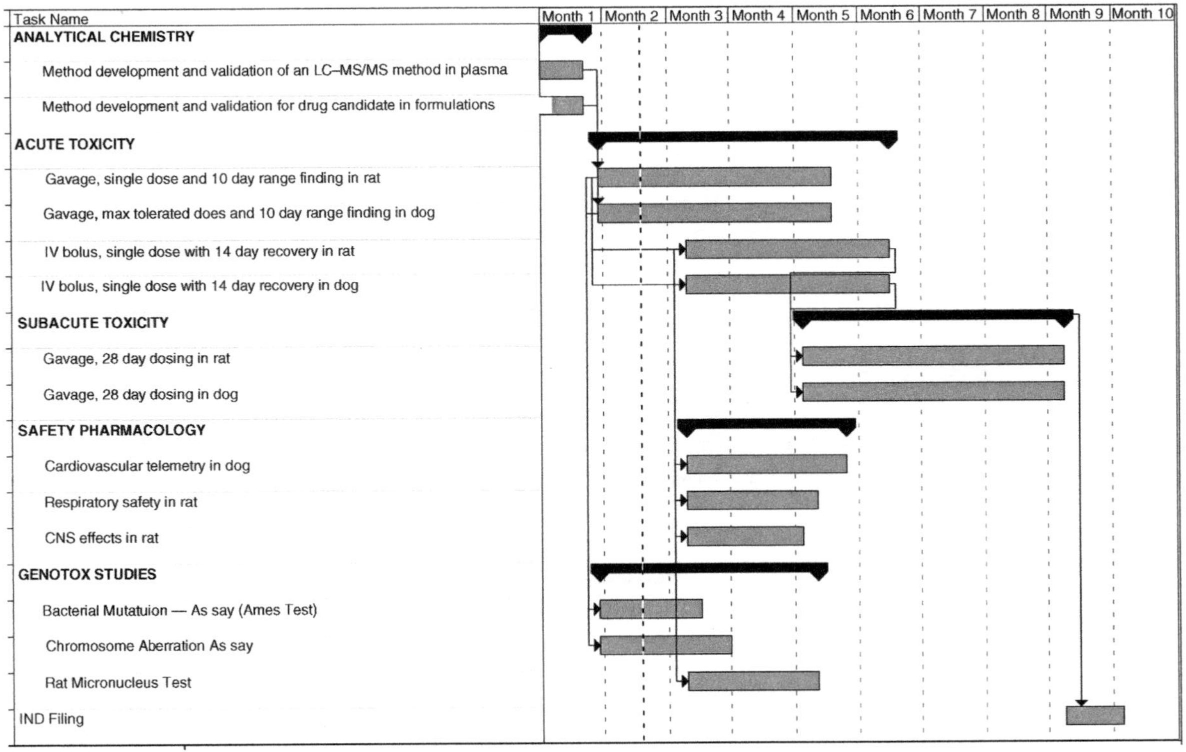

Figure 10.3 Timeline for generic IND enabling studies to support dosing in humans for 1 month.

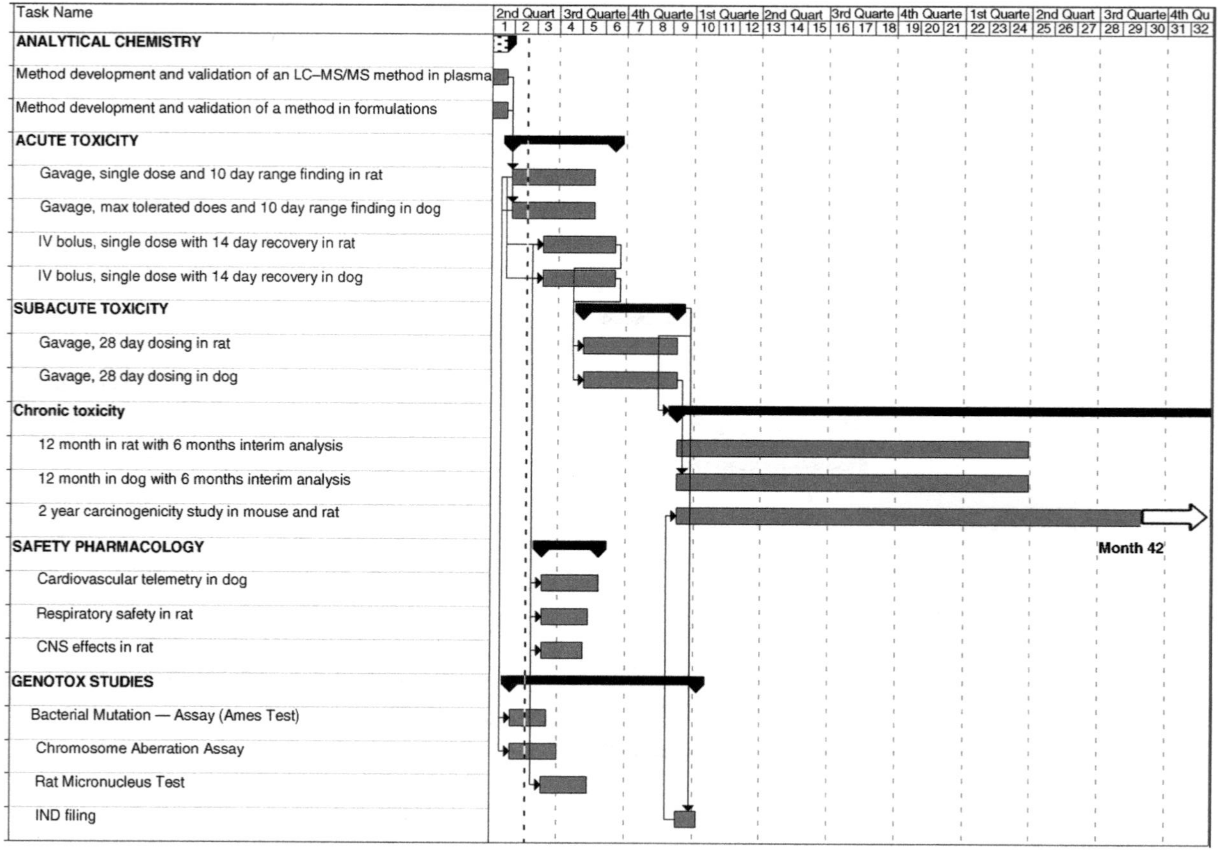

Figure 10.4 Timeline for IND enabling studies required for PPAR agonists to be dosed for >6 months in humans.

TABLE 10.2 Complete Set of Experiments for an IND Enabling Package (Rat and Dog Assumed as Species for Toxicological Assessments)

1. Bioanalytical assay development and validation
   a. Rat
   b. Dog
   c. Human
2. ADME
   a. Protein binding (rat, dog, human)
   b. *In vitro* CYP inhibition (rat, dog, human)
   c. *In vitro* CYP metabolism (rat, dog, human)
   d. Plasma stability (rat, dog, human)
   e. PK
      i. Dose proportionality
      ii. Multiple dose
      iii. Radiolabeled PK/mass balance (rat)
3. GLP safety and toxicology
   a. Method validation of dosing solutions
   b. *In vitro* toxicology
      i. HGPRT forward mutation
      ii. Gene aberration
      iii. Ames
   c. GLP *in vivo* toxicology including toxicokinetics
      i. Escalating single dose in rat
      ii. Escalating single dose in dog
      iii. 4 week rat study including recovery
      iv. 4 week toxicity and toxicokinetic study in dog
      v. Reproductive toxicology (rat and rabbit)
   d. Safety pharmacology
      i. Cardiovascular telemetry—dog
      ii. Respiratory—rat
      iii. CNS effects—rat
4. CMC
   a. Process chemistry/final synthetic route
   b. Develop and validate drug substance and product characterization
   c. Raw material accelerated stability
   d. GMP batch synthesis for drug substance and product
   e. Drug substance and drug product ICH stability
   f. Develop clinical formulation
   g. Synthesis of radiolabeled drug
5. Regulatory
   a. Establish clinical development plan
   b. Produce pre-IND meeting material
   c. Pre-IND meeting with FDA
   d. Phase 1a clinical protocol
   e. Clinical Investigators Brochure

GMP drug substance and product is not required to conduct animal pharmacology and toxicology studies. However, prior to conducting GLP toxicology studies to support an IND, a well-defined batch of drug substance synthesized by the final process chemistry method is recommended. To accelerate the development of a clinical candidate, a research batch of drug substance may be prepared under non-GMP conditions. This non-GMP batch can be used for preliminary stability as well as initial toxicology studies. Concurrently, a GMP batch may be prepared for final animal toxicology and human trials providing a faster development time to clinical trials. The risk associated with this strategy is as follows:

1. GMP batch cannot contain any new impurities compared to the non-GMP batch.
2. GMP batch cannot contain greater levels of impurities than the non-GMP batch tested in preclinical studies.

If the impurity profile of the GMP batch differs from the non-GMP preclinical batch, then another GMP batch of drug substance will need to be prepared or a bridging toxicology study is required which will delay the clinical trial.

In the single-dose escalating toxicological studies, the dose of the drug candidate is increased via the intended therapeutic route of administration until any adverse events are observed or until a predetermined maximum dose is obtained. The goal for selecting dose levels is to demonstrate no observable adverse effect level (NOAEL) at as high dose as possible, since this will set the limit for what can be tested in humans. As an example, if the doses are increased from 1 mg/kg to 10 mg/kg and then finally 100 mg/kg, and adverse events are evident at 100 mg/kg, the NOAEL is 10 mg/kg. Perhaps doses at 10, 30, and 100 mg/kg would again only show adverse events at 100 mg/kg, in which case the NOAEL now is 30 mg/kg. To ensure a good safety margin, the NOAEL should be at a dose 50- to 100-fold greater than the efficacious dose.

Repeated dosing for 4 weeks at doses expected to produce efficacy and below the maximum tolerated dose in the escalating single-dose study will detect any adverse effects upon repeat systemic exposure. A recovery period will provide information regarding reversal of any side effects noticed. In both single-dose escalating and repeat-dose toxicology studies, toxicokinetic (TK) data should be collected for systemic exposure.

The reproductive toxicology studies administered in rat and rabbit are designed to detect any adverse effects on the ability to reproduce as well as effects on the developing embryo. Safety pharmacology studies are designed to detect effects on the cardiovascular, respiratory, and central nervous system. As previously discussed, safety pharmacology studies of respiratory and central nervous systems for Sibutramine were favorable, but the drug is severely limited in dose due to heart rate and blood pressure effects [10].

10.6.5 Regulatory

It is important to meet with the FDA as early as possible to discuss whether the proposed preclinical plan provides sufficient safety information for the proposed clinical studies, and to discuss the design of the clinical study. Proper timing of this meeting is based upon two factors: (1) a company's strategy for interacting and communicating with the FDA; (2) the Division of the FDA (cardiovascular and renal, neurology, metabolism and endocrinology, etc.) for submission of the application. Different companies will provide the FDA a different preclinical data package for their review and guidance. Differences in the data package may include varying toxicology studies, GLP versus non-GLP, use of GMP drug product, etc. The advice of an experienced consultant is very valuable to decide which data to present including a Phase 1 protocol draft.

Typically in the pre-IND request meeting letter, the Sponsor will submit questions that will allow FDA to guide a Sponsor in the studies that will be required to design and initiate a Phase 1 trial. Data to provide a sense of the maximum tolerated dose, generated in the early pilot toxicological studies, is usually included in the briefing document.

A Phase 1 protocol is prepared while the nonclinical pharmacology and toxicology studies are being conducted. Once the Phase 1 protocol, CMC data, and nonclinical pharmacology and toxicology studies are completed, the clinical Investigator's Brochure (IB) may be prepared. The IB summarizes the CMC, nonclinical pharmacology and toxicology, and clinical data of the drug candidate for the clinical investigators selected to conduct the clinical studies.

10.7 CONCLUSIONS

As discussed, there are a multitude of factors influencing the selection of a preclinical candidate as well as a variety of development paths once a candidate has been selected. The disease area will greatly influence the studies that need to be performed, and also to a large extent determine the side effects that are acceptable for a drug candidate. Given the significant cost associated with generating a preclinical data package, a candidate should be selected with great care and the development plan should be discussed with the FDA at an early stage to insure that the data will support an IND filing.

REFERENCES

1. Guidance for Industry: Content and Format of Investigational New Drug Applications (INDs) for Phase 1 Studies of Drugs, Including Well-Characterized, Therapeutic, Biotechnology-Derived Products. Available at http://www.fda.gov/cder/guidance/phase1.pdf.
2. Clinical Trial. Available at http://en.wikipedia.org/wiki/Clinical_trials.
3. Wang, J. and Urban, L. The impact of early ADME profiling on drug discovery and development strategy. *Drug Discov. World* 2004, *5(Fall)*,73–86.
4. Guidance for Industry. Developing Products for Weight Management. Available at http://www.fda.gov/cder/guidance/7544dft.pdf.
5. Kola, I. and Landis, J. Can the pharmaceutical industry reduce attrition rates? *Nat. Rev. Drug Discov.* 2004, *3(8)*, 711–715.
6. Baycol Information. Available at http://www.fda.gov/cder/drug/infopage/baycol/default.htm.
7. Neuvonen, P. J., Backman, J. T., and Niemi, M. Pharmacokinetic comparison of the potential over-the-counter statins simvastatin, lovastatin, fluvastatin and pravastatin. *Clin. Pharmacokinet.* 2008, *47,463–474.*
8. Neuvonen, P. J., Niemi, M., and Backman, J. T. Drug interactions with lipid-lowering drugs: mechanisms and clinical relevance. *Clin. Pharmacol. Ther.* 2006, *80(6)*, 565–581.
9. Babbs, A. J., Smyth, D. J., and Thomas, G. H. PSN602: A Novel Monoamine Reuptake Inhibitor and 5-HT1A Agonist that, in Rats, Exhibits Equivalent Weight Loss to Sibutramine with a Superior Cardiovascular Profile. *Proceedings of the American Diabetes Association 68th Scientific Sessions*, 2008, 1744 p.

10. Product Monograph, Meridia. Available at http://www.abbott.ca/static/content/document/Meridia-PM-15JAN09.pdf.
11. Pipeline MBX-2982. Available at http://www.metabolex.com/MBX-2982.html.
12. Overton, H. A., Babbs, A. J., Doel, S. M., Fyfe, M. C., Gardner, L. S., Griffin, G., Jackson, H. C., Procter, M. J., Rasamison, C. M., Tang-Christensen. M., Widdowson, P. S., Williams, G. M., and Reynet, C. Deorphanization of a G protein-coupled receptor for oleoylethanolamide and its use in the discovery of small-molecule hypophagic agents. *Cell Metab.* 2006, *3(3)*, 167–175.
13. Summary Basis of Decision (SBD): Pr Sutent. Available at http://www.hc-sc.gc.ca/dhp-mps/prodpharma/sbd-smd/phase1-decision/drug-med/sbd_smd_2007_sutent_101319-eng.php.
14. Turpeinen, M., Korhonen, L. E., Tolonen, A., Uusitalo, J., Juvonen, R., Raunio, H., and Pelkonen. O. Cytochrome P450 (CYP) inhibition screening: comparison of three tests. *Eur J Pharm Sci.* 2006; *29(2)*, 130–138.
15. Madsen, K., Bjerre Knudsen, L., Agersø, H., Nielsen, P.F., Thøgersen, H., Wilken, M., and Johansen, N. L. Structure activity and protraction relationship of long acting glucagon like peptide 1 derivatives: importance of fatty acid length, polarity and bulkiness. *J. Med. Chem.* 2007, *50, 6126–6132.*
16. Guidance for Industry. Diabetes Mellitus—Evaluating Cardiovascular Risk in New Antidiabetic Therapies to Treat Type 2 Diabetes. Available at http://www.fda.gov/cder/guidance/8576fnl.pdf.
17. Davies, N.M., Teng, X.W., and Skjodt, N.M. Pharmacokinetics of rofecoxib: a specific cyclo-oxygenase-2 inhibitor. *Clin. Pharmacokinet.* 2003, *42, 545–556.*
18. Big Problem for BioStratum: Company spends millions on drug, then finds central compound on Internet. Available at http://triangle.bizjournals.com/triangle/stories/2005/10/17/story2.html.
19. Guidance Document. Available at http://www.fda.gov/cder/guidance.
20. Melosky B., Burkes, R., Rayson, D., Alcindor, T., Shear, N., and Lacouture, M. Management of skin rash during egfr-targeted monoclonal antibody treatment for gastrointestinal malignancies: Canadian recommendations. *Curr. Oncol.* 2009, *16(1)*, 16–26.
21. Guidance for Industry. Diabetes Mellitus: Developing Drugs and Therapeutic Biologics for Treatment and Prevention. Available at http://www.fda.gov/cder/guidance/7630dft.pdf.

11

FRAGMENT-BASED DRUG DESIGN: CONSIDERATIONS FOR GOOD ADME PROPERTIES

HAITAO JI

11.1 INTRODUCTION

The development of a new therapeutic drug creates many challenges as a drug has to possess many attributes for it to be an effective medicine, which includes potency, target selectivity, bioavailability, appropriate duration of action, and lack of toxicity. Historically, most drugs have been discovered either based on an already existing therapeutic agent or by random screening of compound collections [1]. Modern technologies for the synthesis and screening of large numbers of compounds have provided unique opportunities and challenges in drug discovery. The onset of combinatorial chemistry and the development of screen miniaturization and automation have resulted in much larger compound collections and vastly enhanced high-throughput screening (HTS) capabilities. These developments have taken the discovery of hits to a new level over the last several decades, enabling the screening of collections of hundreds of thousands of compounds in a matter of days, and allowing high-throughput screening of corporate compound collections the predominant approach for hit discovery in large pharmaceutical companies.

Nevertheless, despite several success stories [2], HTS has not, so far, been able to completely fulfill the original expectations of being able to bring medicines to the marketplace more rapidly [3], because HTS has some inherent fundamental issues that limit its scope. First, even in an ideal world where reliable assays can be developed against all targets, HTS will only be capable of identifying compounds

ADMET for Medicinal Chemists: A Practical Guide, Edited by Katya Tsaioun and Steven A. Kates

that already exist in corporate or commercial collections. This not only puts a strain on novelty and downstream intellectual property of the hits themselves but also limits medicinal chemistry to existing themes and knowledge; exploration of compound chemical space in truly new directions does not, by definition, automatically ensue. Second, different estimates exist in the literature as to the number of possible chemical structures with lead-like sizes, all of them being larger than the number of atoms on earth. Typically, in a HTS campaign, targets are interrogated with approximately 10^6 discrete compounds in parallel, which falls far short of potential chemical diversity space, estimated to be upward of 10^{60} molecules containing up to 30 nonhydrogen atoms [4]. Third, corporate libraries are continuously being filled with compounds that have been synthesized in late-phase discovery projects, and hence have drug-like rather than lead-like properties. The good hits identified from historical compound collections usually have moderate biological activity (K_i or K_d: 1–10 μM), but with relatively high-molecular weights (the average molecular weight is 400 Da) and excessive lipophilicity [5], which are frequently not amenable for lead optimization to generate compounds with drug-like properties. Finally, for many targets, suitable lead molecules will simply be absent from the compound collections or the HTS hit rate is very low, which results in few good chemical starting points for inhibitor optimization [2e].

The adoption of concepts such as *leadlikeness* [6] and *druglikeness* [7], as well as an increased awareness of the importance of more general physicochemical properties of compound collections, will undoubtedly lead to improved success rates in HTS-based lead generation [8]; however, it is generally accepted that there is a need for alternative, complementary approaches for lead generation. The analysis of HTS hits by Hann and coworkers shows that bad ligand–receptor interactions increase exponentially with the size and complexity of the molecule. As a consequence, the probability that small and simple molecules will bind to the protein, albeit with low affinity, is much higher than HTS-size compounds [9]. Indeed, ligand-efficiency (LE) calculations [10] of HTS hit compounds show that the average contribution to binding per atom can be rather modest. This supports the use of molecular fragments to anchor the drug design process rather than complex and large molecules.

11.2 FRAGMENT-BASED SCREENING

Stimulated by the introduction of Lipinski's "rule of five" [11], many research programs filter compound collections and retain those with lower average molecular weights, which have a smaller chance for mismatches with receptor-binding sites. This trend led to the generation of fragment-based screening [12], which was first described in 1997 with the advent of SAR by NMR [13], but has only become practical in recent years because of significant advances in technology.

Fragment-based screening relies on the identification of low-molecular weight and simple (low complexity) compounds that (weakly) bind to a chosen target and attempts to construct drugs from these small-molecular pieces to achieve the desired biological activity and molecular properties. This important approach is largely complementary to HTS as a technique that aids the hit-to-lead processes [14]. The technologies that have played a major role in driving the development of fragment discovery are nuclear magnetic resonance (NMR) spectroscopy [15], X-ray crystallography [16], mass spectrometry [17], and surface plasmon resonance [18]. These methods are also sometimes used in a synergistic way [19].

Fragment-based screening offers a number of attractive features compared with HTS. First, compounds from HTS libraries are more restricted in their rotational degrees of freedom, and thus less able to be adapted to a given target site. Conversely, a high proportion of atoms of a fragment hit are directly involved in the desired receptor–ligand interactions, which allows for optimal positioning within the receptor pocket. Therefore, a fragment is generally a more efficient binder (high binding energies per unit molecular mass) [20]. Second, a fragment-based strategy provides a combinatorial advantage. The number of fragments screened is in the range of only hundreds to a few thousands, but a larger chemical space than a preassembled large compound library may be explored. On the contrary, developing and maintaining a small set of fragments with simpler structures is easier than maintaining a massive HTS library. Third, when the binding of a fragment is identified, the subsequent structural optimization can benefit from extensive design and may result in a higher success rate and greater flexibility for generating novel chemical entities. Finally, starting with a low-molecular mass fragment is likely to produce leads with rather small and simple structures, which allows for molecular mass increases during the lead optimization process. Fragment-based screening provides chemical starting points that have no or few unnecessary structural elements, and therefore allows the addition of groups that can reduce the risk of toxicity or metabolic instability.

11.2.1 Fragment Library Design

The molecules in the library for fragment-based screening should be of a lower complexity than those typically screened by HTS. Since the throughput of fragment-based screening is generally low, typically only about 500–1000 molecules per target are screened. Therefore, a carefully designed library is essential.

The basic principles for the design of fragment libraries have been discussed [21]. One selection strategy to build a generic fragment library is to analyze current drugs, since they have already passed toxicity and ADME studies [22]. Databases such as the MDL comprehensive medicinal chemistry (CMC) [23], the Maccs drug data report (MDDR) [24], and the world drug index (WDI) [25] containing drugs or molecules in development are analyzed to identify interesting structural elements that can be used for library design. When applying this strategy, one must be aware that this is a retrospective analysis and this approach is then biased toward what is known.

To limit the complexity of the fragments, the "rule of three" was introduced for fragments on the basis of Lipinski's "rule of five" [26], stating that the molecular weight of screening fragments should be <300, Clog $P \leq 3$, the number of H-bond donors ≤ 3, the number of H-bond acceptors ≤ 3, the number of rotatable bonds ≤ 3, and polar surface area (PSA) ≤ 60 Å^2. The retrospective analysis of 18 different drug leads confirmed that fragments should not be larger than 20 heavy atoms or about 300 Da (for some targets, the upper limit to the molecular weight of fragment was set to 250 Da). However, a lower limit to the molecular weight should also be taken into account in a fragment library [27]. A lower limit of approximately 150 Da minimizes the chance that a fragment reorients on the target on elaboration [28], because smaller, less complex fragments that only contain single rings with small substituents have a greater likelihood of binding in multiple orientations [29].

Effective molecular recognition elements need to be packed into fragments with low-molecular complexity. Hydrophobic and electrostatic interactions are two important forces that describe the molecular recognition between ligand and protein. Most structures in a generic fragment library should include a hydrophobic group [30] and a strong hydrogen bonding or charged group [21c]. Restrictions to the numbers of substituents are important so as not to miss attractive binders for a particular target [31]. The active chemical functionalities of the fragments have to be masked to avoid potential false positives or negatives due to unwanted reactions with the target enzyme and working buffers. Each fragment should preferably possess at least one masked linker group that can be used for further structural elaboration.

In fragment-based screening, water solubility of fragments is of paramount importance since they are screened at high concentration (0.2–1.0 mM) in aqueous buffer. A 500 μM concentration of compounds in 95% phosphate-buffered saline and 5% DMSO is the typical standard solution to determine whether a fragment is appropriate for fragment-based screening.

Substructural analysis and filtering can be used to evenly select fragments that are dispersed to the different subregions of chemical space. The measure of molecular similarity (2D and 3D fingerprints, physicochemical properties, electrostatic fields, and molecular shape) can be accommodated within this design paradigm [32].

11.2.2 Detection and Characterization of Weakly Binding Ligands

Fragments typically are unable to derive substantial free energies from interactions with protein-binding sites because of their small size and limited functionality, and as a result display equilibrium dissociation constants in the range of 10^{-4}–10^{-2} M. Therefore, fragment-based screening must be able to detect binding that is 2–3 orders of magnitude weaker than that for typical HTS campaigns. Because most detection technologies require a level of binding site occupancy of >20% for reliable identification of a binding event, fragments must be screened at high concentration, and this places severe demands on the assay. Functional biochemical assays, particularly those that have been miniaturized for compatibility with HTS formats, cannot always give reliable results under such conditions. However, biophysics-based detection methods, which give a direct readout of ligand binding to a target protein, are often preferred for fragment-based screening. Biophysical methods tend to have significant robustness and resistance to artifacts, and additionally, some afford a high level of information content that can assist the downstream exploitation of fragment hits.

11.2.2.1 Nuclear Magnetic Resonance NMR has become a favored technique for screening fragment libraries following the pioneering work of SAR by NMR at Abbott Laboratories [15b, 33]. Not only is it capable of detecting weak interactions with high reliability, it may also provide information about the site of interaction, assisting in the ranking and exploitation of the fragment hits. Furthermore, it monitors binding of both partners directly in free solution, without interference from immobilization or detection artifacts, by following the change of intrinsic NMR spectral parameters that are highly sensitive and selective to the binding event between ligand and receptor. Ligand binding can be monitored by observing the effects on the NMR spectra either of the target [34] or of the ligand itself [35].

Target-based NMR screening relies on the detection of perturbations of target resonances on ligand binding [36]. The most well-known technique is the SAR by NMR method. Ligands are identified by monitoring alterations of target signals in a 2D ^{1}H–^{15}N correlation spectrum. This method requires large quantities of isotopically (^{15}N)-labeled protein (50–200 mg, with protein solubility between 0.1 and 1 mM) [37]. This method has the benefit (provided that sequence-specific resonance assignments have been obtained) of high reliability, being able to identify the binding site on the target, offering K_d information, readily distinguishing specific from nonspecific interactions, and assessing whether any significant conformational changes occur upon binding. The incorporation of ^{13}C into the target protein may also be used for the detection of binding of small molecules to targets [38].

Another method for screening larger protein targets is site-selective screening with labeled amino acid pairs [39], which relies on the sequence-specific labeling technique [40]. Using this labeling strategy, it is possible to selectively screen the ligand without sequence-specific assignments, and the chemical shift perturbations upon binding of a potential ligand are easily detected.

The limitation of target-based NMR screening is that the size of targets that can be observed to molecular weights is usually <100 kDa even if techniques like transverse relaxation optimized spectroscopy (TROSY) [41] or cross-relaxation induced polarization transfer (CRIPT) [42] are applied.

Ligand-based NMR screening relies on changes of the ligand signals when binding to the target [35, 43]. Several methods have been developed. One is the detection of an altered hydrodynamic property (i.e., molecular tumbling rate or diffusion rate) upon target binding [44]. When a small ligand binds to a macromolecule, its apparent rates of diffusion and reorientation are decreased. Such decreased diffusion rates can be measured by gradient-enhanced NMR spectroscopy. The decreased rate of molecular tumbling (increased rotational correlation time) is directly manifested in an increased transverse relaxation rate of the NMR signals, which can also be easily measured. The transferred nuclear overhauser enhancement (NOE) technique also falls into this class [45]. It relies on detecting intraligand NOEs that develop in the bound state, where the dipole–dipole interaction caused by the decreased molecular tumbling rate is much stronger than in a free state of a free ligand.

A second ligand-based NMR screening method involves detection of the transfer of an NMR signal between target and ligand. Methods that represent this class of experiments are NOE pumping [46], saturation transfer difference (STD) [47], and water–ligand observed via gradient spectroscopy (waterLOGSY) [48]. These techniques are closely related in that they all rely on dipole–dipole interactions between ligand–target spins. NOE pumping and waterLOGSY represent coherent methods because net magnetization is transferred. In this context, STD is considered an incoherent method because it relies on the transfer of saturation. This set of experiments represents the most attractive NMR-based techniques for binding detection currently available because it enables a lower protein concentration than other techniques.

A third ligand-based method is NMR fragment screening detecting interligand NOEs [49]. This method solely detects the signals between two small-molecule fragments. When two fragments bind to the target at neighboring sites, such that their hydrogen atoms are less than 5–6 Å apart, a transferred NOE can be detected between the hydrogen atoms by 2D NMR spectroscopy. Another ligand-based method involves the use of paramagnetic spin labels, such as 2,2,6,6-tetramethyl piperidine-1-oxyl, to increase the relaxation of nearby spins [50]. The spin label is covalently attached to either a ligand with a known binding site or a reactive amino acid side chain at the edge of the desired binding pocket. When another fragment binds to the target within a distance of less than 15–20 Å from the spin label, its ^{1}H signals can be selectively weakened. The fifth ligand-based method uses ^{19}F NMR to detect binding of fluorinated compounds to a target [51]. The wide chemical shift range and the simple signal pattern for the fluorinated molecules can facilitate the direct assignment of compounds within a mixture that bind to a protein. However, this technique suffers from intrinsic low sensitivity. It can be overcome by the use of an optimized cryogenic ^{19}F probe and the incorporation of magnetically equivalent fluorine atoms in ligands through the use of ^{19}F label of the CF_3 group [52]. The last ligand-based method described here is target-immobilized NMR screening, which immobilizes a target on a solid support and allows rapid characterization of the ligand-binding site [53]. This approach holds the potential for fragment screening of integral membrane proteins.

Contrast to target-based NMR, the protein concentration in ligand-based NMR screening is in the low micrometer range; therefore, the protein consumption is substantially lower. Ligand-based methods do not require protein labeling, so there is no upper limit on the size of the protein. However, the information content is lower (there is, e.g., no direct information on the site of binding, although this can sometimes be obtained indirectly) [54]. Most ligand-detection methods are usually limited to low and medium affinities because of the need to suppress the signals of the target molecule. Ligands that bind too tightly are indistinguishable from the target, and thus are suppressed as well, resulting in a false negative. In contrast, nonspecific binding can result in the appearance of false positives, so having access to a positive control (a known competing ligand) is almost a prerequisite to allow for the discrimination between specific and nonspecific effects [37].

11.2.2.2 X-Ray Crystallography X-ray crystallography can yield the most complete picture of fragment binding to its target. Similar to NMR, crystallography has the advantages of defining the ligand-binding sites and the binding orientations of the molecular fragment with more certainty. With advances in protein production and crystallization, and the degree of automation associated with crystal manipulation, X-ray data collection, and data processing [55], solving crystal structures is increasingly high throughput in recent years [16]. The use of synchrotron radiation sources to generate high-intensity X-rays has enabled many novel structures to be determined at unprecedented rates [56]. The improvement of these techniques has allowed X-ray crystallography to become a primary screening tool for fragment libraries.

Ringe and coworkers alleviated an initial concern that small weakly binding fragments might have insufficient affinity to yield well-solved electron density in a crystallographic structure by demonstrating that even simple organic solvent molecules could bind to specific sites on protein surfaces [57]. Stroud and coworkers demonstrated that individual fragments of the substrate dUMP bound to the enzyme thymidylate synthase in a position similar to that of the full substrate [58]. A survey of the Protein Data Bank has concluded that two structurally similar ligands belonging to the same series in a drug design project can safely be assumed to occupy the same 3D position in the binding site [59].

One of the first research groups to address fragment-based crystallography screening was Verlinde and coworkers. They described a successful fragment-based design of an inhibitor for triose phosphate isomerase (TIM) from *Trypanosoma brucei* [60]. Nienaber and coworkers described a CrystaLEADS (crystallographic screening for lead compound fragments) approach, which uses a library of 10,000 compounds divided into cocktails of 100 compounds [61]. The cocktails were assembled such that each obtained compounds of diverse shapes. SAR by X-ray was proposed by a group at Aventis [62]. A group at Astex developed a fragment-based crystallographic screening procedure, Pyramid™, which has been widely used in the generation of their lead structures [63].

Crystallography-based screening requires 10–50 mg of target protein with a purity of >95% [64]. Efficient fragment screening requires the soaking of a mixture of fragments (a cocktail) into the preexisting crystals of the target protein at high concentration (>10 mM) in the presence of organic solvents (usually DMSO) [65]. The fragments in each cocktail are usually selected to be both highly soluble and also shape diverse to assist interpretation of electron density. The crystals typically need to be able to tolerate cosolvents and high-solute concentrations. After collection of the X-ray data, the identification of the active fragments from the cocktail can be automated and accelerated by software tools such as Quanta from Accelrys [66] and AutoSolve from Astex [67].

Despite many challenges, a crystallographic fragment screen can be very powerful because it directly furnishes the structural information required for the medicinal chemistry elaboration of the identified fragment hits. Today many labs have made crystallographic screening a core component of the fragment-based lead generation platforms [62, 68]. The major drawback to this method is that it can only be applied to targets that form crystals suitable for cocrystallization or soaking experiments, and this level of robustness is not easy to achieve for many protein targets. This limitation also means that important membrane-bound targets (such as GPCRs) require different methodologies. High concentrations of ligands sometimes used in soaking can give false positives, as most compounds (including very weak binders) might bind to target proteins.

*11.2.2.3 **Mass Spectrometry*** The speed and high sensitivity of mass spectrometry (MS) make it an attractive approach to protein–ligand binding studies. Two main approaches have been applied to the discovery of weak binding ligands. A method, called SAR by MS, was developed to detect the binding of noncovalent weak binding fragments to DNA or RNA by electrospray ionization mass spectrometry (ESI-MS) [69]. Complexes with nucleotides are rich in H-bond interactions, making them stable in the gas phase and ideal for study by MS. By optimizing the ionization and desolvation processes, the researchers were able to characterize low-affinity complexes (in the millimolar range) formed between RNA/DNA and small molecules. On the basis of the observed mass and abundance of the complexes, the researchers were further able to directly determine both binding affinity and stoichiometry.

Another technique utilizing MS, called tethering, has also been used to identify low-molecular weight fragments that interact with a protein target at a specific site [70]. The technique relies on the formation of a disulfide bond (e.g., a tether) between the fragment and a cysteine residue in the target protein. If a native cysteine does not exist in the region of interest, one can be inserted by site-directed mutagenesis. The target protein is exposed to a library of disulfide-containing fragments and fragments with the greatest affinity for protein sites in the vicinity of the cysteine form the most stable disulfide bonds. Disulfides are rapidly detected and identified by mass spectrometry, such as ESI-MS which is sufficiently gentle for a sulfur–sulfur bond to remain intact during ionization. Performing the screening experiments under partially reducing conditions ensures that the intrinsic binding properties between fragment and target, rather than thiol reactivity, drive the selection process. However, this method requires *a priori* knowledge of the binding site, because the cysteine has to be located in or close to the active site. The demand to generate cysteine-containing mutant proteins may have potential limitations for the application.

*11.2.2.4 **Surface Plasmon Resonance*** Surface plasmon resonance (SPR) is an optical technique that uses the evanescent wave phenomenon to measure changes in the refractive index in the immediate vicinity of the surface layer of a sensor chip [71]. SPR is observed as a sharp shadow in the reflected light from the surface at an angle that is dependent on the mass of the material at the surface. The SPR angle shifts when molecules bind to the surface and change the mass of the surface layer. This change in resonant angle can be monitored noninvasively as a plot of resonance signal (proportional to the mass change) versus time, which allows the study of the interaction of proteins with ligands in real time.

A typical SPR-binding experiment consists of two phases: the binding of the soluble analyte to the sensor and the dissociation of the analyte on rinsing with analyte-free solution. By fitting kinetics from the association and dissociation phase to appropriate binding models, the corresponding kinetic rate constants k_{on} and k_{off} (and, hence, K_d, which equals k_{off}/k_{on}) may be calculated. Another approach is the direct determination of K_d by analyzing equilibrium-binding data generated at different analyte concentrations.

Because of the high sensitivity of modern SPR sensors, SPR has been shown to be suitable for the detection of low-molecular weight analytes and low-affinity interactions, which is a necessary condition for screening of fragment–protein interactions [72].

One often-discussed issue of SPR-based biosensors is the necessary immobilization of one of the binding partners and the tethering of molecules to surfaces may affect the binding constants measured. However, it has been evident that equilibrium, thermodynamic, and kinetic data from surface experiments can mirror those obtained in solution, if SPR biosensor experiments are carefully designed [73]. Numerous immobilization schemes for the formation of SPR sensor surfaces and their applications have been designed [74]. For example, the use of mediating sensor layers, such as streptavidin layers on gold and the subsequent attachment of biotinylated molecules, such as antibodies or DNA, have been successfully applied. Monoclonal antibodies can be covalently attached to the solid support. A fusion protein containing an antigen tag and a target protein can couple to the surface through the antibody–antigen interaction. The direct immobilization of DNA sequences on gold via the thiol moieties has been demonstrated.

Commercially available SPR sensors for coupling of target proteins include protein A surfaces, carboxymethylated dextran surfaces for covalently coupling to a variety of analytes exhibiting active groups, lipid bilayers [75] for the immobilization of membrane proteins, and nitrilotriacetic acid-coupled surfaces to immobilize His-tagged proteins.

Low consumption of the target protein and the convenient accessibility to experiments are the advantages of fragment-based SPR screening, coupling the target protein onto the solid support. However, the potential drawback of this methodology is that the background signal from unspecific binding might be strong because the binding of low-molecular weight fragments to protein does not change the SPR angle shifts much.

Both the target protein and the ligands (fragments) have been immobilized on the sensor surface [18]. One of the most successful immobilization strategies for biomolecules on sensor surfaces is the formation of self-assembled monolayers on gold or glass surfaces and subsequent covalent attachment of ligands (or fragment) of interest using appropriate linker chemistry. The advantage of this methodology is that the highly ordered monolayers allow precise control over the density of immobilized ligands and can be designed to minimize unspecific protein adsorption. However, the orientations of ligands have been predefined during coupling to the solid support, which might not be able to produce the optimal binding event with the target protein. Furthermore, this method limits to the opportunity to design a fragment library for a specific target because all ligands have to be coupled to the solid support.

11.2.2.5 Biochemical Assays

High Concentration Screening Inherited from HTS, high concentration screening (HCS) is a HTS application to the identification of fragment hits with low-molecular weights. Due to the low binding affinity to its target, fragments are generally required to be used at high compound concentrations, typically 0.1–2 mM, which is close to the aqueous solubility limit for a substantial number of compounds. The value of biochemical assays for fragment screening has been initially questioned based on experience with the traditional HTS, where compound concentrations of $\geq$10 μM can be associated with false positive (or negative) hits. Four typical sources of false positive (or negative) hits in the HTS functional assays are (1) readout distortion by colored, autofluorescent, or quenching compounds [76], (2) readout distortion by a limited compound solubility in aqueous solution with resulting precipitation [77], (3) target inhibition due to nonspecific aggregation [78], and (4) irreversible inactivation of the protein target [79].

In spite of these problems and challenges, HCS is attractive to many fragment-based ligand discovery campaigns because the HTS facilities have been established, and HCS is fast, convenient, and its outcome is actually the endpoint of the biological assays (such as K_i or IC_{50}). HCS can be cost- and resource-effective, provided that the assay platform remains robust and trustworthy. An increasing number of attempts using bioassays to screen fragment collections have been reported. The standard assay and screening techniques such as ELISA [80], absorbance [81], and radiometry [68c, 82] have been reported successfully to screen fragment collections. Among them, ELISA-based fragment screening is of particular interest because it may be advantageous, as the excessive compound concentration is significantly reduced by the washing steps before detection. However, these studies have only been conducted on very small collections of fragments, and the selection of fragment hits is primarily based on the medicinal chemistry-driven hypothesis.

High-sensitivity microscopic fluorescence techniques such as confocal fluorescence correlation spectroscopy have been adopted for fragment-based HCS, which can allow hit thresholds lowering to 10–20% inhibition [83]. This technique has successfully identified inhibitors of Hsp90 [84].

There is no inherent approach to judge the authenticity of a target-specific active compound because there are a number of pitfalls that need to be considered when running a HCS campaign. False positives must be removed as quickly as possible to minimize the risk of carrying them forward. The methods to support their removal include (1) ensuring that the screening library is of a high standard (removal of promiscuous hits and ensuring high solubility), (2) using additional well-designed assays to weed out false hits and confirming the functional biological data, (3) subsequently using structural biology or biophysics-based screenings to determine the binding constants, (4) using mutant information if reachable, and (5) further analog screening to confirm SARs.

Substrate Activity Screening Ellman and coworkers developed a substrate-based fragment identification method, called substrate activity screening (SAS) [85]. This method addresses two key challenges in fragment-based screening (1) the accurate and efficient identification of weak binding fragments and (2) the rapid optimization of the initial weak binding fragments into high-affinity compounds. A typical SAS has three steps (1) a library of substrates consisting of the substrate–catalytic functionalities and diverse, low-molecular weight fragments are screened using a single-step, high-throughput fluorescence-based assay; (2) the activity of the substrate is rapidly optimized by rapid analog synthesis and evaluation; and (3) the optimized substrates are converted to inhibitors by direct replacement of the substrate–catalytic functionalities with inhibitor pharmacophores, which match the catalytic residues in the active site.

In SAS, both an active enzyme and productive active-site binding are required for the catalytic function. The electronic and steric effects of the substituents in the vicinity of the catalytic site have to be compatible with the catalytic function of the target enzyme so that the enzyme is able to identify the substrates. However, SAS has some prominent advantages such as (1) being able to detect weak binding fragments, (2) being high throughput and straightforward to perform, and (3) the catalytic substrate turnover results in signal amplification, and therefore even very weak substrates can be identified at concentrations where only minimal binding to the enzyme occurs.

11.2.3 Approaches from Fragment to Lead Structures

In HTS screening, the transformation of a hit into an attractive lead compound is often achieved by adding the more likely potency-retaining (or increasing) hydrophobic substituents [9, 86]. This leads to increases in molecular weight and often also lipophilicity, which frequently result in negative effects on molecular properties, such as solubility or metabolic stability. Fragment hits derived from fragment-based screening are of high quality in terms of physicochemical properties; therefore, these hits often have superior molecular and ADME/Tox properties compared with hits from HTS. After the fragment hits are identified, the next step is to convert fragment(s) into a lead structure and maintain the drug-like properties of the generated molecule. There are three general strategies for converting fragments into a drug-like lead structure: fragment evolution, fragment linking, and *in situ* fragment assembly (Figure 11.1).

11.2.3.1 Fragment Evolution *Fragment evolution* (Figure 11.1a) is analogous to the standard hit-to-lead medicinal chemistry optimization process, requiring addition of other functionalities to a preexisting template to improve the interactions with the target. The basic requirement for fragment evolution is that the preexisting template should be a small molecule (called "anchor") that has plenty of diverse opportunities for increasing potency before exceeding the boundaries defined by Lipinski's "rules of five."

After the initial fragment hit is identified, there are two common strategies used for fragment evolution (1) if the target three-dimensional structure is accessible, X-ray crystallography or NMR spectroscopy can be used to determine the binding information of the initial hit to its target. Structure-based ligand design approaches are used to accelerate the evolution progress [87]; and (2) when the structural information of the target is unavailable, the screening of appropriate analogs of the original hit would be performed to establish a structure–activity relationship (SAR) to guide the medicinal chemistry efforts.

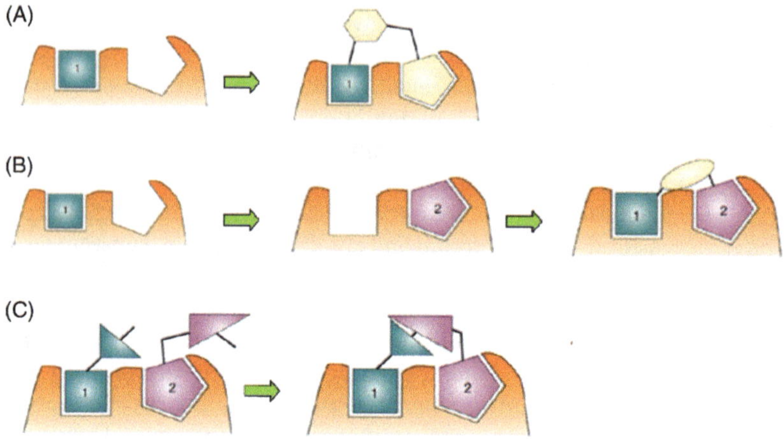

Figure 11.1 Three general strategies for converting fragments into a lead structure. (a) *Fragment evolution.* Fragment 1 binds to the receptor at one site. It is evolved by the addition of more fragments to create good contacts with the active site surface and then grow into a second pocket of the active site. (b) *Fragment linking.* Fragment 1 binds to the receptor at one site. Fragment 2 binds to the receptor at an adjacent site. The two fragments are joined together by a linking group that allows the lead molecule to span both sites. (c) *In situ fragment assembly.* Fragments 1 and 2 bind to receptor sites simultaneously with two reactive groups positioned within conformational reach of each other. The lead molecule is formed in the active site by the chemical reaction between the two reactive groups.

Fragment evolution has proved to be the most popular and effective approach from fragment to lead. One particular application of fragment evolution is to enhance properties other than the inherent potency of the original molecule or to deal with some specific issue, for example, an ADME liability.

11.2.3.2 Fragment Linking *Fragment linking* (Figure 11.1) involves joining two fragments that have been identified to bind at adjacent sites in a given target protein. The potency increase achievable from optimally linking two fragments can be an approximate of an additive effect of two fragments (i.e., the free energy of binding of the joined molecule is approximately equal to the sum of the free binding energies of the binding of two fragments) [58, 88], or in some cases, it can even exceed the sum of the component fragments (Figure 11.2) [89]. In these cases, although the linkers do not bind to the target protein directly, they assist the optimal binding of fragment hits to the target receptor. One extreme case is biotin–avidin binding [90]. In either of these cases, it requires the negative contribution from the linkers to be minimal and the loss in rigid-body entropy on binding of all fragment hits to the enzyme to be very small. An analysis of the experimental energetics associated with optimally linked fragments has suggested that the rigid-body entropy loss on protein binding constitutes a barrier of around three orders of magnitude to the binding affinity. This barrier is essentially independent of molecular mass that implies that there should be

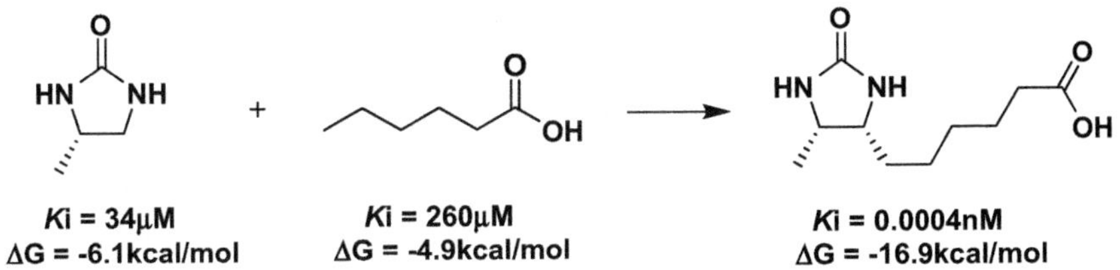

Figure 11.2 Nonadditive effect of fragment linking/merging on the binding affinity.

a superadditive effect when two small molecular-mass fragments are linked in an optimal fashion [91].

However, the linking step can be very difficult to achieve. The linker has to be of just the right length and the right conformation to be able to link fragments so that they can reach their respective binding sites in an optimal way. Access to structural information is essential for this approach to succeed since it can avoid the otherwise necessary and very large combinatorial and random search to find the effective linking scheme. As a consequence of these complications, there are relatively few examples of successful fragment linking in the literature that have resulted in lead-like hits with reasonable compound physicochemical properties and biological activity.

11.2.3.3 In Situ Fragment Assembly *In situ fragment assembly* (Figure 11.1c) entails the use of reactive fragments that link together to form an active inhibitor in the presence of a protein target. This approach can be considered in a wider context of target-guided synthesis (TGS), an umbrella term that covers a variety of systems that feature small-molecule synthesis orchestrated by a large biomolecule. The essence of *in situ* fragment assembly is that the protein serves as a template for synthesis and thermodynamically selects the combinations of fragments that can be converted to a larger and more potent ligand. The biological activities of the larger ligand are then confirmed using the standard biochemical assays. Currently, there are three *in situ* fragment assembly techniques: (1) dynamic combinatorial chemistry (DCC) [92], (2) tethering with extenders [17a], and (3) *in situ* click chemistry [93]. Among them, dynamic combinatorial chemistry and tethering with extenders are the thermodynamically controlled processes, while *in situ* click chemistry is a kinetically controlled process.

Dynamic Combinatorial Chemistry DCC was developed from combinatorial chemistry. The principal difference between DCC and the conventional combinatorial chemistry is that the reaction linking the building blocks together in DCC is reversible causing an ongoing interchange between the different members of the dynamic combinatorial library under thermodynamic control. A dynamic combinatorial library is able to respond to a molecular recognition event owing to the presence of the target protein, which can stabilize a particular member of the library and induce a shift in the equilibrium, favoring the formation of the selected species [94]. The amplification of the desired compound can be efficient to enable isolation of the molecule from the library on a preparative scale and in a high yield.

The processes involved in DCC include (1) preparation of a mixture of interconverting building blocks, (2) amplification of the best binder(s) through noncovalent interactions with a template, and (3) isolation and characterization of the best binder(s).

The chemical reaction that can be used in DCC must meet three sets of exacting criteria: (1) does not disrupt the function or structure of the target, (2) must proceed under the near physiological conditions required by the protein target (e.g., aqueous media, physiologically compatible temperatures, and pH value), and (3) fulfils the thermodynamic condition of reversibility. The concept of a preequilibrated dynamic combinatorial library can be used if the reversible exchange is stopped between generation and screening. In this case, reversible covalent reactions are employed to reversibly form and open a chemical bond without the assistance of the protein target. The target protein is used to preferentially select the desired ligands [95]. The set of chemical reactions that have been successfully applied to the construction of a dynamic combinatorial library are imine bond formation between carbonyls and amines [96] or hydrazide [95c, 97], amide bond formation and hydrolysis [98], disulfide bond formation between two thiols [95b, 99], sulfide bond formation between thiols and enones [100], and alkene bond formation by olefin metathesis [101]. The development of techniques to carefully analyze the library composition of a DCC is necessary [102]. An approach called dynamic combinatorial X-ray crystallography was established to visualize ligand–receptor interactions [103].

Tethering with Extenders Tethering with extenders is a technique for extension by tethering [70]. In this approach, a fragment that binds to the target protein is identified first by biophysics- or bioassaybased methods. This fragment is called an extender. The extender is modified to carry a reactive group and a protected thiol group. The reactive functionality is used to covalently bind to the protein and to fit the fragment into the active site. The thiol group is deprotected and used for tethering to a fragment that binds nearby. A new molecule linking the extender and the new identified fragment using a similar binder as that formed in the tethering study can be generated and tested for activity.

Similar to dynamic combinatorial chemistry, tethering with extenders uses a disulfide bond to explore optimal binders between two fragments. Tethering with extenders has been used to identify inhibitors of cysteine aspartyl proteases (caspase-1 [104] and caspase-3 [105]).

In Situ Click Chemistry Click chemistry was defined as a modular reaction with wide scope, giving very high yields, stereospecific, and generating only innocuous by-products that are easily separated. The process must include simple reaction conditions, readily available starting materials and reagents, the use of no solvent, or a solvent that is benign or easily removed, and simple product isolation [93]. In contrast to dynamic combinatorial chemistry, *in situ* click chemistry is a kinetically controlled TGS that irreversibly generates the products that are unable to revert to the starting materials.

Irreversible TGS was pioneered by Benkovic and coworkers [106]. They developed multisubstrate adduct inhibitors by an irreversible reaction, in which the enzyme glycinamide ribonucleotide transformylase templated the alkylation of its substrate glycinamide ribonucleotide thiol analog with a folate-derived bromide. Wilson and coworkers described an enzyme-templated epoxide opening reaction of folate-derived epoxide with glycinamide ribonucleotide to generate a tight-binding inhibitor [107]. Huc and Nguyen described a similar approach in which inhibitors of carbonic anhydrase (CAII) were generated via a reaction of a thiol with different α-chloroketones in the presence of the Zn(II) metalloenzyme [108].

To date, the most popular *in situ* click chemistry, developed by Sharpless et al., is the 1,3-dipolar cycloaddition reaction, also known as Huisgen cycloaddition [109] between an azide and an alkyne to afford the 1,2,3-triazole moiety [93]. Totally different from the other highly reactive reagents mentioned previously (e.g., aldehydes, hydrazine, thiols, epoxides, and α-chloroketones), the azide and alkyne groups are low-reactive functional groups in organic chemistry and are inert to biological molecules and living systems. The cycloaddition reaction of an azide and an alkyne is extremely slow at room temperature. However, the maximally unsaturated azide and alkyne bonds store a large amount of energy. When these two groups are arranged in close proximity, such as in the active site of a target protein [110], the 1,3-dipolar cycloaddition reaction is accelerated remarkably.

Besides the reliability of the linking reaction between the azide and alkyne groups, the newly formed 1,2,3-triazole ring has favorable physicochemical properties for the biological system, which has been regarded as a nonclassical bioisotere of the amide group. The 1,2,3-triazole ring possesses a large dipole moment of ~5 Debye, and the nitrogen atoms on the triazole ring are weak hydrogen bond acceptors. The successful application of *in situ* azide and alkyne click chemistry has been reported for the inhibitor design of acetylcholinesterase [111], carbonic anhydrase [112], and HIV protease [113].

11.3 CASE STUDIES OF FRAGMENT-BASED SCREENING FOR BETTER BIOAVAILABILITY

11.3.1 Adenosine Kinase

Adenosine kinase [114] is a 39 kDa protein that is primarily responsible for the intracellular metabolism of adenosine. Inhibitors of adenosine kinase have potential use as anticonvulsant and antinociceptive agents. Compound **1** has poor solubility. On the basis of known SARs, **2** was chosen as an anchoring pharmacophore, and NMR-based screening (SAR by NMR) was used to identify alternative companion fragments that bound to adenosine kinase in the presence of 1 mM **1** (Scheme 11.1). Indole **3** was found bound to the bromobenzene-binding pocket with a K_d of 3 mM. The merging of **3** with **1** generated **4**, which showed lower potency than **1**, but had better pharmacokinetic properties.

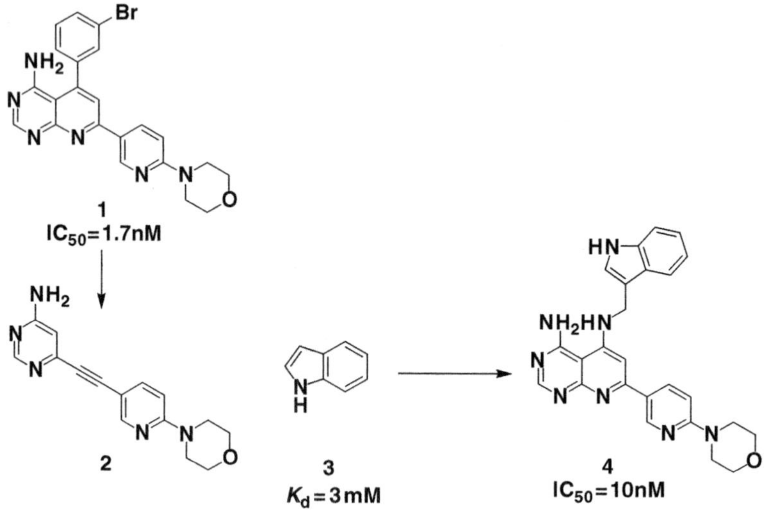

Scheme 11.1 NMR-based fragment screening for adenosine kinase inhibitors.

11.3.2 Leukocyte Function-Associated Antigen-1

Leukocyte function-associated antigen-1 (LFA-1) [115] is a heterodimeric transmembrane glycoprotein expressed on all leukocytes. An interaction between LFA-1 and its counterreceptors, the intracellular adhesion molecules (ICAM)-1, -2, and -3, cause immune responses. Therapeutic prevention of LFA-1 from binding to ICAMs has the potential for the treatment of inflammatory diseases and graft rejection after transplantation. Diaryl sulfide lead compound **5** ($IC_{50} = 44$ nM) was found by NMR spectroscopy to bind to an allosteric site on the I domain of LFA-1. However, the solubility of this compound is very low (0.9 μg/mL), and this compound shows no oral bioavailability (Scheme 11.2). NMR-based fragment screening (SAR by NMR) was used to identify new fragments in the presence of the substructure of **5** (i.e., 6, $IC_{50} = 80$ μM). A number of fragments were found to coexist with **6**. Two of them, **7** and **8**, have K_d values of 300 μM and 10 mM, respectively. The merging of **7** or **8** with **6** generated **9** ($IC_{50} = 20$ nM) or 10 ($IC_{50} = 40$ nM). The solubility of **10** is fourfold better than **5** and shows oral bioavailability.

11.3.3 Matrix Metalloproteinase 3 (Stromelysins)

Matrix metalloproteinases (MMPs) are a family of zinc-dependent endoproteinases. The inhibitors of MMPs-3 (also called stromelysins) have been implicated in the treatment of cancer. Potent peptide-based inhibitors designed on the basis of substrate specificity had been discovered; however, many of these compounds exhibit poor bioavailability. A previous HTS of 115,000 compounds had failed to identify any nonpeptide inhibitors with a potency better than 10 μM. Acetohydroxamic acid (**11**) was selected as an initial fragment based on its known ability to serve as a zinc chelator

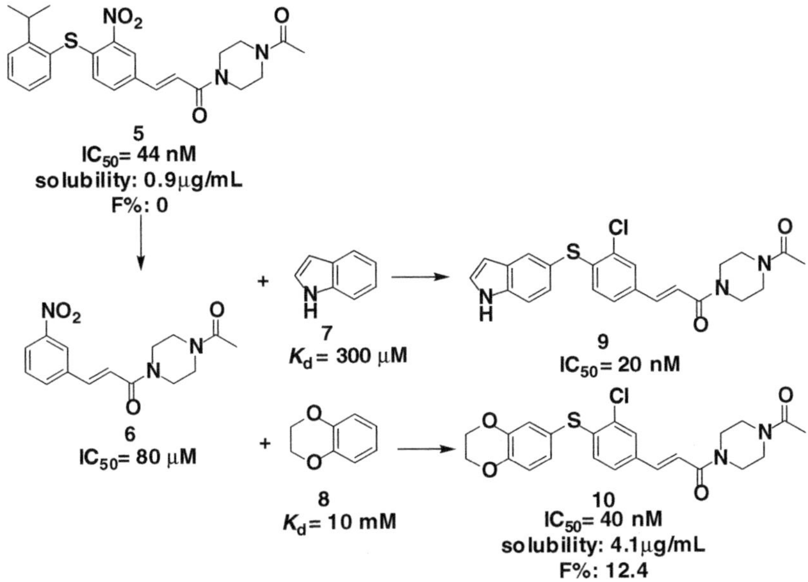

Scheme 11.2 NMR-based fragment screening for leukocyte function-associated antigen-1 inhibitors.

(Scheme 11.3). A NMR-based screening (SAR by NMR) was conducted in the presence of **11**, and the biphenyl binders **12** and **13** were identified. The linking of **11** with **12** or **13** generated **14** ($IC_{50} = 25$ nM) or **15** ($IC_{50} = 15$ nM). However, due to the lability of the hydroxamate moiety to hydrolysis, **14** and **15** lack oral bioavailability [116].

Further structural modifications targeting to the hydroxamate analogs were made. A SAR by NMR screen in the presence of **12** and **13** identified **16** with a K_d of 50 μM. The merging of **16** to **14** and **15** led to **17** and **18**, having IC_{50} values with stromelysin of 340 and 62 nM, respectively. Compound **17** exhibits a C_{max} of 28 μM and a $t_{1/2}$ of about 2 h [117].

11.3.4 Protein Tyrosine Phosphatase 1B

Protein tyrosine phosphatase 1B (PTP1B) regulates phosphorylation of the insulin receptor and is a promising target for diabetes and obesity therapy. However, finding small-molecule inhibitors for this target has been recognized to be challenging. PTP1B has two adjacent phosphotyrosine-binding sites. One is the catalytic pocket. The other one is on the substrate recognition surface. NMR-based screening (SAR by NMR) was used to identify a potential lead series that occupies both sites (Scheme 11.4). Compound **19** was identified as a weak binder that showed inhibition of PTP1B with a $K_i = 293$ μM. A simple optimization led to **20**, which was shown to be a competitive and reversible inhibitor ($K_i = 39$ μM). Structure-based optimization led to **21** ($K_i = 1.1$ μM), which extended a pentyl chain toward the

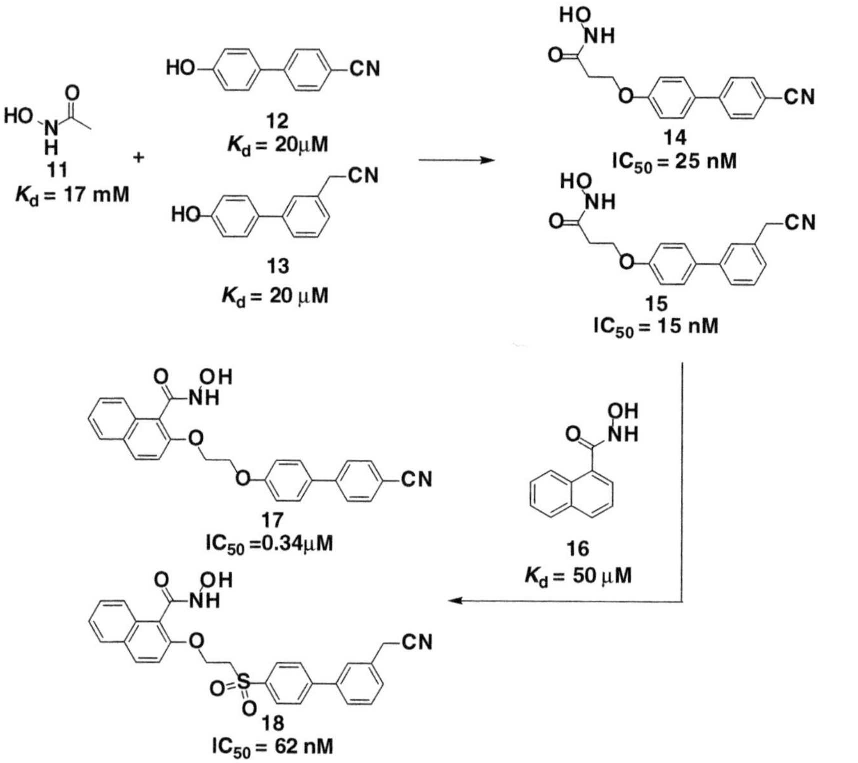

Scheme 11.3 NMR-based screening for matrix metalloproteinase 3 (MMP-3, stromelysis) inhibitors.

second phosphotyrosine-binding site. NMR-based screening to the second phosphotyrosine-binding site identified a weak binder (**22**). A closely related analog of **22** was appended to **21** to generate **23**, which exhibited a K_i of 22 nM [118].

Starting with fragment **19**, structure-based optimization led to **24** and **25**, with K_i values of 1.2 and 1.5 μM respectively [119]. NMR-based screening (SAR by NMR) of the second phosphotyrosine-binding site identified **26**. The linking of **26** to **24** led to **27** with a K_i of 42 nM. The methyl ester (**28**) exhibited better potency [120]. Unfortunately, **23**, **27**, and **28** show no cell permeability. To increase the cell permeability of the inhibitors, heterocyclic monocarboxylic acids were screened by NMR spectroscopy, and fragment **29** was found to bind to the active site (Scheme 11.5). Limited optimization led to **30**. The linking of modified **30** and **26** generated **31**, which displayed low micromolar potency; however, it displayed cell permeability in a Caco-2 permeability assay and cell-based activity in a phosphorylation assay [121].

Mass spectrometry-based approach (tethering) was also used to search monocarboxylic acid fragments that can bind to the catalytic binding site [122]. Because the catalytic binding site of PTP1B is deep and highly conserved, the introduction of

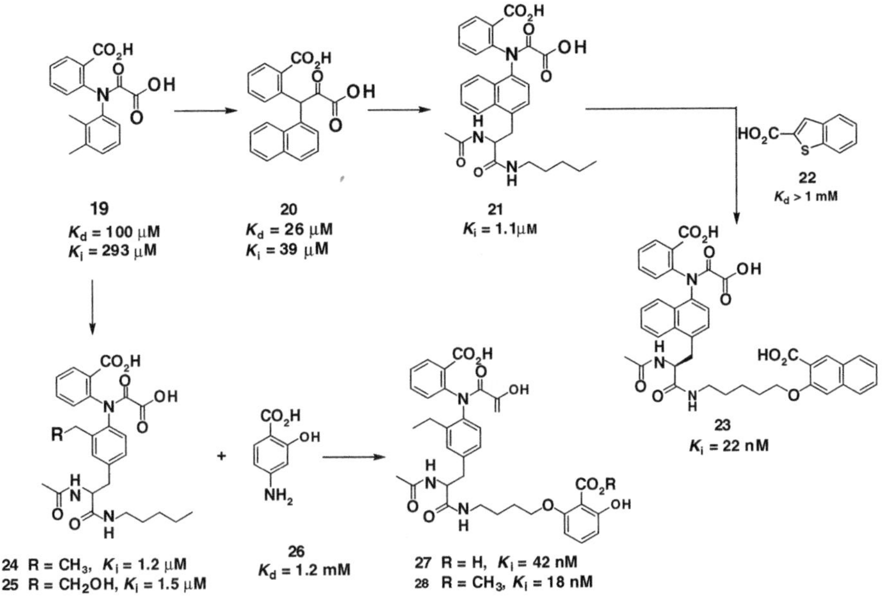

Scheme 11.4 NMR-based screening for protein tyrosine phosphatase 1B (PTP1B) inhibitors.

a cysteine mutation within the active site itself is not desirable. A technology called breakaway tethering was developed [122]. In this method, a cysteine is introduced outside the active site and alkylated with a spacer that has a thiol group positioned toward the catalytic site (Figure 11.3). This thiol group is used to interrogate fragment libraries. In the case of PTP1B, an R47C mutation was introduced, and a 2-mercaptoethylcarbamoyl spacer group was appended (Figure 11.3). Fragment **32** was identified by breakaway tethering. It is a competitive inhibitor with a K_i of 4.1 mM. The binding affinity for **32** is comparable to pTyr (K_m = 4.9 mM). An X-ray crystal structure of PTP1B with **32** showed that **32** binds to the catalytic site. This fragment forces a loop that lines the active site to adopt a new open conformation, which can be utilized to design selective inhibitors.

An X-ray crystallography-based method (Pyramid) was also used to search monocarboxylic acid fragments to solve the problem that PTP1B generally recognizes

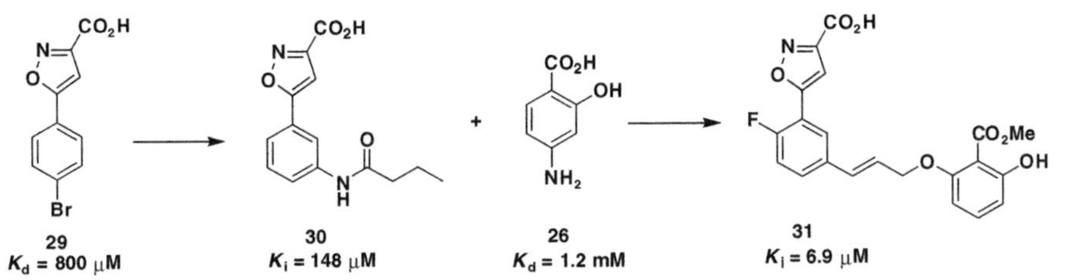

Scheme 11.5 NMR-based screening for protein tyrosine phosphatase 1B (PTP1B) inhibitors with improved Caco-2 permeability.

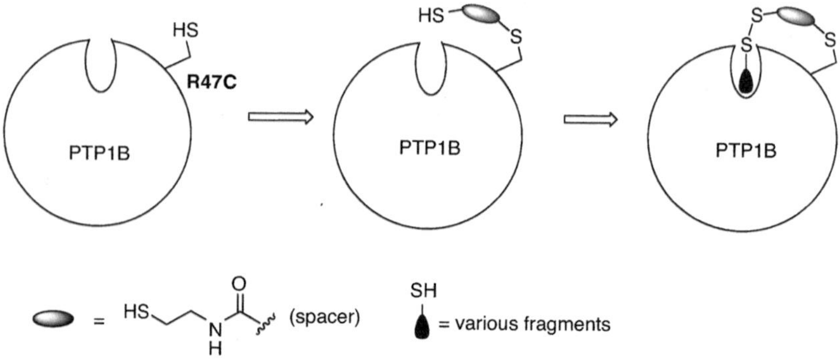

Figure 11.3 Breakaway tethering on PTP1B.

doubly anionic groups in the phosphate-binding pocket [67] (Figure 11.4). Compound **33** was identified with a K_i of 86 μM. This fragment can be used as a starting point to design new lead structures with superior physical and pharmacokinetic properties.

11.3.5 β-Secretase (BACE-1)

β-Secretase is a membrane-associated aspartyl protease that cleaves the membrane-associated amyloid precursor protein (APP) at an extracellular membrane site. Subsequently, γ-secretase cleaves APP within the transmembrane site, which generates the β-amyloid peptide. The aggregation of β-amyloid peptides forms neurofibrillary plaques. The accumulation of amyloid plaques and neurofibrillary tangles is thought to cause Alzheimer's disease. Since β-secretase cleavage is the rate-limiting step in the process from the membrane-associated APP to β-amyloid peptide, β-secretase is considered an important target for the treatment of Alzheimer's disease. However, HTS of several different compound collections and traditional medicinal chemistry to convert peptidic inhibitors to peptidomimetic or nonpeptidic inhibitors failed to provide a suitable hit (**31**). An X-ray crystallography screen (Pyramid) identified two initial fragment hits, **34** and **35**, which exhibited approximately 30–40% inhibition at 1 mM (Scheme 11.6) [123]. Fragment evolution of **34** led to **36** with an IC_{50} of 94 μM. Further optimization led to **37** with an IC_{50} of 25 μM [124]. On the basis of the structure of **35**, virtual screening of fragment libraries generated **38** as a primary hit with an IC_{50} of 310 μM. Further fragment evolution led to **39**–**41**. The introduction of an indole moiety led to **42** with an IC_{50} of 9.1 μM. Further modification of **42** led to **43** with an IC_{50} of 0.69 μM.

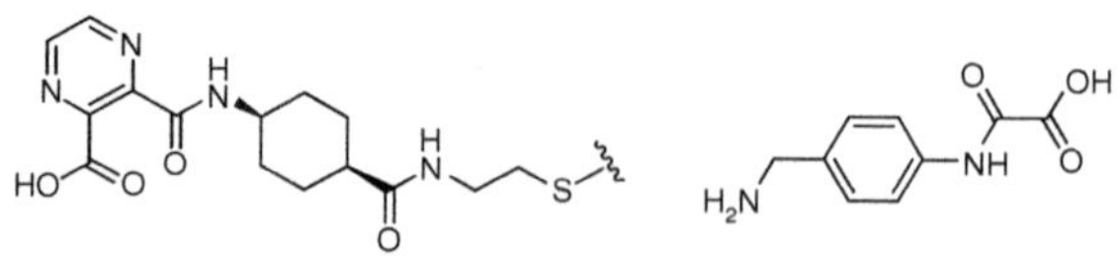

32
K_i = 4.1 mM

33
K_i = 86 μM

Figure 11.4 Two monocarboxylic acid inhibitors of PTP1B.

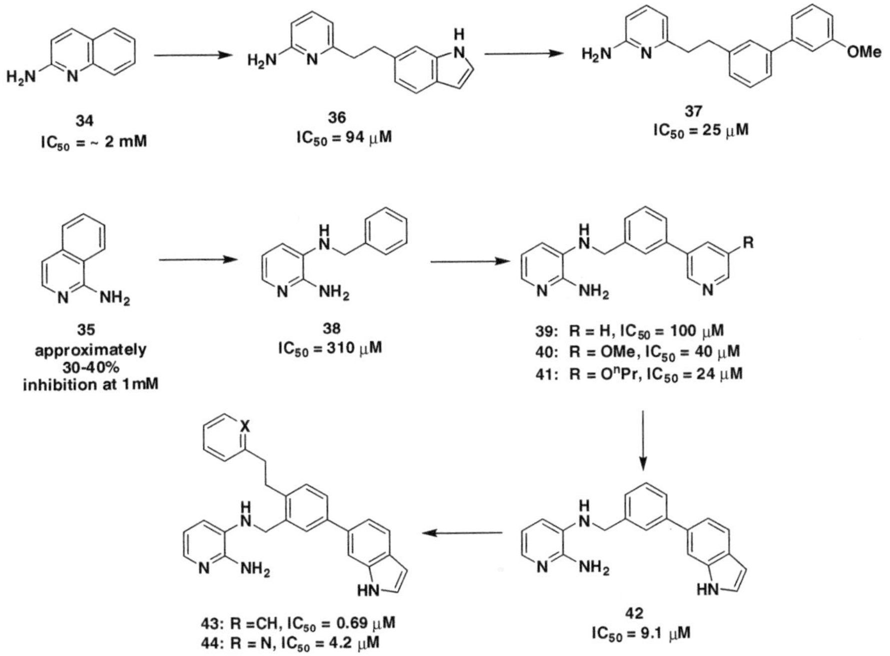

Scheme 11.6 X-ray crystallography screen (pyramid) for β-secretase (BACE-1) inhibitors.

Ligand-based NMR spectroscopy (waterLOGSY) was also used to screen fragment libraries (Scheme 11.7). Fragment **45** was identified as a hit with a K_d of 4.45 mM. Database mining around **45** resulted in the identification of **46**, with a sevenfold increase of affinity [125]. X-ray crystallography, SPR, and two highly sensitive bioassay techniques, fluorescence resonance energy transfer (FRET) and electrochemiluminescence-based assay (referred as IGEN), were used to drive the optimization of the primary fragment hit. To increase solubility and exploit potential hydrogen-bonding interactions with the enzyme, fragment evolution identified **47**, which had an IC_{50} of 86 μM in the SPR assay, and an IC_{50} of 130 μM in the FRET assay. The X-ray crystal structure of β-secretase in complex with **46** suggested an ^3N-methylation, which led to **48**. The SPR, FRET, and IGEN IC_{50} values for **48** were 180, 220, and 150 μM, respectively. Further fragment evolution led to **50** with a SPR, FRET, and IGEN IC_{50} of 5.7, 5.9, and 5.3 μM, respectively. In consideration of the possible metabolic oxidation of the dihydroisocytosine ring of **50, 51** was designed with the aid of the crystal structure, resulting in IC_{50} values of 80 and 470 nM in the FRET assay and cell-based assay [126].

Tethering also successfully identified new primary fragment hit **52** for β-secretase where V332C was introduced as the tethering site (Scheme 11.8). The optimization of the fragment hit generated **53**. The conversion of tethered ligand to nonconvalent inhibitors led to the nonpeptidic compound **55** with a K_i of 74 μM [127].

Surface plasmon resonance was used to identify the primary fragment hit for β-secretase (Scheme 11.9) [128]. The tyrosine metabolite tyramine **56** was found to

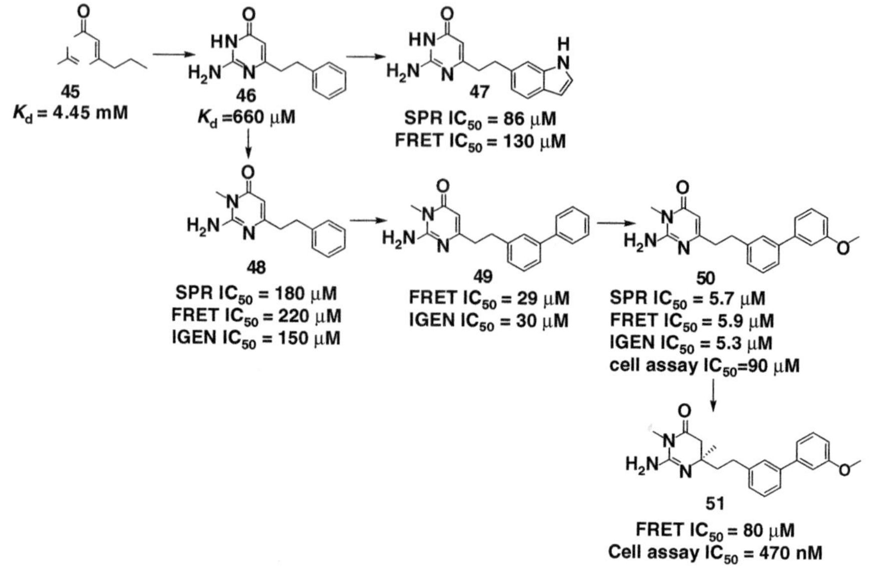

Scheme 11.7 Ligand-based NMR spectroscopy (waterLOGSY) for β-secretase (BACE-1) inhibitors.

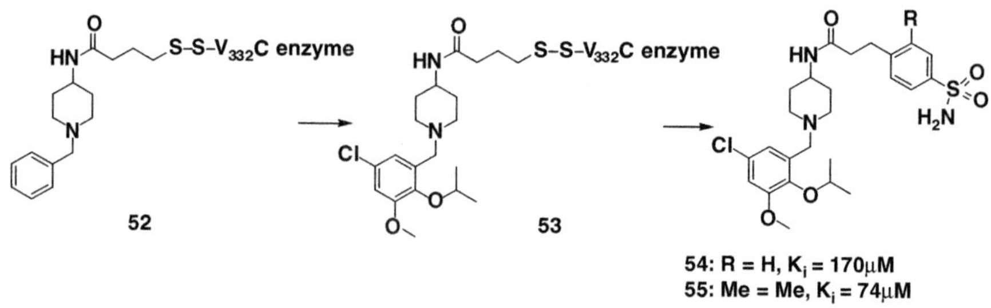

Scheme 11.8 Tethering strategy for β-secretase (BACE-1) inhibitors.

have a K_d of 2 mM for β-secretase. 2-Ethyl substitution (**57**) resulted in increased binding affinity (K_d = 660 μM). The replacement of the 2-ethyl group with a *para*-toluene group (**59**) led to an increase of binding affinity by more than one order of magnitude.

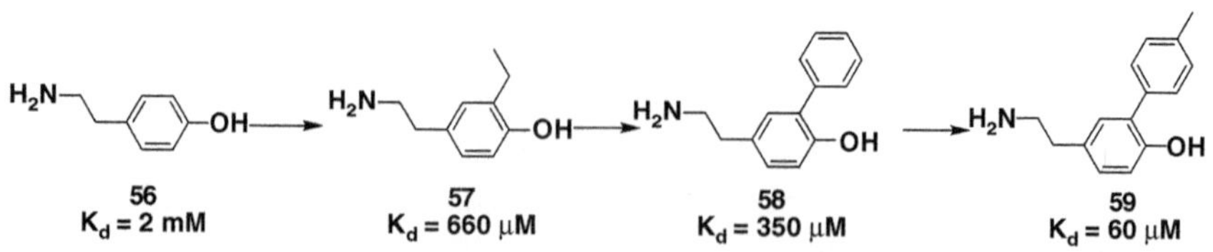

Scheme 11.9 Surface plasmon resonance for β-secretase (BACE-1) inhibitors.

11.3.6 SH2 Domain of pp60Src [62, 129]

^{pp60}Src is involved in signal transduction and plays an essential role in bone resorption. The selective binder of the SH2 domain of ^{pp60}Src can inhibit bone resorption and could be useful for the treatment of osteoporosis. Structure-based medicinal chemistry has identified **60** as an inhibitor with an IC_{50} of 9 nM (Scheme 11.10). However, the phosphate group of **60** has a high rate of hydrolysis by phosphatases, and the high charge property of the phosphate group of **60** precludes cell penetration. The $t_{1/2}$ in rat plasma of **60** is reported to be 0.6 h in rat plasma. X-ray crystallography-based screening (SAR by X-ray) identified **61** with an IC_{50} of 2.5 mM, which occupies the binding site of the phosphate group. The merging of **61** with **60** generated **62** with an IC_{50} of 3 nM. This compound shows superior rat and human plasma stability (it is stable in rat and human plasma over 24 h).

11.3.7 Thrombin

Thrombin, a serine protease, which plays a central role in the blood coagulation cascade, is an important target for thrombosis-related diseases such as deep vein thrombosis, stroke, and myocardial infarction. The majority of the known thrombin inhibitors are characterized by the presence of highly charged guanidine or benzamidine functionalities binding to the enzyme's S1 pocket. While this feature promotes inhibitory potency, it is detrimental to oral bioavailability. One challenge for the thrombin inhibitor design is the identification of nonbasic groups that can bind to the thrombin S1 pocket. Ligand-based surface plasmon resonance screening was used to identify new fragment hits that can bind to the thrombin S1 pocket. On-array competition experiments with a known thrombin inhibitor showed that not only the charged fragments **63** and **64** but also the nonbasic fragments **65–68** are among the top ranked fragment hits (Figure 11.5)) [130].

The linking of **64** and **66** generated **69** with a K_i of 200 μM (Scheme 11.11). X-ray crystallography revealed that the 4-chlorophenylthioether moiety, but not the guanidinophenyl moiety, binds to the thrombin S1 pocket. Incorporation of a known diphenylalanine proline dipeptide (**70**) scaffold led to **71** with a K_i of 5 μM. On the basis of computer modeling, cyclization of the thioether substructure with the chlorophenyl ring generated **72** ($K_i = 2$ nM). Incorporation of the pyrazinone acetamide scaffold from a known thrombin inhibitor led to **73** with a K_i of 20 nM. The

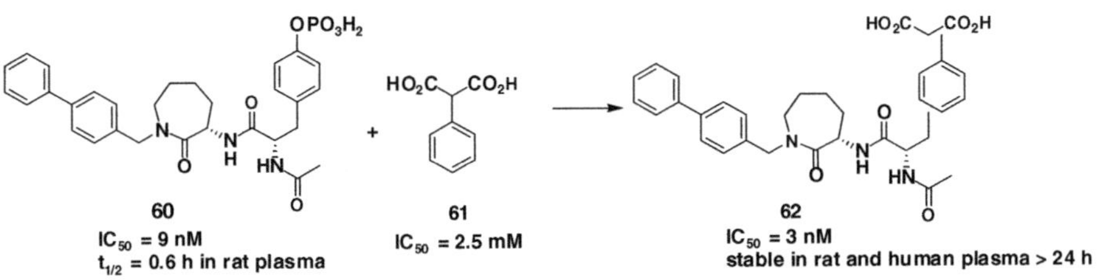

Scheme 11.10 X-ray crystallography-based screening for SH2 domain of ^{pp60}Src inhibitors.

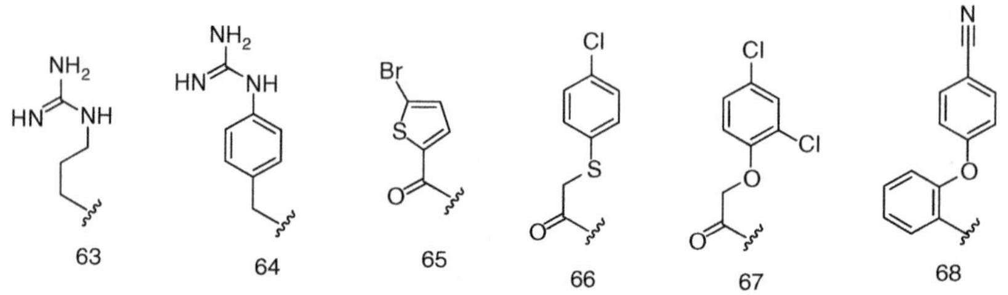

Figure 11.5 Six fragment binders for thrombin identified by surface plasmon resonance.

substitution of the phenyl group in **73** with a pyridyl group led to **74** with an order of magnitude increase in potency. However, intrinsically low aqueous solubility is an inherent problem for the pyrazinone acetamide scaffold. When the amide group of **74** was changed to a secondary amine (**75**), the aqueous solubility was increased 10-fold while retaining the potency at the same level ($K_i = 3$ nM) [131].

X-ray crystallography-based fragment screening (Pyramid) was also used to identify new fragment hits for thrombin (Scheme 11.12). Fragments **76–78** were found to bind to the thrombin S1 pocket, where the guanidine or benzamidine functionalities of most thrombin inhibitors bind. The linking of **78** ($IC_{50} = 330\ \mu M$) with **79** ($IC_{50} = 12\ \mu M$) led to **80** with an IC_{50} of 1.4 nM [67, 132].

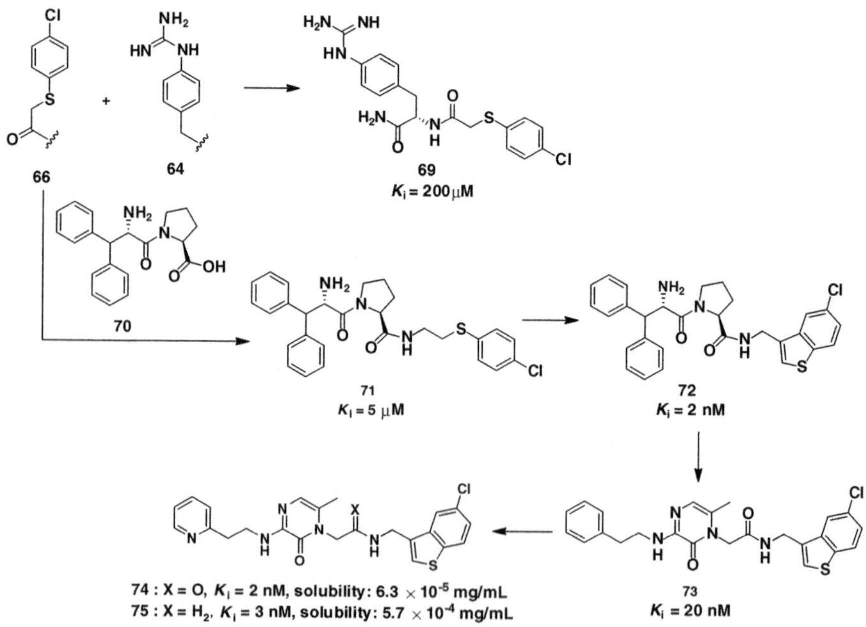

Scheme 11.11 Surface plasmon resonance for thrombin inhibitors.

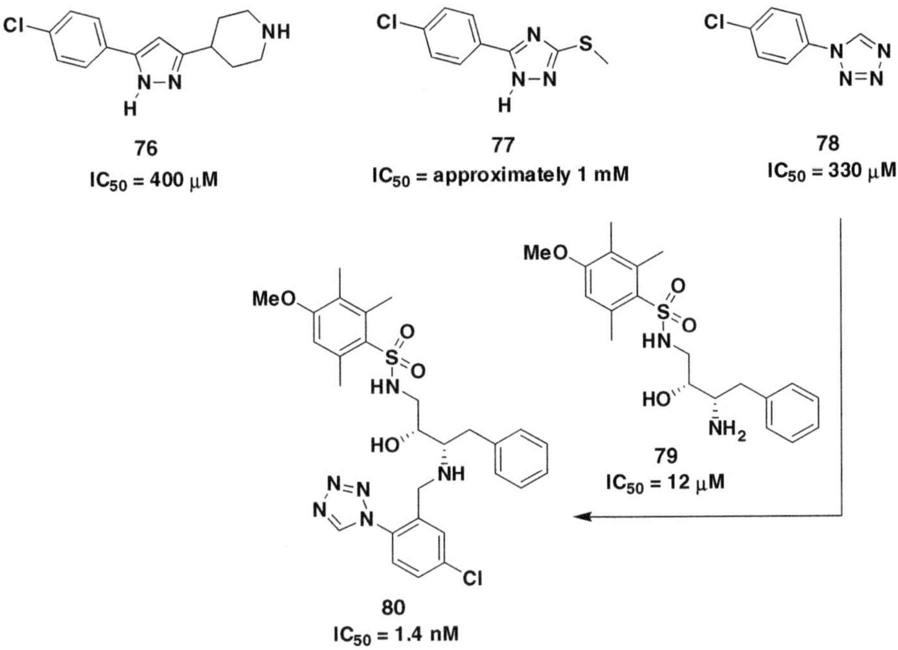

Scheme 11.12 X-ray crystallography-based fragment screening (pyramid) for thrombin inhibitors.

11.3.8 Urokinase

Urokinase is an activator of plasminogen. Its inhibitors can inhibit tumor metastasis and slow cancer growth. However, inhibitors of urokinase usually contain a highly basic amidine or guanidine group ($pK_a > 9$), and this positively charged moiety is unfavorable for bioavailability. A previously discovered inhibitor (**81**) exhibits a K_i of 0.03 μM but with no oral bioavailability (Scheme 11.13). X-ray crystallography-based screening (CrystaLEAD) identified **82** with a K_i of 56 μM ($pK_a = 7.3$). An overlay of the crystal structures of **81** and **82** in complex with urokinase revealed that **82** bound to the same site as the naphthyl moiety of **81**. The merging of **82** with **81**

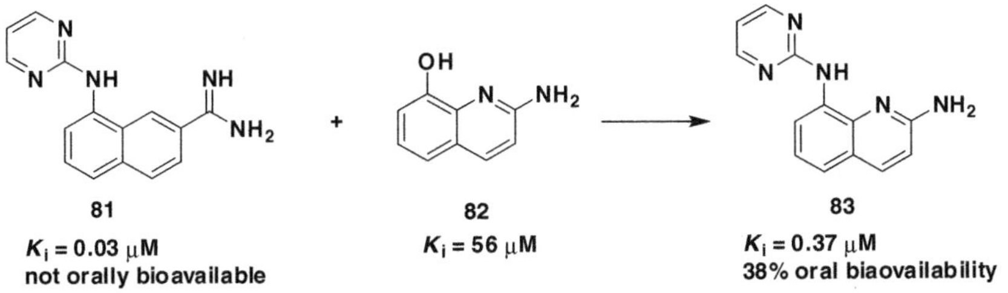

Scheme 11.13 X-ray crystallography-based screening (CrystaLEAD) for urokinase inhibitors.

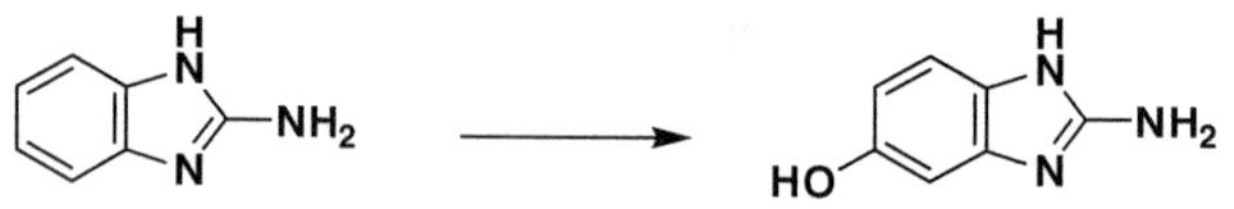

Scheme 11.14 NMR screen (SAR by NMR) for urokinase inhibitors.

generated **83**, which exhibited a dramatic improvement in oral bioavailability relative to **81** [61].

With the same target, an NMR screen (SAR by NMR) of more than 3000 compounds led to the identification of **84** as a weak ($IC_{50} = 200\,\mu M$) but competitive inhibitor that binds to the same site on urokinase as the traditional amidine or guanidine derivatives (Scheme 11.14). The compound is less ionized at physiological pH ($pK_a = 7.5$). A fragment evolution led to **85** with an IC_{50} of 10 μM and a pK_a of 7.4 [133].

11.3.9 Cathepsin S

Cathepsin S degrades the major histocompatibility complex class II-associated invariant chain that is required for productive loading of antigen onto this complex. Inhibition of cathepsin S can attenuate antigen presentation in autoimmune disease. Oral bioavailability of antiautoimmune agents is an important consideration in inhibitor design due to the long-term treatment. SAS was employed to identify nonpeptidic cathepsin S inhibitors (Scheme 11.15). The *N*-acyl aminocoumarin library was designed, and **86** was recognized by the enzyme as a substrate ($k_{cat}/K_m = 1$). The structural optimization of **86** led to **87** with a much better binding affinity ($k_{cat}/K_m = 8200$). The replacement of the aminocoumarin moiety by a hydrogen atom provided aldehyde **88** that exhibited a K_i of 9 nM [85a]. Replacement of the aldehyde with a nitrile moiety led to **89** with a K_i of 420 nM. The structural optimization of **87** led to a better substrate (**90**; $k_{cat}/K_m = 27{,}000$). The corresponding nitrile derivative (**91**) has a K_i of 15 nM [134].

SAS also identified **92** as a primary hit (Scheme 11.16). The optimization of **92** led to **93** and **95**. The conversion of the substrates into inhibitors by SAS generated **94** and **96**. Nonpeptidic **96** has a K_i of 9.6 nM [135].

11.3.10 Caspase-3

Caspases (cysteinyl aspartate-specific proteases) play key roles in both cytokine maturation and programmed cell death (apoptosis). Caspase-3 lies at a key junction in the apoptotic cascade. The inhibition of caspase-3 has been investigated as a valuable therapeutic approach for the treatment of diseases ranging from Alzheimer's and Parkinson's to myocardial infarction and sepsis. As do all members of the caspase family, caspase-3 has a linear peptide-binding site that nearly accommodates four

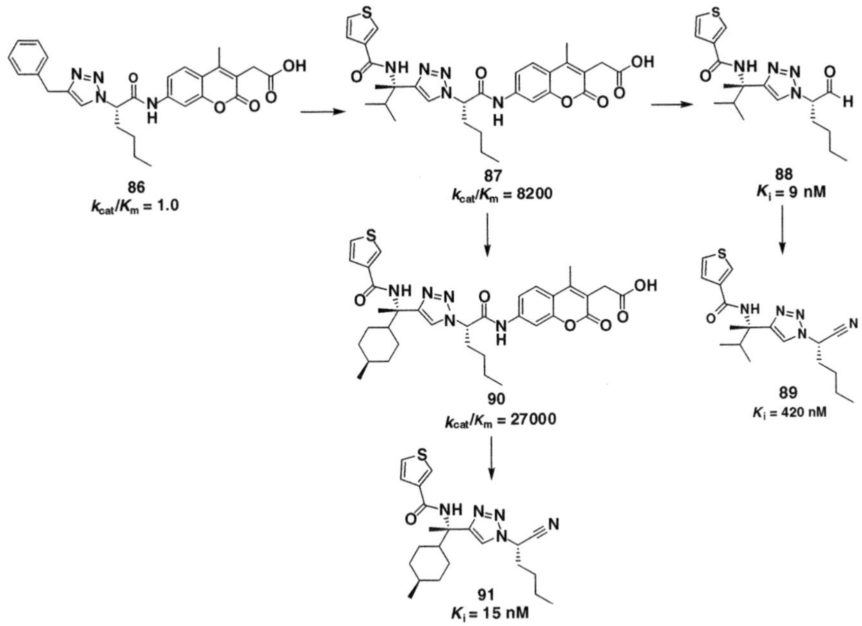

Scheme 11.15 Substrate activity screening (SAS) for cathepsin S inhibitors.

residues. Not surprisingly, most inhibitors of caspase-3 are linear peptides or peptidomimetics, which are not bioavailable. *In situ* fragment assembly using tethering with extender was conducted to identify reversible small-molecule inhibitors (Scheme 11.17) [105a]. An irreversible tetrapeptide inhibitor **97** was used as a starting point. A derivative of **97** (**98**) was treated with the enzyme to generate **99**. The deprotection of the thioester moiety generated extender **100**, which was used to

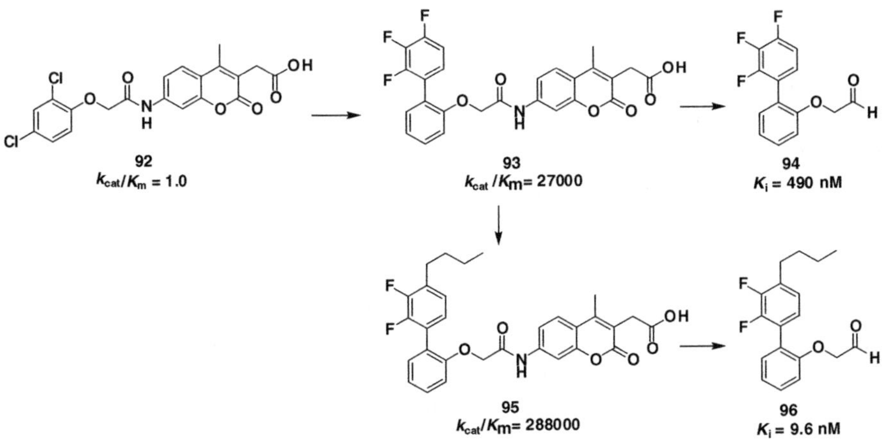

Scheme 11.16 Substrate activity screening (SAS) for cathepsin S inhibitors.

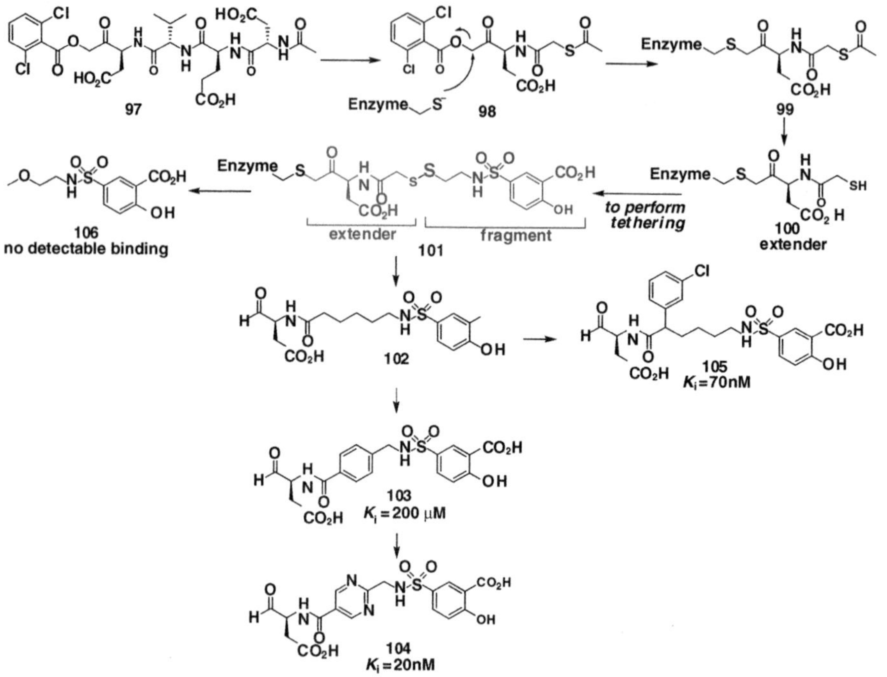

Scheme 11.17 *In situ* fragment assembly using tethering with extender for caspase-3 inhibitors.

interrogate fragment libraries (tethering). A salicylic acid was identified as important fragment hit **101**. The resulting molecule **102** exhibited a K_i of 2.8 μM. Simple conversion of the flexible linker in **102** to rigid aromatic linker **103** increased the potency by more than one order of magnitude. The functionalization of **103** afforded **104**, which added another order of magnitude in increased affinity [105b]. Compound **105** shows another way to increase the binding affinity ($K_i = 70$ nM) by addition of a phenyl group onto the linker [136]. Both **104** and **105** are small-molecule inhibitors that could be developed into drug candidates with better bioavailability compared with peptides or peptidomimetics. The simple salicyclic acid fragment **106** does not inhibit the enzyme demonstrating that this fragment would not be detected by other fragment-based technologies, supporting the advantages of tethering with extender.

11.3.11 HIV-1 Protease

HIV-1 protease has been recognized as an important target for anti-AIDS treatment. Although several inhibitors have been approved, the alarming rate at which strains of HIV-1 are resistant to the currently available drugs underscores the urgent need for new inhibitors that are effective against the new mutants as well as the wild-type virus. *In situ* click chemistry has been applied to discover new nonpeptidic compounds that inhibit HIV-1 protease (Scheme 11.18) [113]. Azide (**107**, $IC_{50} = 4.2$ μM) was

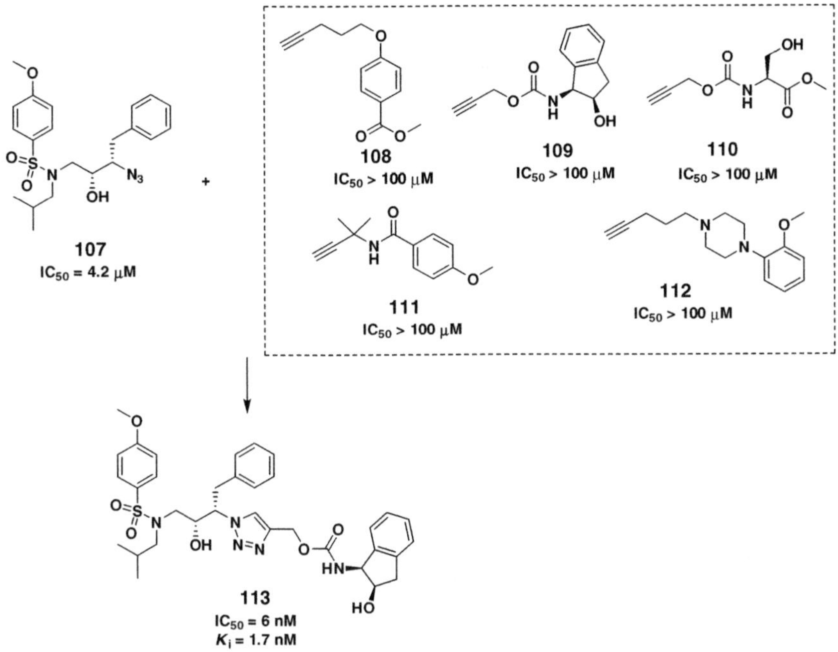

Scheme 11.18 *In situ* click chemistry for HIV-1 protease inhibitors.

incubated with alkynes (**108–112**, IC_{50} of all of these alkynes >100 μM) in the presence of HIV protease. Only **109** was selectively picked up by the enzyme to react with **107** to generate **113** ($IC_{50} = 6$ nM, $K_i = 1.7$ nM). This strategy provides the possibility to generate other bioavailable nonpeptidic inhibitors for HIV-1 protease.

11.4 *DE NOVO* DESIGN

In addition to experimental screening approaches, computational methods have also shown value in fragment-based drug discovery. *De novo* ligand design is a computation-based approach to design bioactive compounds that do not exist in known compound libraries. It, therefore, provides an opportunity to utilize other areas of chemical space. *De novo* design has been proposed since the 1980s. To date, 45 computation-based *de novo* design programs have been reported [137]. Primarily, *de novo* design can be divided into receptor- and ligand-based approaches. In the former case, the 3D structure of the receptor is known or can be modeled by homology modeling, and the *de novo* design is based on the structural information of the target. In the latter case, the structure of the target is unknown, and the pharmacophore information of ligands is used to guide the design of new structures.

Five different approaches have been developed for the receptor-based *de novo* design according to the method of structure sampling [137a]: (1) planar structure

TABLE 11.1. Receptor-Based *De Novo* Design Programs

Structure Sampling	*De Novo* Design Programs
Planar structure fitting	HSITE/2D [138]
Atom or fragment growing	3D Skeletons [139], LEGEND [140], LUDI [141], GenStar [142], GroupBuild [143], SPROUT [144], GrowMol [145], PRO_LIGAND [146], SMoG [147], RASSE [148], PRO_SELECT [149], LigBuilder [150], BREED [151], GROW [152], LeapFrog [153], Pellegrini & Field [154], and BOMB [155]
Fragment linking	LUDI, NEWLEAD [156], SPLICE [157], SPROUT, MCSS/HOOK [158], PRO_LIGAND, LigBuilder, BREED, CAVEAT [159], COREGEN [160], MCSS/SEED/CCLD [161], FlexNovo [162], Flux/CATS [163], and GRANDI [164]
Target protein lattice-based sampling	Diamond Lattice [165], BUILDER [166], MCDNLG [167], MCSS/DLD [168], SkelGen [169], ADAPT [170], CLIX [171], and Chemical Genesis [172]
Molecular dynamics simulation-based sampling	CONCEPTS [173], CONCERTS [174], DycoBlock [175], and F-DycoBlock [176]

fitting, (2) atom or fragment growing, (3) fragment linking, (4) target protein lattice-based sampling, and (5) molecular dynamics simulation-based sampling. The corresponding *de novo* design programs are shown in Table 11.1.

Two approaches are used in ligand-based *de novo* design according to the method of structure sampling: (1) topological molecular graphs-based sampling and (2) molecular physicochemical properties-based sampling. The corresponding *de novo* design programs are shown in Table 11.2.

In conventional computation-based *de novo* design strategies, the output structures obtained from computer programs can be problematic with regard to synthetic accessibility [183] and binding affinity predictions [184]. Analyses of conventional computation-based *de novo* design techniques indicate that it is rare to generate novel lead structures with nanomolar activity initially [137b]. Synthetic feasibility problems can be controlled during the buildup of ligands. This can be done by using commercially available or easy to synthesize building blocks or by connecting them via common reaction schemes. This feature has already been incorporated into more

TABLE 11.2. Ligand-Based *De Novo* Design Programs

Structure Sampling	*De Novo* Design Programs
Topological molecular graphs-based sampling	Chemical Genesis, SkelGen, Nachbar [177], Globus [178], TOPAS [179], CoG [180], and BREED
Molecular physicochemical properties-based sampling	LEA [181], Pellegrini & Field, SYNOPSIS [182], and PRO_LIGAND

recent *de novo* design programs such as CAESA for SPOUT [185], SEEDS for LEGEND [186], RECAP [187], SYNOPSIS [182], and Flux [163a, 163b].

The prediction of binding affinity is a real problem [188]. *De novo* design utilizes various scoring functions to evaluate each step of the design process. Unfortunately, available scoring functions are limited in their abilities to accurately predict experimental binding affinities. Rigorous approaches based on free energy perturbation and thermodynamic integration have been applied to predict binding energies [189]. However, the sampling and convergence problems prevent them from being used routinely in ligand screening. Moreover, it is very difficult to handle large structural diversity between ligands during screening, for example, in the case of completely different core structures. Currently, the best that can be done is to model the complexes in the presence of hundreds or thousands of explicit water molecules using Monte Carlo (MC) statistical mechanics or molecular dynamics [190]. Several semiempirical methods based on linear approximations to the free energy such as linear response theory [191] and molecular mechanics/Poisson–Boltzmann surface area [192] have been introduced and used with success.

In concomitance with the development of experimentally fragment-based screening, fragment-based *de novo* design has been an active field in *de novo* ligand design in recent years. Two computation-based strategies for lead identification have been extensively reported: one is *in silico* fragment screening and assembly, and the other one is scaffold hopping.

11.4.1 *In Silico* Fragment Screening

In silico fragment screening is conceptually related to the experimental fragment-based screening methodology. A typical protocol for *in silico* fragment screening consists of docking a fragment into the binding site, choosing a best orientation, and using it as the starting point for fragment evolution and fragment linking. The *in silico* fragment screening has obvious advantages over experimental methods because they are very fast, cost efficient, and much more applicable across a wide range of targets.

However, to reliably calculate the affinity of a fragment, its binding site and binding mode need to be predicted correctly. Furthermore, a reliable scoring function is required to score the protein–ligand complex. Both tasks are particularly challenging for fragments for two concerns (1) a weakly binding small fragment has more possibilities of multiple binding modes to the receptor than a tightly binding ligand that fits well in the binding pocket; (2) the existing scoring functions have been elaborately calibrated with data from tightly binding ligands; therefore, the range of prediction is outside the typical fragment-binding affinities, that is, in the range from $K_d = 100\ \mu M$ to $K_d = 100\ mM$ [193]. Shoichet and coworkers recently reported an *in silico* screen of 300,000 fragments using DOCK3.5.54 to test the concerns of this approach [164]. Among them, 69 top-ranking fragments were tested, and 10 inhibitors in the millimolar range were successfully identified [194a]. An X-ray crystallographic study showed that the docking poses matched very well with the experimentally determined structures, which highlights the liability of the DOCK program in *in silico* fragment screening.

An integrated approach of experimental fragment-based screening and *in silico* fragment-based screening offers huge advantages. An experimental investigation of the affinity and the binding mode of a fragment with biophysics- or bioassay-based methods can substantially increase the reliability of *in silico* design. These validated binders can be used as the starting points for *in silico de novo* design. *In silico* design can give quick feedback about the possible binding modes of fragments in the active site, which helps to evaluate the proposed ligands and guide the hit-to-lead process. Furthermore, the new design ligands can be verified experimentally.

Two different scenarios for the integrated *in silico* fragment design process and experimental fragment-based screening are briefly outlined. The design cycle could start either from an existing fragment library or from an *in silico* fragment screen, which needs to be synthesized initially. The latter approach has the advantage that novel starting points can be utilized, whereas the first approach relies on existing molecules. The first approach is beneficial since experimental data (affinity and structure) can be incorporated from the beginning, therefore increasing the reliability of the method. In both cases, the crucial step is the biological screening of fragments, which will give direct input to the design cycle. These data not only allow one to focus on the most promising fragments on which to follow up but also aid in the calibration of the scoring functions. Alternatively, constraints derived from the experimental data reduce the number of (possibly false) solutions generated by the algorithm.

11.4.2 Scaffold Hopping

In drug design programs, biological active molecules often show severe limitations, and this prevents these compounds from moving toward clinical development. Such limitations can include an inherently low solubility, metabolic instability, or the absence of binding selectivity. On the basis of the concept that biologically active compounds for a specific target are discontinuous points in the vast chemical space, scaffold hopping (also termed lead hopping, leapfrogging, scaffold searching, and chemotype switching) has been proposed to identify those compounds that have similar biological activities, but totally different scaffolds [195].

The starting point of scaffold hopping is the selection of a template structure followed by hopping isofunctional, but structurally dissimilar, substructures (scaffolds) into different parts of the template structure. In contrast to *de novo* design, which aims to generate entire ligands, scaffold hopping is an attempt to replace only the core motif of a known ligand, while conserving key substituents. Scaffold hopping can be viewed as a special case of *de novo* design.

Three different approaches for scaffold hopping have been proposed (1) pharmacophore-driven approach [196], (2) the use of reduced graphs for the identification of scaffold [197], and (3) shape-based similarity searching [198]. The programs for different categories of scaffold hopping are shown in Table 11.3.

In pharmacophore-driven scaffold hopping, various pharmacophore descriptors have been proposed to determine the correlation between the newly generated scaffold and the original scaffold. Beside the common 2D and 3D pharmacophoric

TABLE 11.3 Scaffold Hopping Programs

	Scaffold Hopping Programs
Pharmacophore-driven approaches	CATS descriptors (CATS, CATS3D, and SURFCATS) [199], Charge3D and TripleCharge3D [200], FEPOPS [201], the Similog pharmacophoric keys [202], SQUID [199c, 203], and LIQUID [204]
Reduced graph-based approaches	Clique detection [205], ErG [206], centroid connecting path [207], structural unit analysis [208], Recore [209]
Shape-based approaches	GRID molecular interaction field-based approaches [210] (such as MOLPRINT3D [211], FLAP [212], and SHOP [213]), ROCS [214], FieldScreen [215], extended electric distribution [216], field-based similarity search [217], Surflex-Sim [218], Topomer [219], KIN [220], and ParaFrag [221]

fingerprints [222], specific pharmacophore descriptors for scaffold hopping have been designed, as shown in Table 11.3.

Reduced graph representation has been employed to identify related structural classes, rather than related compounds. In this method, entire substructures of a molecule, according to the defined scheme, are collapsed into single nodes resulting in a reduced graph that is smaller and less complex, and only the important features of a molecule are retained. This allows the identification of a diverse set of structures starting from a single reference structure. There have been several programs proposed to implement this general concept (Table 11.3). Among them, Recore is a reduced graph-based method for identifying suitable scaffold based on the X-ray crystal structure conformations that emphasize ligand similarity in the 3D space. Some approaches that are at the interface of reduced graph and pharmacophore-driven methods have also been proposed, including feature tree algorithm [223] and MED-SuMoLig [224].

Shape-based scaffold hopping has been intensively addressed recently. It has been demonstrated that the use of shape and electrostatics for similarity searching is superior to the traditional 2D fingerprints [225]. The important programs in this field are summarized in Table 11.3. The important approaches in this field including SQUIRREL take into account both molecular shape and potential pharmacophore points [226].

These methods can decrease the risks of molecular construction or synthetic accessibility, increase the hit rates for lead generation, and offer certain structural diversity. However, the skeleton of the newly designed molecules is confined to the basic architecture of the template structure, which usually comes from a known drug or drug candidate. Moreover, mimicking the different parts of the template structure with scaffolds often does not optimize the interaction between ligand and receptor to the maximal extent, because the scaffold is quite large and rigidity of the template structure sometimes does not allow an optimal match between ligand and receptor.

11.5 CASE STUDIES OF *DE NOVO* DESIGN FOR BETTER BIOAVAILABILITY

11.5.1 DNA Gyrase

DNA gyrase is a prokaryotic type-II DNA topoisomerase that is involved in the vital processes of DNA replication, transcription, and recombination. Because there is no direct mammalian counterpart, DNA gyrase is an attractive and well-established antibacterial target. The enzyme consists of two subunits, A and B; subunit B catalyzes the hydrolysis of ATP. The known classes of DNA inhibitors for the ATP recognition site include coumarins and cyclothialidines. However, the coumarins suffer from low membrane permeability, high toxicity, and a rapidly developing resistance. The limitation on cyclothialidines is their rapid and extensive glucuronidation of the essential phenol moiety. *In silico* fragment screening of an initial pool of 350,000 fragments revealed 600 compounds as potential hits. High concentration assays of these fragments were carried out, and analytical ultracentrifuge, surface plasmon resonance, NMR, and X-ray crystallography were used to discard nonspecific inhibitors and further characterize useful fragments. Compounds **114** and **115** were identified as the primary fragment hits (Scheme 11.19). The maximal noneffective concentration (MNEC) of **115** is 41 μM. Structural optimization, guided by X-ray crystallography, led to the discovery of **117** with an MNEC of 62 nM [81b]. This study is one of the earliest examples using *in silico* fragment screening prior to an enzyme assay. This strategy allows an early focus on the most promising candidates in a compound library, increases the hit rate, and is highly time- and cost-efficient. It has also been noted that fragment-based drug discovery provides chemical starting points that do not have unnecessary structural elements, and therefore reduces the risk of toxicity or metabolic instability.

11.5.2 Factor Xa

Factor Xa lies at the junction of the intrinsic and extrinsic pathways of the coagulation cascade. It converts prothrombin into thrombin. The inhibition of factor Xa can offer antithrombotic treatment. It has been claimed that factor Xa is a better antithrombotic target than thrombin because there is evidence that factor Xa inhibitors may have less propensity to cause bleeding side effects. Fragment-based *de novo* design by

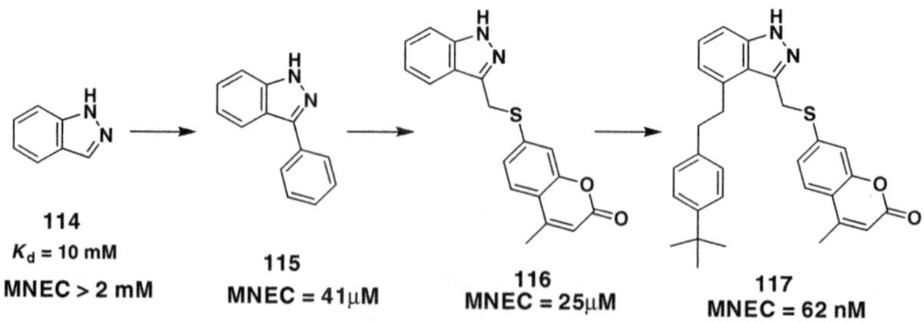

Scheme 11.19 *In silico* fragment screening for DNA gyrase inhibitors.

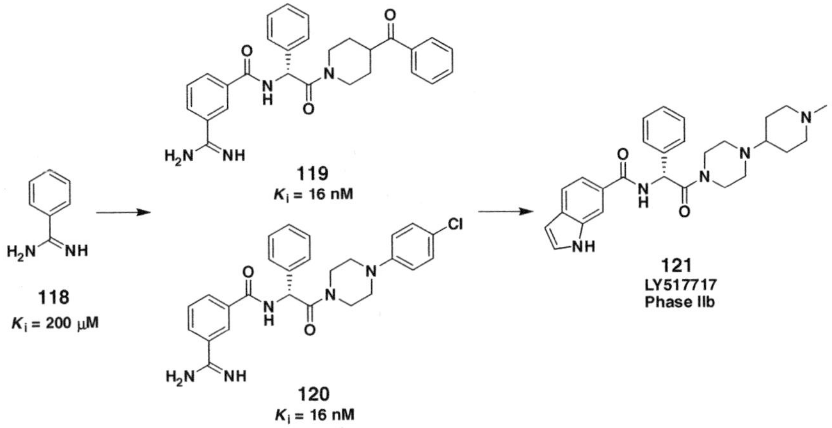

Scheme 11.20 Fragment-based *de novo* design of factor Xa inhibitors.

PRO_SELECT identified **118** as the primary hit, which binds to the S1 pocket of factor Xa ($K_i = 200\,\mu M$, Scheme 11.20). *In silico* screening of combinatorial fragment libraries led to the discovery of **119** and **120**. Both of these compounds have a K_i of 16 nM, which is 10,000 times more potent than the initial fragment [149d]. A combination of medicinal chemistry and structure-based drug design led to the replacement of the benzamidine, a moiety that is associated with poor oral bioavailability, and provided LY517717 (in Phase 2 clinical trials). This is a remarkable example demonstrating that fragment-based *de novo* design and *in silico* fragment screening can lead to the discovery of a drug candidate.

11.5.3 X-Linked Inhibitor of Apoptosis Protein

The baculovirus IAP repeat 3 domain of the X-linked inhibitors of apoptosis protein binds directly to the *N*-terminus of caspase-9, thus inhibiting programmed cell death. The blockage of this interaction has an implication in anticancer therapy. It has been found that in the cell this interaction can be displaced by the protein second mitochondrial activator of caspases (SMAC) and that *N*-terminal tetrapeptides (AVPI) of SMAC are responsible for this binding. The synthetic SMAC-derived peptides or peptidomimetics as therapeutic compounds suffer from problems of cell permeability, proteolytic instability, and poor pharmacokinetics. *In silico* screening of fragment libraries of alanine derivatives identified **122** as a weak binder ($K_d = 200\,\mu M$, Scheme 11.21). Further structural optimization led to **123** with a K_d of 1.2 μM. This compound exhibits cellular activity and has better human plasma stability and metabolic stability compared to AVPI [227].

11.5.4 Activator Protein-1 [196b]

Activator protein-1 (AP-1) is a transcription factor that is responsible for the induction of a number of genes involved in cell proliferation, differentiation, and immune and

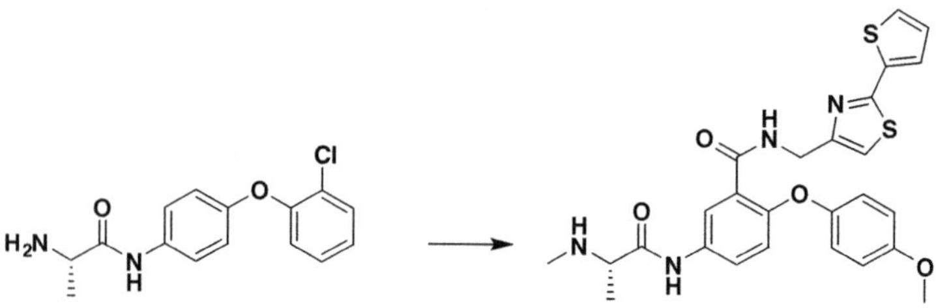

122
K_d = 200 μM

123
K_d = 1.2 μM
cell-based assay IC_{50} = 16.4 μM
human plasma stability > 120 min
$t_{1/2}$ = 14.5 min

Scheme 11.21 *In silico* screening fragment libraries for X-linked inhibitors of apoptosis protein inhibitors.

inflammatory responses. Inhibitors of AP-1 have been implicated in the treatment of rheumatoid arthritis. On the basis of the pharmacophore of cyclic disulfide decapeptide inhibitor **124** (IC_{50} = 64 μM), scaffold hopping was used to discover two nonpeptidic inhibitors **125** and **126** with IC_{50} values of 610 and 420 μM, respectively (Scheme 11.22).

11.6 MINIMAL PHARMACOPHORIC ELEMENTS AND FRAGMENT HOPPING

11.6.1 Minimal Pharmacophoric Elements

Current fragment-based screening has several internal problems and challenges. First, a fragment-based strategy can provide a combinatorial advantage relative to preassembled large chemical libraries. A collection of 10^3 fragments can typically probe the chemical diversity space of 10^9 molecules, a tremendous increase relative to HTS; however, this is still a small fraction of the total diversity space [228]. Second, most fragments have low binding affinities as a result of limited interactions with the target. Although many affinity-based assay techniques have been developed, the identification of relevant fragments and determination of how to link them productively in 3D

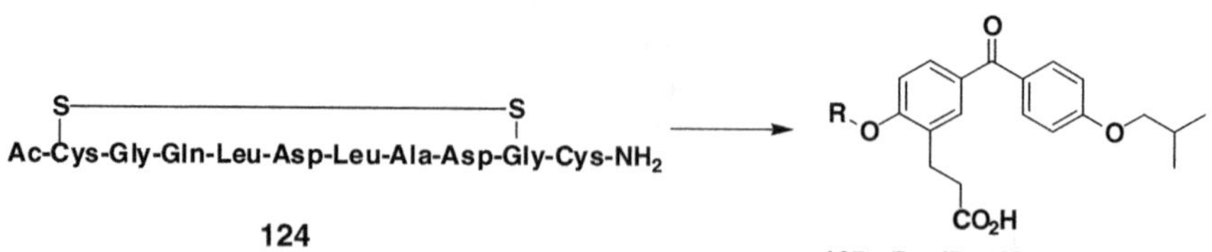

124
IC_{50} = 64 μM

125 : R = iBu, IC_{50} = 610 μM
126 : R = Bn, IC_{50} = 420 μM

Scheme 11.22 Scaffold hopping for activator protein-1 (AP-1) inhibitors.

space are still quite intractable problems, Third, ligand specificity for its targets is a particularly important goal of drug discovery in the postgenomic era because a myriad of functional proteins has been characterized. The enzymatic pockets within a target family/or superfamily, which execute the same or similar metabolic reactions and functions, are often quite similar. An important challenge in modern medicine is how to design compounds that can modulate a specific enzyme while leaving related isozymes unaffected. Known fragment-based approaches, however, are only able to identify and characterize fragment-binding sites of the target protein (often called "hot spots," that is, the regions of a protein surface that are major contributors to the ligand-binding free energy [63, 229]). In fact, many binding sites in the active site that are responsible for target selectivity are not included in these "hot spots."

In *de novo* ligand design, the accurate prediction of binding free energy is a major problem. In *in silico* fragment screening how to effectively identify fragment hits is still a concern. In scaffold hopping, the skeleton of the newly designed molecules is confined to the basic architecture of the template structure. Scaffold rigidities sometimes prevent an optimal binding event.

The concept of minimal pharmacophoric elements has recently been proposed [230]. The minimal pharmacophoric element is smaller than a fragment. It can be an atom, a cluster of atoms, a virtual graph or vector(s). The focused (or targeted) fragment libraries that match the requirement of minimal pharmacophoric elements are generated on the basis of various fragment libraries. Various fragments with different chemotypes, but containing the same minimal pharmacophoric elements, can be derived and a wider chemical space can be explored. Conversely, in many cases, the region in the active site responsible for ligand selectivity is rather delicate. Although conventional fragment-based approaches are able to identify and characterize those fragments located in the "hot spot" of the active site [231], the fragments that are responsible for isozyme selectivity are generally not located in these "hot spots." The mapping of minimal pharmacophoric elements can preferentially consider the regions in the active site responsible for isozyme selectivity; thus, better isozyme selectivity can be incorporated in the inhibitor design.

11.6.2 Fragment Hopping

Fragment hopping, a pharmacophore-driven strategy for fragment-based inhibitor design, is represented in Figure 11.6. The first step of the strategy is to determine the pharmacophoric sites of a specific drug target. If the target structure can be determined by X-ray crystallography or NMR spectroscopy, various experimental approaches can be used to determine the potential pharmacophoric sites. The multiple solvent crystal structures method [57a, 232] and various affinity-based biophysical techniques mentioned above are efficacious tools for understanding how small molecules bind to the active site of the enzymes. The energetic hot spots of enzymes for ligand binding can be elucidated in combination with alanine scanning [233]. The computational methods for active site analysis are useful when the receptor structure is known or, if unknown, the structure can be constructed by homology modeling [234]. Two of the most popular and venerable algorithms are GRID [235], and multiple copy

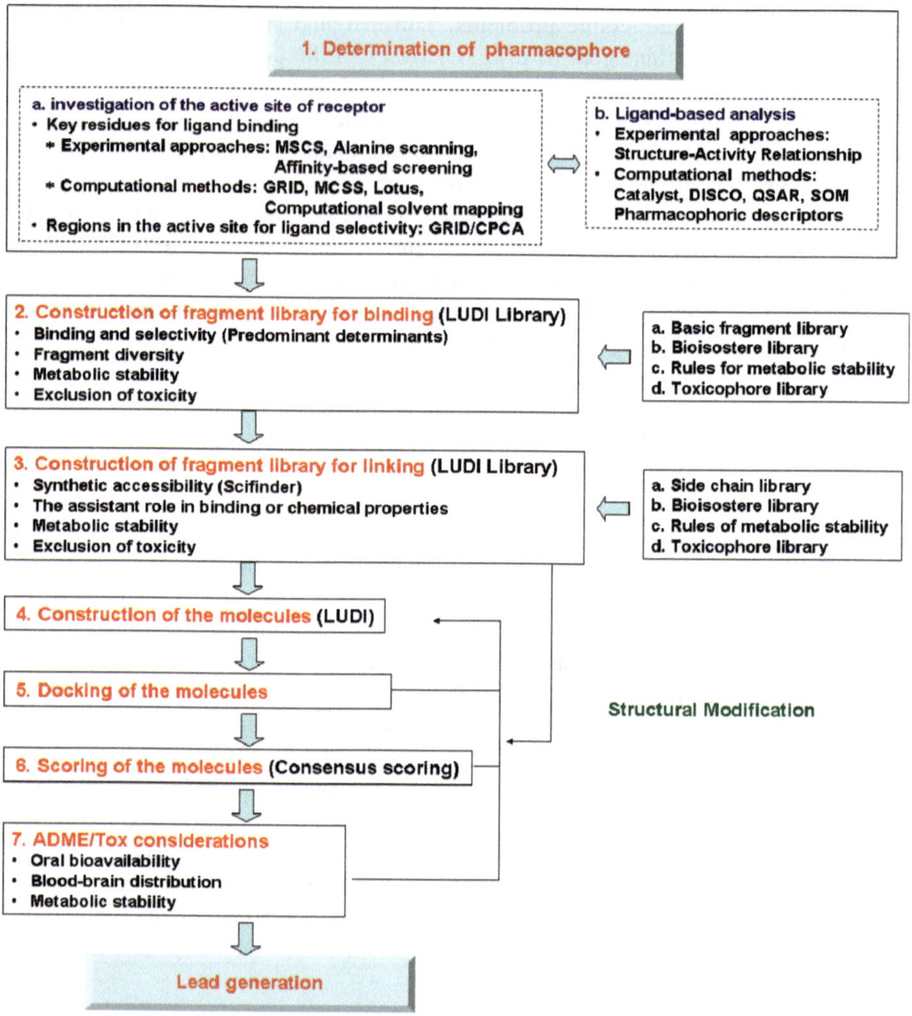

Figure 11.6 Schematic flow diagram for fragment hopping, the pharmacophore-driven strategy for fragment-based *de novo* design.

simultaneous search [236] (MCSS). GRID calculates 3D energy maps around protein-binding sites, thus highlighting favorable sites for small functional groups. MCSS randomly places thousands of copies of small functional groups into the binding site and subjects them to energy minimization. The copies with the lowest energies highlight hot spots of ligand binding. Many other computational methods such as the knowledge-based equivalents of GRID (X-SITE [237] and SuperStar [238]) and energy-based approaches (PocketFinder [239], Q-SiteFinder [240]) also can be used to explore sensitive and specific hot spots in the active site. Computational solvent mapping [241] and binding site determination technology (Lotus™) [190b, 229a, 242], can be regarded as an important new breakthrough in this field.

GRID/CPCA is an excellent tool for understanding the selectivity of inhibitors for a specific target over the other structure-related enzymes [243]. If the structure of the receptor is unknown, the pharmacophoric sites can be identified by structure–activity analysis of ligands, various pharmacophoric, molecular shape, or field descriptors, or by various computational methods, such as Catalyst, DISCO, and GASP [244]. Self-organizing maps can be used as a ligand-based approach to predict compound selectivity [245].

Three- or four-point pharmacophore models can be generated from the above analyses [246]. However, the key essential for the above pharmacophore investigation is to derive the minimal pharmacophoric elements for each pharmacophore, which requires a combinatorial application of different pharmacophore identification methods to provide as much information as possible. On the basis of the derived minimal pharmacophoric elements, the second step of this approach is to query two main general-purpose libraries: (1) a basic fragment library, constructed from fragments extracted directly from known drugs and/or drug candidates. The fragments are either from well-known libraries, such as the MDL CMC database, the WDI, the MDDR, or from the literature [65, 81b, 247]; (2) a bioisostere library, constructed from known bioisosteric principles reported in the literature [248]. The basic fragment library is initially searched to find all of the possible fragments that are able to match the requirements of the minimal pharmacophoric elements for each pharmacophore. The bioisostere library is then utilized to generate a focused fragment library with diverse structures.

The generated focused fragment library is then interrogated with the rules for metabolic stability (Figure 11.7) [79a, 249] and a toxicophore library (Figure 11.8) [250] to provide a focused library for a specific pharmacophore. The focused library is then converted into a LUDI fragment library, and the LUDI program is used to search the optimal binding position for each fragment of each pharmacophore [141a, 251].

The third step of this approach is to link these fragments. A constructed side-chain library is used for this purpose, in which the synthetic accessibility is considered [187, 252]. SciFinder Scholar [253], in conjunction with the bioisostere library, also plays a key role in securing the synthetic accessibility of the formed chemical bond. The bioisostere library plays an assistant role in enhancing the binding capabilities and optimizing the chemical properties of the generated ligands. The generated ligands are interrogated again with the rules for metabolism stability and the toxicophore library.

The ligands generated by this iterative process are then docked into the active site (using AutoDock3.0 [254]), scored with consensus scoring functions [255], and filtered with absorption, distribution, metabolism, excretion, and toxicity (ADME/Tox) considerations [256]. If the ligands generated are not satisfactory, the molecule is reconstructed using the generated focused fragment libraries, the side chain library, and the bioisostere library (Figure 11.6).

Fragment hopping determines the minimal pharmacophoric elements for each pharmacophore that is important for ligand selectivity. Fragments are generated to match the requirement of minimal pharmacophoric elements based on the basic

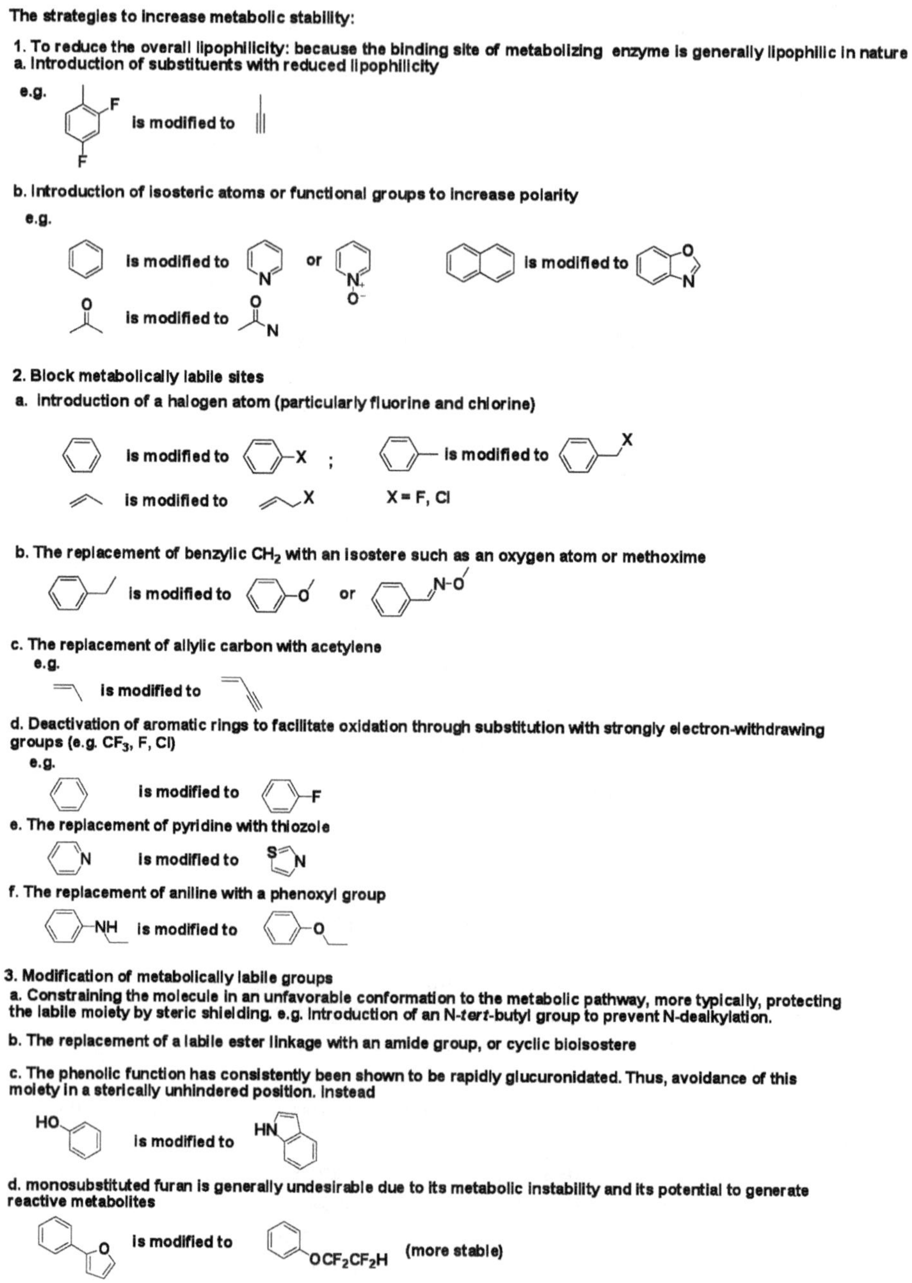

Figure 11.7 An example of the rules for metabolic stability.

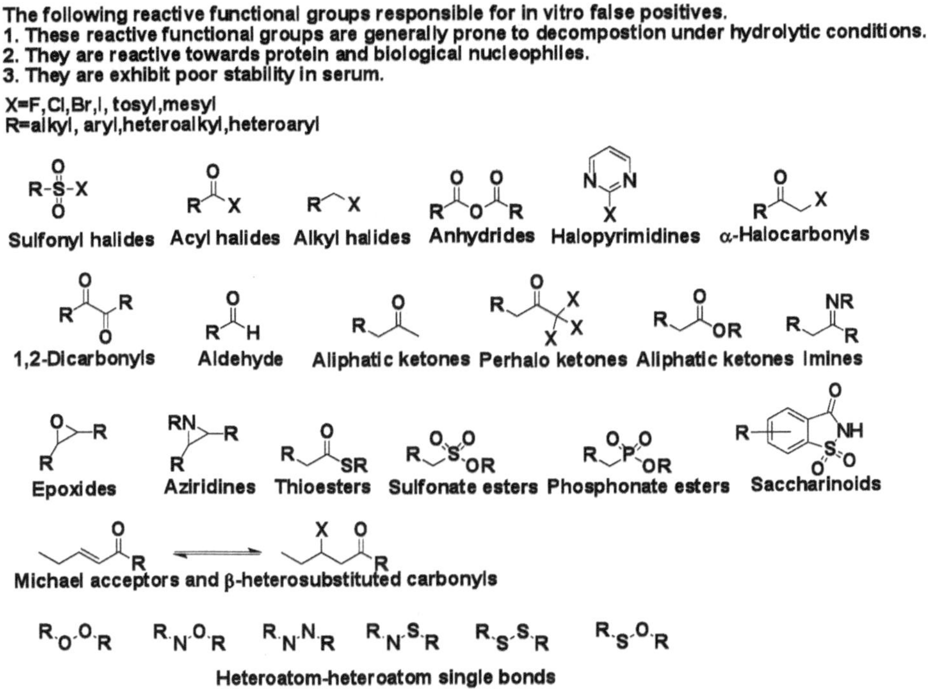

Figure 11.7 (Continued)

fragment and bioisostere libraries. After the focused fragment library is generated for each pharmacophore, other fragment-based approaches, such as NMR-based and/or X-ray crystallography-based fragment screening techniques, click chemistry, and dynamic combinatorial chemistry, can be utilized to investigate the binding mode of the above-generated fragments within the active site of the enzyme. The interaction of the generated fragments with the selective regions of the active site can be analyzed further by tethering or tethering with an extender. Therefore, fragment hopping as a pharmacophore-driven strategy is an open system that can incorporate other techniques and provide a more efficient pathway to generate more potent and more selective inhibitors.

11.6.3 Case Study: Nitric Oxide Synthase

Nitric oxide synthase (NOS) catalyzes the five-electron, two-step oxidation of L-arginine to produce L-citrulline and NO. NOS consists of three isozymes: neuronal NOS (nNOS), endothelial NOS (eNOS), and inducible NOS (iNOS). Overproduction of NO from nNOS has been associated with harmful effects in the central nervous system, including stroke, various neurodegenerative diseases, and cerebral palsy. The minimal pharmacophoric elements were extracted according to the binding mode of peptidic inhibitor **127** ($K_i = 130$ nM) with nNOS (Scheme 11.23). Fragment hopping led to the generation of **128** with a K_i of 388 nM [230]. The structural optimization of

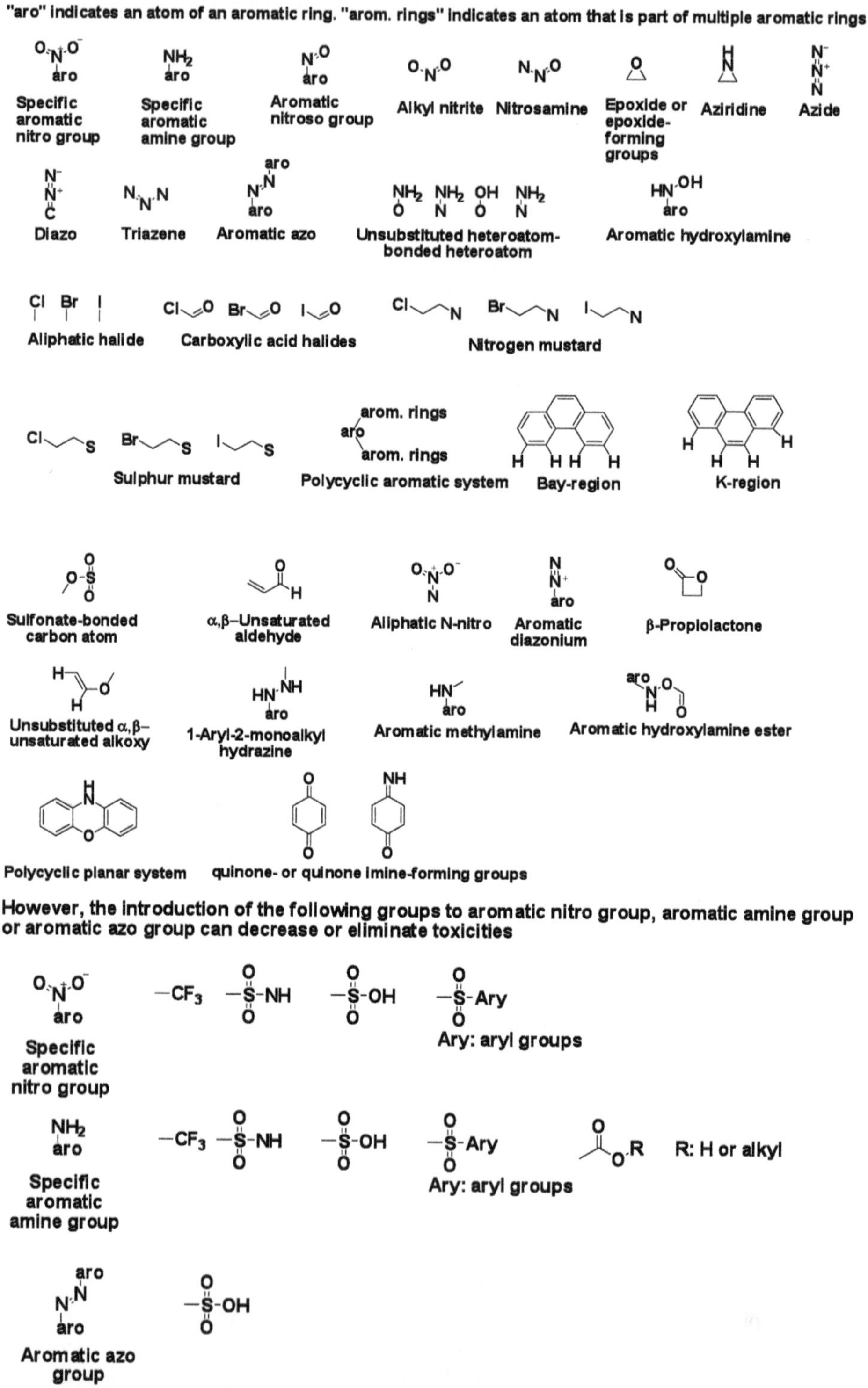

Figure 11.8 An example of toxicophores.

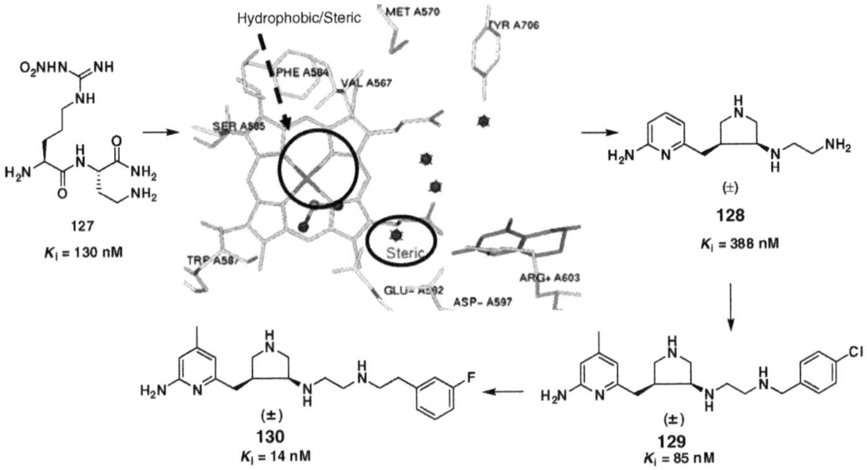

Scheme 11.23 Fragment hopping for nitric oxide synthase (NOS) inhibitors.

128 using fragment hopping led to **129** and **130** with K_i values of 85 and 14 nM, respectively [257]. These compounds were then tested in a rabbit model for cerebral palsy and were found to prevent hypoxiaischemia-induced deaths of the fetuses and to reduce the number of newborn kits exhibiting symptoms of cerebral palsy. Following maternal administration of **129** and **130** in a rabbit model, the compounds were found to distribute to fetal brain, to be nontoxic, without cardiovascular effects, and inhibit fetal brain NOS activity *in vivo* [258].

11.7 CONCLUSIONS AND FUTURE PERSPECTIVES

The techniques of fragment-based drug discovery are orthogonal to those of HTS on the basis of screening techniques, binding affinities, compound size and weight, size of compound libraries, and the strategies for hit-to-lead optimization. It has been widely accepted in large pharmaceutical companies that fragment-based drug design is an effective complement to HTS. In academic and biotechnological laboratories, these methods have emerged as the major approaches to obtain new chemical structures. Fragment-based drug discovery has successfully identified new hits when an HTS campaign has failed to yield useful results with difficult targets.

Compared with HTS, fragment-based drug discovery can generate new leads with better physicochemical properties that are more amenable to structural optimization for the generation of compounds with better drug-like properties. Fragment-based methods also provide chemical starting points that have no or fewer unnecessary structural elements, and therefore leave more chemical space to reduce the risk of toxicity or metabolic instability. In most current cases, the integration of early ADME considerations in fragment-based design is dependent on random ideas with a lack of systematic approaches. Fragment hopping utilizes the concept of minimal pharmacophoric elements to provide an open system that can efficiently incorporate early

"ADME/Tox" considerations. However, to draw a complete picture for incorporation of early ADME considerations into fragment-based drug discovery, a comprehensive survey and analysis of metabolic stability and the bioactivation and biotransformation of fragments *in vivo* are urgently needed.

Similar to structure-based drug design, computational chemistry and computer modeling, and combinatorial chemistry and HTS, fragment-based drug design is and will not be a panacea. It is only one of many key weapons in the drug design arsenal that can be used to discover new ligands for a particular target. However, it is also noteworthy that with continuing breakthroughs in structural biology, particularly a better understanding of the active site of receptors, further developments in molecular modeling and computational chemistry might be able to place fragment-based drug discovery into a priority position for the practice of standard medicinal chemistry.

ACKNOWLEDGMENTS

The author would like to thank Professor Richard B. Silverman of the Department of Chemistry, Northwestern University for support and encouragement in this work, and also for his critical reading of the manuscript and thoughtful discussions.

REFERENCES

1. (a) Abou-Gharbia, M. Discovery of innovative small molecule therapeutics. *J. Med. Chem.* 2009, *52(1)*, 2–9; (b) Davis, A. M., Keeling, D. J., Steele, J., Tomkinson, N. P., and Tinker, A. C. Components of successful lead generation. *Curr. Top. Med. Chem.* 2005, *5(4)*, 421–439; (c) Lombardino, J. G. and Lowe, J. A. III., The role of the medicinal chemist in drug discovery—then and now. *Nat. Rev. Drug Discov.* 2004, *3 (10)*, 853–862.
2. (a) Snowden, M. and Green, D. V. The impact of diversity-based, high-throughput screening on drug discovery: "chance favours the prepared mind". *Curr. Opin. Drug Discov. Devel.* 2008, *11(4)*, 553–558; (b) Golebiowski, A., Klopfenstein, S. R., and Portlock, D. E. Lead compounds discovered from libraries. *Curr. Opin. Chem. Biol.* 2001, *5*, 273–284; (c) Golebiowski, A., Klopfenstein, S. R., and Portlock, D. E. Lead compounds discovered from libraries: Part 2. *Curr. Opin. Chem. Biol.* 2003, *7*, 308–325; (d) Fox, S., Farr-Jones, S., Sopchak, L., Boggs, A., Nicely, H. W., Khoury, R., and Biros, M. High-throughput screening: update on practices and success. *J. Biomol. Screen.* 2006, *11(7)*, 864–869; (e) Posner, B. A. High-throughput screening-driven lead discovery: meeting the challenges of finding new therapeutics. *Curr. Opin. Drug Discov. Devel.* 2005, *8(4)*, 487–494.
3. (a) Bender, A., Bojanic, D., Davies, J. W., Crisman, T. J., Mikhailov, D., Scheiber, J., Jenkins, J. L., Deng, Z., Hill, W. A., Popov, M., Jacoby, E., and Glick, M. Which aspects of HTS are empirically correlated with downstream success? *Curr. Opin. Drug Discov. Devel.* 2008, *11(3)*, 327–337; (b) Review Lahana, R. How many leads from HTS? *Drug Discov. Today* 1999, *4(10)*, 447–448; (c) Shelat, A. A. and Guy, R. K. The interdependence between screening methods and screening libraries. *Curr. Opin. Chem. Biol.* 2007,

11(3), 244–251; (d) Bender, A., Bojanic, D., Davies, J. W., Crisman, T. J., Mikhailov, D., Scheiber, J., Jenkins, J. L., Deng, Z., Hill, W. A., Popov, M., Jacoby, E., and Glick, M. Which aspects of HTS are empirically correlated with downstream success? *Curr. Opin. Drug Discov. Devel.* 2008, *11(3)*, 327–337.

4. Bohacek, R. S., McMartin, C., and Guida, W. C. The art and practice of structure-based drug design: a molecular modeling perspective. *Med. Res. Rev.* 1996, *16(1)*, 3–50.
5. Teague, S. J., Davis, A. M., Leeson, P. D., and Oprea, T. The design of leadlike combinatorial libraries. *Angew. Chem. Int. Ed. Engl.* 1999, *38(24)*, 3743–3748.
6. (a) Hann, M. M. and Oprea, T. I. Pursuing the leadlikeness concept in pharmaceutical research. *Curr. Opin. Chem. Biol.* 2004, *8(3)*, 255–263; (b) Rishton, G. M. Molecular diversity in the context of leadlikeness: compound properties that enable effective biochemical screening. *Curr. Opin. Chem. Biol.* 2008, *12(3)*, 340–351.
7. (a) Wenlock, M. C., Austin, R. P., Barton, P., Davis, A. M., and Leeson, P. D. A comparison of physiochemical property profiles of development and marketed oral drugs. *J. Med. Chem.* 2003, *46(7)*, 1250–1256; (b) Vieth, M. and Sutherland, J. J. Dependence of molecular properties on proteomic family for marketed oral drugs. *J. Med. Chem.* 2006, *49(12)*, 3451–3453.
8. Leeson, P. D. and Springthorpe, B. The influence of drug-like concepts on decision-making in medicinal chemistry. *Nat. Rev. Drug Discov.* 2007, *6(11)*, 881–890.
9. Hann, M. M., Leach, A. R., and Harper, G. Molecular complexity and its impact on the probability of finding leads for drug discovery. *J. Chem. Inf. Comp. Sci.* 2001, *41(3)*, 856–864.
10. Hopkins, A. L., Groom, C. R., and Alex, A. Ligand efficiency: a useful metric for lead selection. *Drug Discov. Today* 2004, *9(10)*, 430–431.
11. Lipinski, C. A., Lombardo, F., Dominy, B. W., and Feeney, P. J. Experimental and computational approaches to estimate solubility and permeability in drug discovery and development settings. *Adv. Drug Deliv. Rev.* 1997, *23(1–3)*, 3–25.
12. (a) Erlanson, D. A., McDowell, R. S., and O'Brien T. *Fragment-based drug discovery. J. Med. Chem.* 2004, *47(14)*, 3463–3482; (b) Rees, D. C., Congreve, M., Murray, C. W., and Carr, R. Fragment-based lead discovery. *Nat. Rev. Drug Discov.* 2004, *3(8)*, 660–672; (c) Erlanson, D. A. Fragment-based lead discovery: a chemical update. *Curr. Opin. Biotechnol.* 2006, *17(6)*, 643–652; (d) Hajduk, P. J. and Greer, J. A decade of fragment-based drug design: strategic advances and lessons learned. *Nat. Rev. Drug Discov.* 2007, *6 (3)*, 211–219; (e) Congreve, M., Chessari, G., Tisi, D., and Woodhead, A. J. Recent developments in fragment-based drug discovery. *J. Med. Chem.* 2008, *51(13)*, 3661–3680.
13. Shuker, S. B., Hajduk, P. J., Meadows, R. P., and Fesik, S. W. Discovering high-affinity ligands for proteins: SAR by NMR. *Science* 1996, *274(5292)*, 1531–1534.
14. Keserü, G. M. and Makara, G. M. Hit discovery and hit-to-lead approaches. *Drug Discov. Today* 2006, *11(15–16)*, 741–748.
15. (a) Pellecchia, M., Bertini, I., Cowburn, D., Dalvit, C., Giralt, E., Jahnke, W., James, T. L., Homans, S. W., Kessler, H., Luchinat, C., Meyer, B., Oschkinat, H., Peng, J., Schwalbe, H., and Siegal, G. Perspectives on NMR in drug discovery: a technique comes of age. *Nat. Rev. Drug Discov.* 2008, *7(9)*, 738–745; (b) Lepre, C. A., Moore, J. M. and Peng, J. W. Theory and application of NMR-based screening in pharmaceutical research. *Chem. Rev.* 2004, *104(8)*, 3641–3675; (c) Meyer, B. and Peters, T. NMR spectroscopy techniques for

screening and identifying ligand binding to protein receptors. *Angew. Chem. Int. Ed. Engl.* 2003, *42(8)*, 864–890; (d) Pellecchia, M., Sem, D. S., and Wüthrich, K. NMR in drug discovery. *Nat. Rev. Drug Discov.* 2002, *1(3)*, 211–219.

16. (a) Jhoti, H., Cleasby, A., Verdonk, M., and Williams, G. Fragment-based screening using X-ray crystallography and NMR spectroscopy. *Curr. Opin. Chem. Biol.* 2007, *11(5)*, 485–493; (b) Blundell, T. L. and Patel, S. High-throughput X-ray crystallography for drug discovery. *Curr. Opin. Pharmacol.* 2004, *4(5)*, 490–496; (c) Blundell, T. L., Jhoti, H., and Abell, C. High-throughput crystallography for lead discovery in drug design. *Nat. Rev. Drug Discov.* 2002, *1(1)*, 45–54; (d) Kuhn, P., Wilson, K., Patch, M. G., and Stevens, R. C. The genesis of high-throughput structure-based drug discovery using protein crystallography. *Curr. Opin. Chem. Biol.* 2002, *6(5)*, 704–710.
17. (a) Erlanson, D. A. and Hansen, S. K. Making drugs on proteins: site-directed ligand discovery for fragment-based lead assembly. *Curr. Opin. Chem. Biol.* 2004, *8(4)*, 399–406; (b) Hofstadler, S. A. and Sannes-Lowery, K. A. Applications of ESI-MS in drug discovery: interrogation of noncovalent complexes. *Nat. Rev. Drug Discov.* 2006, *5 (7)*, 585–595.
18. Neumann, T., Junker, H.-D., Schmidt, K., and Sekul, R. SPR-based fragment screening: advantages and applications. *Curr. Top. Med. Chem.* 2007, *7(16)*, 1630–1642.
19. Ciulli, A. and Abell, C. Fragment-based approaches to enzyme inhibition. *Curr. Opin. Biotechnol.* 2007, *18(6)*, 489–496.
20. Hesterkamp, T. and Whittaker, M. Fragment-based activity space: smaller is better. *Curr. Opin. Chem. Biol.* 2008, *12(3)*, 260–268.
21. (a) Jacoby, E., Davies, J., and Blommers, M. J. Design of small molecule libraries for NMR screening and other applications in drug discovery. *Curr. Top. Med. Chem.* 2003, *3 (1)*, 11–23; (b) Lepre, C. A. Library design for NMR-based screening. *Drug Discov. Today* 2001, *6(3)*, 133–140; (c) Schuffenhauer, A., Ruedisser, S., Marzinzik, A. L., Jahnke, W., Blommers, M., Selzer, P., and Jacoby, E. Library design for fragment based screening. *Curr. Top. Med. Chem.* 2005, *5(8)*, 751–762; (d) Baurin, N., Aboul-Ela, F., Barril, X., Davis, B., Drysdale, M., Dymock, B., Finch, H., Fromont, C., Richardson, C., Simmonite, H., and Hubbard, R. E. Design and characterization of libraries of molecular fragments for use in NMR screening against protein targets. *J. Chem. Inf. Comput. Sci.* 2004, *44(6)*, 2157–2166.
22. Siegel, M. G. and Vieth, M. Drugs in other drugs: a new look at drugs as fragments. *Drug Discov. Today* 2007, *12(1–2)*, 71–79.
23. MDL Comprehensive Medicinal Chemistry, (CMC). Available at http://www.symyx.com/.
24. Maccs drug data report (MDDR). Available at http://www.symyx.com/.
25. World Drug Index (WDI). Available at http://www.thomsonreuters.com/.
26. Congreve, M., Carr R., Murray, C., and Jhoti, H. A 'rule of three' for fragment base discovery. *Drug Discov. Today*, 2003, *8(19)*, 876–877.
27. Hajduk, P. J. Fragment-based drug design: how big is too big? *J. Med. Chem.* 2006, *49 (24)*, 6972–6976.
28. Siegal, G., AB, E., and Schultz, J. Integration of fragment screening and library design. *Drug Discov. Today* 2007, *12(23–24)*, 1032–1039.
29. Babaoglu, K. and Shoichet, B. K. Deconstructing fragment-based inhibitor discovery. *Nat. Chem. Biol.* 2006, *2(12)*, 720–723.

30. Hajduk, P. J., Huth, J. R., and Fesik, S. W. Druggability indices for protein targets derived from NMR-based screening data. *J. Med. Chem.* 2005, *48(7)*, 2518–2525.

31. Albert, J. S., Blomberg, N., Breeze, A. L., Brown, A. J., Burrows, J. N., Edwards, P. D., Folmer, R. H., Geschwindner, S., Griffen, E. J., Kenny, P. W., Nowak, T., Olsson, L. L., Sanganee, H., and Shapiro, A. B. An integrated approach to fragment-based lead generation: philosophy, strategy and case studies from AstraZencca's drug discovery programmes. *Curr. Top. Med. Chem.* 2007, *7(16)*, 1600–1629.

32. (a) Willett, P. Similarity methods in chemoinformatics. *Annu. Rev. Inform. Sci. Technol.* 2009, *43*, 3–71; (b) Bender, A. and Glen, R. C. Molecular similarity: a key technique in molecular informatics. *Org. Biomol. Chem.* 2004, *2(22)*, 3204–3218; (c) Nikolova, N. and Jaworska, J. Approaches to measure chemical similarity—a review. *QSAR Comb. Sci.* 2003, *22(9–10)*, 1006–1026.

33. (a) Moore, J. M. NMR screening in drug discovery. *Curr. Opin. Biotech.* 1999, *10(1)*, 54–58.

34. Zartler, E. R. and Shapiro, M. J. Protein NMR-based screening in drug discovery. *Curr. Pharm. Des.* 2006, *12(31)*, 3963–3972.

35. Diercks, T., Coles, M., and Kessler, H. Applications of NMR in drug discovery. *Curr. Opin. Chem. Biol.* 2001, *5(3)*, 285–291.

36. Hajduk, P. J., Gerfin, T., Boehlen, J. M., Häberli, M., Marek, D., and Fesik, S. W. High-throughput nuclear magnetic resonance-based screening. *J. Med. Chem.* 1999, *42(13)*, 2315–2317.

37. Klages, J., Coles, M., and Kessler, H. NMR-based screening: a powerful tool in fragment-based drug discovery. *Mol. Biosyst.* 2006, *2(6–7)*, 318–331.

38. Hajduk, P. J., Augeri, D. J., and Mack, J., Mendoza, R., Yang, J., Betz, S. F., and Fesik, S. W. NMR-based screening of proteins containing ^{13}C-labeled methyl groups. *J. Am. Chem. Soc.* 2000, *122(33)*, 7898–7904.

39. Weigelt, J., van Dongen, M., Uppenberg, J., Schultz, J., and Wikström, M. Site-selective screening by NMR spectroscopy with labeled amino acid pairs. *J. Am. Chem. Soc.* 2002, *124(11)*, 2446–2447.

40. Yabuki, T., Kigawa, T., Dohmae, N., Takio, K., Terada, T., Ito, Y., Laue, E. D., Cooper, J. A., Kainosho, M., and Yokoyama, S. Dual amino acid-selective and site-directed stable-isotope labeling of the human c-Ha-Ras protein by cell-free synthesis. *J. Biomol. NMR* 1998, *11(3)*, 295–306.

41. Pervushin, K., Riek, R., Wider, G., and Wüthrich, K. Attenuated T2 relaxation by mutual cancellation of dipole–dipole coupling and chemical shift anisotropy indicates an avenue to NMR structures of very large biological macromolecules in solution. *Proc. Natl. Acad. Sci. USA* 1997, *94(23)*, 12366–12371.

42. Riek, R., Wider, G., Pervushin, K., and Wüthrich, K. Polarization transfer by cross-correlated relaxation in solution NMR with very large molecules. *Proc. Natl. Acad. Sci. USA* 1999, *96(9)*, 4918–4923.

43. Peng, J. W., Lepre, C. A., Fejzo, J., Abdul-Manan, N., and Moore, J. M. Nuclear magnetic resonance-based approaches for lead generation in drug discovery. *Methods Enzymol.* 2002, *338*, 202–230.

44. (a) Hajduk, P. J., Olejniczak, E. T., and Fesik, S. W. One-dimensional relaxation- and diffusion-edited NMR methods for screening compounds that bind to macromolecules. *J. Am. Chem. Soc.* 1997, *119(50)*, 12257–12261; (b) Lin, M., Shapiro, M. J., and Wareing,

J. R. Diffusion-edited NMR—affinity NMR for direct observation of molecular interactions. *J. Am. Chem. Soc.* 1997, *119(22)*, 5249–5250.

45. (a) Meyer, B., Weimar, T., and Peters, T. Screening mixtures for biological activity by NMR. *Eur. J. Biochem.* 1997, *246(3)*, 705–709; (b) Inooka, H., Ohtaki, T., Kitahara, O., Ikegami, T., Endo, S., Kitada, C., Ogi, K., Onda, H., Fujino, M., and Shirakawa, M. Conformation of a peptide ligand bound to its G-protein coupled receptor. *Nat. Struct. Biol.* 2001, *8(2)*, 161–165.
46. (a) Chen, A. and Shapiro, M. J. NOE pumping as high-throughput method to determine compounds with binding affinity to macromolecules by NMR. *J. Am. Chem. Soc.* 2000, *122(2)*, 414–415; (b) Chen, A. and Shapiro, M. J. NOE pumping: a novel NMR technique for identification of compounds with binding affinity to macromolecules. *J. Am. Chem. Soc.* 1998, *120(39)*, 10258–10259.
47. (a) Mayer, M. and Meyer, B. Characterization of ligand binding by saturation transfer difference NMR spectroscopy. *Angew. Chem. Int. Ed.* 1999, *38(12)*, 1784–1788; (b) Mayer, M. and Meyer, B. Group epitope mapping by saturation transfer difference NMR to identify segments of a ligand in direct contact with a protein receptor. *J. Am. Chem. Soc.* 2001, *123(25)*, 6108–6117.
48. (a) Dalvit, C., Pevarello, P., Tato, M., Veronesi, M., Vulpetti, A., and Sundstrom, M. Identification of compounds with binding affinity to proteins via magnetization transfer from bulk water. *J. Biomol. NMR* 2000, *18(1)*, 65–68; (b) Dalvit, C., Fogliatto, G., Stewart, A., Veronesi, M., and Stockman, B. WaterLOGSY as a method for primary NMR screening: practical aspects and range of applicability. *J. Biomol. NMR.* 2001, *21(4)*, 349–359.
49. Becattini, B., Sareth, S., Zhai, D., Crowell, K. J., Leone, M., Reed, J. C., and Pellecchia, M. Targeting apoptosis via chemical design: inhibition of bid-induced cell death by small organic molecules. *Chem. Biol.* 2004, *11(8)*, 1107–1117.
50. (a) Jahnke, W., Perez, W. B., Paris, C. G., Strauss, A., Fendrich, G., and Nalin, C. M. Second-site NMR screening with a spin-labeled first ligand. *J. Am. Chem. Soc.* 2000, *122 (30)*, 7394–7395; (b) Jahnke, W., Rdisser, S., and Zurini, M. Spin label enhanced NMR screening. *J. Am. Chem. Soc.* 2001, *123(13)*, 3149–3150.
51. Dalvit, C., Ardini, E., Flocco, M., Fogliatto, G. P., Mongelli, N., and Veronesi, M. A general NMR method for rapid, efficient, and reliable biochemical screening. *J. Am. Chem. Soc.* 2003, *125(47)*, 14620–14625.
52. (a) Dalvit, C., Mongelli, N., Papeo, G., Giordano, P., Veronesi, M., Moskau, D., and Kümmerle, R. Sensitivity improvement in ^{19}F NMR-based screening experiments: theoretical considerations and experimental applications. *J. Am. Chem. Soc.* 2005, *127(38)*, 13380–13385; (b) Forino, M., Johnson, S., Wong, T. Y., Rozanov, D. V., Savinov, A. Y., Li, W., Fattorusso, R., Becattini, B., Orry, A. J., Jung, D., Abagyan, R. A., Smith, J. W., Alibek, K., Liddington, R. C., Strongin, A. Y., and Pellecchia, M. Efficient synthetic inhibitors of anthrax lethal factor. *Proc. Natl. Acad. Sci. USA* 2005, *102 (27)*, 9499–9504.
53. Vanwetswinkel, S., Heetebrij, R. J., van Duynhoven, J., Hollander, J. G., Filippov, D. V., Hajduk, P. J., and Siegal, G. TINS, target immobilized NMR screening: an efficient and sensitive method for ligand discovery. *Chem. Biol.* 2005, *12(2)*, 207–216.
54. (a) Jahnke, W., Floersheim, P., Ostermeier, C., Zhang, X., Hemmig, R., Hurth, K., and Uzunov, D. P. NMR reporter screening for the detection of high-affinity ligands. *Angew. Chem. Int. Ed. Engl.* 2002, *41(18)*, 3420–3423; (b) Dalvit, C., Fasolini, M., Flocco, M., Knapp, S., Pevarello, P., and Veronesi, M. NMR-Based screening with competition water-

ligand observed via gradient spectroscopy experiments: detection of high-affinity ligands. *J. Med. Chem.* 2002, *45(12)*, 2610–2614.

55. (a) Muchmore, S. W., Olson, J., Jones, R., Pan, J., Blum, M., Greer, J., Merrick, S. M., Magdalinos, P., and Nienaber, V. L. Automated crystal mounting and data collection for protein crystallography. *Structure* 2000, *8(12)*, R243–R246; (b) Sharff, A. and Jhoti, H. High-throughput crystallography to enhance drug discovery. *Curr. Opin. Chem. Biol.* 2003, *7(3)*, 340–345.
56. Hendrickson, W. A. Synchrotron crystallography. *Trends Biochem. Sci.* 2000, *25(12)*, 637–643.
57. (a) Mattos, C. and Ringe, D. Locating and characterizing binding sites on proteins. *Nat. Biotechnol.* 1996, *14(5)*, 595–599; (b) Mattos, C. and Ringe, D. Proteins in organic solvents. *Curr. Opin. Struct. Biol.* 2001, *11(6)*, 761–764.
58. Stout, T. J., Sage, C. R. and Stroud, R. M. The additivity of substrate fragments in enzyme–ligand binding. *Structure* 1998, *6(7)*, 839–848.
59. Boström, J., Hogner, A., and Schmitt, S. Do structurally similar ligands bind in a similar fashion? *J. Med. Chem.* 2006, *49(23)*, 6716–6725.
60. Verlinde, C. L., Rudenko, G., and Hol, W. G. In search of new lead compounds for trypanosomiasis drug design: a protein structure-based linked-fragment approach. *J. Comput. Aided Mol. Des.* 1992, *6(2)*, 131–147.
61. Nienaber, V. L., Richardson, P. L., Klighofer, V., Bouska, J. J., Giranda, V. L., and Greer, J. Discovering novel ligands for macromolecules using X-ray crystallographic screening. *Nat. Biotechnol.* 2000, *18(10)*, 1105–1108.
62. Lesuisse, D., Lange, G., Deprez, P., Bénard, D., Schoot, B., Delettre, G., Marquette, J. P., Broto, P., Jean-Baptiste, V., Bichet, P., Sarubbi, E., and Mandine, E. SAR and X-ray. A new approach combining fragment-based screening and rational drug design: application to the discovery of nanomolar inhibitors of Src SH2. *J. Med. Chem.* 2002, *45(12)*, 2379–2387.
63. Verdonk, M. L. and Hartshorn, M. J. Structure-guided fragment screening for lead discovery. *Curr. Opin. Drug Discov. Devel.* 2004, *7(4)*, 404–410.
64. Gill, A. New lead generation strategies for protein kinase inhibitors—fragment based screening approaches. *Mini. Rev. Med. Chem.* 2004, *4(3)*, 301–311.
65. Carr, R. and Jhoti, H. Structure-based screening of low-affinity compounds. *Drug Discov. Today* 2002, *7(9)*, 522–527.
66. Accelrys, Inc. 10188 Telesis Court, Suite 100. San Diego, CA 92121, USA. Phone: (858)799-5000. Fax: (858)799-5100. Available at http://www.accelrys.com.
67. Hartshorn, M. J., Murray, C. W., Cleasby, A., Frederickson, M., Tickle, I. J., and Jhoti, H. Fragment-based lead discovery using X-ray crystallography. *J. Med. Chem.* 2005, *48(2)*, 403–413.
68. (a) Gill, A., Cleasby, A., and Jhoti, H. The discovery of novel protein kinase inhibitors by using fragment-based high-throughput X-ray crystallography. *ChemBioChem* 2005, *6(3)*, 506–512; (b) Sanders, W. J., Nienaber, V. L., Lerner, C. G., McCall, J. O., Merrick, S. M., Swanson, S. J., Harlan, J. E., Stoll, V. S., Stamper, G. F., Betz, S. F., Condroski, K. R., Meadows, R. P., Severin, J. M., Walter, K. A., Magdalinos, P., Jakob, C. G., Wagner, R., and Beutel, B. A. Discovery of potent inhibitors of dihydroneopterin aldolase using CrystaLEAD high-throughput X-ray crystallographic screening and structure-directed lead optimization. *J. Med. Chem.*

2004, *47(7)*, 1709–1718; (c) Card, G. L., Blasdel, L., England, B. P., Zhang, C., Suzuki, Y., Gillette, S., Fong, D., Ibrahim, P. N., Artis, D. R., Bollag, G., Milburn, M. V., Kim, S.-H., Schlessinger, J., and Zhang, K. Y. J. A family of phosphodiesterase inhibitors discovered by cocrystallography and scaffold-based drug design. *Nat. Biotechnol.* 2005, *23(2)*, 201–207.

69. (a) Seth, P. P., Miyaji, A., Jefferson, E. A., Sannes-Lowery, K. A., Osgood, S. A., Propp, S. S., Ranken, R., Massire, C., Sampath, R., Ecker, D. J., Swayze, E. E., and Griffey, R. H. SAR by MS: discovery of a new class of RNA-binding small molecules for the hepatitis C virus: internal ribosome entry site IIA subdomain. *J. Med. Chem.* 2005, *48(23)*, 7099–7102; (b) Swayze, E. E., Jefferson, E. A., Sannes-Lowery, K. A., Blyn, L. B., Risen, L. M., Arakawa, S., Osgood, S. A., Hofstadler, S. A., and Griffey, R. H. SAR by MS: a ligand based technique for drug lead discovery against structured RNA targets. *J. Med. Chem.* 2002, *45(18)*, 3816–3819.

70. Erlanson, D. A., Wells, J. A., and Braisted, A. C. Tethering: fragment-based drug discovery. *Annu. Rev. Biophys. Biomol. Struct.* 2004, *33*, 199–223.

71. (a) Huber, W. and Mueller, F. Biomolecular interaction analysis in drug discovery using surface plasmon resonance technology. *Curr. Pharm. Des.* 2006, *12(31)*, 3999–4021; (b) Baird, C. L. and Myszka, D. G. Current and emerging commercial optical biosensors. *J. Mol. Recognit.* 2001, *14(5)*, 261–268.

72. Pröll, F., Fechner, P., and Proll, G. Direct optical detection in fragment-based screening. *Anal. Bioanal. Chem.* 2009, *393(6–7)*, 1557–1562.

73. Day, Y. S., Baird, C. L., Rich, R. L., and Myszka, D. G. Direct comparison of binding equilibrium, thermodynamic, and rate constants determined by surface- and solution-based biophysical methods. *Protein Sci.* 2002, *11(5)*, 1017–1025.

74. Cooper, M. A. Optical biosensors in drug discovery. *Nat. Rev. Drug Discov.* 2002, *1(7)*, 515–528.

75. Cooper, M. A. Advances in membrane receptor screening and analysis. *J. Mol. Recognit.* 2004, *17(4)*, 286–315.

76. Gribbon, P. and Sewing, A. Fluorescence readouts in HTS: no gain without pain? *Drug Discov. Today.* 2003, *8(22)*, 1035–1043.

77. Dai, W.-G., Pollock-Dove, C., Dong, L. C., and Li, S. Advanced screening assays to rapidly identify solubility-enhancing formulations: high-throughput, miniaturization and automation. *Adv. Drug Deliv. Rev.* 2008, *60(6)*, 657–672.

78. (a) McGovern, S. L., Caselli, E., Grigorieff, N., and Shoichet, B. K. A common mechanism underlying promiscuous inhibitors from virtual and high-throughput screening. *J. Med. Chem.* 2002, *45(8)*, 1712–1722; (b) McGovern, S. L., Helfand, B. T., Feng, B., and Shoichet, B. K. A specific mechanism of nonspecific inhibition. *J. Med. Chem.* 2003, *46(20)*, 4265–4272.

79. (a) Rishton, G. M. Reactive compounds and *in vitro* false positives in HTS. *Drug Discov. Today* 1997, *2(9)*, 382–384; (b) Huth, J. R., Mendoza, R., Olejniczak, E. T., Johnson, R. W., Cothron, D. A., Liu, Y., Lerner, C. G., Chen, J., and Hajduk, P. J. ALARM NMR: a rapid and robust experimental method to detect reactive false positives in biochemical screens. *J. Am. Chem. Soc.* 2005, *127(1)*, 217–224.

80. (a) Maly, D. J., Choong, I. C., and Ellman, J. A. Combinatorial target-guided ligand assembly: identification of potent subtype-selective c-Src inhibitors. *Proc. Natl. Acad. Sci. USA* 2000, *97(6)*, 2419–2424; (b) He, M. M., Smith, A. S., Oslob, J. D., Flanagan, W.

M., Braisted, A. C., Whitty, A., Cancilla, M. T., Wang, J., Lugovskoy, A. A., Yoburn, J. C., Fung, A. D., Farrington, G., Eldredge, J. K., Day, E. S., Cruz, L. A., Cachero, T. G., Miller, S. K., Friedman, J. E., Choong, I. C., and Cunningham, B. C. Small-molecule inhibition of TNF-α. *Science* 2005, *310(5750)*, 1022–1025.

81. (a) Wang, X., Choe, Y., Craik, C. S., and Ellman, J. A. Design and synthesis of novel inhibitors of gelatinase B. *Bioorg. Med. Chem. Lett.* 2002, *12(16)*, 2201–2204; (b) Boehm, H.-J., Boehringer, M., Bur, D., Gmuender, H., Huber, W., Klaus, W., Kostrewa, D., Kuehne, H., Luebbers, T., Meunier-Keller, N., and Mueller, F. Novel inhibitors of DNA gyrase: 3D structure based biased needle screening, hit validation by biophysical methods, and 3D guided optimization. A promising alternative to random screening. *J. Med. Chem.* 2000, *43(14)*, 2664–2674; (c) Black, E., Breed, J., Breeze, A. L., Embrey, K., Garcia, R., Gero, T. W., Godfrey, L., Kenny, P. W., Morley, A. D., Minshull, C. A., Pannifer, A. D., Read, J., Rees, A., Russell, D. J., Toader, D., and Tucker, J. Structure-based design of protein tyrosine phosphatasc-1B inhibitors. *Bioorg. Med. Chem. Lett.* 2005, *15(10)*, 2503–2507; (d) Schilling, S., Niestroj, A. J., Rahfeld, J. U., Hoffmann, T., Wermann, M., Zunkel, K., Wasternack, C., and Demuth, H. U. Identification of human glutaminyl cyclase as a metalloenzyme. Potent inhibition by imidazole derivatives and heterocyclic chelators. *J. Biol. Chem.* 2003, *278(50)*, 49773–49779; (e) Buchholz, M., Heiser, U., Schilling, S., Niestroj, A. J., Zunkel, K., and Demuth, H. U. The first potent inhibitors for human glutaminyl cyclase: synthesis and structure–activity relationship. *J. Med. Chem.* 2006, *49(2)*, 664–677.

82. Kehoe, J. W., Maly, D. J., Verdugo, D. E., Armstrong, J. I., Cook, B. N., Ouyang, Y. B., Moore, K. L., Ellman, J. A., and Bertozzi, C. R. Tyrosylprotein sulfotransferase inhibitors generated by combinatorial target-guided ligand assembly. *Bioorg. Med. Chem. Lett.* 2002, *12(3)*, 329–332.

83. Hesterkamp, T., Barker, J., Davenport, A., and Whittaker, M. Fragment based drug discovery using fluorescence correlation: spectroscopy techniques: challenges and solutions. *Curr. Top. Med. Chem.* 2007, *7(16)*, 1582–1591.

84. Barker, J. J., Barker, O., Boggio, R., Chauhan, V., Cheng, R. K., Corden, V., Courtney, S. M., Edwards, N., Falque, V. M., Fusar, F., Gardiner, M., Hamelin, E. M., Hesterkamp, T., Ichihara, O., Jones, R. S., Mather, O., Mercurio, C., Minucci, S., Montalbetti, C. A., Müller, A., Patel, D., Phillips, B. G., Varasi, M., Whittaker, M., Winkler, D., and Yarnold, C. J. Fragment-based identification of Hsp90 inhibitors. *ChemMedChem* 2009, *4(6)*, 963–966.

85. (a) Wood, W. J. L., Patterson, A. W., Tsuruoka, H., Jain, R. K., and Ellman, J. A. Substrate activity screening: a fragment-based method for the rapid identification of nonpeptidic protease inhibitors. *J. Am. Chem. Soc.* 2005, *127(44)*, 15521–15527; (b) Brak, K., Doyle, P. S., McKerrow, J. H., and Ellman, J. A. Identification of a new class of nonpeptidic inhibitors of cruzain. *J. Am. Chem. Soc.* 2008, *130(20)*, 6404–6410; (c) Soellner, M. B., Rawls, K. A., Grundner, C., Alber, T., and Ellman, J. A. Fragment-based substrate activity screening method for the identification of potent inhibitors of the Mycobacterium tuberculosis phosphatase PtpB. *J. Am. Chem. Soc.* 2007, *129(31)*, 9613–9635.

86. (a) Oprea, T. I., Davis, A. M. Teague, S. J., and Lesson, P. D. Is there a difference between leads and drugs? A historial perspective. *J. Chem. Inf. Comput. Sci.* 2001, *41(5)*, 1308–1315; (b) Baurin, N., Baker, R., Richardson, C., Chen, I., Foloppe, N., Potter, A., Jordan, A., Roughley, S., Parratt, M., Greaney, P., Morley, D., and Hubbard, R. E. Drug-like annotation and duplicate analysis of a 23-supplier chemical database totalling 2.7 million compounds. *J. Chem. Inf. Comput. Sci.* 2004, *44(2)*, 643–651.

87. Scapin, G. Structural biology and drug discovery. *Curr. Pharm. Des.* 2006, *12(17)*, 2087–2097.

88. (a) Jencks, W. P. On the attribution and additivity of binding energies. *Proc. Natl. Acad. Sci. USA* 1981, *78(7)*, 4046–4050; (b) Saxty, G., Woodhead, S. J., Berdini, V., Davies, T. G., Verdonk, M. L., Wyatt, P. G., Boyle, R. G., Barford, D., Downham, R., Garrett, M. D., and Carr, R. A. Identification of inhibitors of protein kinase B using fragment-based lead discovery. *J. Med. Chem.* 2007, *50(10)*, 2293–2296.

89. Patel, Y., Gillet, V. J., Howe, T., Pastor, J., Oyarzabal, J., and Willett, P. Assessment of additive/nonadditive effects in structure–activity relationships: implications for iterative drug design. *J. Med. Chem.* 2008, *51(23)*, 7552–7562.

90. Green, N. M. Avidin. *Adv. Protein Chem.* 1975; *29*, 85–133.

91. Murray, C. W. and Verdonk, M. L. The consequences of translational and rotational entropy lost by small molecules on binding to proteins. *J. Comput. Aided Mol. Des.* 2002, *16(10)*, 741–753.

92. (a) Ganesan, A. Strategies for the dynamic integration of combinatorial synthesis and screening. *Angew. Chem. Int. Ed.* 1998, *37(20)*, 2828–2831; (b) Otto, S., Furlan, R. L., and Sanders, J. K. Recent developments in dynamic combinatorial chemistry. *Curr. Opin. Chem. Biol.* 2002, *6(3)*, 321–327; (c) Ramström, O. and Lehn, J.-M. Drug discovery by dynamic combinatorial libraries. *Nat. Rev. Drug Discov.* 2002, *1(1)*, 26–36.

93. Kolb, H. C., Finn, M. G., and Sharpless, K. B. Click chemistry: diverse chemical function from a few good reactions. *Angew. Chem. Int. Ed. Engl.* 2001, *40(11)*, 2004–2021.

94. Lehn, J.-M. and Eliseev, A. V. Dynamic combinatorial chemistry. *Science* 2001, *291 (5512)*, 2331–2332.

95. (a) Eliseev, A. V. and Nelen, M. I. Use of molecular recognition to drive chemical evolution. 1. Controlling the composition of an equilibrating mixture of simple arginine receptors. *J. Am. Chem. Soc.* 1997, *119(5)*, 1147–1148; (b) Ramström, O. and Lehn J.-M. *In situ* generation and screening of a dynamic combinatorial carbohydrate library against concanavalin A. *ChemBioChem* 2000, *1(1)*, 41–48; (c) Bunyapaiboonsri, T., Ramström, O., Lohmann, S., Lehn, J.-M., Peng, L., and Goeldner, M. Dynamic deconvolution of a pre-equilibrated dynamic combinatorial library of acetylcholinesterase inhibitors. *ChemBioChem* 2001, *2(6)*, 438–444; (d) Edwards, P. Fragment-based drug discovery of carbonic anhydrase II inhibitors by dynamic combinatorial chemistry. *Drug Discov. Today* 2007, *12(11/12)*, 497–498.

96. (a) Huc, I. and Lehn, J.-M. Virtual combinatorial libraries: dynamic generation of molecular and supramolecular diversity by self-assembly. *Proc. Natl. Acad. Sci. USA* 1997, *94(6)*, 2106–2110; (b) Hochgürtel, M., Kroth, H., Piecha, D., Hofmann, M. W., Nicolau, C., Krause, S., Schaaf, O., Sonnenmoser, G., and Eliseev, A. V. Target-induced formation of neuraminidase inhibitors from *in vitro* virtual combinatorial libraries. *Proc. Natl. Acad. Sci. USA* 2002, *99(6)*, 3382–3387; (c) Hochgürtel, M., Biesinger, R., Kroth, H., Piecha, D., Hofmann, M. W., Krause, S., Schaaf, O., Nicolau, C., and Eliseev, A. V. Ketones as building blocks for dynamic combinatorial libraries: highly active neuraminidase inhibitors generated via selection pressure of the biological target. *J. Med. Chem.* 2003, *46(3)*, 356–358; (d) Zameo, S., Vauzeilles, B., and Beau, J.-M. Dynamic combinatorial chemistry: lysozyme selects an aromatic motif that mimics a carbohydrate residue. *Angew. Chem. Int. Ed. Engl.* 2005, *44(6)*, 965–969; (e) Bugaut, A., Bathany, K., Schmitter, J.-M., and Rayner, B. Target-induced selection of ligands from a dynamic combinatorial library of mono- and bi-conjugated oligonucleotides. *Tetrahedron Lett.* 2005, *46(4)*, 687–690.

97. (a) Cousins, G. R. L., Poulsen, S.-A., and Sanders, J. K. M. Dynamic combinatorial libraries of pseudo-peptide hydrazone macrocycles. *Chem. Commun.* 1999, *(16)*, 1575–1576; (b) Bunyapaiboonsri, T., Ramström, H., Ramström, O., Haiech, J., and Lehn, J.-M. Generation of bis-cationic heterocyclic inhibitors of *Bacillus subtilis* HPr kinase/phosphatase from a ditopic dynamic combinatorial library. *J. Med. Chem.* 2003, *46(26)*, 5803–5811; (c) Ramström, O., Lohmann, S., Bunyapaiboonsri, T., and Lehn, J.-M. Dynamic combinatorial carbohydrate libraries: probing the binding site of the concanavalin A lectin. *Chem. Eur. J.* 2004, *10(7)*, 1711–1715.

98. (a) Swann, P. G., Casanova, R. A., Desai, A., Frauenhoff, M. M., Urbancic, M., Slomczynska, U., Hopfinger, A. J., Le Breton, G. C., and Venton, D. L. Nonspecific protease-catalyzed hydrolysis/synthesis of a mixture of peptides: product diversity and ligand amplification by a molecular trap. *Biopolymers* 1996, *40(6)*, 617–625; (b) Burger, M. T., and Bartlett, P. A. Enzymatic, polymer-supported formation of an analog of the trypsin inhibitor A90720A: a screening strategy for macrocyclic peptidase inhibitors. *J. Am. Chem. Soc.* 1997, *119(51)*, 12697–12698.

99. (a) Nicolaou, K. C., Hughes, R., Cho, S. Y., Winssinger, N., Smethurst, C., Labischinski, H., and Endermann, R. Target-accelerated combinatorial synthesis and discovery of highly potent antibiotics effective against vancomycinn-resistant bacteria. *Angew. Chem. Int. Ed.* 2000, *39(21)*, 3823–3828; (b) Ladame, S., Whitney, A. M., and Balasubramanian S. Targeting nucleic acid secondary structures with polyamides using an optimized dynamic combinatorial approach. *Angew. Chem. Int. Ed. Engl.* 2005, *44(35)*, 5736–5739; (c) Hotchkiss, T., Kramer, H. B., Doores, K. J., Gamblin, D. P., Oldham, N. J., and Davis, B. G. Ligand amplification in a dynamic combinatorial glycopeptide library. *Chem. Commun.* 2005, *(34)*, 4264–4266.

100. (a) Shi, B. and Greaney, M. F. Reversible Michael addition of thiols as a new tool for dynamic combinatorial chemistry. *Chem. Commun.* 2005, *(7)*, 886–888; (b) Shi, B., Stevenson, R., Campopiano, D. J., and Greaney, M. F. Discovery of glutathione *S*-transferase inhibitors using dynamic combinatorial chemistry. *J. Am. Chem. Soc.* 2006, *128(26)*, 8459–8467.

101. Poulsen, S. A. and Bornaghi, L. F. Fragment-based drug discovery of carbonic anhydrase II inhibitors by dynamic combinatorial chemistry utilizing alkene cross metathesis. *Bioorg. Med. Chem.* 2006, *14(10)*, 3275–3284.

102. Liénard, B. M. R., Selevsek, N., Oldham, N. J., and Schofield, C. J. Combined mass spectrometry and dynamic chemistry approach to identify metalloenzyme inhibitors. *ChemMedChem* 2007, *2(2)*, 175–179.

103. Congreve, M. S., Davis, D. J., Devine, L., Granata, C., O'Reilly, M., Wyatt, P. G., and Jhoti, H. Detection of ligands from a dynamic combinatorial library by X-ray crystallography. *Angew. Chem. Int. Ed. Engl.* 2003, *42(37)*, 4479–4482.

104. (a) O'Brien, T., Fahr, B. T., Sopko, M. M., Lam, J. W., Waal, N. D., Raimundo, B. C., Purkey, H. E., Pham, P., and Romanowski, M. J. Structural analysis of caspase-1 inhibitors derived from Tethering. *Acta Crystallogr. Sec. F Struct. Biol. Cryst. Commun.* 2005, *61 (5)*, 451–458; (b) Fahr, B. T., O'Brien, T., Pham, P., Waal, N. D., Baskaran, S., Raimundo, B. C., Lam, J. W., Sopko, M. M., Purkey, H. E., and Romanowski, M. J. Tethering identifies fragment that yields potent inhibitors of human caspase-1. *Bioorg. Med. Chem. Lett.* 2006, *16(3)*, 559–62.

105. (a) Erlanson, D. A., Lam, J. W., Wiesmann, C., Luong, T. N., Simmons, R. L., DeLano, W. L., Choong, I. C., Burdett, M. T., Flanagan, W. M., Lee, D., Gordon, E. M., and O'Brien, T.

In situ assembly of enzyme inhibitors using extended tethering. *Nat. Biotechnol.* 2003, *21 (3)*, 308–314; (b) Choong, I. C., Lew, W., Lee, D., Pham, P., Burdett, M. T., Lam, J. W., Wiesmann, C., Luong, T. N., Fahr, B., DeLano, W. L., McDowell, R. S., Allen, D. A., Erlanson, D. A., Gordon, E. M., and O'Brien, T. Identification of potent and selective small-molecule inhibitors of caspase-3 through the use of extended tethering and structure-based drug design. *J. Med. Chem.* 2002, *45(23)*, 5005–5022.

106. Inglese, J., Blatchly, R. A., and Benkovic, S. J. A multisubstrate adduct inhibitor of a purine biosynthetic enzyme with a picomolar dissociation constant. *J. Med. Chem.* 1989, *32(5)*, 937–940.

107. Greasley, S. E., Marsilje, T. H., Cai, H., Baker, S., Benkovic, S. J., Boger, D. L., and Wilson, I. A. Unexpected formation of an epoxide-derived multisubstrate adduct inhibitor on the active site of GAR transformylase. *Biochemistry* 2001, *40(45)*, 13538–13547.

108. Nguyen, R. and Huc, I. Using an enzyme's active site to template inhibitors. *Angew. Chem. Int. Ed. Engl.* 2001, *40(9)*, 1774–1776.

109. Huisgen, R. In *1,3-Dipolar Cycloaddition Chemistry*, Vol. 1, Padwa, A. (ed.), Wiley, New York, 1984, pp. 1–176.

110. (a) Kolb, H. C. and Sharpless, K. B. The growing impact of click chemistry on drug discovery. *Drug Discov. Today* 2003, *8(24)*, 1128–1137; (b) Moorhouse, A. D. and Moses, J. E. Click chemistry and medicinal chemistry: a case of "cyclo-addiction". *ChemMedChem* 2008, *3(5)*, 715–723; (c) Tron, G. C., Pirali, T., Billington, R. A., Canonico, P. L., Sorba, G., and Genazzani, A. A. Click chemistry reactions in medicinal chemistry: applications of the 1, 3-dipolar cycloaddition between azides and alkynes. *Med. Res. Rev.* 2008, *28(2)*, 278–308.

111. (a) Lewis, W. G., Green, L. G., Grynszpan, F., Radić, Z., Carlier, P. R., Taylor, P., Finn, M. G., and Sharpless, K. B. Click chemistry *in situ*: acetylcholinesterase as a reaction vessel for the selective assembly of a femtomolar inhibitor from an array of building blocks. *Angew. Chem. Int. Ed. Engl.* 2002, *41(6)*, 1053–1057; (b) Manetsch, R., Krasiński, A., Radić, Z., Raushel, J., Taylor, P., Sharpless, K. B., and Kolb, H. C. *In situ* click chemistry: enzyme inhibitors made to their own specifications. *J. Am. Chem. Soc.* 2004, *126(40)*, 12809–12818; (c) Krasiński, A., Radić, Z., Manetsch, R., Raushel, J., Taylor, P., Sharpless, K. B., and Kolb, H. C. *In situ* selection of lead compounds by click chemistry: target-guided optimization of acetylcholinesterase inhibitors. *J. Am. Chem. Soc.* 2005, *127(18)*, 6686–6692.

112. Mocharla, V. P., Colasson, B., Lee, L. V., Röper, S., Sharpless, K. B., Wong, C. H., and Kolb, H. C. *In situ* click chemistry: enzyme-generated inhibitors of carbonic anhydrase II. *Angew. Chem. Int. Ed Engl.* 2004, *44(1)*, 116–120.

113. Whiting, M., Muldoon, J., Lin, Y. C., Silverman, S. M., Lindstrom, W., Olson, A. J., Kolb, H. C., Finn, M. G., Sharpless, K. B., Elder, J. H., and Fokin, V. V. Inhibitors of HIV-1 protease by using *in situ* click chemistry. *Angew. Chem. Int. Ed. Engl.* 2006, *45(9)*, 1435–1439.

114. Hajduk, P. J., Gomtsyan, A., Didomenico, S., Cowart, M., Bayburt, E. K., Solomon, L., Severin, J., Smith, R., Walter, K., Holzman, T. F., Stewart, A., McGaraughty, S., Jarvis, M. F., Kowaluk, E. A., and Fesik, S. W. Design of adenosine kinase inhibitors from the NMR-based screening of fragments. *J. Med. Chem.* 2000, *43(25)*, 4781–4786.

115. Liu, G., Huth, J. R., Olejniczak, E. T., Mendoza, R., DeVries, P., Leitza, S., Reilly, E. B., Okasinski, G. F., Fesik, S. W., and von Geldern, T. W. Novel *p*-arylthio cinnamides as antagonists of leukocyte function-associated antigen-1/intracellular adhesion molecule-1 interaction. 2. Mechanism of inhibition and structure-based improvement of pharmaceutical properties. *J. Med. Chem.* 2001, *44(8)*, 1202–1210.

116. Hajduk, P. J., Sheppard, G., Nettesheim, D. G., Olejniczak, E. T., Shuker, S. B., Meadows, R. P., Steinman, D. H., Carrera, G. M., Jr., Marcotte, P. A., Severin, J., Walter, K., Smith, H., Gubbins, E., Simmer, R., Holzman, T. F., Morgan, D. W., Davidsen, S. K., Summers, J. B., and Fesik, S. W. Discovery of potent nonpeptide inhibitors of stromelysin using SAR by NMR. *J. Am. Chem. Soc.* 1997, *119(25)*, 5818–5827.

117. Hajduk, P. J., Shuker, S. B., Nettesheim, D. G., Craig, R., Augeri, D. J., Betebenner, D., Albert, D. H., Guo, Y., Meadows, R. P., Xu, L., Michaelides, M., Davidsen, S. K., and Fesik, S. W. NMR-based modification of matrix metalloproteinase inhibitors with improved bioavailability. *J. Med. Chem.* 2002, *45(26)*, 5628–5639.

118. Szczepankiewicz, B. G., Liu, G., Hajduk, P. J., Abad-Zapatero, C., Pei, Z., Xin, Z., Lubben, T. H., Trevillyan, J. M., Stashko, M. A., Ballaron, S. J., Liang, H., Huang, F., Hutchins, C. W., Fesik, S. W., and Jirousek, M. R. Discovery of a potent, selective protein tyrosine phosphatase 1B inhibitor using a linked-fragment strategy. *J. Am. Chem. Soc.* 2003, *125(14)*, 4087–4096.

119. Liu, G., Szczepankiewicz, B. G., Pei, Z., Janowick, D. A., Xin, Z., Hajduk, P. J., Abad-Zapatero, C., Liang, H., Hutchins, C. W., Fesik, S. W., Ballaron, S. J., Stashko, M. A., Lubben, T., Mika, A. K., Zinker, B. A., Trevillyan, J. M., and Jirousek, M. R. Discovery and structure–activity relationship of oxalylarylaminobenzoic acids as inhibitors of protein tyrosine phosphatase 1B. *J. Med. Chem.* 2003, *46(11)*, 2093–2103.

120. Liu, G., Xin, Z., Liang, H., Abad-Zapatero, C., Hajduk, P. J., Janowick, D. A., Szczepankiewicz, B. G., Pei, Z., Hutchins, C. W., Ballaron, S. J., Stashko, M. A., Lubben, T. H., Berg, C. E., Rondinone, C. M., Trevillyan, J. M., and Jirousek, M. R. Selective protein tyrosine phosphatase 1B inhibitors: targeting the second phosphotyrosine binding site with non-carboxylic acid-containing ligands. *J. Med. Chem.* 2003, *46 (16)*, 3437–3440.

121. Liu, G., Xin, Z., Pei, Z., Hajduk, P. J., Abad-Zapatero, C., Hutchins, C. W., Zhao, H., Lubben, T. H., Ballaron, S. J., Haasch, D. L., Kaszubska, W., Rondinone, C. M., Trevillyan, J. M., and Jirousek, M. R. Fragment screening and assembly: a highly efficient approach to a selective and cell active protein tyrosine phosphatase 1B inhibitor. *J. Med. Chem.* 2003, *46(20)*, 4232–4235.

122. Erlanson, D. A., McDowell, R. S., He, M. M., Randal, M., Simmons, R. L., Kung, J., Waight, A., and Hansen, S. K. Discovery of a new phosphotyrosine mimetic for PTP1B using breakaway tethering. *J. Am. Chem. Soc.* 2003, *125(19)*, 5602–5603.

123. Murray, C. W., Callaghan, O., Chessari, G., Cleasby, A., Congreve, M., Frederickson, M., Hartshorn, M. J., McMenamin, R., Patel, S., and Wallis, N. Application of fragment screening by X-ray crystallography to β-secretase. *J. Med. Chem.* 2007, *50(6)*, 1116–1123.

124. Congreve, M., Aharony, D., Albert, J., Callaghan, O., Campbell, J., Carr, R. A., Chessari, G., Cowan, S., Edwards, P. D., Frederickson, M., McMenamin, R., Murray, C. W., Patel, S., and Wallis, N. Application of fragment screening by X-ray crystallography to the discovery of aminopyridines as inhibitors of β-secretase. *J. Med. Chem.* 2007, *50(6)*, 1124–1132.

125. Geschwindner, S., Olsson, L.-L., Albert, J. S., Deinum, J., Edwards, P. D., de Beer, T., and Folmer, R. H. A. Discovery of a novel warhead against β-secretase through fragment-based lead generation. *J. Med. Chem.* 2007, *50(24)*, 5903–5911.

126. Edwards, P. D., Albert, J. S., Sylvester, M., Aharony, D., Andisik, D., Callaghan, O., Campbell, J. B., Carr, R. A., Chessari, G., Congreve, M., Frederickson, M., Folmer, R. H. A., Geschwindner, S., Koether, G., Kolmodin, K., Krumrine, J., Mauger, R. C., Murray, C. W., Olsson, L.-L., Patel, S., Spear, N., and Tian, G. Application of fragment-based lead generation to the discovery of novel, cyclic amidine β-secretase inhibitors with nanomolar potency, cellular activity, and high ligand efficiency. *J. Med. Chem.* 2007, *50(24)*, 5912–5925.

127. Yang, W., Fucini, R. V., Fahr, B. T., Randal, M., Lind, K. E., Lam, M. B., Lu, W., Lu, Y., Cary, D. R., Romanowski, M. J., Colussi, D., Pietrak, B., Allison, T. J., Munshi, S. K., Penny, D. M., Pham, P., Sun, J., Thomas, A. E., Wilkinson, J. M., Jacobs, J. W., McDowell, R. S., and Ballinger, M. D. Fragment-based discovery of nonpeptidic BACE-1 inhibitors using tethering. *Biochemistry* 2009, *48(21)*, 4488–4496.

128. Kuglstatter, A., Stahl, M., Peters, J. U., Huber, W., Stihle, M., Schlatter, D., Benz, J., Ruf, A., Roth, D., Enderle, T., and Hennig, M. Tyramine fragment binding to BACE-1. *Bioorg. Med. Chem. Lett.* 2008, *18(4)*, 1304–1307.

129. Lange, G., Lesuisse, D., Deprez, P., Schoot, B., Loenze, P., Bénard, D., Marquette, J.-P., Broto, P., Sarubbi, E., and Mandine, E. Requirements for specific binding of low affinity inhibitor fragments to the SH2 domain of ^{pp60}Src are identical to those for high affinity binding of full length inhibitors. *J. Med. Chem.* 2003, *46(24)*, 5184–5195.

130. Neumann, T., Junker, H.-D., Keil, O., Burkert, K., Ottleben, H., Gamer, J., Sekul, R., Deppe, H., Feurer, A., Tomandl, D., and Metz, G. Discovery of thrombin inhibitor fragments from chemical microarray screening. *Lett. Drug Des. Discov.* 2005, *2(8)*, 590–594.

131. Bulat, S., Bosio, S., Papadopoulos, M. A., Cerezo-Gálvez, S., Grabowski, E., Rosenbaum, C., Matassa, V. G., Ott, I., Metz, G., Schamberger, J., Sekul, R., and Feurer, A. Design and discovery of novel, potent pyrazinone-based thrombin inhibitors with a solubilizing amino P_1_P_2-linker. *Lett. Drug Des. Discov.* 2006, *3(5)*, 289–292.

132. Howard, N., Abell, C., Blakemore, W., Chessari, G., Congreve, M., Howard, S., Jhoti, H., Murray, C. W., Seavers, L. C. A., and van Montfort, R. L. M. Application of fragment screening and fragment linking to the discovery of novel thrombin inhibitors. *J. Med. Chem.* 2006, *49(4)*, 1346–1355.

133. Hajduk, P. J., Boyd, S., Nettesheim, D., Nienaber, V., Severin, J., Smith, R., Davidson, D., Rockway, T., and Fesik, S. W. Identification of novel inhibitors of urokinase via NMR-based screening. *J. Med. Chem.* 2000, *43(21)*, 3862–3866.

134. Patterson, A. W., Wood, W. J. L., Hornsby, M., Lesley, S., Spraggon, G., and Ellman, J. A. Identification of selective, nonpeptidic nitrile inhibitors of cathepsin S using the substrate activity screening method. *J. Med. Chem.* 2006, *49(21)*, 6298–6307.

135. Inagaki, H., Tsuruoka, H., Hornsby, M., Lesley, S. A., Spraggon, G., and Ellman, J. A. Characterization and optimization of selective, nonpeptidic inhibitors of cathepsin S with an unprecedented binding mode. *J. Med. Chem.* 2007, *50(11)*, 2693–2699.

136. Allen, D. A., Pham, P., Choong, I. C., Fahr, B., Burdett, M. T., Lew, W., DeLano, W. L., Gordon, E. M., Lam, J. W., O'Brien, T., and Lee, D. Identification of potent and novel small-molecule inhibitors of caspase-3. *Bioorg. Med. Chem. Lett.* 2003, *13(21)*, 3651–3655.

137. (a) Schneider, G., and Fechner, U. Computer-based *de novo* design of drug-like molecules. *Nat. Rev. Drug Discov.* 2005, *4(8)*, 649–663; (b) Honma, T. Recent advances in *de novo* design strategy for practical lead identification. *Med. Res. Rev.* 2003, *23(5)*, 606–632; (c) Böhm, H.-J. Current computational tools for *de novo* ligand design. *Curr. Opin. Biotechnol.* 1996, *7(4)*, 433–436; (d) Bohacek, R. S. and McMartin, C. Modern computational chemistry and drug discovery: structure generating programs. *Curr. Opin. Chem. Biol.* 1997, *1(2)*, 157–161.

138. (a) Danziger, D. J. and Dean, P. M. Automated site-directed drug design: a general algorithm for knowledge acquisition about hydrogen-bonding regions at protein surfaces. *Proc. R. Soc. Lond. B Biol. Sci.* 1989, *236(1283)*, 101–113; (b) Danziger, D. J. and Dean, P. M. Automated site-directed drug design: the prediction and observation of ligand point positions at hydrogen-bonding regions on protein surfaces. *Proc. R. Soc. Lond. B Biol. Sci.* 1989, *236(1283)*, 115–124; (c) Lewis, R. A. and Dean, P. M. Automated site-directed drug design: the concept of spacer skeletons for primary structure generation. *Proc. R. Soc. Lond. B Biol. Sci.* 1989, *236(1283)*, 125–140; (d) Lewis, R. A. and Dean, P. M. Automated site-directed drug design: the formation of molecular templates in primary structure generation. *Proc. R. Soc. Lond. B Biol. Sci.* 1989, *236(1283)*, 141–162.

139. Gillet, V. J., Johnson, A. P., Mata, P., and Sike, S. Automated structure design in 3D. *Tetrahedron Comput. Methodol.* 1990, *3(6)*, 681–696.

140. (a) Nishibata, Y. and Itai, A. Automatic creation of drug candidate structures based on receptor structure. Starting point for artificial lead generation. *Tetrahedron* 1991, *47(43)*, 8985–8990; (b) Nishibata, Y. and Itai, A. Confirmation of usefulness of a structure construction program based on three-dimensional receptor structure for rational lead generation. *J. Med. Chem.* 1993, *36(20)*, 2921–2928.

141. (a) Böhm, H.-J. The computer program LUDI: a new method for the *de novo* design of enzyme inhibitors. *J. Comput. Aided Mol. Des.* 1992, *6(1)*, 61–78; (b) Böhm, H.-J. LUDI: rule-based automatic design of new substituents for enzyme inhibitor leads. *J. Comput.-Aided Mol. Des.* 1992, *6(6)*, 593–606; (c) Böhm, H.-J. Towards the automatic design of synthetically accessible protein ligands: peptides, amides and peptidomimetics. *J. Comput. Aided Mol. Des.* 1996, *10(4)*, 265–272.

142. Rotstein, S. H. and Murcko, M. A. GenStar: a method for *de novo* drug design. *J. Comput. Aided Mol. Des.* 1993, *7(1)*, 23–43.

143. Rotstein, S. H. and Murcko, M. A. GroupBuild: a fragment-based method for *de novo* drug design. *J. Med. Chem.* 1993, *36(12)*, 1700–1710.

144. (a) Gillet, V., Johnson, A. P., Mata, P., Sike, S., and Williams, P. SPROUT: a program for structure generation. *J. Comput. Aided Mol. Des.* 1993, *7(2)*, 127–153; (b) Gillet, V. J., Newell, W., Mata, P., Myatt, G., Sike, S., Zsoldos, Z., and Johnson, A. P. SPROUT: recent developments in the *de novo* design of molecules. *J. Chem. Inf. Comput. Sci.* 1994, *34(1)*, 207–217; (c) Mata, P., Gillet, V. J., Johnson, A. P., Lampreia, J., Myatt, G. J., Sike, S., and Stebbings, A. L. SPROUT: 3D Structure Generation Using Templates. *J. Chem. Inf. Comput. Sci.* 1995, *35(3)*, 479–493.

145. Bohacek, R. S. and McMartin, C. Multiple highly diverse structures complementary to enzyme binding sites: results of extensive application of a *de novo* design method incorporating combinatorial growth. *J. Am. Chem. Soc.* 1994, *116(13)*, 5560–5571.

146. (a) Clark, D. E., Frenkel, D., Levy, S. A., Li, J., Murray, C. W., Robson, B., Waszkowycz, B., and Westhead, D. R. PRO-LIGAND: an approach to *de novo* molecular design. 1. Application to the design of organic molecules. *J. Comput. Aided Mol. Des.* 1995, *9(1)*,

13–32; (b) Waszkowycz, B., Clark, D. E., Frenkel, D., Li, J., Murray, C. W., Robson, B., and Westhead, D. R. PRO_LIGAND: an approach to *de novo* molecular design. 2. Design of novel molecules from molecular field analysis (MFA) models and pharmacophores. *J. Med. Chem.* 1994, *37(23)*, 3994–4002; (c) Westhead, D. R., Clark, D. E., Frenkel, D., Li, J., Murray, C. W., Robson, B., and Waszkowycz, B. PRO-LIGAND: an approach to *de novo* molecular design. 3. A genetic algorithm for structure refinement. *J. Comput. Aided Mol. Des.* 1995, *9(2)*, 139–148; (d) Frenkel, D., Clark, D. E., Li, J., Murray, C. W., Robson, B., Waszkowycz, B., and Westhead, D. R. PRO_LIGAND: an approach to *de novo* molecular design. 4. Application to the design of peptides. *J. Comput. Aided Mol. Des.* 1995, *9(3)*, 213–225; (e) Clark, D. E. and Murray, C. W. PRO_LIGAND: an approach to *de novo* molecular design. 5. Tools for the analysis of generated structures. *J. Chem. Inf. Comput. Sci.* 1995, *35(5)*, 914–923; (f) Murray, C. W., Clark, D. E., and Byrne, D. G. PRO_LIGAND: an approach to *de novo* molecular design. 6. Flexible fitting in the design of peptides. *J. Comput. Aided Mol. Des.* 1995, *9(5)*, 381–395.

147. (a) DeWitte, R. S. and Shakhnovich, E. I. SMoG: *de novo* design method based on simple, fast, and accurate free energy estimates. 1. Methodology and supporting evidence. *J. Am. Chem. Soc.* 1996, *118(47)*, 11733–11744; (b) DeWitte, R. S., Ishchenko, A. V., and Shakhnovich, E. I. SMoG: *de novo* design method based on simple, fast, and accurate free energy estimates. 2. Case studies in molecular design. *J. Am. Chem. Soc.* 1997, *119(20)*, 4608–4617; (c) Ishchenko, A. V. and Shakhnovich, E. I. SMall Molecule Growth 2001 (SMoG2001): an improved knowledge-based scoring function for protein–ligand interactions. *J. Med. Chem.* 2002, *45(13)*, 2770–2780; (d) Grzybowski, B. A., Ishchenko, A. V., Kim, C.-Y., Topalov, G., Chapman, R., Christianson, D. W., Whitesides, G. M., and Shakhnovich, E. I. Combinatorial computational method gives new picomolar ligands for a known enzyme. *Proc. Natl. Acad. Sci. USA* 2002, *99(3)*, 1270–1273; (e) Grzybowski, B. A., Ishchenko, A. V., Shimada, J., and Shakhnovich, E. I. From knowledge-based potentials to combinatorial lead design *in silico*. *Acc. Chem. Res.* 2002, *35(5)*, 261–269.

148. Luo, Z., Wang, R., and Lai, L. RASSE: a new method for structure-based drug design. *J. Chem. Inf. Comput. Sci.* 1996, *36(6)*, 1187–1194.

149. (a) Murray, C. W., Clark, D. E., Auton, T. R., Firth, M. A., Li, J., Sykes, R. A., Waszkowycz, B., Westhead, D. R., and Young, S. C. PRO_SELECT: combining structure-based drug design and combinatorial chemistry for rapid lead discovery. 1. Technology. *J. Comput. Aided Mol. Des.* 1997, *11(2)*, 193–207; (b) Eldridge, M. D., Murray, C. W., Auton, T. R., Paolini, G. V., and Mee, R. P. Empirical scoring functions: I. The development of a fast empirical scoring function to estimate the binding affinity of ligands in receptor complexes. *J. Comput. Aided Mol. Des.* 1997, *11(5)*, 425–445; (c) Murray, C. W., Auton, T. R., and Eldridge, M. D. Empirical scoring functions. II. The testing of an empirical scoring function for the prediction of ligand-receptor binding affinities and the use of Bayesian regression to improve the quality of the model. *J. Comput. Aided Mol. Des.* 1998, *12(5)*, 503–519; (d) Liebeschuetz, J. W., Jones, S. D., Morgan, P. J., Murray, C. W., Rimmer, A. D., Roscoe, J. M. E., Waszkowycz, B., Welsh, P. M., Wylie, W. A., Young, S. C., Martin, H., Mahler, J., Brady, L., and Wilkinson, K. PROSELECT: combining structure-based drug design and array-based chemistry for rapid lead discovery. 2. The development of a series of highly potent and selective factor Xa inhibitors. *J. Med. Chem.* 2002, *45(6)*, 1221–1232.

150. Wang, R., Gao, Y., and Lai, L. LigBuilder: a multi-purpose program for structure-based drug design. *J. Mol. Model.* 2000, *6(7–8)*, 498–516.

151. Pierce, A. C., Rao, G., and Bemis, G. W. BREED: Generating novel inhibitors through hybridization of known ligands. Application to CDK2, p38, and HIV protease. *J. Med. Chem.* 2004, *47(11)*, 2768–2775.

152. Moon, J. B. and Howe, W. J. Computer design of bioactive molecules: a method for receptor-based *de novo* ligand design. *Proteins* 1991, *11(4)*, 314–328.

153. LeapFrog, *SYBYL version 8.1*, Tripos, Inc., St. Louis, MO, Available at http://www.tripos.com.

154. Pellegrini, E. and Field, M. J. Development and testing of a *de novo* drug-design algorithm. *J. Comput. Aided Mol. Des.* 2003, *17(10)*, 621–641.

155. Jorgensen, W. L. Efficient drug lead discovery and optimization. *Acc. Chem. Res.* 2009, *42(6)*, 724–733.

156. Tschinke, V. and Cohen, N. C. The NEWLEAD program: a new method for the design of candidate structures from pharmacophoric hypotheses. *J. Med. Chem.* 1993, *36(24)*, 3863–3870.

157. (a) Ho, C. M. W. and Marshall, G. R. Cavity search: an algorithm for the isolation and display of cavity-like binding regions. *J. Comput. Aided Mol. Des.* 1990, *4(4)*, 337–354; (b) Ho, C. M. W. and Marshall, G. R. SPLICE: a program to assemble partial query solutions from three-dimensional database searches into novel ligands. *J. Comput. Aided Mol. Des.* 1993, *7(6)*, 623–647; (c) Ho, C. M. W. and Marshall, G. R. DBMAKER: a set of programs to generate three-dimensional databases based upon user-specified criteria. *J. Comput. Aided Mol. Des.* 1995, *9(1)*, 65–86.

158. Eisen, M. B., Wiley, D. C., Karplus, M., and Hubbard, R. E. HOOK: a program for finding novel molecular architectures that satisfy the chemical and steric requirements of a macromolecule binding site. *Proteins* 1994, *19(3)*, 199–221.

159. Lauri, G. and Bartlett, P. A. CAVEAT: a program to facilitate the design of organic molecules. *J. Comput. Aided Mol. Des.* 1994, *8(1)*, 51–66.

160. Aronov, A. M. and Bemis, G. W. A minimalist approach to fragment-based ligand design using common rings and linkers: application to kinase inhibitors. *Proteins* 2004, *57(1)*, 36–50.

161. (a) Caflisch, A. Computational combinatorial ligand design: application to human α-thrombin. *J. Comput. Aided Mol. Des.* 1996, *10(5)*, 372–396; (b) Majeux, N., Scarsi, M., Apostolakis, J., Ehrhardt, C., and Caflisch, A. Exhaustive docking of molecular fragments with electrostatic solvation. *Proteins* 1999, *37(1)*, 88–105; (c) Majeux, N., Scarsi, M., Tenette-Souaille, C., and Caflisch, A. Hydrophobicity maps and docking of molecular fragments with solvation. *Perspect. Drug Discov. Des.* 2000, *20*, 145–169; (d) Majeux, N., Scarsi, M., and Caflisch, A. Efficient electrostatic solvation model for protein-fragment docking. *Proteins* 2001, *42(2)*, 256–268.

162. Degen, J. and Rarey, M. FlexNovo: structure-based searching in large fragment spaces. *ChemMedChem* 2006, *1(8)*, 854–868.

163. (a) Fechner, U. and Schneider, G. Flux (1): a virtual synthesis scheme for fragment-based *de novo* design. *J. Chem. Inf. Model.* 2006, *46(2)*, 699–707; (b) Fechner, U. and Schneider, G. Flux (2): comparison of molecular mutation and crossover operators for ligand-based *de novo* design. *J. Chem. Inf. Model.* 2007, *47(2)*, 656–667; (c) Schüller, A., Suhartono, M., Fechner, U., Tanrikulu, Y., Breitung, S., Scheffer, U., Göbel, M. W., and Schneider, G. The concept of template-based *de novo* design from drug-derived molecular fragments and its application to TAR RNA. *J. Comput. Aided Mol. Des.* 2008, *22(2)*, 59–68.

164. Dey, F. and Caflisch, A. Fragment-based *de novo* ligand design by multiobjective evolutionary optimization. *J. Chem. Inf. Model.* 2008, *48(3)*, 679–690.

165. Lewis, R. A. Automated site-directed drug design: approaches to the formation of 3D molecular graphs. *J. Comput. Aided Mol. Des.* 1990, *4(2)*, 205–210.

166. (a) Lewis, R. A., Roe, D. C., Huang, C., Ferrin, T. E., Langridge, R., and Kuntz, I. D. Automated site-directed drug design using molecular lattices. *J. Mol. Graph.* 1992, *10(2)*, 66–78, 106; (b) Roe, D. C. and Kuntz, I. D. BUILDER v.2: improving the chemistry of a *de novo* design strategy. *J. Comput. Aided Mol. Des.* 1995, *9(3)*, 269–282.

167. Gehlhaar, D. K., Moerder, K. E., Zichi, D., Sherman, C. J., Ogden, R. C., and Freer, S. T. *De novo* design of enzyme inhibitors by Monte Carlo ligand generation. *J. Med. Chem.* 1995, *38(3)*, 466–472.

168. (a) Miranker, A. and Karplus, M. An automated method for dynamic ligand design. *Proteins* 1995, *23(4)*, 472–490; (b) Stultz, C. M. and Karplus, M. Dynamic ligand design and combinatorial optimization: designing inhibitors to endothiapepsin. *Proteins* 2000, *40(2)*, 258–289.

169. (a) Todorov, N. P. and Dean, P. M. Evaluation of a method for controlling molecular scaffold diversity in *de novo* ligand design. *J. Comput. Aided Mol. Des.* 1997, *11(2)*, 175–192; (b) Todorov, N. P. and Dean, P. M. A branch-and-bound method for optimal atom-type assignment in *de novo* ligand design. *J. Comput. Aided Mol. Des.* 1998, *12(4)*, 335–349; (c) Stahl, M., Todorov, N. P., James, T., Mauser, H., Boehm, H.-J, and Dean, P. M. A validation study on the practical use of automated *de novo* design. *J. Comput. Aided Mol. Des.* 2002, *16(7)*, 459–478.

170. Pegg, S. C.-H., Haresco, J. J., and Kuntz, I. D. A genetic algorithm for structure-based *de novo* design. *J. Comput. Aided Mol. Des.* 2001, *15(10)*, 911–933.

171. Lawrence, M. C. and Davis, P. C. CLIX: a search algorithm for finding novel ligands capable of binding proteins of known three-dimensional structure. *Proteins* 1992, *12(1)*, 31–41.

172. Glen, R. C. and Payne, A. W. R. A genetic algorithm for the automated generation of molecules within constraints. *J. Comput. Aided Mol. Des.* 1995, *9(2)*, 181–202.

173. Pearlman, D. A. and Murcko, M. A. CONCEPTS: new dynamic algorithm for *de novo* drug suggestion. *J. Comput. Chem.* 1993, *14(10)*, 1184–1193.

174. Pearlman, D. A. and Murcko, M. A. CONCERTS: dynamic connection of fragments as an approach to *de novo* ligand design. *J. Med. Chem.* 1996, *39(8)*, 1651–1663.

175. (a) Liu, H., Duan, Z., Luo, Q., and Shi, Y. Structure-based ligand design by dynamically assembling molecular building blocks at binding site. *Proteins* 1999, *36(4)*, 462–470; (b) Zhu, J., Yu, H., Fan, H., Liu, H., and Shi Y. Design of new selective inhibitors of cyclooxygenase-2 by dynamic assembly of molecular building blocks. *J. Comput. Aided Mol. Des.* 2001, *15(5)*, 447–463.

176. Zhu, J., Fan, H., Liu, H., and Shi, Y. Structure-based ligand design for flexible proteins: application of new F-DycoBlock. *J. Comput. Aided Mol. Des.* 2001, *15(11)*, 979–996.

177. Nachbar, R. B. Molecular evolution: automated manipulation of hierarchical chemical topology and its application to average molecular structures. *Genet. Program. Evolv. Mach.* 2000, *1*, 57–94.

178. Globus, A., Lawton, J., and Wipke, T. Automatic molecular design using evolutionary techniques. *Nanotechnology* 1999, *10(3)*, 290–299.

179. (a) Schneider, G., Clément-Chomienne, O., Hilfiger, L., Schneider, P., Kirsch, S., Böhm, H.-J., and Neidhart, W. Virtual screening for bioactive molecules by evolutionary *de novo* design. *Angew. Chem. Int. Ed. Engl.* 2000, *39(22)*, 4130–4133; (b) Schneider, G., Lee, M.-L., Stahl, M., and Schneider, P. *De novo* design of molecular architectures by evolutionary assembly of drug-derived building blocks. *J. Comput. Aided Mol. Des.* 2000, *14(5)*, 487–494; (c) Alig, L., Alsenz, J., Andjelkovic, M., Bendels, S., Bénardeau, A., Bleicher, K., Bourson, A., David-Pierson, P., Guba, W., Hildbrand, S., Kube, D., Lübbers, T., Mayweg, A. V., Narquizian, R., Neidhart, W., Nettekoven, M., Plancher, J.-M., Rocha, C., Rogers-Evans, M., Röver, S., Schneider, G., Taylor, S., and Waldmeier, P. Benzodioxoles: novel cannabinoid-1 receptor inverse agonists for the treatment of obesity. *J. Med. Chem.* 2008, *51(7)*, 2115–2127.

180. Brown, N., McKay, B., Gilardoni, F., and Gasteiger, J. A graph-based genetic algorithm and its application to the multiobjective evolution of median molecules. *J. Chem. Inf. Comput. Sci.* 2004, *44(3)*, 1079–1087.

181. (a) Douguet, D., Thoreau, E., and Grassy, G. A genetic algorithm for the automated generation of small organic molecules: drug design using an evolutionary algorithm. *J. Comput. Aided Mol. Des.* 2000, *14(5)*, 449–466; (b) Douguet, D., Munier-Lehmann, H., Labesse, G., and Pochet, S. LEA3D: a computer-aided ligand design for structure-based drug design. *J. Med. Chem.* 2005, *48(7)*, 2457–2468.

182. Vinkers, H. M., de Jonge, M. R., Daeyaert, F. F. D., Heeres, J., Koymans, L. M. H., van Lenthe, J. H., Lewi, P. J., Timmerman, H., Van Aken, K., and Janssen, P. A. SYNOPSIS: SYNthesize and OPtimize System *in Silico*. *J. Med. Chem.* 2003, *46(13)*, 2765–2773.

183. (a) Boda, K., Seidel, T., and Gasteiger, J. Structure and reaction based evaluation of synthetic accessibility. *J. Comput. Aided Mol. Des.* 2007, *21(6)*, 311–325; (b) Baber, J. C., and Feher, M. Predicting synthetic accessibility: application in drug discovery and development. *Mini. Rev. Med. Chem.* 2004, *4(6)*, 681–692.

184. (a) Jorgensen, W. L. The many roles of computation in drug discovery. *Science* 2004, *303 (5665)*, 1813–1818; (b) Shoichet, B. K. Virtual screening of chemical libraries. *Nature* 2004, *432(7019)*, 862–865.

185. Gillet, V. J., Myatt, G., Zsoldos, Z., and Johnson, A. P. SPOUT, HIPPO and CAESA: tools for de novo structure generation and estimation of synthetic accessibility. *Perspect. Drug Discov. Des.* 1995, *3*, 34–50.

186. (a) Honma, T., Hayashi, K., Aoyama, T., Hashimoto, N., Machida, T., Fukasawa, K., Iwama, T., Ikeura, C., Ikuta, M., Suzuki-Takahashi, I., Iwasawa, Y., Hayama, T., Nishimura, S., and Morishima, H. Structure-based generation of a new class of potent Cdk4 inhibitors: new *de novo* design strategy and library design. *J. Med. Chem.* 2001, *44 (26)*, 4615–4627; (b) Honma, T., Yoshizumi, T., Hashimoto, N., Hayashi, K., Kawanishi, N., Fukasawa, K., Takaki, T., Ikeura, C., Ikuta, M., Suzuki-Takahashi, I., Hayama, T., Nishimura, S., and Morishima, H. A novel approach for the development of selective Cdk4 inhibitors: library design based on locations of Cdk4 specific amino acid residues. *J. Med. Chem.* 2001, *44(26)*, 4628–4640.

187. Lewell, X. Q., Judd, D. B., Watson, S. P., and Hann, M. M. RECAP—retrosynthetic combinatorial analysis procedure: a powerful new technique for identifying privileged molecular fragments with useful applications in combinatorial chemistry. *J. Chem. Inf. Comput. Sci.* 1998, *38(3)*, 511–522.

188. (a) Leach, A. R., Shoichet, B. K., and Peishoff, C. E. Prediction of protein–ligand interactions. Docking and scoring: successes and gaps. *J. Med. Chem.* 2006, *49(20)*, 5851–5855; (b) Gohlke, H. and Klebe, G. Approaches to the description and prediction of the binding affinity of small-molecule ligands to macromolecular receptors. *Angew. Chem. Int. Ed. Engl.* 2002, *41(15)*, 2644–2676.

189. (a) Kollman, P. A., Massova, I., Reyes, C., Kuhn, B., Huo, S., Chong, L., Lee, M., Lee, T., Duan, Y., Wang, W., Donini, O., Cieplak, P., Srinivasan, J., Case, D. A., and Cheatham, T. E. III., Calculating structures and free energies of complex molecules: combining molecular mechanics and continuum models. *Acc. Chem. Res.* 2000, *33(12)*, 889–897; (b) Jorgensen, W. L. and Thomas, L. L. Perspective on free-energy perturbation calculations for chemical equilibria. *J. Chem. Theory Comput.* 2008, *4(6)*, 869–876.

190. (a) Jorgensen, W. L. and Tirado-Rives, J. Molecular modeling of organic and biomolecular systems using BOSS and MCPRO. *J. Comput. Chem.* 2005, *26(16)*, 1689–1700; (b) Clark, M., Guarnieri, F., Shkurko, I., and Wiseman, J. Grand canonical Monte Carlo simulation of ligand–protein binding. *J. Chem. Inf. Model.* 2007, *46(1)*, 231–242.

191. (a) Åqvist, J., Medina, C., and Samuelsson, J.-E. A new method for predicting binding affinity in computer-aided drug design. *Protein Eng.* 1994, *7(3)*, 385–391; (b) Hansson T, Marelius J, and Åqvist J. Ligand binding affinity prediction by linear interaction energy methods. *J. Comput. Aided Mol. Des.* 1998, *12(1)*, 27–35.

192. (a) Kuhn, B. and Kollman, P. A. Binding of a diverse set of ligands to avidin and streptavidin: an accurate quantitative prediction of their relative affinities by a combination of molecular mechanics and continuum solvent models. *J. Med. Chem.* 2000, *43(20)*, 3786–3791; (b) Pearlman, D. A. Evaluating the molecular mechanics Poisson–Boltzmann surface area free energy method using a congeneric series of ligands to p38 MAP kinase. *J. Med. Chem.* 2005, *48(24)*, 7796–7807; (c) Barreiro, G., Guimarães, C. R. W., Tubert-Brohman, I., Lyons, T. M., Tirado-Rives, J., and Jorgensen, W. L. Search for non-nucleoside inhibitors of HIV-1 reverse transcriptase using chemical similarity, molecular docking, and MM-GB/SA scoring. *J. Chem. Inf. Model.* 2007, *47(6)*, 2416–2428.

193. Marcou, G. and Rognan, D. Optimizing fragment and scaffold docking by use of molecular interaction fingerprints. *J. Chem. Inf. Model.* 2007, *47(1)*, 195–207.

194. (a) Chen, Y. and Shoichet, B. K. Molecular docking and ligand specificity in fragment-based inhibitor discovery. *Nat. Chem. Biol.* 2009, *5(5)*, 358–364; (b) Teotico, D. G., Babaoglu, K., Rocklin, G. J., Ferreira, R. S., Giannetti, A. M., and Shoichet, B. K. Docking for fragment inhibitors of AmpC β-lactamase. *Proc. Natl. Acad. Sci. USA* 2009, *106(18)*, 7455–7460.

195. (a) Böhm, H.-J., Flohr, A., and Stahl, M. Scaffold hopping. *Drug Discov. Today Technol.* 2004, *1(3)*, 217–224; (b) Brown, N. and Jacoby, E. On scaffolds and hopping in medicinal chemistry. *Mini. Rev. Med. Chem.* 2006, *6(11)*, 1217–1229; (c) Mauser, H. and Guba, W. Recent developments in *de novo* design and scaffold hopping. *Curr. Opin. Drug Discov. Devel.* 2008, *11(3)*, 365–374; (d) Krueger, B. A., Dietrich, A., Baringhaus, K. H., and Schneider, G. Scaffold-hopping potential of fragment-based *de novo* design: the chances and limits of variation. *Comb. Chem. High Throughput Screen.* 2009. *12(4)*, 383–396.

196. (a) Schneider, G., Schneider, P., and Renner, S. Scaffold-hopping: how far can you jump? *QSAR Comb. Sci.* 2006, *25(12)*, 1162–1171; (b) Tsuchida, K., Chaki, H., Takakura, T., Kotsubo, H., Tanaka, T., Aikawa, Y., Shiozawa, S., and Hirono, S. Discovery of

nonpeptidic small-molecule AP-1 inhibitors: lead hopping based on a three-dimensional pharmacophore model. *J. Med. Chem.* 2006, *49(1)*, 80–91.

197. (a) Takahashi, Y., Sukekawa, M., and Sasaki, S.-i. Automatic identification of molecular similarity using reduced-graph representation of chemical structure. *J. Chem. Inf. Comput. Sci.* 1992, *32(6)*, 639–643; (b) Gillet, V. J., Willett, P., and Bradshaw, J. Similarity searching using reduced graphs. *J. Chem. Inf. Comput. Sci.* 2003, *43(2)*, 338–345; (c) Barker, E. J., Gardiner, E. J., Gillet, V. J., Kitts, P., and Morris, J. Further development of reduced graphs for identifying bioactive compounds. *J. Chem. Inf. Comput. Sci.* 2003, *43(2)*, 346–356.

198. Cramer, R. D. Leadhopping—and beyond. *Expert Opin. Drug Discov.* 2006, *1(4)*, 311–321.

199. (a) Schneider, G., Neidhart, W., Giller, T., and Schmid, G. "Scaffold-Hopping" by topological pharmacophore search: a contribution to virtual screening. *Angew. Chem. Int. Ed. Engl.* 1999, *38(19)*, 2894–2896; (b) Renner, S., Noeske, T., Parsons, C. G., Schneider, P., Weil, T., and Schneider, G. New allosteric modulators of metabotropic glutamate receptor 5 (mGluR5) found by ligand-based virtual screening. *ChemBioChem* 2005, *6(4)*, 620–625; (c) Renner, S., Ludwig, V., Boden, O., Scheffer, U., Göbel, M., and Schneider, G. New inhibitors of the Tat-TAR RNA interaction found with a "fuzzy" pharmacophore model. *ChemBioChem* 2005, *6(6)*, 1119–1125; (d) Renner, S. and Schneider, G. Scaffold-hopping potential of ligand-based similarity concepts. *ChemMedChem* 2006, *1(2)*, 181–185; (e) Renner, S., Schwab, C. H., Gasteiger, J., and Schneider, G. Impact of conformational flexibility on three-dimensional similarity searching using correlation vectors. *J. Chem. Inf. Model.* 2006, *46(6)*, 2324–2332; (f) Franke, L., Schwarz, O., Müller-Kuhrt, L., Hoernig, C., Fischer, L., George, S., Tanrikulu, Y., Schneider, P., Werz, O., and Steinhilber, D., Schneider, G. Identification of natural-product-derived inhibitors of 5-lipoxygenase activity by ligand-based virtual screening. *J. Med. Chem.* 2007, *50(11)*, 2640–2646.

200. Hofmann, B., Franke, L., Proschak, E., Tanrikulu, Y., Schneider, P., Steinhilber, D., and Schneider, G. Scaffold-hopping cascade yields potent inhibitors of 5-lipoxygenase. *ChemMedChem* 2008, *3(10)*, 1535–1538.

201. Jenkins, J. L., Glick, M., and Davies, J. W. A 3D similarity method for scaffold hopping from known drugs or natural ligands to new chemotypes. *J. Med. Chem.* 2004, *47(25)*, 6144–6159.

202. Schuffenhauer, A., Floersheim, P., Acklin, P., and Jacoby, E. Similarity metrics for ligands reflecting the similarity of the target proteins. *J. Chem. Inf. Comput. Sci.* 2003, *43(2)*, 391–405.

203. Renner, S. and Schneider, G. Fuzzy pharmacophore models from molecular alignments for correlation-vector-based virtual screening. *J. Med. Chem.* 2004, *47 (19)*, 4653–4664.

204. (a) Tanrikulu, Y., Nietert, M., Scheffer, U., Proschak, E., Grabowski, K., Schneider, P., Weidlich, M., Karas, M., Göbel, M., and Schneider, G. Scaffold hopping by "fuzzy" pharmacophores and its application to RNA targets. *ChemBioChem* 2007 *8(16)*, 1932–1936; (b) Tanrikulu, Y., Rau, O., Schwarz, O., Proschak, E., Siems, K., Müller-Kuhrt, L., Schubert-Zsilavecz, M., and Schneider, G. Structure-based pharmacophore screening for natural-product-derived PPARγ agonists. *ChemBioChem* 2009, *10(1)*, 75–78.

205. Barker, E. J., Buttar, D., Cosgrove, D. A., Gardiner, E. J., Kitts, P., Willett, P., and Gillet, V. J. Scaffold hopping using clique detection applied to reduced graphs. *J. Chem. Inf. Model.* 2006, *46(2)*, 503–511.

206. Stiefl, N., Watson, I. A., Baumann, K., and Zaliani, A. ErG: 2D pharmacophore descriptions for scaffold hopping. *J. Chem. Inf. Model.* 2006, *46(1)*, 208–220.

207. Bohl, M., Loeprecht, B., Wendt, B., Heritage, T., Richmond, N. J., and Willett, P. Unsupervised 3D ring template searching as an ideas generator for scaffold hopping: use of the LAMDA, RigFit, and field-based similarity search (FBSS) methods. *J. Chem. Inf. Model.* 2006, *46(5)*, 1882–1890.

208. Wolohan, P. R. N., Akella, L. B., Dorfman, R. J., Nell, P. G., Mundt, S. M., and Clark, R. D. Structural unit analysis identifies lead series and facilitates scaffold hopping in combinatorial chemistry. *J. Chem. Inf. Model.* 2006, *46(3)*, 1188–1193.

209. Maass, P., Schulz-Gasch, T., Stahl, M., and Rarey, M. Recore: a fast and versatile method for scaffold hopping based on small molecule crystal structure conformations. *J. Chem. Inf. Model.* 2007, *47(2)*, 390–399.

210. Ahlström, M. M., Ridderström, M., Luthman, K., and Zamora, I. Virtual screening and scaffold hopping based on GRID molecular interaction fields. *J. Chem. Inf. Model.* 2005, *45(5)*, 1313–1323.

211. Bender, A., Mussa, H. Y., Gill, G. S., and Glen, R. C. Molecular surface point environments for virtual screening and the elucidation of binding patterns (MOLPRINT 3D). *J. Med. Chem.* 2004, *47(26)*, 6569–6583.

212. Baroni, M., Cruciani, G., Sciabola, S., Perruccio, F., and Mason, J. S. A common reference framework for analyzing/comparing proteins and ligands. Fingerprints for Ligands and Proteins (FLAP): theory and application. *J. Chem. Inf. Model.* 2007, *47(2)*, 279–294.

213. (a) Bergmann, R., Linusson, A., and Zamora, I. SHOP: scaffold HOPping by GRID-based similarity searches. *J. Med. Chem.* 2007, *50(11)*, 2708–2717; (b) Fontaine, F., Cross, S., Plasencia, G., Pastor, M., and Zamora, I. SHOP: a method for structure-based fragment and scaffold hopping. *ChemMedChem* 2009, *4(3)*, 427–439; (c) Bergmann, R., Liljefors, T., Sørensen, M. D., and Zamora, I. SHOP: receptor-based scaffold HOPping by GRID-based similarity searches. *J. Chem. Inf. Model.* 2009, *49(3)*, 658–669.

214. (a) Rush, T. S. III, Grant, J. A., Mosyak, L., and Nicholls, A. A shape-based 3-D scaffold hopping method and its application to a bacterial protein–protein interaction. *J. Med. Chem.* 2005, *48(5)*, 1489–1495; (b) Kirchmair, J., Ristic, S., Eder, K., Markt, P., Wolber, G., Laggner, C., and Langer, T. Fast and efficient *in silico* 3D screening: toward maximum computational efficiency of pharmacophore-based and shape-based approaches. *J. Chem. Inf. Model.* 2007, *47(6)*, 2182–2196; (c) Oyarzabal, J., Howe, T., Alcazar, J., Andrés, J. I., Alvarez, R. M., Dautzenberg, F., Iturrino, L., Martínez, S., and Van der Linden, I. Novel approach for chemotype hopping based on annotated databases of chemically feasible fragments and a prospective case study: new melanin concentrating hormone antagonists. *J. Med. Chem.* 2009, *52(7)*, 2076–2089.

215. (a) Cheeseright, T., Mackey, M., Rose, S., and Vinter, A. molecular field extrema as descriptors of biological activity: definition and validation. *J. Chem. Inf. Model.* 2006, *46 (2)*, 665–676; (b) Cheeseright, T. J., Mackey, M. D., Melville, J. L., and Vinter, J. G. FieldScreen: virtual screening using molecular fields. Application to the DUD data set. *J. Chem. Inf. Model.* 2008, *48(11)*, 2108–2117.

216. (a) Kalindjian, S. B., Buck, I. M., Davies, J. M. R., Dunstone, D. J., Hudson, M. L., Low, C. M. R., McDonald, I. M., Pether, M. J., Steel, K. I., Tozer, M. J., and Vinter, J. G. Non-peptide cholecystokinin-B/gastrin receptor antagonists based on bicyclic, heteroaromatic skeletons. *J. Med. Chem.* 1996, *39(9)*, 1806–1815; (b) Low, C. M. R., Buck, I. M., Cooke,

T., Cushnir, J. R., Kalindjian, S. B., Kotecha, A., Pether, M. J., Shankley, N. P., Vinter, J. G., and Wright, L. Scaffold hopping with molecular field points: identification of a cholecystokinin-2 (CCK2) receptor pharmacophore and its use in the design of a prototypical series of pyrrole- and imidazole-based CCK2 antagonists. *J. Med. Chem.* 2005, *48(22)*, 6790–6802.

217. (a) Wild, D. J. and Willett, P. Similarity searching in files of three-dimensional chemical structures. Alignment of molecular electrostatic potential fields with a genetic algorithm. *J. Chem. Inf. Comput. Sci.* 1996, *36(2)*, 159–167; (b) Thorner, D. A., Wild, D. J., Willett, P., and Wright, P. M. Similarity searching in files of three-dimensional chemical structures: flexible field-based searching of molecular electrostatic potentials. *J. Chem. Inf. Comput. Sci.* 1996, *36(4)*, 900–908; (c) Schuffenhauer, A., Gillet, V. J., and Willett, P. Similarity searching in files of three-dimensional chemical structures: analysis of the BIOSTER database using two-dimensional fingerprints and molecular field descriptors. *J. Chem. Inf. Comput. Sci.* 2000, *40(2)*, 295–307; (d) Bohl, M., Dunbar, J., Gifford, E. M., Heritage, T., Wild, D. J., Willett, P., and Wilton, D. J. Scaffold searching: automated identification of similar ring systems for the design of combinatorial libraries. *Quant. Struct. Act. Relat.* 2002, *21(6)*, 590–597.

218. Jain, A. N. Ligand-based structural hypotheses for virtual screening. *J. Med. Chem.* 2004, *47(4)*, 947–961.

219. (a) Cramer, R. D., Patterson, D. E., Clark, R. D., Soltanshahi, F., and Lawless, M. S. Virtual compound libraries: a new approach to decision making in molecular discovery research. *J. Chem. Inf. Comput. Sci.* 1998, *38(6)*, 1010–1023; (b) Cramer, R. D., Poss, M. A., Hermsmeier, M. A., Caulfield, T. J., Kowala, M. C., and Valentine, M. T. Prospective identification of biologically active structures by topomer shape similarity searching. *J. Med. Chem.* 1999, *42(19)*, 3919–3933; (c) Andrews, K. M. and Cramer, R. D. Toward general methods of targeted library design: topomer shape similarity searching with diverse structures as queries. *J. Med. Chem.* 2000, *43(9)*, 1723–1740; (d) Jilek, R. J. and Cramer, R. D. Topomers: a validated protocol for their self-consistent generation. *J. Chem. Inf. Comput. Sci.* 2004, *44(4)*, 1221–1227; (e) Cramer, R. D., Jilek, R. J., Guessregen, S., Clark, S. J., Wendt, B., and Clark, R. D. "Lead hopping". Validation of topomer similarity as a superior predictor of similar biological activities. *J. Med. Chem.* 2004, *47(27)*, 6777–6791.

220. Good, A. C. Novel DOCK clique driven 3D similarity database search tools for molecule shape matching and beyond: adding flexibility to the search for ligand kin. *J. Mol. Graph. Model.* 2007, *26(3)*, 656–666.

221. Jakobi, A. J., Mauser, H., and Clark, T. ParaFrag—an approach for surface-based similarity comparison of molecular fragments. *J. Mol. Model.* 2008, *14(7)*, 547–558.

222. (a) Zhang, Q. and Muegge, I. Scaffold hopping through virtual screening using 2D and 3D similarity descriptors: ranking, voting, and consensus scoring. *J. Med. Chem.* 2006, *49(5)*, 1536–1548; (b) Nair, P. C. and Sobhia, M. E. Fingerprint directed scaffold hopping for identification of CCR2 antagonists. *J. Chem. Inf. Model.* 2008, *48(9)*, 1891–1902; (c) Yamazaki, K., Kusunose, N., Fujita, K., Sato, H., Asano, S., Dan, A., and Kanaoka, M. Identification of phosphodiesterase-1 and 5 dual inhibitors by a ligand-based virtual screening optimized for lead evolution. *Bioorg. Med. Chem. Lett.* 2006, *16(5)*, 1371–1379; (d) Byvatov, E., Sasse, B. C., Stark, H., and Schneider, G. From virtual to real screening for D3 dopamine receptor ligands. *ChemBioChem* 2005, *6(6)*, 997–999; (e) Shoda, M., Harada, T., Kogami, Y., Tsujita, R., Akashi, H., Kouji, H., Stahura, F. L., Xue, L., and Bajorath, J. Identification of structurally diverse growth hormone secreta-

gogue agonists by virtual screening and structure–activity relationship analysis of 2-formylaminoacetamide derivatives. *J. Med. Chem.* 2004, *47(17)*, 4286–4290; (f) Franke, L., Byvatov, E., Werz, O., Steinhilber, D., Schneider, P., and Schneider, G. Extraction and visualization of potential pharmacophore points using support vector machines: application to ligand-based virtual screening for COX-2 inhibitors. *J. Med. Chem.* 2005, *48 (22)*, 6997–7004.

223. (a) Rarey, M. and Dixon, J. S. Feature trees: a new molecular similarity measure based on tree matching. *J. Comput. Aided Mol. Des.* 1998, *12(5)*, 471–490; (b) Rarey, M. and Stahl, M. Similarity searching in large combinatorial chemistry spaces. *J. Comput. Aided Mol. Des.* 2001, *15(6)*, 497–520; (c) Boehm, M., Wu, T.-Y., Claussen, H., and Lemmen, C. Similarity searching and scaffold hopping in synthetically accessible combinatorial chemistry spaces. *J. Med. Chem.* 2008, *51(8)*, 2468–2480.

224. Sperandio, O., Andrieu, O., Miteva, M. A., Vo, M.-Q., Souaille, M., Delfaud, F., and Villoutreix, B. O. MED-SuMoLig: a new ligand-based screening tool for efficient scaffold hopping. *J. Chem. Inf. Model.* 2007, *47(3)*, 1097–1110.

225. Jennings, A. and Tennant, M. Selection of molecules based on shape and electrostatic similarity: proof of concept of "electroforms". *J. Chem. Inf. Model.* 2007, *47(5)*, 1829–1838.

226. (a) Proschak, E., Zettl, H., Tanrikulu, Y., Weisel, M., Kriegl, J. M., Rau, O., Schubert-Zsilavecz M, and Schneider G. From molecular shape to potent bioactive agents I: bioisosteric replacement of molecular fragments. *ChemMedChem* 2009, *4(1)*, 41–44; (b) Proschak, E., Sander, K., Zettl, H., Tanrikulu, Y., Rau, O., Schneider, P., Schubert-Zsilavecz, M., Stark, H., and Schneider, G. From molecular shape to potent bioactive agents II: fragment-based *de novo* design. *ChemMedChem* 2009, *4(1)*, 45–48.

227. Huang, J.-W., Zhang, Z., Wu, B., Cellitti, J. F., Zhang, X., Dahl, R., Shiau, C.-W., Welsh, K., Emdadi, A., Stebbins, J. L., Reed, J. C., and Pellecchia, M. Fragment-based design of small molecule X-linked inhibitor of apoptosis protein inhibitors. *J. Med. Chem.* 2008, *51*(22), 7111–7118.

228. Dobson, C. M. Chemical space and biology. *Nature* 2004, *432(7019)*, 824–828.

229. (a) Vajda, S. and Guarnieri, F. Characterization of protein–ligand interaction sites using experimental and computational methods. *Curr. Opin. Drug Discov. Devel.* 2006, *9(3)*, 354–362; (b) Landon, M. R., Lancia, D. R. Jr., Yu, J., Thiel, S. C., and Vajda, S. Identification of hot spots within druggable binding regions by computational solvent mapping of proteins. *J. Med. Chem.* 2007, *50(6)*, 1231–1240.

230. Ji, H., Stanton, B. Z., Igarashi, J., Li, H., Martásek, P., Roman, L. J., Poulos, T. L., and Silverman, R. B. Minimal pharmacophoric elements and fragment hopping, an approach directed at molecular diversity and isozyme selectivity. Design of selective neuronal nitric oxide synthase inhibitors. *J. Am. Chem. Soc.* 2008, *130(12)*, 3900–3914.

231. Böhm, M. and Klebe, G. Development of new hydrogen-bond descriptors and their application to comparative molecular field analyses. *J. Med. Chem.* 2002, *45(8)*, 1585–1597.

232. Mattos, C., Bellamacina, C. R., Peisach, E., Pereira, A., Vitkup, D., Petsko, G. A., and Ringe, D. Multiple solvent crystal structures: probing binding sites, plasticity and hydration. *J. Mol. Biol.* 2006, *357(5)*, 1471–1482.

233. DeLano, W. L. Unraveling hot spots in binding interfaces: progress and challenges. *Curr. Opin. Struct. Biol.* 2002, *12(1)*, 14–20.

234. Ji, H., Zhang, W., Zhang, M., Kudo, M., Aoyama, Y., Yoshida, Y., Sheng, C., Song, Y., Yang, S., Zhou, Y., Lu, J., and Zhu, J. Structure-based *de novo* design, synthesis, and biological evaluation of non-azole inhibitors specific for lanosterol 14α-demethylase of fungi. *J. Med. Chem.* 2003, *46(4)*, 474–485.

235. (a) Goodford, P. J. A computational procedure for determining energetically favorable binding sites on biologically important macromolecules. *J. Med. Chem.* 1985, *28(7)*, 849–857; (b) von Itzstein, M., Wu, W.-Y., Kok, G. B., Pegg, M. S., Dyason, J. C., Jin, B., Van Phan, T., Smythe, M. L., White, H. F., Oliver, S. W., Colman, P. M., Varghese J. N., Ryan, D. M., Woods, J. M., Bethell, R. C., Hotham, V. J., Cameron, J. M., and Penn, C. R. Rational design of potent sialidase-based inhibitors of influenza virus replication. *Nature* 1993, *363(6428)*, 418–423.

236. (a) Miranker, A. and Karplus, M. Functionality maps of binding sites: a multiple copy simultaneous search method. *Proteins* 1991, *11(1)*, 29–34; (b) Zoete, V., Meuwly, M., and Karplus, M. Study of the insulin dimerization: binding free energy calculations and per-residue free energy decomposition. *Proteins* 2005, *61(1)*, 79–93.

237. Laskowski, R. A., Thornton, J. M., Humblet, C., Singh, J. X-SITE: use of empirically derived atomic packing preferences to identify favourable interaction regions in the binding sites of proteins. *J. Mol. Biol.* 1996, *259(1)*, 175–201.

238. Boer, D. R., Kroon, J., Cole, J. C., Smith, B., and Verdonk, M. L. SuperStar: comparison of CSD and PDB-based interaction fields as a basis for the prediction of protein–ligand interactions. *J. Mol. Biol.* 2001, *312(1)*, 275–287.

239. An, J., Totrov, M., and Abagyan, R. Pocketome via comprehensive identification and classification of ligand binding envelopes. *Mol. Cell. Proteomics* 2005, *4(6)*, 752–761.

240. Laurie, A. T., Jackson, R. M. Q-SiteFinder: an energy-based method for the prediction of protein–ligand binding sites. *Bioinformatics* 2005, *21(9)*, 1908–1916.

241. (a) Dennis, S., Kortvelyesi, T., and Vajda, S. Computational mapping identifies the binding sites of organic solvents on proteins. *Proc. Natl. Acad. Sci. USA* 2002, *99(7)*, 4290–4295; (b) Silberstein, M., Dennis, S., Brown, L., Kortvelyesi, T., Clodfelter, K., and Vajda, S. Identification of substrate binding sites in enzymes by computational solvent mapping. *J. Mol. Biol.* 2003, *332(5)*, 1095–1113.

242. Moore, W. R. Jr., Maximizing discovery efficiency with a computationally driven fragment approach. *Curr. Opin. Drug Discov. Devel.* 2005, *8(3)*, 355–364.

243. Kastenholz, M. A., Pastor, M., Cruciani, G., Haaksma, E. E. J., and Fox, T. GRID/CPCA: a new computational tool to design selective ligands. *J. Med. Chem.* 2000, *43*(16), 3033–3044.

244. Patel, Y., Gillet, V. J., Bravi, G., and Leach, A. R. A comparison of the pharmacophore identification programs: Catalyst, DISCO and GASP. *J. Comput. Aided Mol. Des.* 2002, *16(8–9)*, 653–681.

245. Noeske, T., Sasse, B. C., Stark, H., Parsons, C. G., Weil, T., and Schneider, G. Predicting compound selectivity by self-organizing maps: cross-activities of metabotropic glutamate receptor antagonists. *ChemMedChem* 2006, *1(10)*, 1066–1068.

246. Mason, J. S., Good, A. C., and Martin, E. J. 3-D pharmacophores in drug discovery. *Curr. Pharm. Des.* 2001, *7(7)*, 567–597.

247. (a) Muller, G. Medicinal chemistry of target family-directed masterkeys. *Drug Discov. Today* 2003, *8(15)*, 681–691; (b) Lewell, X. Q., Jones, A. C., Bruce, C. L., Harper, G., Jones, M. M., McLay, I. M., and Bradshaw, J. Drug rings database with web interface. A

tool for identifying alternative chemical rings in lead discovery programs. *J. Med. Chem.* 2003, *46(15)*, 3257–3274.

248. (a) Patani, G. A. and LaVoie, E. J. Bioisosterism: a rational approach in drug design. *Chem. Rev.* 1996, *96(8)*, 3147–3176; (b) Lima, L. M., and Barreiro, E. J. Bioisosterism: a useful strategy for molecular modification and drug design. *Curr. Med. Chem.* 2005, *12 (1)*, 23–49; (c) Thornber, C. W. Isosterism and molecular modification in drug design. *Chem. Soc. Rev.* 1979, *8*, 563–580; (d) Olesen, P. H. The use of bioisosteric groups in lead optimization. *Curr. Opin. Drug Discov. Devel.* 2001, *4(4)*, 471–478; (e) Wermuth, C. G. *The Practice of Medicinal Chemistry*, 2nd Edition. Academic Press, San Diego, 2003; Chapter 13. Wermuth C. G. "Molecular variations based on isosteric replacements." pp. 189–214; (f) Abraham D. J. *Burger's Medicinal Chemistry and Drug Discovery*, Vol. 1 Drug Discovery, 6th Edition, Wiley, New York, 2003; Chapter 16. Cannon J. G. "Analog Design" pp. 687–714.

249. (a) van de Waterbeemd, H., Smith, D. A., Beaumont, K., and Walker, D. K. Property-based design: optimization of drug absorption and pharmacokinetics. *J. Med. Chem.* 2001, *44(9)*, 1313–1333; (b) Nassar, A.-E. F., Kamel, A. M., and Clarimont, C. Improving the decision-making process in the structural modification of drug candidates: enhancing metabolic stability. *Drug Discov. Today 2004 9(23)*, 1020–1028; (c) Rishton, G. M. Nonleadlikeness and leadlikeness in biochemical screening. *Drug Discov. Today* 2003, *8 (2)*, 86–96.

250. (a) Kazius, J., McGuire, R., Bursi, R. Derivation and validation of toxicophores for mutagenicity prediction. *J. Med. Chem.* 2005, *48(1)*, 312–320; (b) Nassar, A.-E. F., Kamel, A. M., and Clarimont, C. Improving the decision-making process in structural modification of drug candidates: reducing toxicity. *Drug Discov. Today, 2004 9(24)*, 1055–1064; (c) Williams, D. P., and Naisbitt, D. J. Toxicophores: groups and metabolic routes associated with increased safety risk. *Curr. Opin. Drug Discov. Devel.* 2002, *5(1)*, 104–115; (d) Llorens, O., Perez, J. J., and Villar, H. O. Toward the design of chemical libraries for mass screening biased against mutagenic compounds. *J. Med. Chem.* 2001, *44(17)*, 2793–2804.

251. Böhm, H.-J., Banner, D. W., and Weber, L. Combinatorial docking and combinatorial chemistry: design of potent non-peptide thrombin inhibitors. *J. Comput. Aided Mol. Des.* 1999, *13(1)*, 51–56.

252. (a) Bemis, G. W. and Murcko, M. A. Properties of known drugs. 2. Side chains. *J. Med. Chem.* 1999, *42(25)*, 5095–5099; (b) Ertl, P. Cheminformatics analysis of organic substituents: identification of the most common substituents, calculation of substituent properties, and automatic identification of drug-like bioisosteric groups. *J. Chem. Inf. Comput. Sci.* 2003, *43(2)*, 374–380.

253. Wagner, A. B. SciFinder Scholar 2006: An empirical analysis of research topic query processing. *J. Chem. Inf. Model.* 2006, *46(2)*, 767–774.

254. Morris, G. M., Goodsell, D. S., Halliday, R. S., Huey, R., Hart, W. E., Belew, R. K., and Olson, A. J. Automated docking using a Lamarckian genetic algorithm and an empirical binding free energy function. *J. Comp. Chem.* 1998, *19(14)*, 1639–1662.

255. Charifson, P. S., Corkery, J. J., Murcko, M. A., and Walters, W. P. Consensus scoring: A method for obtaining improved hit rates from docking databases of three-dimensional structures into proteins. *J. Med. Chem.* 1999, *42(25)*, 5100–5109.

256. (a) Norinder, U. and Haeberlein, M. Computational approaches to the prediction of the blood–brain distribution. *Adv. Drug Deliv. Rev.* 2002, *54(3)*, 291–313; (b) Cruciani, G.,

Carosati, E., De Boeck, B., Ethirajulu, K., Mackie, C., Howe, T., and Vianello, R. MetaSite: understanding metabolism in human cytochromes from the perspective of the chemist. *J. Med. Chem.* 2005, *48(22)*, 6970–6979.

257. Ji, H., Li, H., Martásek, P., Roman, L. J., Poulos, T. L., and Silverman, R. B. Discovery of highly potent and selective inhibitors of neuronal nitric oxide synthase by fragment hopping. *J. Med. Chem.* 2009, *52(3)*, 779–797.

258. Ji, H., Tan, S., Igarashi, J., Li, H., Derrick, M., Martásek, P., Roman, L. J., Vásquez-Vivar, J., Poulos, T. L., and Silverman, R. B. Selective neuronal nitric oxide synthase inhibitors and the prevention of cerebral palsy. *Ann. Neurol.* 2009, *65(2)*, 209–217.

INDEX

ADMET for Medicinal Chemists: A Practical Guide, Edited by Katya Tsaioun and Steven A. Kates

Printed in the USA/Agawam, MA
September 16, 2026

910661.183